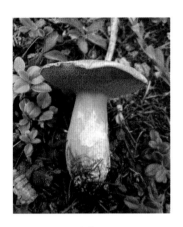

The
Fungal Pharmacy

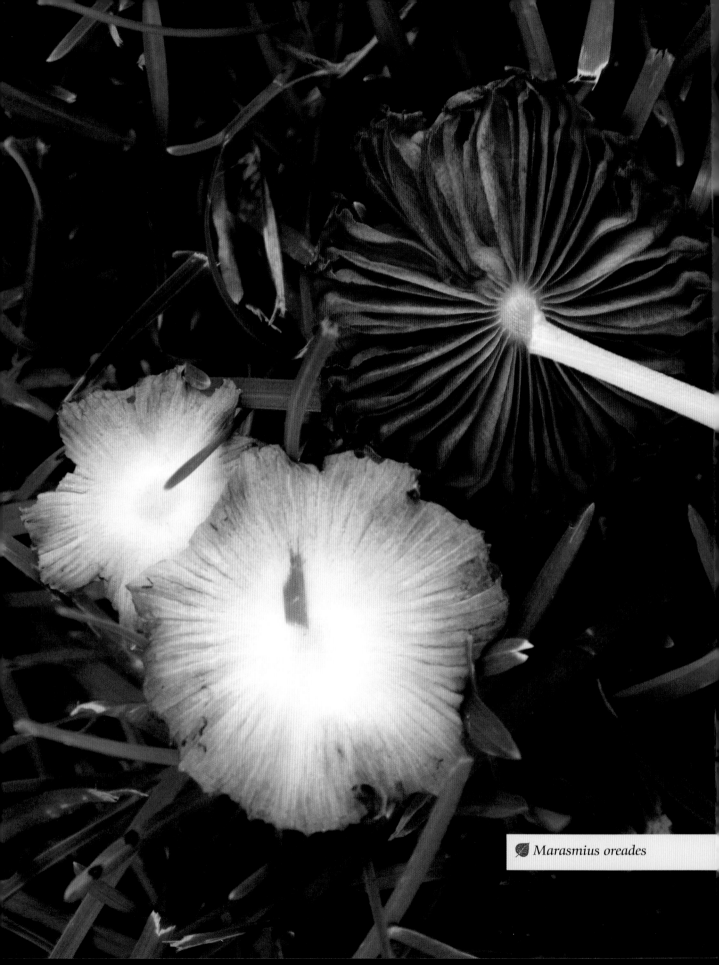

Marasmius oreades

The
Fungal Pharmacy

The Complete Guide to Medicinal Mushrooms and Lichens of North America

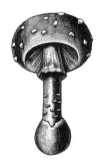

Robert Rogers

BSc, RH (AHG), FICN

Foreword by Solomon P. Wasser

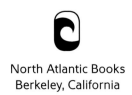

North Atlantic Books
Berkeley, California

Published by
North Atlantic Books
Huichin, unceded Ohlone land
Berkeley, California

Cover photos by Robert Rogers
Cover and book design by Brad Greene
Printed in the United States of America

The Fungal Pharmacy: The Complete Guide to Medicinal Mushrooms and Lichens of North America is sponsored and published by North Atlantic Books, an educational non-profit based in the unceded Ohlone land Huichin (Berkeley, CA) that collaborates with partners to develop cross-cultural perspectives; nurture holistic views of art, science, the humanities, and healing; and seed personal and global transformation by publishing work on the relationship of body, spirit, and nature.

North Atlantic Books's publications are distributed to the US trade and internationally by Penguin Random House Publisher Services. For further information, visit our website at www.northatlanticbooks.com.

Library of Congress Cataloging-in-Publication Data

Rogers, Robert Dale, 1950–
    The fungal pharmacy : the complete guide to medicinal mushrooms and lichens of North America / Robert Dale Rogers.
        p. ; cm.
    Includes bibliographical references and index.
    Summary: "A compendium of more than three hundred species of medicinal mushrooms and lichens, including their historic and modern-day usage, active chemical components, appropriate preparation methods, and cultural significance"—Provided by publisher
    ISBN 978-1-55643-953-7 (pbk.)
    1. Mushrooms—Therapeutic use—North America. I. Title.
    [DNLM: 1. Agaricales—North America. 2. Lichens—North America.
3. Phytotherapy—methods—North America. QW 180.5.B2]
    RM666.M87R64 2011
    615'.329—dc23   2011012688

10 11 12 13 VERSA 26 25 24 23

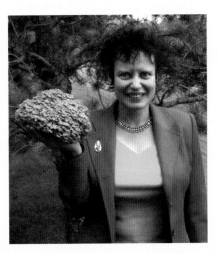

This book is dedicated to Laurie,
my best friend
and love of my life.

Acknowledgments

I would like to acknowledge the trailblazing work of Paul Stamets and Solomon Wasser.

I greatly appreciate the fungal contributions of David Arora, Robert Blanchette, Ken Jones, Christopher Hobbs, Terry Willard, Andrew Weil, Clark Heinrich, David Law, Adrian Morgan, Bruno Boulet, Jim Ginns, Paul Kroeger, Leonard Hutchison, Michael Beug, Larry Evans, Bryce Kendrick, Britt Bunyard, Tom Volk, Gary Lincoff, Michael Kuo, and numerous other mycologists, herbalists, authors, and generally all-round fun guys and fun gals.

I would also like to thank fellow members of NAMA and the Alberta Mycological Society for their warm welcome and significant contributions to my mushroom studies over the past eight years. There are many to thank, but special appreciation should be given to Martin Osis, who has patiently mentored me and become a very special friend and forest forayer. Thank you. Please check out the Alberta Mycological Society's website at www.wildmushrooms.ws.

Thanks to Doug Reil, associate publisher at North Atlantic Books, and my editors, Erin Wiegand and Robin Donovan.

Thanks to all the photographers, especially John Plischke III, for their keen eyes and contributions.

A special thanks to researchers all over the world who have labored and studied and published papers that have contributed so much to our knowledge of the Fifth Kingdom.

Thank you.

While the fungi described in this book can be found throughout North America, the reader will note a regional tone, as my personal experience with fungi does not extend past western Canada. The reader will also note that information on inedible and poisonous mushrooms is included. These species contain medicinal compounds and are included for educational purposes only. This book is meant to encourage more research into medicinal mushrooms; it is not a how-to for picking and eating wild mushrooms. (Those interested in doing so can refer to the bibliography.) Remember, identification is critical, and it is best for amateurs to walk and learn with an experienced picker. Between fifty and three hundred people die every year around the world from misidentified specimens, especially from the *Amanita* genus. Please do not allow yourself to be added to the list.

This book is for educational purposes only and is not meant to replace the advice of a qualified health professional or diagnosis from a physician or medical mycologist or herbalist. The fact that a mushroom contains an interesting compound does not mean it is safe to ingest. Recipes are noted for historical record only. The author takes no responsibility nor encourages anyone to ingest, in any form, any mushroom based solely on information in this volume. The author and publisher are not responsible for any adverse effects or consequences resulting from the use of the information in this book.

> I am the doctor. I am the man of medicines. I am. I am he who cures. . . . I am the remedy and the medicine man. I am the mushroom. I am the fresh mushroom. I am the large mushroom. I am the fragrant mushroom.
> I am the mushroom of spirit.
> — Mazatec Shaman

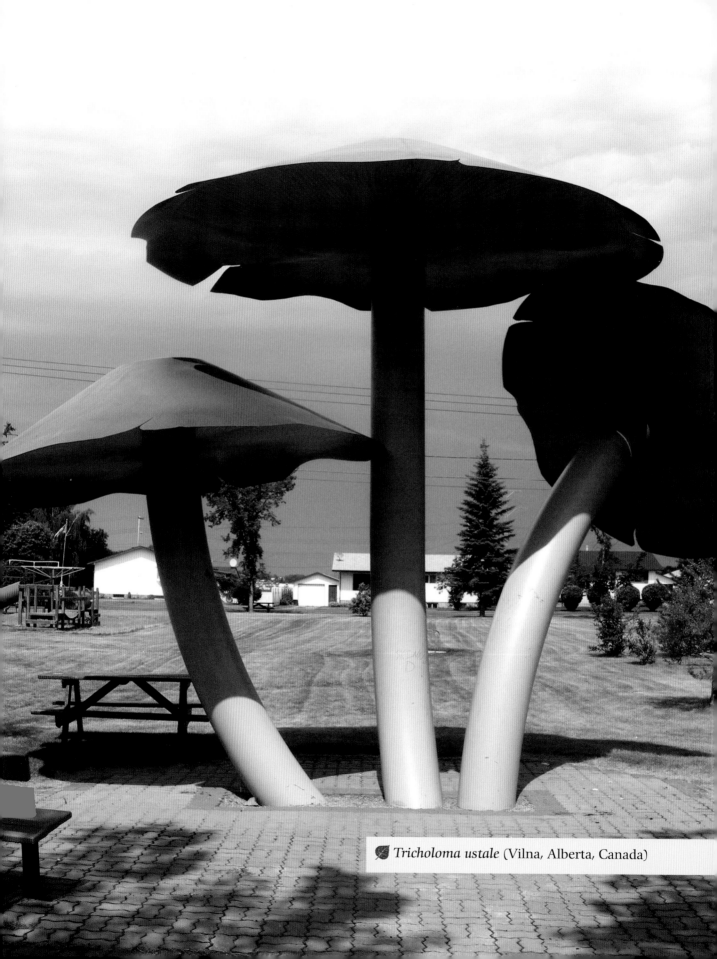

Tricholoma ustale (Vilna, Alberta, Canada)

Contents

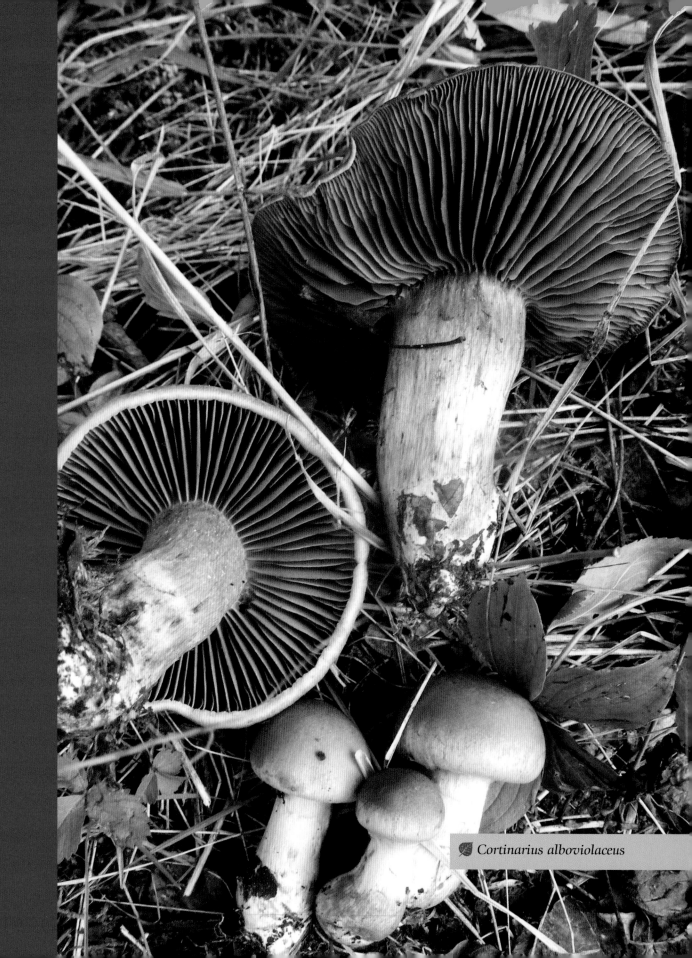

Cortinarius alboviolaceus

Medicinal mushrooms have an established history of use in traditional and ancient therapies. Contemporary research has validated and documented much of the ancient knowledge. In the past three decades, the interdisciplinary field of science that studies medicinal mushrooms has demonstrated the potent and unique properties of compounds extracted from a range of mushroom species. Modern clinical practice in Japan, China, Korea, Russia, and several other countries rely on mushroom-derived preparations.

Ancient oriental traditions have stressed the importance of several mushroom species, especially the lingzhi or reishi mushroom *(Ganoderma lucidum)* and shiitake mushroom *(Lentinus edodes)*. Mushrooms have also played an important role in the treatment of ailments affecting rural populations of eastern European countries. The most important species in these countries were *Inonotus obliquus* (Pers.:Fr.) or chaga, *Fomitopsis officinalis* (Vill.:Fr.) Bond. et Singer (Wood Conk or Agaricon), *Piptoporus betulinus* (Bull.:Fr.) P.Karst. (Birch Polypore), and *Fomes fomentarius* (Fr.:Fr) or tinder bracket. These species were used in the treatment of gastrointestinal disorders, various forms of cancers, bronchial asthma, night sweats, etc. There is also a long history of traditional use of mushrooms as curatives in Mesoamerica (especially for species of the genus *Psilocybe*), in Africa (Yoruba populations in Nigeria and Benin), Algeria, and Egypt. A very special role was found in fly agaric (*Amanita muscaria;* L.:Fr.;Pers.) in Siberia and Tibetan shamanism, Buddhism, and Celtic myths.

Meanwhile, mushrooms comprise an extremely abundant and diverse world of fungi. The number of mushroom species on Earth is currently estimated at a hundred and fifty thousand, yet perhaps only 10 percent (approximately fifteen thousand named species) are known to science. Mushrooms are being evaluated for their nutritional value and acceptability as well as for their pharmacological properties. They make up a vast and yet largely untapped source of powerful new pharmaceutical products. In particular, and most importantly for modern medicine, mushrooms present an unlimited source of polysaccharides and polysaccharide–protein complexes with anticancer and immunostimulating properties. Many, if not all, higher basidiomycetes mushrooms contain biologically active polysaccharides in their fruit bodies, cultured mycelia, and cultured broth. The data on mushroom polysaccharides today include 670 species and intraspecific taxa from 182 genera of higher hetero- and homobasidiomycetes.

Polysaccharides with antitumor and immunostimulating properties are particularly important for modern medicine. Several of the mushroom polysaccharide compounds have proceeded through Phase I, II, and III clinical trials and are used extensively and successfully in Asia to treat various cancers and other diseases. A total of 126 medicinal functions are thought to be produced by medicinal mushrooms and fungi including antitumor, immunomodulating, antioxidant, radical scavenging, cardiovascular, anti-hypercholesterolemia, antiviral, antibacterial, anti-parasitic, antifungal, detoxification, hepatoprotective, and antidiabetic effects.

The Fungal Pharmacy begins with a short historical perspective on how mushrooms have been used through time and in cultures from ancient Greece and Rome to the Far East and beyond. Many of the species discussed are found throughout the boreal forests of North America, Europe, and Asia. Robert Rogers has researched the unique properties of various fungi used in ancient times in these parts of the world and incorporated their contributions into the text.

Rogers explores the diverse uses of mushrooms, ranging from those that inspire musical compositions to those that have application in biological fuel cells. Medical research of fungi exhibiting *in vivo* and *in vitro* activity on bacteria, viruses, and pathogenic fungi is extensive and includes a number of both edible and poisonous species with the potential for present and future research. Mycoremediation, which could help reduce toxic materials presently related to disposal facilities, helps decontaminate and minimize road and farm runoff, creates buffer zones, reduces agricultural waste, reduces pollution in watersheds, reduces the risk of forest fire, and cleans up contaminated pathogenic bacteria such as *Escherichia coli*. The author pays special attention to the use of fungi to clean up the contamination produced by the Athabasca Oil Sands in northern Alberta, one of the largest petroleum deposits in the world.

The book delves into mythology as well as medicine. The chapter on *Amanita muscaria*, for example, is filled with Celtic, Egyptian, and First Nation mythology to inspire the imagination and is guaranteed to surprise the reader with medicinal uses for various neuromuscular and psychosomatic conditions.

Many unusual species including *Boschniakia rossica, Collybia maculata, Cortinarius* spp., *Echinodontium tinctorium, Haploporus odorus, Hydnum repandum, Leccinum* spp., *Mycena* spp., *Phallus impudicus, Pholiota* spp., *Plectania nigrella, Polyporus tuberaster, Rozites caperata, Tricholoma magnivelare,* and a wide variety of *Russula* species, are mentioned.

The author's main interest is in polypore mushrooms. This is evidenced throughout the book by the inclusion of extensive chapters on *Fomes fomentarius* (Amadou or German Tinder), *Fomitopsis officinalis* (quinine conk or agaricon), *F. pinicola* (red belted conk), *Ganoderma applanatum* (artist's conk), *G. tsugae* (varnished conk), *Inonotus obliquus* (chaga), *Lenzites betulina* (white gilled polypore), and *Piptoporus betulinus* (razor strop or birch conk). The author lives on the edge of the boreal forest and mentions that millions of tons of these medicinal conks are available for harvest from public lands. He explains that the northern part of Canada has a number of economically marginalized communities that could benefit from cooperative collection and extraction of these medicinal mushrooms. Robert Rogers' appreciation of the medicine of the people of the First Nations shows through his numerous descriptions of traditional uses of fungi.

The Fungal Pharmacy is timely and welcomed and will be of interest to mycologists, taxonomists, biotechnologists, mushroom producers, researchers, medical doctors and specialists in alternative medicine, environmentalists, ecologists, wild-crafters, scientists, and anyone else interested in medicinal mushrooms. From folklore to modern scientific analysis, this book presents inspiration and hope for increasing the health and wellbeing of humans and other inhabitants of our planet.

— SOLOMON P. WASSER, PhD, DR. SCI. (BIOLOGY); PROFESSOR OF BOTANY AND MYCOLOGY AT THE UNIVERSITY OF HAIFA—MT. CARMEL, ISRAEL; EDITOR-IN-CHIEF, *INTERNATIONAL JOURNAL OF MEDICINAL MUSHROOMS*

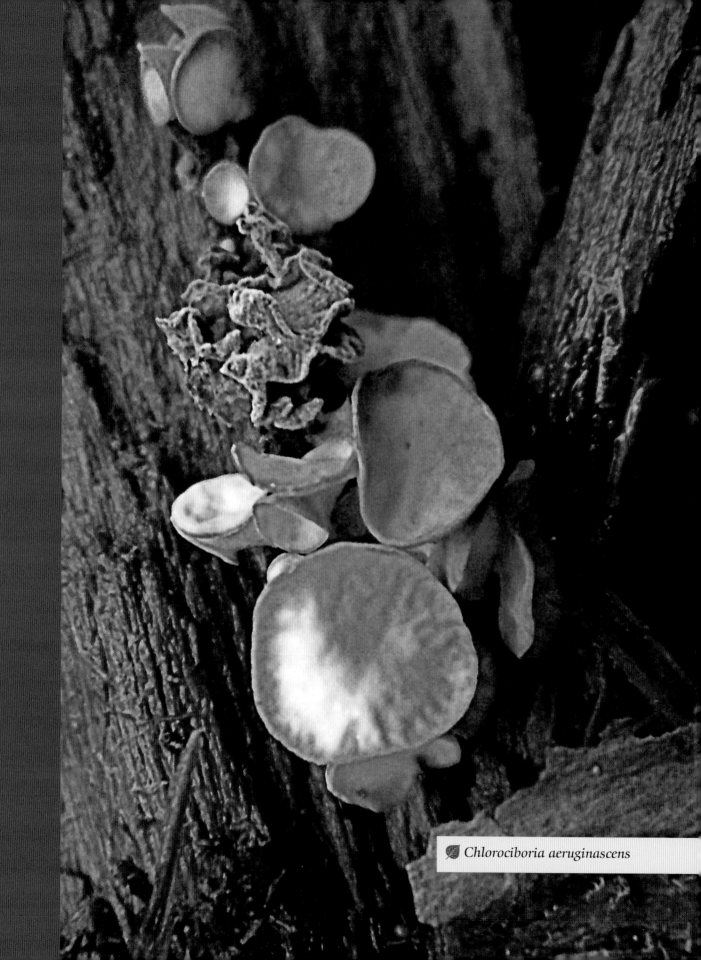

Chlorociboria aeruginascens

This book, like many projects, has been a long process. It was originally self-published as a thirty-two-page manuscript in April of 1999. It is not meant to be an academic contribution but rather a starting point for this ongoing exploration.

My background is in bioregional herbalism, and for whatever reason, I did not look seriously at mushrooms and lichens for the first fifty years of my life. I picked and enjoyed morels and ink caps from the shores of Lesser Slave Lake, Alberta, back in the early 1970s. In my eighteen years of herbal practice in Edmonton, I suggested reishi, shiitake and turkey tail to clients looking to optimize their immune function while undergoing chemotherapy and radiation for various cancers. And I was delighted when oyster, portobello, enoki, and shiitake mushrooms became available year round as a fresh product in my local grocery. But it wasn't until I joined the Edmonton Mycological Society (now the Alberta Mycological Society) and had my senses opened to the delights of mushroom forays that my interest in fungi became keen. I am an amateur mycologist, with no formal training.

This small contribution is an attempt to bring broader awareness to the importance of fungi and the role they play in the health of our planet. Medicinal mushroom uses for human, plant, and animal health are remarkable. Their role in cleaning up our increasingly toxic planet and optimizing Gaia's immune system are yet to be fully realized. I have included the use of fungi in the form of essential oils, homeopathy, and even vibrational essences, as well as their more traditional usage in decoction, powder, or tincture form.

Nomenclature

I have attempted to organize the myconomials as best I can, recognizing that new DNA techniques are helping to reclassify and group mushrooms in their proper place. Whenever possible I have given the most common Latin name first, followed by synonyms that may or may not be useful. I know that in my own research, using only the most up-to-date referenced binomial name would have denied me a wealth of knowledge. Alexander and Ann Shulgin put it well in their book on tryptamines, *Tikhal: The Continuation:*

> I have learned a lot from them (fungi) about the balance of nature, by observing how they propagate and reproduce, but I have learned a lot more from them about the egocentric nature of man, simply by observing how the many experts in the field (called mycologists) seem to disagree, usually with vigor, as to how

fungi should be classified. There are cliques, there are schools, there are societies, there are total philosophies that are convinced that they are completely right, and that all the others are completely wrong.

"This species must be moved to that genus, in yonder family, as noted in my most recent publication in *Applied Mycologia Today*."

"But, Dr. Rasputin, you already have tenure at the University, so let me use this genus for the title of an article in my new journal, *Amanita Northwestica*, and I will make you an Associate Editor. But will you drop your insistence for the renaming of the Pholiota group?"

"Yes, but you must allow me at least one race with my name attached to it, or allow me to identify this group as a new subspecies."

"But Dr. Sanfroid would object to that."

"Probably he would, but I hold Dr. Goodheart to be the defining authority."

"Oh, really? Come to think of it, I'm not sure I have an editorial opening available at the moment."

In short, classification of these organisms has been a nightmare for many years and will, without doubt, remain a nightmare for many years to come. There is no right way. There is not even a currently accepted way.

Couldn't have put it better myself!

How long have mushrooms been on Earth? This is a difficult question. Fossils of microscopic aquatic fungi over 545 million years old have been found in northern Russia. In 1910, at Rhynie in Aberdeenshire, Scotland, a fungal fossil, perhaps associated with cyanobacterium lichen, was uncovered in red sandstone four hundred million years old. These Prototaxites reached heights of nearly thirty feet, and were driven to extinction by either animal grazing or competition from vascular plants.

Mushroom fruiting bodies, similar to modern forms, have been found preserved in amber ninety million years old. Four fossil agarics have been found in amber in the Dominican Republic that are estimated to be fifteen to twenty million years old. A recent discovery from Burma shows an ancient mushroom in amber attacking a parasite that is attacking the fungi.

The number of species in the kingdom Fungi is estimated at 1.4 million species. (It is estimated that the Pacific Northwest region alone contains fifteen to twenty thousand species.) Only eighty thousand have been named, and of the fourteen thousand well-known species only about 50 percent are considered to be edible to any degree. About two thousand are safe edibles, with more than seven hundred species possessing significant pharmacological properties.

Historical Perspectives

"Mushroom" is believed to derive from the French word *mousseron,* as they grow amongst moss *(mousse).* Some authors assume that *mousseron* actually refers to a fly-killing fungus or *moucheron (mouche* means "fly"). More likely it is from the Old English *maes,* "a field," and *rhum,* meaning "a knob." Although some scholars believe it stems from the Gaelic *maes-rhin,* this has not been documented.

One derivation of the word "fungus" is from the Latin *funus,* meaning "a corpse," and *ago* meaning "I make," indicating that the Romans were well aware of the potential danger (and had a good sense of humor). Dioscorides summed it up nicely: "Either they are edible or they are poisonous." Other authors believe it derives from the Greek *spoggos,* meaning "sponge."

Mushrooms have been prized all over the world. The oldest recorded history of mushroom use is a Tassali image from an Algerian cave dating back to 5000 BCE. The mushroom is surrounded with electrified auras outlining a dancing shaman. Ancient Indian, Greek, and Roman myths also suggested that mushrooms sprang from lightning, and in Mexico, the fungi are actually sacred because they are thought to result from the sexual union of a bolt of lightning and Earth.

The ancient Romans feasted on mushrooms; Martial wrote in the first century AD, "It is easy to refuse gold and silver or even attractive ladies, but to refuse mushrooms is difficult." The Romans set aside special silver vessels called *boletaria* to hold and cook mushrooms, and amber knives were reserved for their preparation. Martial also wrote that "gold and silver and dresses may be trusted to a messenger, but not a boletus, because it will be eaten on the way."

Nicandros, a Greek physician of the second century BC, taught mushroom cultivation. Both the Greeks and Romans cultivated *Agrocybe aegerita,* which grows on poplar, "the people's tree."

The Greeks, according to Suetonius, called fungi the "food of the gods," while the Greek philosopher Porphyry called them "sons of the gods," as they were born without seed. In Corinth, humans were believed to have been born from mushrooms.

Avicenna, the famous tenth-century Arabian physician, warned that toadstools green, black, and the color of peacocks were poisonous.

The Chinese have a rich history of fungal interest, dating back some seven thousand years to the Yang Shao culture. *The Mycoflora,* by Chen Jen-yu, written in 1245 AD, was devoted entirely to the development, appearance, harvest, and preparation of eleven species of fungi.

The oldest written record of mushrooms as medicine is an Indian medical treatise from 3000 BC.

In German mythology, on one winter's night, the god Wotan rides through the forest on horseback, pursued by devils. As the horse races faster and faster, blood-specked foam falls from the mouth, producing next spring's beautiful red mushrooms with white specks.

English herbalists called poisonous mushrooms *tode stoles; tode* from the German word meaning "death." This developed into the common name "toadstools" because of the association of the common toad with witchcraft.

Albertus Magnus, in the thirteenth century, said that mushrooms are not really plants but excrescents of earth and plants. "That is why they are generally brittle and owe their poisonous nature to the rotting dampness on which they grow." And thus, for centuries, mushrooms were considered to be the result of decomposition, not the cause. Caesalpinius, the director of the Botanical Gardens in Pisa, Italy, wrote in 1583 that fungi were fruit.

Gerard, the famous English herbalist, did not like mushrooms, leading to the English mycophobia now present in much of North America. This fear did not extend to all Europeans, mind you, as various fungi appear on eighteen coats of arms. Ten are from France, three from Germany, and one each from England, Belgium, Switzerland, Italy, and Poland.

The Russians have a rich and versatile tradition of mushroom feasting, and call their gathering expeditions "the third hunt." An old Russian proverb says, "If you think you are a mushroom, jump into the basket."

A Marketable Product

In Finland, the estimated wild mushroom crop on a good year is five billion kilograms. This follows a government policy, in effect since World War II, to encourage wild harvesting. Slogans about the millions of marks rotting in Finnish forests have helped encourage the industry, as have more than three thousand trained "natural product advisors" who provide advice to commercial mushroom pickers and lead expeditions for those who collect as a hobby. More than fifty thousand pickers were trained between 1969 and 1983, so that by 1979 an estimated 72 percent of Finnish adults were picking mushrooms.

Wild mushrooms were an important foodstuff in wartime. A Russian proverb—"when mushrooms abound, there'll be war around,"— suggests survival rations.

In Lausanne, Switzerland, no fewer than seventy-eight kinds of officially sanctioned fungi are sold in the markets. Certain mushrooms, like the chanterelle, are sold by volume to avoid water soaking to increase their weight; and boletes are cut in half to expose the amount of insect larvae.

In Stockholm, more than three hundred species are permitted in the markets, but in Munich, the largest market for wild fungi, only about thirty species are for sale, largely composed of cepes *(Boletus edulis)*.

In 1927, the French set up a National Inspectorate to ensure the safety of wild fungi. These experts can be found throughout rural France, in town halls or pharmacies, advising edibility and market prices.

In the former Czechoslovakia, government regulations governing the sale were published in 1950, with sixty-four species on the approved list, plus nine *Russulas* that may be used for making mushroom extracts.

Wild mushroom picking is also profitable. A 1993 survey of 10,400 pickers in the Western United States indicate they harvested around four million pounds of wild mushrooms. Morels, chanterelles, and boletes accounted for two-thirds of the take. The matsutake, or pine mushroom *(Tricholoma magnivelare),* harvest was 836,000 pounds, with the whole gross value conservatively estimated at $41 million.

British Columbia leads the export of mushroom harvests in Canada, with most of the product exported to Japan, Europe, and the United States. Seven companies control 90 percent of this export market at the present time.

Cultivation

Today, a wide variety of mushrooms are being cultivated, other than those already available in the grocery store, such as button, enoki, shiitake, and oyster.

Coprinus comatus, Armillaria mellea, Craterullus cornucopioides, and Kuehneromyces mutabilis are additional proven cultivars.

It is estimated that approximately 50 percent of the annual five million metric tons of cultivated edible mushrooms contain functional, medicinal, or nutraceutical properties. The total value of worldwide mushroom production from 1989 to 1991 was about U.S. $7.5 billion. By 2001, the world value of mushroom production (10.32 million metric tons of food plus medicinal mushrooms) was estimated at U.S. $21 billion, the same value as coffee production.

By 1994, medicinal mushrooms were U.S. $2 billion in sales worldwide, and by 1997 had risen to U.S. $3.2 billion or 60 percent in just three years; and $4.5 billion by 1999.

In 2000, the estimated sales of reishi mushrooms alone were U.S. $2.1 billion.

In descending tonnage, the most popular food mushrooms after button are shiitake, oyster *(Pleurotus)*, mu-er *(Auricularia)*, enoki *(Flammulina)*, yin-er *(Tremella)*, hedgehog *(Hericium)*, and maitake *(Grifola)*. They all have various degrees of immune-modulating, lipid-lowering, antitumor, and other therapeutic health properties.

The successful cultivation of *Pleurotus pulmonarius* on water hyacinth and *Lentinula edodes* on coffee wastes will help increase oyster mushroom production.

Sunflower seed hulls can be utilized as a substrate for mushroom production. In 1999, world production of this waste product was 14,073 thousand metric tons, a considerable resource.

Dr. S. T. Chang, director of the Research Center for Food Protein at the Chinese University of Hong Kong, says that "when one considers that they can be produced on waste materials—converting products of little or no market value into food for an over-populated world—then there is no doubt that mushrooms represent one of the world's greatest untapped resources of nutritious and palatable food for the future." Not to mention health and wellness!

Medicinal Qualities

There are more than 270 identified fungal species with known therapeutic properties. These include antioxidants, hypotensives, hypocholesterolemics, liver protectants, antifibrotics, as well as anti-inflammatory, antidiabetic, antiviral, and antimicrobial properties.

Other medicinal properties derived from fungi include immunosuppressants used in organ transplants and as adjuncts to cancer chemotherapy and radiation.

Mushrooms contain bioactive metabolites capable of helping revitalize and modulate our immune systems. These biological response modifiers help activate macrophages and T-cells and produce cytokines, including interleukins as well as tumor necrosis factors (TNF). Medicinal mushrooms may hold the key to much disease and chronic illness on our planet. *The Fungal Pharmacy* may one day become a reality.

Common to every medicinal mushroom is beta-D-glucan, a polysaccharide. Polysaccharides are long sugar chains with oxygen-bearing molecules; in the process of breakdown, this oxygen is released and made available at a cellular level. Polysaccharides are poorly digested and may be acted upon by intestinal bacteria to release oligosaccharides. The main immunological activity is believed to be due to the interaction of the oligosaccharides with gut-associated lymphoid tissue. Immune cells associated with GALT, activated by beta-glucans in the gut, may migrate to other tissue and thereby exert immune-modulating activity. Beta-glucans stimulate interferon, interleukins, TNF, NK, B- and T-lymphocytes, tumor-infiltrating lymphocytes, lymphokine-activated killer cells, macrophages, granulocytes in bone marrow, and production of platelets in bone marrow. Beta-glucans also attach themselves to the receptor sites on the immune cells and activate them, allowing them to recognize cancer cells as "foreign" and create a higher level of response.

We know that dectin-1, on macrophages, is a receptor that mediates beta-glucan activation of phagocytosis and production of cytokines, an action coordinated by the toll-like receptor-2.

Activated complement receptors on natural killer cells, neutrophils, and lymphocytes are associated with tumor cytotoxicity. Scavenger and lactosyl-ceramide bind beta-glucans and mediate a sequence of pathways leading to immune activation.

TNF is a pro-inflammatory cytokine that activates nuclear factor-kB (NFkappaB) and c-Jun N-terminal kinase (JNK). NFkappaB is anti-apoptotic, and JNK contributes to cell death. In cancer, TNF is a double-edged sword. It can be an endogenous tumor-promoter, because TNF stimulates the growth, proliferation, invasion and metastasis, and tumor angiogenesis of cancer cells. On the other hand, TNF is also a cancer-killer, and mushrooms appear to sensitize cancer cells to TNF-induced apoptosis by inhibiting NFkappaB, etc.

In an interview, Paul Stamets explained, "Mushrooms don't like to rot, so they produce natural antibiotics. The mycelium produces these sweats of enzymes, and in these sweats are very potent antibiotics that are antiviral, antibacterial, antiprotozoal, and antifungal." Suzanne McNeary of the marketing firm Tradeworks (quote in Madley 2001) explains further, "The mushroom acquires food outside its cells. During the . . . mycelical stage . . . digestive enzymes are excreted to digest the food outside the cells. Since the mushroom needs to absorb the digested food, it must first deactivate any natural pathogens. The mushroom is also uniquely proficient at expelling undesirable chemicals and contaminants absorbed during the ingestion. Hence, in order for the mushroom to survive and thrive it must possess a remarkably aggressive, proactive, and protective immune system."

One study has shown that post-menopausal women eating mushrooms received more breast cancer protection than women who were still ovulating (S. A. Hong et al. 2008). Sonolight Pharmaceuticals, a company with roots in the University of Alberta, has also conducted research into the use of compounds derived from a bamboo mushroom for use in breast cancer therapy.

Mushrooms can be used medicinally in the form of homeopathy and essences. The former is based upon the use of mother tinctures (one part fungi to one part alcohol or water) and subsequent triturations or dilutions of these in water. This type of healing, based on the work of Samuel Hahnemann, is based on the idea of "similar cures similar" and that symptoms provoked by large material doses are remedied by small, dilute ingestion. Fungal essences are loosely based on the work of Dr. Edward Bach, an English physician who first produced flower essences nearly a century ago. Fungal essences are considered "vibrational medicine," and work on various mental, emotional, and spiritual aspects of a person's health.

The use of mushrooms in animal health medicine, both for pets and livestock, is a growing market. A recent project in British Columbia found shiitake extracts improved the effects of vaccination in farmed salmon (Nikl et al. 1991, 7). Another study found that mushroom extracts helped protect carp from bacterial infections (Yano et al. 1991). A recent phase-one study by Duane Barker and John Holliday (2010) looked at optimal amounts of Fin-Immune™, a proprietary mixture of medicinal mushrooms, on rainbow trout.

Other Uses for Mushrooms

Fungi may be a source of biological fuel cells of the future. Yeasts, growing in sugar, are capable of raising or lowering an electronic charge. By connecting six biological cells in a series and using carbon electrodes, M. C. Potter, in 1911, developed the first man-made "living battery," which gave a current of 1.25 milliamperes. He went on to show the enzymes invertase and diastase are capable of making electricity. A biochemical fuel cell, developed by Dr. Frederick Sisler, has been operating in his laboratory for several months. A Navy project known as "BEEP" (Biological Energy Production) is researching fuel cells based on yeast, algae, bacteria, and enzymes. Microbial electric cells for operating lights, radio receivers, and transmitters have been designed.

An unusual use of fungi is as a dye for wool. To use dry fungi as a dye, simmer with an equal amount of wool by weight for up to one hour in water no hotter than 194 degrees Fahrenheit. In many cases, these dyes are capable of fixing effectively without the use of mordants. *Mushrooms for Dyes, Paper Pigments and Myco-stix™*, by Miriam C. Rice, is a thorough examination of this application.

Fungi for Mycoremediation

Mycoremediation is a process that uses fungi to help reduce toxic materials presently relegated to disposal facilities, decontaminate and minimize road and farm runoff, create buffer zones, reduce agricultural waste, reduce pollution in watersheds, reduce forest fire potential, and clean up contaminated bacterium such as *Escherichia coli* and other pathogenic microbes. The methods are safe and economical, reduce unpleasant odors, and result in clean soil and water. Macrofungi help degrade contaminants into nitrogen, carbon, and oxygen, giving a viable alternative for remediation of agricultural chemicals, petroleum by-products, pesticides, and other industrial and pharmaceutical wastes.

Dr. Janusz Zwiazek at the University of Alberta is looking at fungi-protected trees and seedlings and their resistance to salt damage. The findings of that work could help mycoremediate the oil sands tailings in the Fort McMurray area of northern Alberta. For more information on mycoremediation, I recommend the excellent book *Mycoremediation: Fungal Bioremediation* by Harbhajan Singh, which contains nearly two thousand references related to this growing field.

Fungal Toxicity

Several myths exist regarding differentiation of edible and toxic fungi. As recently as the 1950s, it was believed that a silver spoon used to stir cooking mushrooms would discolor in the presence of toxins. Others believed that a sprinkling of salt would turn poisonous specimens black. Earlier "wisdom" suggested that a mushroom collected while the sun shone on them was bad, or that mushrooms, once seen by human eyes, will stop growing.

An old English rhyme reflects the fungiphobia and misinformation of fungal toxicity:

When the moon is at the full
Mushrooms you may freely pull.
But when the moon is on the wane
Wait ere you think to pluck again.

On the other hand, wild mushrooms are an edible delight, and in their prime they are remarkably tasty and satisfying. Be alert, sensible, and enjoy.

Mushrooms in Popular Culture

I am a mushroom, on whom the dew of heaven drops now and then.

— JOHN FORD

Modern literature, films, and musical compositions make use of fungi to create unearthly or mystical settings. Flying amanitas both grow and shrink in the Disney animated film *Fantasia*. In a Mickey Mouse short film, the hero's home is uprooted by sprouting toadstools. In *Peter Pan,* the nefarious Captain Hook "sat down on one of the enormous forest mushrooms, [for] in Never-Never Land, mushrooms grow to gigantic size." The Smurfs live in mushroom cottages, and mushrooms are one of the favorite foods of Hobbits.

Video games also make great use of mushrooms. "Super Mario" fans will recognize the mushroom that can make them big or small, inspired, according to originator Shigeru Miyamoto, by *Alice in Wonderland*.

The Purple Pileus, by H. G. Wells, is about a mushroom that changes the course of a man's life. *Journey to the Center of the Earth* by Jules Verne included giant subterranean mushrooms. Ray Bradbury and John Wyndham have written science fiction stories featuring frightening fungi. Other great books featuring mushrooms include *I Is for Innocent,* by Sue Grafton; *Acceptable Risk,* by Robin Cook; *The Flounder,* by Nobel Prize-winning author Günter Grass, and *Mr. Bass's Planetoid,* by Eleanor Cameron.

At the young age of twenty-two, Igor Stravinsky composed a six-minute song for voice and piano called "The Mushrooms Going To War." First performed in 1904, this song tells the story of a pine mushroom (*Borovik*) who calls up various mushroom troops to arms. But each group claims entitlement to exemption, with the golden chanterelle (*Opionki*) objecting that they are too frail, with slender legs, and the wrinkled morels (*Smorchki*) too old.

A Czech composer, Vaclav Halek, has written some 1,650 musical compositions inspired by distinct varieties of mushroom. The sixty-seven-year-old picks fungi and hears music. "I know that each mushroom has its own special melody," he says. A book and CD called *The Musical Atlas of Mushrooms,* containing forty of his compositions, is available from www.fontana.ws.

In the rock musical *The Pick of Destiny,* Jack Black's song "Papagenu (He's My Sassafrass)" is inspired by mushrooms.

Interesting Notes

- It is mentioned that to dream of mushrooms denotes fleeting happiness, but to dream that you are gathering them suggests fickleness in a lover or consort.

- First Nations, such as the Thompson of British Columbia, bathed new babies in mushroom infusions to make them strong and independent, since fungi were considered so powerful.
- Curiously, fungi are more closely related to animals than to plants, meaning they are closer to the people who eat them than they are to the dead wood on which they live.
- Mushrooms come in all sizes, from microscopic to giant; one wild mushroom found in France some years back measured fifty feet in circumference and weighed 108 pounds.
- Mushrooms are powerful, some able to lift heavy rocks and even break through cement sidewalks. Fruiting bodies have cells that stretch and act like tiny hydraulic rams creating slow, steady pressure. They have moved through three-inch-thick asphalt, lifted wine casks off a cellar floor, and broken through concrete floors in factories. In England, a stone slab weighing thirty-seven kilograms (about eighty-one pounds) was lifted two inches off the ground by two small meadow mushrooms, which were found balancing the stone in the center.
- Two Italian mycologists heard a loud noise like an exploding firecracker coming from a portico that faced their courtyard. The concrete floor split and rose in the air, revealing several compact agaric mushrooms in the floor opening. Impressive indeed!

Part One
Mushrooms

Acremonium

This ergot fungus establishes itself on various *Stipa* grass species. It appears to contain a first cousin of LSD, in this case lysergic acid amide, which (unlike its infamous relative) is considered a mild sedative. Studies from the Agricultural Research Service (Kaiser et al. 1996) and Indiana University (Clay 1999) describe this fungus in greater detail.

Dose: one microgram of fungus for an average-sized (150-pound) adult.

Agaricus

Agaricus campestris
Psalliota campestris
(FIELD MUSHROOM)
(MEADOW MUSHROOM)
(GHOST EARS)
A. arvensis
P. arvensis
(HORSE MUSHROOM)
A. brunnescens
A. bisporus
A. hortensis
(WILD BUTTON MUSHROOM)
(CULTIVATED MUSHROOM)
(PORTOBELLO)
(CRIMINI)
A. bitorquis
A. rodmanii
(SPRING AGARICUS)
(SIDEWALK MUSHROOM)
A. moelleri
A. placomyces
A. praeclaresquamosus
(FLAT TOP)
A. augustus
(THE PRINCE)
A. crocodilinus
A. macrosporus
(CROCODILE AGARICUS)
A. brasiliensis Wasser et al.
A. blazei ssp. Heinemann
(ROYAL SUN AGARICUS)
(ALMOND PORTOBELLO)

> *The meadow mushrooms are in kind*
> *the best,*
> *It is ill trusting any of the rest.*
> — HORACE

9

To the respectable mushroom hunter, *Agaricus bisporus* is only a poor imitation of a real mushroom, as natural to mycophagists as refined sugar is to health food purists.

— SARA ANN FRIEDMAN

"Mushrooms!" exclaimed Kamba the Tortoise, joyfully. "Do I see mushrooms? REAL mushrooms?" Yes, they were real mushrooms, little, white, satiny buttony mushrooms, with lovely pink underneaths; little white mushrooms that had pushed all night at the dark brown earth above them, and had struggled through its hard crust just in time to see the sun rise, just in time to make a fine breakfast for a hungry Tortoise.

— MALAWI FOLK TALE

Agaricus may derive from *agrarius* meaning "growing in the fields," or from the Greek *agarikon*. *Agaric* is used to describe all mushrooms with gills, and is from the name of a pre-Scythian people, the Agari, who were skilled in the use of medicinal plants, including mushrooms. They used a fungus called *Agaricum,* which was probably a *Fomes* polypore.

The field mushroom was called *Amanitai* by Galen, *Fungi pratenses* by Horace, and *Fungi albi* by Ovid.

Criminy is a seventeenth century minced oath on Christ, and related to crimine and crime.

Bitorquis means "having two rings," for the double annulus that distinguishes this mushroom from its close relatives.

Brasiliensis means "from Brazil." *Blazei* is named after Mr. R. Blaze because it is one of some six hundred and fifty species discovered by the American mycologist William A. Murrill on Blaze's lawn in Gainesville, Florida, in 1945. It was identified as *A. blazei* by the Belgian botanist Heinemann in 1967. The origins of this mushroom can be traced to Piedade, southeast of São Paulo. The mushroom has been consumed for centuries and has gone by several common names, including the sun mushroom, the mushroom of God, and the mushroom of life. Richard Kerrigan suggested that it be named *Agaricus subrufescens* (*sub* meaning "under" and *rufescens* meaning "becoming red"), as new data suggests the medicinal mushroom from Brazil and Japan is biologically and phylogenetically the same species as *Agaricus subrufescens* from North America (Kerrigan 2005). The North American *Agaricus subrufescens* was first described by the New York botanist C.H. Peck in 1893, and if it is in fact the same species as the Brazilian mushroom, the older name should have priority. Work by Colauto et al. (2002) showed little genetic variability, but Da Eira et al. (2002) concluded that *A. blazei* Murrill differs from *A. blazei* ssp. Heinemann in various ways, suggesting that there are, in fact, two distinct species.

The name "button mushroom" is derived from the size and shape of this mushroom, the term being an English slang term for small male genitalia.

Campestris means "campus" or "field." *Horsens* means "in the garden" or "cultivated." *Placomyces* is Greek for "flat cake."

Field or meadow mushrooms can still be found, but they have become far less common due to the widespread use of chemical fertilizers and pesticides. According to noted French

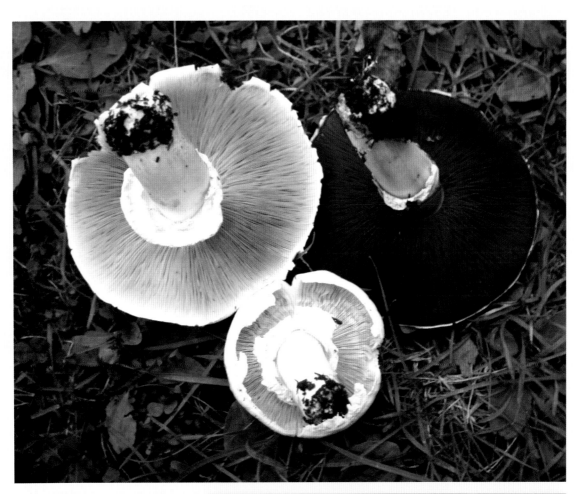

Clockwise from above: *Agaricus campestris,* showing different stages of gill color; *Agaricus bitorquis;* cultivated crimini.

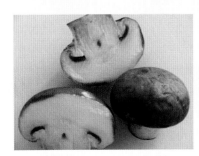

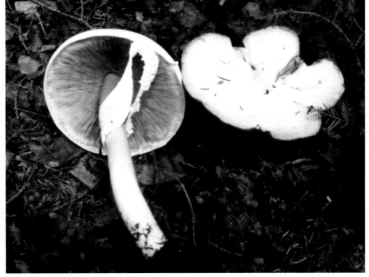

mycologist George Becker, field mushrooms are becoming "nothing more than a memory in the heads of aging mycologists."

There is some controversy regarding the origins of the familiar supermarket mushroom. According to Dr. Malloch, *A. brunnescens* (formerly *A. bisporus*) is the precursor to the common button mushroom. Others believe it was a pure white field mushroom discovered by a farmer in 1926. Today, the cultivated button mushroom can be found in every supermarket in North America. More than 860 million pounds were sold on the American market in 1998. Few are grown organically, and in fact, the industry relies heavily on pesticides, suggesting a new market opportunity. Dipping button mushrooms in a 5 percent hydrogen peroxide solution and storing them at forty degrees Fahrenheit prevents the cap from browning for ten days, and inhibits the growth of bacteria.

Crimini and portobello mushrooms are variations of the button mushroom with a richer, meatier flavor. The portobello is a large brown mushroom previously thought to be unsalable and taken home by mushroom pickers. Today, through good marketing and a growing appetite for variety among consumers, the portobello is available at most supermarkets year round. A relatively new variety called the portobellini is a cremini mushroom that is picked just after the veil has broken. These mushrooms are high in crude protein (43.5 percent) and acid-hydrolyzed fat.

Wild *Agaricus* species tend to be softer, more pliable, and less chalky than their domesticated counterparts. They have a nutty flavor when cooked. The prince mushroom, which leaves a yellow stain, is a very common almond-scented edible found along the Pacific coast.

Agaricus fungi were called "ghost ears" by the Mohawk, who, along with other First Nations people, used them as food and as a flavoring agent. The neighboring Onondaga called them *ananau'tra,* meaning "hat or cap." In parts of India and Afghanistan, they are known by the name *kallulac-div,* meaning "fairy's cap."

Agaricus brasiliensis has recently attracted a lot of attention from the myco-medical community. It looks like a large portobello, bruises yellow, and smells and tastes like almonds. It contains significant quantities of protein (from 33 to 48 percent of dry weight), and up to 14 percent beta-glucans, including beta-1–6 and alpha 1–3 glucans, riboglucans, glucomannans, with nearly 27 percent polysaccharides. It is now cultivated under controlled conditions similar to *A. brunnescens.*

This mushroom is very popular in Japan, where it goes by the commercial name *hime-matsutake* or the common name *kawari-haaratake.*

This mushroom has become the center of a $700 million industry since 1995. The Iwade Strain 101A is most popular; it is named after Dr. Iwade, who spent ten years of trial and error before its cultivation was perfected in 1975. Commercial button mushroom producers will surely be exploring the great opportunity this mushroom presents, as growing techniques are well established for other *Agaricus* species. It is presently cultivated in Japan, Korea, the United States, Denmark, Holland, and Brazil. It grows well on leached cow manure, of which there is no shortage, and can be grown outdoors in northern climates in the summertime or year-round in controlled conditions indoors. Work by Rinker et al. (2002) at the University of Guelph found optimal mycelial growth at pH 5 and 6 at thirty degrees Celsius. A casing of pH 5 and pinning temperature of twenty-four degrees Celsius produced the highest yield.

The flat top mushroom is widespread but not common. It is recognized by its black scales and beige base. It is not a recommended edible, as it causes gastrointestinal upset for some.

Crocodile *Agaricus* is a choice edible when young, with a faint odor of almonds.

Yellow-staining *Agaricus (A. xanthodermus)* and felt-ringed *Agaricus (A. hondensis)* are not recommended as edibles and have phenolic and metallic odors, respectively. The yellow-staining varieties tend to concentrate heavy metals, another reason to avoid them.

The horse mushroom stains lemon yellow when bruised and smells of anise.

The compound lenthionine is believed to be a contributing factor in the flavor of the wild button mushroom.

Spring *Agaricus (A. bitorquis)* is cultivated commercially in warm climates, as it requires a higher temperature by six to eight degrees Celsius over that of its cousin for optimal growth. It is highly resistant to viruses, tolerates higher levels of carbon dioxide, and has a superior shelf life.

It should be noted that manganese added to compost boosted yields of *A. bisporus* by 9.6 to 11.8 percent. (Weil et al. 2006)

Traditional Uses

The use of *Agaricus* mushrooms for medicine was first described in the Byzantine treatise by Orivasios, back in the fourth century AD.

The meadow mushroom is used in Unani medicine as a treatment for sinusitis and to abort coughs and colds. It was used in both Ayurvedic and Unani medicine during the sixteenth century as an aphrodisiac. It was boiled in milk for consumption and debility. In Norfolk, England, it was stewed in milk and used as a treatment for throat cancer.

In China, field mushrooms are believed to be a cure for hypertension.

Culpepper wrote that garden mushrooms (*A. campestris*) were used medicinally. "Roasted and applied in a poultice, or boiled with white lily roots and linseed in milk, they ripen boils and abscesses better than any preparation that can be made."

Horse mushrooms are resistant to both gram-positive and gram-negative bacteria and have been shown to inhibit, or even arrest the growth of certain types of cancer, including sarcoma 180 and Ehrlich carcinoma (Ohtsuka et al. 1973).

In traditional Chinese medicine, the dried mushroom is used as part of the Tendon Easing Powder, which is used for curing lumbago (lower back pain), pain in the legs, numbed limbs and discomfort in the tendons and veins.

Horse mushrooms have one of the highest concentrations (8.7 percent of dry weight) of phosphatidyl serine (a chemical that boosts brain function) of any mushroom, making it of likely interest to formulators.

The button mushroom was traditionally used in China (where it is known as chicken foot or gill fungus mushroom) and Korea to help breastfeeding mothers increase milk production.

In traditional Chinese medicine, the button mushroom is used to regulate body energy, and remove phlegm from the body. Good for the stomach and intestines, it is cooked in soups to ease indigestion and increase appetite. It is often simmered with reishi mushroom *(Ganoderma lucidum)* for treating chronic hepatitis, given daily for two weeks and then three days off. It is also used as a treatment for measles, coughs, and hiccups.

Medicinal Use

The field mushroom *(A. campestris)* contains traces of many valuable vitamins such as A, B1, C, K, and bioflavonoids, and taken regularly helps prevents debility, loss of appetite, indigestion, and insufficient breast milk secretion. It also helps alleviate the rupturing of capillaries, gum and abdominal bleeding, and pellagra, a vitamin deficiency diseases associated with a lack of niacin (vitamin B3).

Iodine is present in trace amounts (130 to 230 micrograms per kilogram), which is somewhat rare for a land-based food.

The mushroom contains campestrin, effective against both gram-positive and gram-negative bacteria and has been used traditionally to treat tuberculosis and sinusitis.

It contains Coenzyme Q10 (ubiquinone), which is associated with energy production on a cellular level. The fruiting body and cultured mycelia contain hetero-auxin that act as a growth inhibitor on higher plants and stimulating in low ones.

The fruiting bodies contain ergosterol, fungisterol, and proteolytic enzymes, which may have anti-coagulative properties.

Retine, or alpha-ketoaldehyde, inhibits the growth of certain types of cancer, including sarcoma 180 and Ehrlich carcinoma.

The species contains lectins that bind with erythrocytes and leukocytes; as well as basidiolipids that are novel immune adjuvants (Jennemann et al. 1999).

Field mushrooms have been shown to possess significant antiviral potential, particularly against poliomyelitis, perhaps due to the presence of (S)-agaridoxin and indigo (Cochran 1978).

Modern research by Gray and Flatt (1998) found that given to diabetic lab mice in drinking water, *A. campestris* countered hyperglycemia. The insulin releasing activity is greatest in the polar fractions, and leads to as many questions as answers.

Work in Poland found the wild field Agaric to concentrate silver at an average of thirty-five milligrams per kilogram of dry weight. Researchers found organic silver accumulation in *Lepista nuda, Boletus edulis, Leccinum scrabum, Cantharellus cibarius,* and *Coprinus comatus,* but at a lower level (Falandysz et al. 1994).

Vitamin D2 derived from mushrooms has been found to increase femur bone mineral density in animal studies (Jasinghe et al. 2006).

Both button and portobello mushrooms inhibit the enzyme aromatase, which is associated with breast cancer, and 5-alpha reductase activity, which is associated with prostate cancer. The conversion of testosterone, an androgen, to dihydrotestosterone increases benign prostatic hypertrophy and promotes the growth of prostate cancers. Over production of DHT is related to hair loss, and fatty acids are believed to be involved.

The button mushroom has been found to contain a polysaccharide, PA3DE, that inhibits the *Helicobacter pylori* bacterium, which is responsible for many stomach ulcers, gastritis, and gastric carcinomas (Kim, D.-H. et al. 1996).

The button mushroom *(A. bisporus)* is resistant to both gram-positive and gram-negative bacteria. Work by Rana et al. (2008) found culture filtrate of *A. bisporus* and *A. bitorquis* active against *Bacillus subtilis.*

Button mushrooms contain aromatase inhibitors and possess anticancer activity, especially against hormone-sensitive cells of the breast and prostate (Grube et al. 2001; Chen, S. et al. 2006).

Shnyreva et al. (2010) found button mushroom treatment of K562 leukemia cell lines promoted transcription of IL-10.

A phase-one clinical trial is underway at City of Hope in Duarte, California. Several funding agencies, including the NIH, American Institute Cancer Research, California Breast Cancer Research Program, and the button mushroom industry are involved. The initial trial involves twenty-four post-menopausal breast cancer survivors taking five to thirteen grams of freeze-dried button mushroom extract daily for twelve weeks.

A study conducted on 2,018 pre- and post-menopausal women, half with diagnosed breast cancer and the other half deemed "healthy," looked at the effects of a daily dose of ten grams of fresh button mushrooms or four grams of dried. Results showed a 64 percent reduction in the risk of breast cancer in the group that consumed the fresh mushrooms and a slightly lower risk reduction for those who consumed the dried version. The decrease in breast cancer risk went up to 90 percent when the women also drank green tea (Zhang, Min et al. 2008).

Button mushrooms have been shown to inhibit proliferation and growth and to induce apoptosis of tumor cells in athymic mice (Adams et al. 2008).

Mushroom lectins have been shown to possess potent anti-proliferative effects on human epithelial cancer cells, without apparent cytotoxicity (Yu, Lugang et al. 1999). This suggests an important therapeutic potential for preventing the development of neoplasms in people receiving chemotherapy treatment for cancer. Still other research has uncovered a lectin in button mushrooms with potent anti-proliferative properties, blocking the uptake of protein by the cell, but no apparent cytotoxicity (Yu, Lugang et al. 1999). Earlier work by the same researcher found this lectin showed reversible inhibition of proliferation of epithelial cell lines (Yu, Lugang et al. 1993).

Work by Jordinson et al. (1999) found *A. bisporus* agglutinin cytotoxic or inhibit tumor cells in LS174T, SW1222 and HT human colon cancer cells.

The lectin inhibits Caco-2 human colorectal cells, Tennon's fibroblasts, retinal pigment endothelial and RPE mediated collagen matrix contraction in vitro (Wenkel et al. 1999). ABL lectins do not exhibit cytotoxicity, compared to wheat germ and other lectins.

Lectin can help repair wounds such as proliferative vitreoretinopathy (the formation of scar tissue in the eye), or modulate wound healing in the subconjunctival space after glaucoma surgery (Kent et al. 2003; Batterbury et al. 2002). It can also prevent keloids, hypertrophic scars, adhesions, and the like.

Button mushrooms may boost both innate and active immune system health. The former system naturally protects against intruders such as viruses, bacteria, and fungi, while the active system springs into activity when the innate system fails.

Button mushrooms given in vitro have been found to enhance maturation of bone marrow dendritic cells and enhance antigen-presenting function. This suggests innate and T-cell-mediated immunity against both microbial and tumor invasion is enhanced by the mushroom.

ABL lectin is immune modulating, inducing up-regulation of IL-1beta and TNF-alpha in splenocytes for up to twenty-four hours (Ooi et al. 2002).

Decoctions of dried button mushrooms have traditionally been used to treat diabetes. In a study by Swanston-Flatt et al. at the University of Surrey, they were found to lower blood sugar and counter the initial reduction in plasma insulin and the reduction in pancreatic insulin concentration, and improve the hypoglycemic effect of exogenous insulin. Gray and Flatt (1998) confirmed the blood sugar reduction.

The active compounds are heat stable, and may be due in part to guanidine, related to the biquanide class of antidiabetic drugs.

The button mushroom's outer skin contains significant amounts of vitamin B12 like that derived from beef, eggs, salmon, and liver (Koyyalamudi et al. 2009).

The purple color observed on some cultivated and washed mushrooms is due to the oxidization of L-dopa by tyrosinase to indol-5,6-quinone, then to melanochrome, and finally to melanin. A number of animal studies have looked at tyrosinase to treat vitiligo, and melanin is responsible for skin pigmentation.

Tyrosinase is a copper-containing enzyme with a number of useful applications, including as a treatment for malignant melanoma in the form of melanocyte-directed enzyme prodrug therapy (MDEPT) and may lead to new treatments.

Tyrosinase is obtained from the mushroom by both hot- and cold-water extraction (Shi, Y.-L. et al. 2002a).

Button mushrooms contain phenolic and quinoid derivatives with antibacterial activity. Studies indicate that ethanol extracts from button mushrooms contain anti-mutagenic substances that are heat stable (Grüter et al. 1990).

Lectins from them were found to proliferate smooth muscle cell growth (Sanford et al. 1990).

Rats fed a diet made up of 5 and 10 percent dried mushrooms showed an accumulation of lipids in the liver and a simultaneous decrease in the circulatory lipids, except for healthy phospholipids, in blood plasma. This could be due, in part, to the content of novel glyco-inositol-phosphingo lipids found in both button and field mushrooms.

According to one report, a polysaccharide from button mushrooms can be used to treat leukocytopenia, inhibit bacterial growth, and reduce blood sugar levels. They can be taken after cancer operations to prevent metastasis.

Experiments by Wardle and Schisler in 1969 showed that the growth of mushroom mycelium in vitro was stimulated by the addition of lipids.

The fungal metabolite 10-oxo-trans-8-decenoic acid may be beneficial in mycelia fermentation of edible and medicinal mushrooms (Mau et al. 2004).

Vitamin D2, or ergocalciferol, is increased in button mushrooms by nearly six times after just two hours of exposure to UV-C rays (Mau et al. 1998).

Based on work by Penn State Research Foundation, pulsed UV light has been found to increase vitamin D2 content of commercial mushrooms by 800 percent after one second of exposure. One second!

Total Nutraceutical Solutions is one company pursuing the commercial viability.

An unusual use of *A. bisporus* was developed by Sezginturk et al. (2005). Fungal tissue homogenate was set on a Clark-type oxygen electrode and used as a biosensor that is both cheap and easy to produce.

Conventional wisdom had held for years that hydrazines were destroyed in cooking, while some authors believe that aromatase, antioxidants, and anticancer polysaccharides neutralize their effects. The mushroom's superoxide dimutase and aromatase inhibitors also may help neutralize some of agaritine's potential danger. It is worth noting, though, that mice fed uncooked button mushrooms developed cancer tumors from the phenylhydrazine derivative agaritine. Mice studies do not always transfer to humans, and recent studies have failed to confirm these observations. One Swiss study suggested that four grams of raw button mushrooms daily led to a lifetime risk of cancer of two cases per hundred thousand lives; another study of agaritine found no known toxicology to healthy humans and, in fact, agaritine derived from *A. blazei* was found to inhibit the growth of various leukemia cell lines (Roupas 2010). Another study found that agaratine neither affected normal cells nor activated the umu gene of *Salmonella,* which reacts to carcinogens (Endo et al. 2010). The data is too limited to be certain one way or the other. Until more conclusive studies are conducted, it is probably a good idea to cook all button mushrooms before eating them, but beware, also, that cooking only reduces the carcinogenic hydrazines by 25 percent.

Tyrosinase, found in button mushrooms, on the other hand, helps lower blood pressure and is used in treating hypertension. It is, however, destroyed by heat.

Both button and portobello mushrooms contain twelve times more of the antioxidant ergothioneine than wheat germ, and four times that of chicken liver, the previous top rated sources of the compound. Shiitake, oyster, and maitake mushrooms contain nearly forty times as much of this compound as wheat germ. Joy Dubost, a doctoral candidate at Penn State, suggests, "ergothioneine, a unique metabolite produced by fungi, has been shown to have strong antioxidant properties and to provide cellular protection within the human body."

When nine common mushrooms were tested for protection against oxidative DNA damage, researchers found that cold-water extracts of *A. bisporus* (button mushrooms) afforded the highest protection, followed by hot-water extraction from *Ganoderma lucidum* (Shi, Y.-L. et al. 2002b). Another study found that ethanol extracts exhibit antioxidant activity at various stages of growth (Tsai et al. 2008).

Ergosterol and ergosterol peroxide suppress LPS induced inflammation via NFkappaB and other pathways. The latter compound also suppresses STAT 1 mediated inflammation by altering redux state in HT29 cells (Kobori et al. 2007).

Nearly all edible and medicinal mushrooms contain ergosterol peroxide. This compound is both anti-inflammatory and anticancer in nature (Kobori et al. 2007).

Dr. Peter Romaine and his company, Agarigen Inc., have been recently awarded $2.2 million under the Accelerated Manufacture of Pharmaceuticals program for the rapid development of vaccines and other therapeutic protein in altered button mushrooms.

"Our immediate research goals are to maximize the level of expression of various biopharmaceuticals and to devise efficient and economical methods for their extractions and purification from mushroom tissue," says Romaine. He and his team at Penn State hold the patent to genetically modify *Agaricus bisporus*. Antibiotics, antivirals, and insulin are also possible applications of this technology.

Work at the University of Warwick is proceeding to sequence the full genome of this mushroom in the near future.

There is a definite need for the development of agaritine-free strains, even if agaritine is weakly mutagenic against *Salmonella typhimurium,* responsible for acute gastroenteritis.

In 1998, the button mushroom accounted for 98 percent of the market with 861 million pounds sold. In 1970, the button mushroom accounted for more than 70 percent of the total global mushroom production, but by the new century, it accounts for only 30 percent, even though production has more than doubled in those years.

Of more concern is the heavy use of malathione and other fungicides used in commercial mushroom cultivation. Organic production has become the new standard.

Work by Sokovic et al. (2006) suggests carvacrol essential oil compounds may be useful in button mushroom cultivation. In France, another fungi, a green mold called *Trichoderma,* is used as a spray-concentrate alternative to the systemic fungicide Benomyl to control *Verticillium fungicola,* a serious pathogen of *A. brunnescens.*

Champex, a patented field mushroom derivative, is a functional foodstuff designed to deodorize the body in the digestive system. It is 400 percent more effective for this purpose than parsley seed extract.

Work by Tamaki et al. (2007) found a button mushroom powder significantly reduced the odor produced by garlic.

As a nutritional supplement, it helps eliminate breath and body odor, improves intestinal function and regularity, helps blood cleansing, and detoxifies the kidney and liver by suppressing the serum levels of creatinine.

It has been clinically proven to repress production of indole and tryptamine in vivo.

In pets, it helps reduce fecal / ammonia odor and suppresses odors internally, resulting in cleaner litter.

Dr. Tatsuo Shiigai, of Toride Kyodo General Hospital, found that serum creatinine levels, a measure of the progress of kidney failure, was significantly suppressed by using *champignon* extract. Six of nine patients with glomerulonephritis that did not respond to low-protein diets were helped by the extract. It is possible that the mushroom extract works, in part, by reducing the production of nephrotoxic substances in the intestines. It is extremely safe, with an LD50 (lethal dose) value of less than 50,185 milligrams per kilogram.

A product containing champex and nettle seed is worthy of human clinical trials due to the significant degree of chronic kidney disease in our society.

A randomized, double-blind study of thirty-eight overweight patients found biscuits containing one and a half grams of dried powder taken for four weeks helped reduce weight. (Donatini and Le Blaye 2007).

Because of its biocompatibility with human tissue, chitosan is effective in all types of dressings, including artificial skin, surgical sutures, dental implants, and rebuilding bones and gums. Corneal contact lenses are currently being developed. Chitosan also helps deliver time-release drugs and supplements.

Work by Hamlyn and Schmidt (1994) examines the potential therapeutic application of fungal filaments in wound management.

Chitosan is produced from shells of crustaceans and shellfish, but because this product is sourced from animals, it is prone to pollution. Furthermore, 3 percent of the population suffers from seafood allergies. Kitozyme is one European company that has launched industrial scale chitosan production for food, agriculture, and medical application. See www.kitozyme.com.

Work by Tao Wu et al. (2004) found the crude chitin isolated from stalks stored at twenty-five degrees Celsius (seventy-seven degrees Fahrenheit) for five days was 27 percent of dry weight and consisted of 46 percent glucosamine and 20.9 percent neutral polysaccharides. The degree of acetylation was from 75 to 87 percent, very similar to commercially available crustacean chitin. Yields of crude fungal chitin of 0.65 to 1.15 percent on a fresh weight basis suggests potential for utilization of these mushroom by-products.

Chitosonium acetate coatings may have application as food coatings, exhibiting protection and biocide activity (Lagaron et al. 2007).

Work by Beelman et al. (2003) favorably compared nutritional and medicinal benefits of portobello mushrooms to shiitake and oyster mushrooms.

Portobello contains significant amounts of mannose, glucose, and sugar alcohols. It also contains significantly high levels of phytase, suggesting that both basidiomata and spent substrate may be useful in mycofiltration of elevated phosphorus levels associated with poultry and swine production. Portobellos also contain significant amounts of chitin, a polysaccharide polymer that has valuable applications in chemistry, biotechnology, agriculture, dentistry, food processing, environmental protection, and textile production.

Studies indicate that the flat top mushroom has antiviral potential and contains the steroid ergosterol.

It inhibits sarcoma 180 and Ehrlich carcinoma by 60 percent (Ohtsuka et al. 1973).

Fermentation cultures of crocodile *Agaricus* have identified agrico-glyceride A, a triglyceride that exhibits a strong activity against neurolysin, a protease involved in the regulation of elynophin and neurotensin metabolism (Stadler et al. 2005).

Yellow-staining *Agaricus* contains psalliotin, active against gram-positive *Salmonella* species (Dornberger et al. 1986).

The yellow-staining *A. xanthodermus* contains the carcinogen, 4,4'-dihydroxy-azobenzene, that is toxic in high doses, and in low doses does not induce tumors (Toth et al. 1989)

Early work by Atkinson (1946) found activity against *Staphylococcus aureus* and *Salmonella typhi (Bacillus typhosus)*.

Extracts made with dichlormethane inhibit the growth of *E. coli, Biomphalaria glabrata,* and *Aedes aegupti* (Keller, C. et al. 2002).

The closely related wine-colored *Agaricus (A. subrutilescens)* is reported to be antifungal. It inhibits sarcoma 180 and Ehrlich carcinoma cells at 100 percent (Ohtsuka et al. 1973).

The related *A. semotus* contains polysaccharides with antitumor activity, as well as moderate activity against *Staphylococcus aureus* (Nano et al. 2002; Suay et al. 2000).

The related *A. sylvaticus* was supplemented at thirty milligrams per kilogram daily for six months to fifty-six colorectal post-surgery patients. This randomized, double-blind, placebo-controlled trial found significant reduction of fasting blood sugar levels (Fortes et al. 2008).

Royal *Agaricus* has been found to contain many of the same polyhydroxysteroids as turkey tail (*Trametes versicolor;* see page 401), with beta-glucan levels from 9 to 14 percent. Its polysaccharides promote natural killer cells that are selective to tumor cells, but the mushroom possesses immune-modulating properties, as well. Modulating the immune system is beneficial in autoimmune disorders such as lupus erythematosus, rheumatoid arthritis, and certain forms of thyroid conditions.

Work by Liang Chen and HanJuan Shao (2006) suggests royal *Agaricus* extracts might provide a strategy to improve the efficacy of DNA vaccines.

Water-soluble proteoglycans found in royal *Agaricus* may be useful in both cancers and immune deficient diseases through the up-regulation of bone marrow-derived dendritic cell maturation (Kim, G. Y. et al. 2005).

Royal *Agaricus* has been widely studied for antitumor and anticancer effect, both from the fruiting body as well as mycelium (Mizuno, T. 1999; Kawagishi et al. 1988; Kawakami et al. 2002.)

The Japan Cancer Association approves use of royal *Agaricus* extracts for sigmoid colon, breast, ovarian, lung, and liver cancers, as well as Ehrlich's ascites carcinoma and solid cancers. Each year in Japan, about three hundred to five hundred thousand cancer patients consume the recommended three to five grams daily of a hot-water extract .

Work by Ahn et al. (2004) found that after six weeks of this treatment, NK cell activity was increased, and improvement in appetite, alopecia, emotional stability, and general weakness were observed.

A study of guinea pigs at the National Cancer Center, Tokyo University, and Tokyo Pharmacology Institute found sarcoma 180 cancers showed a 99.4 percent prevention rate and 90 percent recovery rate with a daily dose of just ten milligrams of royal *Agaricus* extract. The same study showed a prevention rate of only 77.8 percent with a daily dose of thirty milligrams of reishi extract.

Fruiting bodies inhibited the proliferation of human thyroid carcinoma cell line TPC-3 (Shimizu et al. 2002).

A recent study showed water extracts activate apoptosis of gastric epithelial AGS cells through induction of caspase-3 and related cell cycle arrest at the G2/M phase. (Jin, C. Y. et al. 2006).

A study at the Catholic University of Korea in Seoul of one hundred patients with cancers of the cervix, ovary, or endometrial tissue compared immune status and quality of life while undergoing chemotherapy with and without mushrooms. The NK cell activity was significantly greater in the group ingesting mushrooms, but no significant difference was found between the groups' lymphokine activated killer and monocyte activity. Side effects of chemotherapy, such as loss of appetite, alopecia, emotional stabil-

ity, and weakness were improved with mushroom supplementation.

A study at the University of Sorocaba in Brazil supplemented seventy cancer patients with 0.4 grams of Royal *Agaricus* extract four times daily. The majority showed a statistically significant increase in NK cell count, whereas the control group showed unchanged or decreased levels. One interesting aspect is that this particular mushroom stimulates natural killer cells but does not affect T-cell activity. One human study showed the mushroom added to the diet increased NK-cells by 3,000 percent in two to four days.

Natural killer (NK) cells circulate and become active in the body in response to cytokines. Upon activation, they seek out tumor cells, attach themselves, inject a substance, and dissolve them. They then move on and can destroy up to twenty-seven cancer cells before they die themselves. Often forgotten is that the number of NK-cells is not a measure of the body's immune system efficacy. It is their activity, how well they recognize and bind to tumor cells, that is most important. The low molecular weight of some molecules makes them more easily absorbed.

Immune modulators increase the level of function, not the numbers, of NK-cells.

Royal *Agaricus* may be a useful protectant in patients with a family history of breast or prostate cancer.

The mushroom activates granulocytes that help control acute inflammatory reactions. Patents have been filed for its use externally for maintaining skin health and protecting against environmental toxins, pollution, chemicals, and radiation. Extracts may be of value in reducing age spots, stimulating dermal fibroblasts, or preventing benign keratosis.

A recent study found inhibitions of mast cell-mediated anaphylaxis-like reactions with water extracts (Choi, Y. H. et al. 2006).

Mice tumors were initiated and promoted with exposure to UVB light in one experiment. One group was given a topical application of a water extract one hour prior to exposure and fared better than the mice in a control group.

Royal *Agaricus* contains compounds that inhibit aromatase, associated with hormone-sensitive cancers. In one study, one hundred cervical, ovarian, and endometrial cancer patients undergoing chemotherapy were treated with carboplatin and etoposide or carboplatin plus taxol every three weeks. One group also consumed the mushroom extract, with significantly higher NK cell activity. The chemotherapy side effects, such as appetite loss, alopecia, emotional stability, and general weakness were all improved with the mushroom extract.

Immobilizing or neutralizing cancer cells is one aspect, but the body also has to destroy the cells by bursting them open. The activation of the complement process helps punch holes, and the attraction and stimulation of macrophages helps mop up the malignant cells.

A recent study in Japan looked at the activating of C3 complement by a polysaccharide derived from the mycelia. Apparently, no matter what polysaccharide is isolated from either the mycelium or fruiting body, they all have the immune system-modulating and antitumor activity in living organisms.

Shimizu et al. (2002) found fine particles of fruiting body and mycelium activate human complement, enhancing natural immunity in bacterial infections.

The mushroom appears to have prophylactic activity against septicemia that may prove invaluable in peritonitis and other serious intestinal infections. Bernardshaw et al. (2006) found significant protection against septicemia in mice first given a fungal extract.

Sorimachi et al. (2001) showed that ethanol extracts from the mycelium, possess antiviral activity against western equine encephalitis and herpes simplex.

The mushroom possesses antiviral, anti-cholesterol, and blood sugar modulation. Yea Woon Kim et al. (2005) found both beta glucan and oligosaccharides show anti-hyperglycemic, anti-triglyceride, anti-cholesterol, and anti-sclerotic activity, suggesting that it may be useful in the treatment of diabetes.

Kweon et al. (2002) investigated the effects of mycelium extracts on ninety women for eight weeks and found an 11.8 percent decrease in weight and an 11 percent decrease in cholesterol levels.

Toshiro et al. (2003) found GABA-enriched *A. blazei* decreased both systolic and diastolic blood pressure.

Bernardshaw et al. (2005) found antimicrobial activity against *Streptococcus pneumoniae, E. coli, and Salmonella* species.

Dr. Mai Furukawa et al. (2006) found cold-water extracts given orally to diabetic-induced mice increased T-cells versus B-cells and T-cells versus NK-cells more favorably than hot-water extracts or the control. The difference is significant and worthy of further research.

Recent work by Bellini et al. (2006) suggests some extraction methods are genotoxic and caution is advised.

The fruiting body, grown outdoors, was tested on humans and found to lower body and peripheral fat, lower cholesterol and blood sugar levels, and increase NK cell activity (Liu, Ying et al. 2007).

Patients with chronic hepatitis C decreased their viral load slightly, but not significantly, after one week of treatment with the mushroom extract. The beta-glucans did not enter the blood, but the components proposed to have anticancer effects were found active in the blood (Grinde et al. 2006).

Twenty patients with chronic hepatitis C received an extract twice daily for eight weeks. Decreased GTP activity was found in 80 percent of both sexes with no side effects (Inuzuka et al. 2002). Morimoto et al. (2008) found extracts increased interferon gamma and decreased IL-4 production of cytokines from spleen cells. This suggests a Th1 dominance that contributes to cellular immunity.

Immune response in humans is complex. It is thought that tumor-derived chemokines act as inhibitors of antitumor immune responses, as well as autocrine growth factors for the tumors.

In Brazil, a concentrated extract called Agaricus Drops is taken to treat breast cancer, ovarian cancer, lung cancer, gastrointestinal tumors, gastric ulcers, and viral infections.

The time of harvest and best form of extract for optimal benefit are still unknown. The mature fruiting bodies are probably best due to the significant increase in water-soluble 1-4 beta-glucans during maturation (Mizuno, T. et al. 1990). The mycelium contains various 1,6 and 1,4 glucans, as well as glucomannan that inhibit tumorigenesis (Mizuno, M. et al. 1999).

The mushroom extract down-regulates cytochrome P4501A and can be useful in reducing the production of metabolically activated procarcinogens from xenobiotics. On the other hand, it may prolong the duration and intensity of herb-drug interactions.

Three cases of severe hepatic dysfunction in cancer patients have been reported, indicating that more attention is required (Mukai et al. 2006).

Extracts containing up to 45 percent beta 1-6 glucan are on the market.

Homeopathy

Agaricus blazei seems to have the ability to maintain a balance between psoric deficiency and sycotic excess. On the one hand, it revitalizes what has been weakened by stress, poor eating habits, pollution, etc.; on the other hand, it reduces excessive immune reactions, e.g. those resulting in atopic dermatitis, asthma, pollinosis, or rheumatism. It falls into the "psoric" category by activating metabolism and stimulating defenses, and into the "sycotic" category by leveling excesses in blood pressure, blood sugar, and cholesterol.

— FRANS VERMEULEN

Field mushroom *(A. campestris)* may be associated with slight delirium, eyes sunken with livid circles, tongue red and patched, nausea and vomiting, abdominal pain, severe colic, irregular respiration, suppuration and gangrene, formation of abscesses and pus. Skin is cold, covered with cold sweat.

— ALLEN

Essential Oil

Seven volatiles were identified in the fruiting body and sixteen in the mycelia of *A. resiliencies.*

Benzaldehyde was 43 percent by weight, and benzyl alcohol was 29 percent in the fruiting body, with the former compound up to 38 percent in the mycelia. This explains the distinct almond flavor and odor.

Fungi Essences

Agaricus campestris essence is for stubbornness, inflexibility, and nervous behavior. It helps to open both the crown and base chokers. Mushrooms are a valuable future healing system.

— PEGASUS

Horse mushroom essence is for those you are not sure which direction to move into. It will help to remove hard mental patterning, stomach problems, nerves, anxiety, and stress."

— SILVERCORD

Mycoremediation

Rabinovich et al. (2007) found supplementing copper and zinc at four hundred parts per million to mycelium increased copper content by 449 times and zinc by 163 times.

High concentrations of cadmium have been found in this species (Yesil et al. 2004).

The related *A. abruptibulbus* myco-accumulates cadmium, and in fact, the heavy metal

stimulates its growth in laboratories (Meisch et al. 1986).

The button mushroom *(A. bisporus)* contains laccase and manganese peroxide that help lignin degradation (Bonnen et al. 1994; Trejo-Hernandez et al. 2001).

Cosmetics

Royal sun *Agaricus,* in whole or extracted form, can be applied to the skin to protect against environmental toxins, pollution, chemicals, and radiation, as well as prevent or treat malignant neoplasms, melanomas, Kaposi's sarcoma, and mycosis fungoides. Shoji Uchiyama filed a U.S. patent in January 2005 for various cosmetic and medical applications.

Button mushroom extracts, whether in the form of tinctures, concretes, absolutes, essential oils, oleoresins, distillates, or other residues, have application for the cosmetic industry. European companies already incorporate various extracts into products.

Chitosan has application for cosmetics because it forms a protective, moisturizing elastic film on the skin's surface and is capable of binding other ingredients. It has application for skin moisture, treating acne, reducing static electricity in hair, fighting dandruff, and making the hair softer and more supple. Chitosonium salts are used in hair setting products, with several advantages over synthetic polymers.

Mushroom oil derived from this species is used in several Paul Mitchell shampoos and rinses.

Button mushrooms secrete laccase and manganese peroxidase, the latter similar in activity to peroxidases from oyster mushrooms, especially when cultured on wheat and rye bran. Waste ends contain up to a hundred grams of laccase per ton.

Food Industry

When put through a weak acid bath, chitin is transformed into chitosan, a dietary supplement that is used to lower cholesterol and promote weight loss.

Chitosan is commonly used as a preservative and food stabilizer. It is used in Japan to thicken and stabilize sauces and other foods, clarify and remove heavy metals from beverages, and create a protective, antibacterial, fungistatic film for fruits and vegetables.

Work by Werner and Beelman (2002) found selenium-enriched button mushrooms can be produced for the functional food or nutraceutical industry. Work by Mavoungou et al. (1987) showed antitumor activity.

The related *A. paludosa,* found in swampy areas, shows an inhibition rate against sarcoma 180 and Ehrlich carcinoma of 90 percent and 100 percent respectively (Ohtsuka et al. 1973).

Agrocybe praecox

Pholiota praecox
(SPRING AGROCYBE)
A. aegerita
A. cylindracea
P. cylindracea
(PIOPPINO)
(BLACK POPLAR MUSHROOM)

Spring *Agrocybe* is found on forest ground or fields or even roadside lawns in summer and fall, is edible, and has a chocolate brown spore print. The soft flesh is pleasant and mealy in odor, but some specimens may be bitter.

The related *A. cylindracea (A. aergerita)* is not native to this continent. Known as black poplar fungus, or pippin, it is believed that the Greeks and Romans cultivated or encouraged the mushrooms' growth by placing small pieces of poplar wood on land that had been manured. The Greeks called it *Muketes aigeiritai,* and both Pliny and Dioscorides called it *Fungi populi.*

Today it is grown commercially in parts of Europe. China and Japan cultivate the fungi for food and medicine. In Japan it is known as the black poplar mushroom, the swordbelt *Agrocybe,* and *yanagi-matsutake.*

In China, it is called *zhuzhuang-tiantougu,* or south poplar mushroom.

As the name suggests, it grows on hardwood such as poplar, willow, and maple. It grows well in the southeastern United States, and would be a good candidate for field experiments or controlled growing rooms for commercial production.

A. praecox is not as tasty, but definitely edible, and hardy.

Cultivation

Work by Ohga et al. (2004) found an electric impulse of 150 kilovolts discharged directly into the substrate enhanced fruiting in this mushroom and eight others including *Grifola frondosa, Flammulina velutipes, Hypsizygus marmoreus,* and various *Pleurotus* species. A mixture of sawdust with 10 percent wheat bran was found to give 74 percent biological efficiency in cultivation (Sharma and Sharma 2009).

It may be rather easy to introduce the European species into our native poplar for a commercial opportunity, or to explore hybridization potential.

Medicinal Use

Chemical Constituents

■ *A. cylindracea:* **benzastatins A-G, betulinans A and B, indole derivatives, agrocybenine, agrocybin, and illudine sesquiterpenes, palmitic acid, ergosterol, mannitol, trehalose.**

In Fuji, it is used to penetrate dampness, strengthen the spleen, and stop diarrhea.

Research by Jin Won Hyun et al. (1996) found a neutral protein-bound polysaccharide fraction (cylindan) that showed marked antitumor activity, with 70 percent inhibition of sarcoma 180 when a dose of thirty milligrams per kilogram of body weight per day was given to mice.

Yoshida et al. (1996) identified three carboxymethylated alpha D-glucans, which increased immune function by more than 50 percent after administration to lab mice.

Won Gon (1997) showed cylindan increased the life of mice with the ascites form of sarcoma 180 and Lewis lung carcinoma at doses of milligrams per kilogram (about 2.2 pounds) of body weight per day. It was reported to have restored the decreased immune response of the tumor-bearing mice. The same group also discovered two indole compounds with free radical-scavenging potential.

A polysaccharide compound from *A. cylindracea* was found to inhibit skin tumors in mice by 88.2 percent and the percentage of mice with tumors by 30 percent after exposure to tetrachloroterephthalic acid (TPA).

An antitumor lectin (Yang, N. et al. 2005), a novel antigentoxic peptide or protein (Taira et al. 2005), and a lectin that induces apoptosis and expression of DNAse activity (Zhao, C. et al. 2003) have been found in the mushroom.

An ethyl acetate extract of the culture liquid has shown moderate inhibition of both IkB-alpha degradation and phosphorylation (Petrova et al. 2007).

Nine active extracellular enzymes in six different stages of growth from three different strains of *A. aegerita* have been identified (Wang, N. et al. 2000).

A lectin with potent mitogenic activity toward mouse splenocytes has also been identified (Wang, H. et al. 2002).

Cold-water extracts of *A. aegerita,* in vitro, inhibit leukemic U937 cells (Ou et al. 2005).

Ethanol extracts of the mycelium at four to eight milligrams per milliliter exhibit 82.7 percent antioxidant activity (Asatiani et al. 2007).

Researchers have isolated two polysaccharides with hypoglycemic activity (Kiho et al. 1994). This is believed due to AG-HN1 with a high molecular weight composed of glucose, and AG-HN2 with low molecular weight composed of fructose, galactose, glucose, and mannose.

The fungus has been shown to be active against five bacteria including *E. coli, Streptococcus aureus, Bacillus cereus, B. subtilis,* and *Salmonella typhimurium.*

Researchers have isolated a lectin with antiviral activity against tobacco mosaic virus and antifungal peptides from the fresh fruiting bodies (Ngai et al. 2005).

Yanjun Zhang et al. (2003) identified antioxidant compounds and discovered that the fruiting body inhibited both COX-1 and COX-2 enzyme activity, as well as cyclooxygenase activity.

A lectin in *A. aegerita* induces apoptosis in cancer cell through a novel nuclear pathway (Liang et al. 2010).

Recent studies have found ethyl acetate extracts of *A. cylindracea* exhibit strong inhibition of COX-2 enzyme, reflective of anti-inflammatory activity (Elgorashi et al. 2008).

Water-soluble peptides, or proteins, that protect DNA from mitogens have been identified, suggesting anti-genotoxic activity (Taira et al. 2005).

Kyung-Ae Lee et al. (2005) have shown hepatoprotective activity from this mushroom when cultivated on a waxy brown rice substrate.

Spring *Agrocybe* contains anti-carcinogenic substances with inhibition rates of 100 percent for both sarcoma 180 and Ehrlich carcinoma cells.

Hui-Ling Mao et al. (2007) found extraction of polysaccharides optimal at pH 7.5 at ninety degrees Celsius for one hour.

Mycoremediation

The mushroom has shown lacasse activity, suggesting mycoremedial potential. This term will come up again, so it is worth explaining in brief. Laccases are a group of copper-containing, radical-producing oxide reductases found in many white rot basidiomycetes and some ascomycetes. They degrade lignins and detoxify plant phenolic compounds. They can also degrade and detoxify artificially produced phenols to water and carbon dioxide.

Oxidation of endocrine disruptors, like nonylphenol and bisphenol A, by laccase has been reported.

Ullrich et al. (2004) have found the mushroom produces a peroxidase that oxidizes aryl alcohols, such as veratryl and benzyl alcohols in aldehydes and then acids at neutral pH.

Albatrellus

Albatrellus ovinus
Polyporus ovinus
Scutiger ovinus
(SHEEP POLYPORE)
A. confluens
P. confluens
S. confluens
(CONFLUENT POLYPORE)
A. fletti
(BLUE CAPPED POLYPORE)
A. caeruleoporus
(GREENING GOAT'S FOOT)
A. cristatus
(CRESTED POLYPORE)

Sheep polypore is an exception among the polypores, as it grows on the ground and is not woody. It tastes somewhat like oysters, and is harvested from the wild in parts of the Pacific Northwest for commercial sales. Ovinus means "related to sheep." Confluens means "running together."

It is a good nickel accumulator—Jorhem, in trials from Sweden, showed accumulation of nickel as high as 0.72 milligrams per kilogram (about 2.2 pounds) in industrial areas—and could be used as an environmental monitor.

The *Albatrellus* genus appears to be a selenium accumulator.

Sheep polypore is a significant source of carboxyl esterase, protease, and amylase enzymes. Protease is used in cheese-making, meat tenderizers, flavor development, and to treat blood clotting and inflammatory conditions. Amylases digest starch, and are used in the cosmetic and brewing industry, for laundry detergents, wood-pulp bleaching, pharmaceuticals, cleaners, leather, and fur, as well as food and feed products (Goud et al. 2009).

Crested polypore is found from New Brunswick to Florida and westward.

Medicinal Use

Chemical Constituents

- *A. ovinus:* **Novel neogrifolin derivatives, as well as grifolin, scutigeral, ilicicolin B, ovinal, and ovinol.**

- *A. confluens:* **albaconol, (t)-(r)-grifolinone, albatrellin, grifolinone, grifoline, and grifolinone A.**

- *A. caeruleoporus:* **grifolin, neogrifolin, and grifolinones A-B.**

- *A. fletti:* **confluentin, grifolin, and neogrifolin.**

- *A. cristatus:* **grifolic acid.**

Sheep polypore contains grifolin, which has been shown to lower cholesterol levels when fed to rats (Sugiyama et al. 1992).

Grifolin up-regulates the expression of the reporter gene for the farnesoid X receptor that controls bile acid and cholesterol metabolism (Suzuki, T. et al. 2006).

Mycelium polysaccharides have been shown to inhibit both sarcoma 180 and Ehrlich carcinoma cell lines by 100 percent (Ohtsuka et al. 1973).

Research has shown inhibition and induction by apoptosis of various cancer cell lines, including CNE1 (nasopharyngeal), HeLa (cervical), MCF7 (breast), SW480 (colon), K562 (leukemia), Raji (Burkitts lymphoma), and B95-8 (marmoset B lymphblastoid) (Ye et al. 2005). The same lead researcher found grifolin inhibits the ERK1/2 or the ERK5 pathway, inducing G_1 phase of cell cycle arrest (Ye et al. 2007).

Grifolin has been found to inhibit cancer and induce apoptosis of the osteosarcoma cell lines (Choi, J.-S. et al. 2007).

Szallasi et al. (1999) identified scutigeral as a stimulant of dorsal root ganglion neurons via interaction at vanilloid receptors. Although it mimicked capsaicin, it was not pungent on the human tongue. It has an affinity to the brain dopamine D1 receptors and may act as an oral painkiller targeting vanilloid receptors.

This novel compound could lead to the development of orally active, non-pungent vanilloids with potential for nerve and brain influence.

Kawagishi et al. (1996) isolated a novel pyradine derivative from the fungus that promotes melanin synthesis by B16 melanoma cells.

Sheep polypore contains at least three neogrifolin derivatives that possess antioxidant activity more potent than alpha tocopherol or BHA (Nukata et al. 2002).

Anti-inflammatory activity has been shown for grifolin and neogrifolin due to inhibition of nitric oxide production.

Various conditions including rheumatoid arthritis, septic shock, and other inflamed conditions are the result of over production of nitric oxide, suggesting that sheep polypore could be useful in the treatment of these painful pathologies.

Grifolin inhibits *Staphylococcus aureus* and *Bacillus subtilis,* as well as *Mycobacterium avium* and *M. phlei.* The toxicity is low and the activity is heat stable.

Confluent polypore is commonly found under conifers. The infiltrates have been shown to inhibit the growth of *Bacillus cereus, B. subtilis, E. coli,* and *Salmonella typhimurium* (Hirata et al. 1950).

Studies by Takashi Mizuno et al. (1992a) indicate that it contains polysaccharides with antitumor activity and aurovertins B and E, not normally found in basidiomycetes.

The confluent polypore contains albaconol, which breaks strands of pBR322 DNA at relatively high concentrations but has no effect on the macromolecule DNA of K562, suggesting that it specifically targets DNA topo II as one of its mechanisms of antitumor activity against cell lines K562, A549, BGC-823 and Bcap-37 (Qing et al. 2004).

Albaconol, present in the fruiting bodies, is an antagonist at the VR1 receptor with an IC 50 value of five micrometers (Liu, J. 2002).

Albaconol was found to induce contraction and desensitization of guinea pig trachea in vitro (Yang, W.-M. et al. 2003).

Albaconol inhibits lipid peroxidation in a manner comparable to vitamin E and increases the activity of superoxide dismutase (SOD) and butylated hydroxy-anisole (BHA).

Confluetin affects the vanilloid receptors, suggesting pain-relieving ability (Hellwig et al. 2003).

Both ememeterone and 3,6-dibenzyl-2-hydroxy-5-methoxypyradine have been found, the latter pyradine derivative reported to promote melanin synthesis by B16 melanoma cells (Kawagishi et al. 1996).

The related eastern species, *A. caeruleoporus,* contains grifolin and neogrifolin, as well as grifolinones A and B. All show inhibitory effects against the production of nitric oxide stimulated by lipopolysaccharide (Quang et al. 2005).

Grifolin has shown the ability to inhibit growth of cancer cells by induction of apoptosis, inhibiting tumor cell lines CNE1, HeLa, MCF7, SW480, K562, Raji, and B95-8 (Ye et al. 2005). The related *A. pes-caprae* also shows antitumor effects.

Greening goat's foot *(A. ellisii)* contains a glycosphingolipid with an unusual sphingoid base. Sphingolipids play a role in antigen-antibody reactions and cell-to-cell communication.

Grifolin, extracted from the rare *A. dispanus* shows antifungal activity against a variety of plant pathogens (Luo, D.-Q. et al. 2005).

The blue-capped polypore *(A. fletti)* is a beautiful blue to blue-green species found under conifers and mixed woods in western North America. It is edible and, according to David Arora, sold commercially in northern California. It contains confluentin, grifolin, and neogrifolin that exhibit activity against

Bacillus cereus and *Enterococcus faecalis* (Liu, X.-T. et al. 2010).

Crested polypore *(A. cristatus),* found in Bavaria, is active against the *Bacillus* species, hemolytic, and cytotoxic (Zechlin et al. 1981).

The American species contains grifolic acid.

Mycoremediation

Sheep polypore is a rich source of esterase, protease, and amylase enzymes. Esterases, such as lipase and carboxyl esterase, are important in food processing, fats and oleochemicals, cosmetics, leather, and dairy and tea processing, as well as sewage treatment, pulp and paper, oil degradation, and biodiesel production.

Aleuria

Aleuria aurantia
Peziza aurantia
(ORANGE PEEL FUNGUS)
(ORANGE PEEL CUP)
A. rhenana
(STALKED ORANGE PEEL)
(FALSE ORANGE PEEL)

Aurantia means "orange." *Peziza* is from the Greek meaning "living on the land, close to the ground or on foot."

Both fungi are bright orange and cup shaped. The stalked variety is more common in western North America, but both are widespread and common.

Orange peel is often found in summer and fall alongside trails or gravel roads, while its stalked cousin is more familiar in mosses of the boreal forest.

Both are edible, although they are small and it is difficult to gather more than a handful at a time. They can be eaten raw and may be added to salads for texture and color. One author suggests snacking on them with a glass of Kirsch. Why not?

The bright orange color is due to carotenoids, mainly aleuriaxanthin.

Medicinal Use

Chemical Constituents

- **One constituent is a fucose-binding lectin, which may be useful in some diagnostic tests for neoplasms. It is being studied for medicinal properties. Other contents include steroids, fatty acids, quaternary amines, and indole derivatives.**

Fungi Essence

Orange peel cup *(A. aurantia)* essence brings us back into balance between matter and spirit. It can assist both those people who are too attached to the physical and also those who ignore their material needs, escaping into spiritual realms too often.

—KORTE PHI

Agriculture

Orange peel was traditionally decocted in Europe and given to cows suffering from colds and other ailments.

Alnicola melinoides

Naucoria melinoides
(BROWN ALDER MUSHROOM)

Melinoides is from the Greek meaning "looking like grain." It looks like a dirty *Lepiota,* and is found on sandy soil under alder, hence the genus name.

Medicinal Use

Work by Hervey (1947) found agar plate growth active against *Staphylococcus aureus.*

Amanita muscaria

A. muscaria
(FLY AGARIC)
A. gemmata
(GEM STUDDED AMANITA)
A. pantherina
(THE PANTHER)
A. citrina
A. mappa
(FALSE DEATH CAP)
A. rubescens
(THE BLUSHER)
A. vaginata
Vaginata plumbea
Amanitopsis vaginata
(GRISETTE)
A. caesarea
(CAESAR'S MUSHROOM)
A. pseudoceciliae
A. inaurata
A. strangulata
(STRANGULATED AMANITA)

In a few minutes the caterpillar took the hookah out of its mouth, and got down off the mushroom *(Amanita muscaria),* and crawled away into the grass, merely remarking as it went "the top will make you grow taller, and the stalk will make you grow shorter."

"The top of what? The stalk of what?" thought Alice.

"Of the mushroom," said the caterpillar, just as if she had asked it aloud and in another moment was out of sight.

— LEWIS CARROLL, *ALICE'S ADVENTURES IN WONDERLAND*

It is called fungus of flies by reason that, when crushed up in milk, it kills flies.

— ALBERTUS MAGNUS

Teetotalers must be afraid of the *tengu-dake.*

— BENSEKI

Muscaria is derived from the Latin *musci* meaning "fly." *Mucarine* is another obvious derivation. *Amanita* derives from either the Greek *amanitai* meaning "fungus without any details," or from Amanos, a mountain between Syria and Cicilia.

Agaricum was a name originally given to the larch polypores *(Fomes)* native to a region of Sarmatia known as Agraria.

Another name is fly agaric. Many cultures crushed it in water and honey, or boiled it in milk and set a dish on windowsills to attract and kill flies. An English herbal published in 1440 reported, "there is also the sort of fungus that is impure, broad and thick and red with white spots on the top, when mixed with milk, it will kill the flies that are around, this is why it is known as the fly fungi, *muscinery* in Latin."

The German name, *fliegenpilz,* or "fly mushroom," may also derive from the ancient association of flies with madness. Beelzebub, later known as the devil, was originally called Lord of the Flies. In Austria, it is known as *hexenpilz,* or "witches' mushroom." In the Basque region of Spain, it is called *amoroto,* meaning "toad-like thing." From the Fribourg dialect of Switzerland comes *tsapi de diablhou,* or "devil's hat."

Other names include the Russian *mukhomor,* Lithuanian *musiomeris,* Danish *flue-svamp,* Italian *moscario,* and French *tue mouche.* My Polish in-laws refer to the fly agaric as *baramuha,* as *muha* means "fly." The fungus was placed in a cast iron pan, sprinkled with sugar, and gently heated on the wood stove. When removed from heat and cooled, it attracts house flies very effectively.

In France, this mushroom is known as *grapoudin,* meaning "toad thing." The Japanese call it *hayetoritake,* or "fly destroying mushroom" and *aka-haetori,* meaning "red fly catcher." It is sold in Japanese head shops as *beniteng.* In Hungary, the mushroom is called *bolond gomba,* or "mad mushroom."

Fly agaric is common in the birch, pine, and poplar forests of the northern prairies. It cannot be mistaken for any other mushroom with its brilliant orange-red head and white flecks.

This orange red coloring has been used as a red dye. Some authors believe that yellow colored mushrooms are the weakest in psychoactivity, and red the strongest.

DNA sequencing suggests distinct phylgenetic species around the world (Geml et al. 2008).

The mushroom is commonly eaten boiled in France and Italy.

In regions around Hamburg, the mushrooms, with their red skin removed, are made into soup. In some Alpine valleys, fresh fly agaric is sliced and made into an appetizer with vinegar, oil, salt, and pepper, and in Russia, it is added to vodka.

Fly agaric intoxications make up 1 to 2 percent of all cases of mushroom poisoning, and in many areas the species is considered very poisonous. In Finland, the red membrane of the cap is diluted in vodka and used externally to treat painful bruises or taken internally in small amounts for stomach aches or headaches.

Rainwater collected on the inverted caps, a cold-water extract, is called "dwarves' wine" and has definite psychoactive effect.

The concentrations of alkaloids in the panther mushroom are the most powerful in the genus, and often preferred by students and participants of hallucinogenic mushrooms. The ibotenic and muscimol content is much stronger and requires considerable adjustment of dosage.

"Pantherine syndrome" has been used to describe the symptoms of poisoning by this mushroom. The toxins responsible are isoxazole derivatives that interfere with neurotransmission in the brain.

There is one record of death from the fresh mushroom in the United States. According to legend, more than a century ago, Count Vechi, a member of the Italian diplomatic corps, reportedly ate two dozen fresh panther mushrooms for breakfast and died the next day.

False death cap *(A. citrina)* contains 7.5 grams

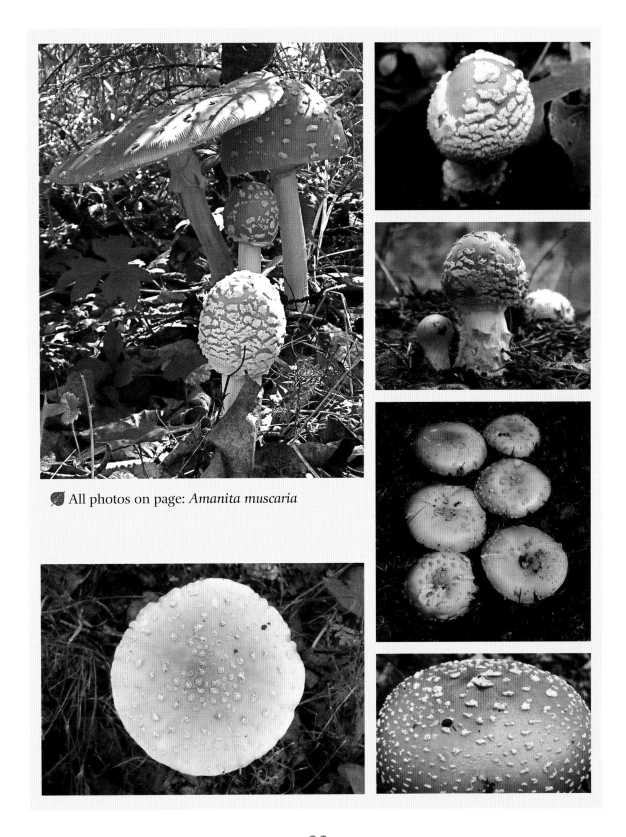

🍂 All photos on page: *Amanita muscaria*

of bufotenin per dry gram. Bufotenin is not centrally active in humans when taken orally at doses below fifty milligrams (Spoerke and Rumack 1994).

Gem-studded *Amanita (A. gemmata)* contains muscimol and ibotenic acid. It has a pale to dark yellow cap with white patches and appears in the Pacific Northwest region from spring to fall.

Purple *Amanita (A. porphyria)* contains trace amounts of bufotenine.

The eastern *A. parcivolvata* contains traces of isoxazole, but is harmless, and has no sac-like volva, or partial veil. It is red to yellow-orange and often mistaken for *A. muscaria.*

Grisette *(A. vaginata)* with its gray color and white fragments is common in my area. I used to throw them away, but now I take them home and eat them.

Pantherina is from the Latin, meaning to resemble a panther. In Japan, it is known as *ibo tengutake* from *ibo* meaning "warted," *tengu* being the proper name, and *take,* for "mushroom."

The panther is found more frequently in boreal forests or in the Rocky Mountains, having a symbiotic relationship with various conifers, including the douglas fir.

Fly agaric has been used for centuries as part of secret religious ceremonies and is thought by many scholars to be the Soma mentioned in the Rig Veda, in which more than 120 hymns are devoted to its praise. Some of the poems describe how priests, having drunk the juice of Soma, "urinate the divine drink." Here is one sample:

Like a stag, come here to drink!
Drink Soma, as much as you like.
Pissing it out day by day, O generous one,
You have assumed your most mighty force.

Soma, Divine Mushroom of Immortality, by Gordon Wasson, is a highly regarded book attempting to prove that Soma of the Riga-Veda was, in fact, fly agaric. Some of the poems describe how priests, having drunk the juice of Soma "urinate the divine drink." Soma literally means "the pressed one." It has been suggested that the name "fly agaric" may allude to the fly of madness, or divine possession.

In the Middle Ages, delirium, drunkenness, and insanity were attributed to insects loose in the head. In English, we speak of "bees in his bonnet"; while in France they say "la mouche lui monte a la tete" meaning "the fly is climbing in this head." In Russian, there is an expression that a drunken man is "with fly."

Add to the fact that Soma was said to lack a root, leaves, or blossoms, and it makes for a very compelling argument.

Wasson traced the mushroom metaphor through other cultures, and coined the term "bemushroomed" to describe fly agaric intoxication.

In Russia, *pup* means "navel," and *pupyry* means "fungal growth." In contemporary Cambodia, *pzat* means both "navel" and "mushroom," suggesting a connection with inner knowledge.

The Sacred Mushroom and the Cross, by John Allegro, a Dead Sea Scroll authority, also endeavored to prove that "Israelistism" was based on the sacred fungus. Allegro deduced that the root words derived from Sumerian were related to the phallic symbol of fertility and the sacred mushroom.

Sara Friedman, in *Celebrating the Wild Mushroom,* speculates: "Could the red-capped resident of the far north who flies through the heavens driving reindeer be anything but a fly agaric-inspired metaphor?"

In northern Europe, the Germanic gods played a role in bringing us mushrooms. On winter solstice night each year, the chief God, Wotan, rides through the forest on horseback, pursued by devils. They ride faster and faster, until blood-specked foam falls from the horse's mouth. The following spring, a beautiful, red-capped mushroom with white specks is found.

In Norse myths, Odin had an eight-legged horse called Sleipnir that he rode into battle. Together they traveled through the nine worlds of gods, giants, elves, men, and the underworld. Because he carried Odin through the skies around Christmas in the Wild Hunt, when fits were left for the faithful under pine trees, some authors have suggested the eight-legged steed gave rise to Santa Claus' eight reindeer.

Thomas Nast's famous portrayal of Santa Claus, with twinkling eyes and cherry nose, driving a sleigh pulled by reindeer flying over treetops, takes on a whole new connotation. His clothing of red and white represents the fly agaric eaten by the shaman, and the Koryak custom of eating mushroomed reindeer is another shamanic journey.

The image of Santa Claus climbing down the chimney resonates of Siberian festivals where the shaman would climb the central post of winter dwellings and exit via the smokehole.

Drying the mushrooms by stringing them like popcorn and hanging them above the fireplace hearth is reminiscent of hanging stockings for Christmas. Decorating the pine or other coniferous tree with dried fungi is similar to our modern day decoration.

Another custom associated with the Celtic harvest festival Samhein is a special tea brewed from the peeled cap picked during a full moon. This holiday is still celebrated by some who drink a cold-water extract of the dried skin before going to bed. The next morning, the dreams are described and interpreted.

According to Wasson, chimney sweeps of central Europe consider the mushroom their emblem.

The Egyptian God of the Underworld, Osiris, rode the sky in a chariot. After his death, Isis found an evergreen had grown overnight in his place, suggesting death and rebirth. The traditional birth of Osiris was December 25, from mythology more than 5,000 years old. Djed was the pillar or phallus of Osiris, and the Eye of Horus was the Djed-Eye.

Esau comes from the Sumerian *E-sh-u-a,* which means "raised canopy" (or cap), and Esau's brother's name, Jacob, or *Ia-a-gub,* refers to the "pillar" or stem.

The Greek *chrisma* means "anointing," suggesting a deeper level to this holy substance.

In the Garden of Eden, the serpent and mushroom become one. "Both emerged from holes in the ground, in a manner reminiscent of the erection of the sexually aroused penis," says Allegro.

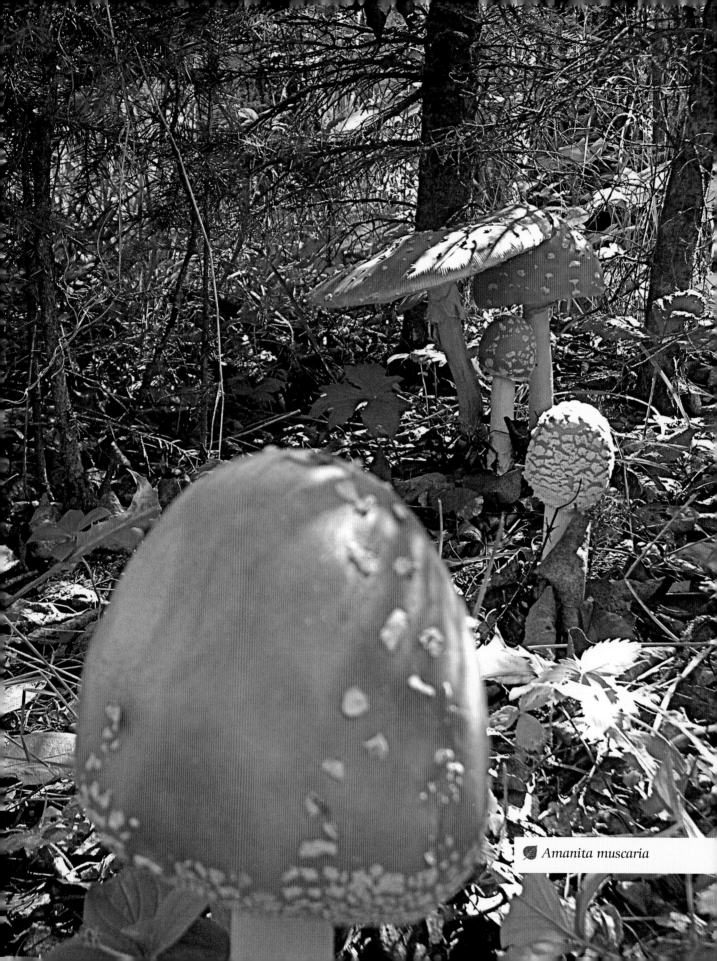

Amanita muscaria

Even Freud, in his *Interpretation of Dreams,* suggests that there are some things that are best left alone.

> Even in the best interpreted dreams, there is often a place that must be left in the dark, because in the process of interpreting one notices a tangle of dream-thoughts arising which resists unraveling but has also made no further contributions to the dream content.
>
> This then is the navel of the dream, the place where it straddles the unknown. The dream-thoughts, to which interpretation leads one, are necessarily interminable and branch out on all sides into the net-like entanglement of our world of thought. Out of one of the denser places in this meshwork, the dream-wish rises like a mushroom out of its mycelium.

Hmmm!

The Cree and other First Nations people made eyewash of *Amanita* to fight infection, but I can find no record of their use of the fungi for spiritual quest. The Algonquin, around the Great Lakes, were familiar with its use (see below). The Jesuit priest Charles l'Allemant wrote back to France in 1626 that natives believed that "after death they go to heaven where they eat mushrooms and have intercourse with each other."

The Dogrib Athabascans, now known as *tåîchô,* still use fly agaric as a hallucinogen. Franz Boas, when studying Siberian tales of Big Raven, noted similar usage.

> Here *Amanita muscaria* is employed as a sacrament in shamanism. A young neophyte reported that whatever the shaman had done to him "he had snatched me. I had no voli-tion, I had no power of sleep, I didn't eat, didn't sleep, I didn't think—I wasn't in my body any longer.
>
> "Cleansed and ripe for vision, I rise, a bursting ball of seeds in space . . . I have sung the note that shatters structure. And the note that shatters chaos, and been bloody. . . . I have been with the dead and attempted the labyrinth."

The Ojibwa, near the Great Lakes, also used fly agaric for hallucinogenic effect. Manabozoh had a twin brother, a wolf, who was killed by the water spirits after luring him onto thin ice. To avenge his brother's death, Manabozoh impersonated a frog shaman before killing the ice spirit, or manitous. He then found consolation in the mushrooms, which he introduced to humans. Other First Nations people, including the Cree, Menomini, and Salteaux, have their own versions of this tale.

Christian Rätsch suggests the Mayan Lacandon know the mushroom as *hkib lu'um,* meaning "the light of the earth." The neighboring Chuj of Northern Guatemala dried the caps and smoked them with tobacco to induce inner journeys of prophecy.

People in the Shutul Valley of Afghanistan call the fungus raven's bread, a term used in ancient Egypt and to this day in Eastern Europe. They boil the ground powder of the mushroom with fresh jewelweed *(Impatiens noli-tangere)* and soured goat cheese brine to produce the well-known extract of Shutul (Bokar). The term *chashm baskon* is used for the mushroom, and means "eye-opener."

In the small village of Qaf-e-Changar in the upper valley, the extract is mixed with calyx tips of henbane for therapeutic massage.

Igorot aborigines of Luzon, Philippines, call the mushroom *ampacao,* and brew six fresh caps into a drink used for rites of passage.

A recent book by Clark Heinrich, called *Magic Mushrooms in Religion and Alchemy,* is a fascinating exploration of the historical use of fly agaric, in both written and painted form. He traces mushroom use through the Vedic verses, as well as the Bible, the Holy Grail, and Alchemy with scholarly examination; making much sense of the hidden meanings in various cultures. It is a superb contribution to our knowledge of the ritual use of this fascinating fungus! A fresco in a Roman Catholic church in Plaincouralt, France, depicts Adam and Eve on either side of a tree of knowledge that is unequivocally a branched *Amanita muscaria.*

Another fresco found on the wall of a basilica of Aquileia in northern Italy may be left over from a former Roman temple.

A painted ceiling of St. Michael's Church in Hildescheim, Germany, dated to 1192 AD, shows a large *Amanita* with Adam and Eve each holding a mushroom bud.

In magical use, the mushroom was placed on altars or in the bedroom for fertility purposes.

Laplanders make use of the reindeer's fondness for the dried agaric by sprinkling it on the snow to help in herding. More potent is the muscimol-rich urine that is saved to help round up reindeer, or for their own intoxication.

Head twitching is noted in deer, squirrels, and chipmunks who nibble on the mushroom. In some areas of the boreal forest, dried *Amanita muscaria* caps are found set on spruce branches by squirrels for winter use. Assorted dried mushrooms may make up as much as 25 percent of their winter diet. In Alaska and Yukon, caribou have been observed munching the fungi.

Fly agaric use is sprinkled throughout folk literature in legend, songs, and poems. One German folk song, "Ein Männlein steht im Walde," meaning "a little man stands in the forest," is found in the children's opera *Hansel and Gretel.*

It is highly likely that the Celts used the mushroom as well. Derg Corra, a hero of the Celtic otherworld, is famed for his power of leaping, a trait associated in Siberia with ingestion of fly agaric. The epithet Derg Corra means "red-peaked" or "red-pointed," like the cap.

Brigid, the goddess of poets, was depicted with fires around her head, representing agaric intoxication and the inspiration of poetry and songs.

It is believed by some Celtic and Gaelic scholars that the often-cited hazelnut is a metaphor for *A. muscaria.* In Celtic legend, hazelnuts are known as *cuill crimaind,* "the hazels of knowledge," or *bolg fis,* "bubbles of wisdom." This refers to bubbles caused by the nuts falling into the well of wisdom. *Bolg* is found in both Irish and Scots Gaelic names of mushrooms.

According to Christian Rätsch, there is some evidence that the Beaker People of Stonehenge, and later the Celts, used fly agaric in cult rituals.

The shamans of Siberia and parts of Scandinavia used a drink from *mukhumor* to induce visions, communicate with the supernatural, divine the future, diagnose illness, and celebrate festive occasions like weddings.

The shaman would control harmful beings, called *nimvits,* and communication could take place only at night with the mushroom's aid.

The Chukchee believed the mushrooms to be another tribe and that the visions personified the mushroom and the "mushroom men." These beings accompanied a person on a voyage through their world, and to visit places where the dead reside.

Both Chukchee and Koryak shamans could be openly homosexual or transvestite. These transvestite shamans, as well as the Pima *ber-ache,* were considered most powerful. They revered a deity called "the big raven," a transformer of the world and an ancestor of men.

The Yurk Samoyed reported man-like creatures that appeared before them in a dream. They would run down a path that the sun follows in the evening, and the intoxicated person would follow.

On the journey, the fly agaric spirits would tell him what he wanted to know, and when he returned to the light, he would find a pole with seven holes and cords. When he tied up the spirits, he would awaken. Then he would sit down, taking a symbol of the pillar of the world, a four-sided staff with seven slanting crosses cut into each side, and sing about what he had seen.

The Ostyaks filled their huts with smoke from tree resins, and the shaman took three to seven dried caps, after fasting all day.

Cortez observed Amanita mushrooms being consumed during the coronation of Montezuma. Natives of Mexico believe it comes from drops of God's sperm and grows from the vulva of Mother Earth, appearing like an erect penis becoming more and more aroused and the cap (woman) penetrated by the stipe.

The Huichol practice wolf shamanism revolving around *A. muscaria* as "wolf-peyote." Mark Hoffman posts his analysis at http://homepage.mac.com/photomorphose/ethno.html.

In Guatemala, *Amanita* is believed to appear when lightning strikes the earth.

The Tzeltal call it "red thunderbolt mushroom" and dry the red skins, combining them with tobacco as a smoke for prophecy and disease diagnosis.

Adrian Morgan, in his book *Toads and Toadstools,* which is highly recommended, shares his own experience with *Amanita,* including the ingestion of his own urine, which he found produced the strongest effect.

The Japanese call it *beni tengu take,* or "scarlet goblin fungus." According to folklore the *tengu* were flying wood spirits that took the form of birds or long-nosed humans. Tengu is the spirit of the fly agaric and one of the most popular figures in Japanese mythology. The mushrooms can represent bird-like demons, wild reclusive monks, or transformed shamans.

Male *tengu* have a phallic nose and are regarded as tricksters or sexual demons, and sometimes benefactors. Mountain shrines have been built in their honor, with fossilized shark teeth considered reminders of their passing. These "claws of *tengu*" are sold as amulets or talismans.

Tengu carry magical fans or leaves, some of which resemble hemp. The Japanese red kite is identified with tengu. They favor drinking sake, of course.

People in the Sanada region of Nagano are said to use dried *A. muscaria* as a condiment in food to add the umami flavor to food, or as a base or soup stock. A recent article by Rubel and Arora (2008) has an attached appendix with a recipe for safely preparing *A. muscaria* for the dinner table.

We cannot be sure that Lewis Carroll knew about the various reports out of Siberia regarding distortion of the senses, but the scarlet and white spotted *Amanita muscaria* illustrated in *Alice's Adventures in Wonderland* make me think he did. There are scattered reports in English literature of the late nineteenth and early twentieth centuries that the hallucinogenic properties of *Amanita muscaria* were explored by upper-class opium eaters.

The Documents in the Case by Dorothy Sayer is a sixty-year-old whodunit in which a mushroom collector is found dead, apparently mistaking this mushroom for *A. rubescens*. Although small amounts of muscarine are present in the fungi, the victim's son refused to believe his father would make such a glaring mistake, and through his sleuthing determined poisoning by synthetic muscarine. A good mushroom mystery!

Herbalist Christopher Hobbs suggests that perhaps it was the original "electric Kool-Aid," after the adventures of Ken Kesey, Timothy Leary, and others.

Tom Robbins wrote about his experiences with the mushroom in 1976:

> I have eaten the fly agaric three times. . . .
> Euphoric energy was mine aplenty, but at both the onset and the termination of the intoxication I fell fitfully asleep . . . if not actually the godhead, is holistic awareness of the godhead. But it does not do this gently.
>
> Instead of slipping one into the cosmic fabric like a silver needle, it drives one in like a wooden stake. And of course, a stake is blunted in the driving. It was not mere psychedelic fickleness that prompted both the olden Greeks and the Mexicans to drop *Amanita muscaria* cold when they discovered that the innocuous looking little Psilocybe made up in grace what it lacked in flamboyance.

A recent book by Andy Letcher, *Shroom: A Cultural History of the Magic Mushroom,* is a nice addition to the debate. In his chapter on the fly agaric, he weaves a wonderful journey of the mushroom through art and literature. It is noted that the book was widely embraced in Europe, but critically reviewed and debunked by a number of ethnomycologists on this side of the pond. I enjoyed it.

Amanita Muscaria: Herb of Immortality, an e-book published by Donald E. Teeter, contains some very interesting ideas concerning preparation and resurrection of mycelium from dried caps.

Myths and Legends

A Koryak legend tells of Big Raven. He had caught a whole whale and cold not send it home because he was unable to lift the bag containing its traveling provisions. He appealed to the Existence to help him. The deity said "find the white soft stalks with the spotted hats—these are the spirits Wa'pag." Big Raven found and ate the fungus, lifted the bag, and sent the whale home.

— CRUNWELL

There were two brothers who were very hungry, their stomachs empty. Since there were mountains, they climbed up the rocky slopes looking for food. At last they came to a great cave high in the mountainside. It seemed to them that light came out of the cave opening, and when they peered through, they saw a beautiful meadow in which there grew many tall red and white mushrooms—handsome *wajaskwedeg*—turning and revolving, buzzing and murmuring, singing a strange song of happiness.

Younger brother ran to the tallest, strongest, and reddest mushroom. White fluffs like tuft feathers of a forest war bonnet, waved across the shining cap.

The younger brother became fused to the stipe, and began to grow a bright red cap. Slowly at first, then faster and faster, he began to spin in the sun.

The elder brother ran back to his village to consult the medicine people, about how to rescue his younger sibling. . . . Which he did!

Many days and nights went by. The elder brother awoke in the morning with a heavy and sad heart, the younger brother, smiling and his heart filled with happiness.

Elder brother noticed that the younger brother went very frequently to urinate behind the wigwam, particularly at full moon. One time, he went to look and his brother was not there. He follows his trail, and sees him standing in the center of an open space with a large number of people around him. The younger brother's arms are open wide, spread like the umbrella of a mushroom. His robes are beautiful, glowing red, and tufts of white feathers adorn his head. He sings to the people:

Because of my supernatural experience,
in the land of the Miskwedo,

I have a cure to alleviate your ills,
To take away all your unhappiness.
If only you will come to my penis
And take the quickening waters flowing from it
You, too, can be forever happy.

Every time the clouds darken the moon, he urinates. The people catch his urine in birch bark containers. They drink this liquid that has been given to them as a great boon by the Miskwedo spirits.

Poor elder brother! He did not understand the ways of the red-topped mushroom. He worried and was unhappy.

Younger brother did not understand the workings of the Sacred Mushroom. But he went on being happy, and all the people following him continued in a state of bliss. They drink the Elixir of the Great Miskwedo, and much is revealed of the supernatural and other knowledge in this way. It is the *kesuwabo*—the liquid "Power of the Sun."

— Keewaydinoquay, Anishinauberb Medicine Woman and Storyteller (Vermeulen 2007)

Traditional Uses

Often a brew of dried amanita, fireweed, and cow parsnip were made into fermented ale; or the dried mushrooms were soaked in fireweed must. Some authors mention it works synergistically with unripe bog blueberry (*V. uliginosum*) juice for vision quests.

An expedition led by Dane Vitus Bering, who gave his name to the strait between Russia and Alaska, traveled with the botanist Stefan Krasheninnikov to explore Kamchatka. He wrote that the dried mushrooms were sold for feasts where

The landlords entertain their guests with great bowls of opanga, 'til they are all set a vomiting; sometimes they use a liquor made of a large mushroom, with which the Russians kill flies. This they prepare with the juice of Epilobium.

Georg Steller, on the same expedition, said that when the Koryak find a reindeer intoxicated on fly agaric, they slaughter it, and all those who eat the flesh also become intoxicated.

Scottish poachers would drink a mixture of fly Agaric and fireweed *(Epilobium angustifolium)* to stay awake for nighttime jobs. This mixture was known as Cathies, named after Catherine the Great, the lusty Empress of Russia, who was said to enjoy the same drink before her well-known conquests. Drinking the urine of those who ingested the drink resulted not only in a stronger effect, but also removed the toxic effects. This could be repeated up to five times before the drug began to lose its potency.

This knowledge may have come about from observations of reindeer being attracted to human urine. When these animals eat the mushroom they acquire a special craving for the urine of human beings, and will frequent dwellings to drink this special urine.

Every Koryak man carries a sealskin vessel, suspended from his belt, to collect urine. The reindeer will be attracted from far pastures to eat this yellow snow. During a festival that is associated with reindeer herding, the dried mushroom is mixed with fresh reindeer blood and drunk to strange music that lasts for three to four days.

One common name in the Kamchatka peninsula is woodpecker of Mars, due to its increase in strength and stamina. In that part of the world, the mushroom is so highly regarded that the words for trance, daze, and drunkenness are derived from the noun meaning "fungus, fly agaric."

A cold-water extract of the fungus was traditionally rubbed onto the legs of patients suffering snakebite in Siberia.

Physicians of the nineteenth century used it to treat fever and epilepsy.

W. Schneider wrote that "only the lower portion of the stalk is chosen . . . the fly agaric, in powder form, is administered internally in small doses (ten to thirty grains) against falling sickness, etc., and is sprinkled externally onto malignant tumors, gangrene, etc. Meinhard gives a tincture to treat favus and other persistent eruptions."

A tincture of the crumbled, dry fungi soaked in vodka for two weeks has been used traditionally in Russia to alleviate joint pain by external application.

In Kamchatka, three small fresh pieces of the mushroom are used to treat sore throat and cancer.

The related strangulated *Amanita (A. pseudoceciliae)* has been used in Chinese medicine to cure eczema.

Medicinal Use

Chemical Constituents

- *A. muscaria:* **ibotenic acid (0.08–0.1 percent), which converts to muscimol or pantherine; muscarine; muscazone, muscasophine, stizololic, and tricholomic acid, 1,3-diolein,** amavadine, R4-hydroxy-pyrrolidone-(2), 1,2,3,4-tetrahydro-l-methyl-B-carboline-carboxylic acid, B-N-b-Butyl-D-glucopyranoside, stizolobic and stixolobinic acids, (-)-4-hydroxypyrrolidine, two hundred milligrams per kilogram of vanadium, betalains, muscaaurins muscapurpurin, and muscaflavins pigments in the cap skin. Muscimol content of fall fungi is 0.05 percent.

- *Mycelium:* muscarine, epi-muscarine, allo-muscarine, and possibly, epiallo-muscarine; psychoactive tryptamines; MAO inhibitors; harmine and harmaline; and atropine and scopolamine, albeit in very small amounts.

- *A. pantherina:* same as above, as well as stizolobic, stizolobinic acids, and several unidentified alkaloids and muscimol/ibotenic acid 0.46 percent.

Muscimol is a central nervous system hallucinogen, muscarine a highly toxic hallucinogen. Ironically, they are physiological "opposites"—one is food for the spiritual body and the other poison to the physical. The kidneys detoxify muscarine, but allow muscimol to pass through largely intact. This can be repeated four to five times. Only 30 to 35 percent of muscimol is excreted unchanged, unlike ibotenic acid, which is cleared from the body in ninety minutes.

Muscarine is found in the fresh mushroom at very low concentrations of 0.0003 percent. Much larger amounts are found in many species of *Inocybe* and *Clitocybe* mushrooms. In fact, it would take 110,000 kilograms of fresh *A. muscaria* to deliver a dose of muscarine large enough to be dangerous to humans.

Muscimol and ibotenic acid cross the blood-brain barrier more readily than glutamic acid or GABA. Ibotenic acid excites or stimulates neurons, while muscimol is inhibitory. GABA is an inhibitory neurotransmitter, active at 40 percent of brain synapses, and appears to function, in part, by opening channels in the neuronal membrane specific to chloride ions.

Much of the recorded medical effect with *Amanita muscaria* comes from Germany. Dr. Reinhard used it successfully to treat cases of paralysis, epilepsy, and chronic catarrh conditions. Dr. M. Paulet used external applications of the plant for cancer and other ulcerous conditions of the skin.

Professor Scudder suggested that a tincture of *Amanita muscaria* is best for "involuntary twitching of the muscles of the face, forehead, and even the eyes." He suggested its use for "pressing pain in the occiput and an inclination to fall backwards."

Felter and Lloyd wrote, "The principal use that has been made of this fungus is to control night sweats from debilitating diseases and profuse sweating during the daytime."

Dr. Culbreth, another Eclectic physician, says that *Amanita* "reduces force and frequency of pulse, contracts muscles of intestine and bladder, increases abdominal secretions that lead to paralysis and death." Obviously great care must be taken with this remedy.

Theodore G. Schurr (1995), an anthropologist and molecular biologist, suggests that "once ingested, the psychoactive alkaloids and substances acted as agonists of normal neurotransmitter function, disrupting the coordinate action between the catecholaminergic and serotoninergic systems and producing hallucinogenic effects similar to those generated by LSD and harmine."

Ethanol extracts of the fruiting bodies significantly inhibit growth of sarcoma 180.

It is worth noting that some Parkinson's patients experience symptomatic relief from the homeopathic preparation below. It is interesting that in 1991, a research team at the University of Lausanne, Switzerland, isolated DOPA, 4,5-dioxygenase from *Amanita muscaria*.

Muscimol, obtained from the decarboxylation of ibotenic acid, more potently activates GABA receptors as a selective GABA-A agonist than GABA itself. Muscimol is very active in displacing bicuculline or GABA.

Although a valuable medicine, it can be toxic when fresh. As few as two to four dried mushrooms can alter awareness, while twenty can be neurotoxic. Muscarine stimulates post-ganglionic cholinergic neuroeffector junctions. The isoxazole constituents are psychoactive.

Muscimol appears to pass the blood-brain barrier, with up to 27 percent of muscimol injected into lab mice recovered from urine.

Muscimol is a GABA agonist, with effect at very low dosage. Different parts of the brain, from the cerebral cortex, to hippocampus and cerebellum, appear to possess different sensitivities to muscimol.

It does, however, induce long-term depression in the CA1 region of the hippocampus at concentrations of only ten micromoles.

Ibotenic acid and muscimol are related structurally to glutamate, the main excitatory neurotransmitter, and activate NMDA receptors.

Ibotenic acid is also a potent agonist at group I and group II metabotrophic glutamate receptors, and, like glutamate, it stimulates the production of inositol triphosphates through a G-protein mediated mechanism. It also stimulates phosphorylation of protein kinase C substrates and increases phospholipase D activity, as well as increasing the release of glutamate.

Ibotenate creates neurotoxic and phosphoinositide effect through distinct receptors, which are prevented by MK-801 and enhanced by glycine, further implying NMDA involvement.

Although they differ in mechanism of action, both ibotenic acid and muscimol produce similar subjective and behavioral states. Muscimol is, however, five times as potent as ibotenic acid.

Muscimol increases levels of serotonin, dopamine and acetylcholine, and decreases noradrenaline.

Moldavan et al. (1999) found Amanita extracts two to four times more exciting to brain tissue than L-glutamic acid, with the neuron frequency of spike discharge twice as high in *A. pantherina,* as compared to *A. muscaria.*

Amavadine is a vanadyl compound, which accounts for the unusually high vanadium content in the fungus ash.

An enzyme involved in the metabolism of betalain pigments was discovered in Switzerland in 1991. Various cosmetic companies in Russia use fly agaric in creams and lotions, but there is no evidence of efficacy.

Ibotenic acid was patented as a flavor enhancer in 1969, but has never reached grocery store shelves. The closely related monosodium glutamate (MSG), however, is found in many products and is a neurotoxin and excitotoxin with similar activity.

The panther contains stizolobic and stizolobinic acids that exhibit an excitatory action on isolated spinal-cord tissue (Ishida, M. and H. Shinozaki 1988).

The edible Caesar's mushroom (*A. caesarea*) fruiting body shows activity against *Bacillus subtilis* and *Staphylococcus aureus* (Yamac and Bilgili 2006). Ethanol extracts inhibit sarcoma 180 in mice.

Homeopathy

Waldschmidt, a physician who uses the homeopathic mother tincture in his practice reports "one portion (15 to 20 percent) of the patients I have treated with *Amanita muscarius* had altered dreams during or after the therapy. Especially: dreams of flying with positive contents, dreams reminiscent of *Alice in Wonderland,* and other pleasant dream experiences. In no case did nightmares occur . . . following the prescription of fly agaric, almost all of the patients exhibited increased motivation, improved mood, and improved mental and physical well being. Here again it is the dosage that determines that something is not a poison."

Amanita muscaria is used to treat various neuralgic and spasmodic afflictions, including skin troubles. It is a cerebral excitant with many mental manifestations, including vertigo from sunlight.

One of the predominant characteristics of ingestion is that the slightest pressure causes pain.

Headaches are like icy needles with the desire to keep the head warm. It is best for fevers that are low with a tendency to collapse, with great weakness and spasms of lower limbs.

Typed words seem to move or swim about, or there are floaters in the eye. The eyes and eyeballs twitch with redness and itching.

The menses are early and frequent with severe bearing down pain especially after menopause. The nipples itch and burn, and sex may be painful. Vaginal itching and discharge frequently occur.

There is paralysis and numbness of the extremities with skin itching and burning, and yet the feet are ice cold with poor peripheral circulation. Heartbeat may be irregular or weak, with skipping.

Use 30C for skin that is itchy, red or burning from frostbite.

There may also be dejection, irritability, and reluctance for any form of activity or work, with lack of initiative and mood of despair.

Hyper-excitability of sex drive is accompanied by lack of ability, and great exhaustion following coitus.

The symptoms are made worse in the open, with cold air, after eating, and after sex. Slow movement is the only relief.

Dosage: 3C to 30C potency, and in some cases up to 200C. In skin and mental concerns stick to the lower potencies (Boericke).

Amanita citrina is related to laziness and unconsciousness, coma and lethargy, violent true cholera, and deep stupor.
— ALLEN

Amanita pantherina is related to tingling of the extremities, drowsiness, dizziness with inability to focus eyes, feeling of going to die but unafraid, and very disoriented. Inability to grasp and remember the minor details of everyday life.

— Spoerke and Rumack

The blusher *(A. rubescens)* is related to vomiting, thirst, cramps, albuminaria, disturbance of sensory function, and anemia.

— Blyth

Essential Oils

Ether extracts of *Amanita muscaria* contain, in addition to fatty oils, an essential oil characterized by a strong odor peculiar to edible fungi. Distillation of the dry fungi with water vapor produces a small amount of a camphor-like substance called amanitol. It constitutes fine white flocculi, which melt at forty degrees Celsius. The odor is peculiar and somewhat like parsley.

The spores contain 1.4 percent fat, consisting of about 10 percent palmitic and 90 percent oleic acids.

Fungi Essence

Amanita muscaria essence is for those who have difficulties with self-expression. They include the singer that holds back, or the teacher that finds it difficult to share of self. This essence enables those who are resistant, due to fear of criticism from others.

— Prairie Deva

Fly agaric essence aids in expanding awareness through the mystery schools of sacrificial love, also for psychotherapy. Can be used for energy levels, vitality, muscle cramps, M.E. and sexual problems. Use after stroke or paralysis.

— Silvercord

Fliieenpilz fly agar *(A. muscaria)* essence intensely affects the sixth (third eye) chakra and above. It helps cleanse both our physical and subtle bodies of the residues of psychiatric drugs and similar substances. It can help us gain positive access to higher dimensions."

— Korte Phi

Fly Agaric essence helps identify relationships and gives power to withdraw from entanglements. It helps solve the Gordian Knot."

— Mariana

Mycoremediation

Colpaert and Assche (1992) exposed seven species to cadmium. *Scleroderma citrinum* and *Paxillus involtus* were strongly inhibited at even one part per million, while *A. muscaria* was not affected at even fifty parts per million. Willenborg et al. (1990) showed the fungi more tolerant of cadmium and mercury than other species tested. Other work showed thorium is also accumulated (Seeger and Schweinshaut 1981).

Braun-Lullemann et al. (1999) tested the ability of *Amanita muscaria* to degrade polycyclic aromatic hydrocarbons (PAHs) and found that it utilized about 50 percent of phenanthrene and 35 percent of chrysene. The related *A. excelsa* removed the same amount of benzopyrene in four weeks.

S. Keller et al. (1996) identified streptomyces strain AcH 505 to encourage the development of auxofuran that helps the growth of ectomycorrhizal connection between this mushroom and spruce.

Insecticide

Linnaeus described in 1751 how residents of Sweden used it to banish bedbugs. The fresh specimens were pulped and the juice painted with a feather around the corners and cracks where the bugs were believed to hide.

The compound that attracts flies is called 1,3-diolein. After the flies have dined on the juices of the mushroom, the main isoxazole toxin, ibotenic acid, stuns or kills them. A whole mushroom was often suspended from the ceiling in parts of France as a natural insecticide.

Frans Vermeulen, in his fascinating book *Fungi,* writes "[*Amanita muscaria*] in potency also attracts and kills flies. While waiting for a few granules of … 200C to dissolve in a glass of water, a patient saw three flies, which seemed to appear out of nowhere, dive into the water and drown."

Recipes and Dosage

Tincture of dried fungus: one part dried cap to five parts 40 percent alcohol.

Extract: five drops of a 1:100 preparation.

Dried powder: three and a half to five grams for 150-pound individual.

Smoking: crumble the dried skin with a small amount of marijuana and smoke for pleasant alteration.

Soup: cut the *A. muscaria* cap and stalk into thin slices (one-eighth-inch thick) to hasten dissolving of the active constituents. For each 110 grams (four ounces) of mushroom, use one liter or quart of water with one teaspoon of salt. Garlic and bay leaf may be added to the water for flavoring. Bring the water to a rolling boil, then add the sliced mushrooms. Begin timing the cooking once the water returns to a boil. Boil for ten to fifteen minutes, until the mushroom is soft, then drain and rinse (Rubel and Arora 2008).

Special preparation: slice fresh mushrooms vertically into one-centimeter segments and place in a 110-degree Fahrenheit oven until dry. The muscarine will largely evaporate, and the ibotenic acid will be converted into muscimol.

The correct dosage for an adult is three medium-sized dried mushrooms, or approximately five to ten grams.

These are best soaked in warm water to reconstitute. Both the liquid and the reconstituted mushrooms are ingested. The ingestion of one's own urine will accentuate the experience.

Fasting is critical. Do not eat for four to six hours before ingestion.

Some research suggests that two to three tablespoons of butter or oil will help to mitigate the effects if too much agaric has been ingested, but I don't think that would help.

According to Donald E. Teeter, carbonated beverages should not be consumed before or after ingesting the mushroom because they may cause muscimol to be re-converted into ibotenic acid, reversing the drying effect and inducing unpleasant symptoms of nausea, cramps, and vomiting, and inhibiting hallucinogenic activity.

For nausea, a single toke of marijuana will give quick relief.

The intake of more than ten grams of fresh mushrooms can lead to loss of coordination, confusion, illusions, and manic attacks. More than a hundred grams can lead to unconsciousness, asphyxiation, and coma. No record of death has ever been recorded, although fifteen caps is considered by some authors, at least in theory, to be a toxic dose. Spring and summer mushrooms have higher concentrations of active compounds, with the fully mature mushroom after sporulation the optimum choice for drying. The August mushrooms are more powerful than those collected in September, but the physical symptom of nausea is more marked and the narcotic and visionary effects less pronounced.

In cases of overdose, use vomiting and sedatives. In case of shock, use a plasma volume expander. Artificial respiration may be needed. Additionally, milk thistle seeds may help prevent *Amanita* liver poisoning. Many hospitals want to administer atropine, which would potentiate and aggravate the condition.

Personality Traits

Amanita are the aristocrats of fungi. Their noble bearing, their beauty, their power for good or evil, and above all their perfect structure, have placed them first in their realm; and they proudly bear the three badges of their clan and rank—the volva or sheath from which they spring, the kid-like apron encircling their waists, and patch-marks of their high birth upon their caps.

— CHARLES MCILVAINE

[*Agaricus muscarius*] don't like to be told what to do or to take orders; it's an extremely awkward inner state of stupid rage showing up as a heroic defiance covering an extremely vulnerable interior.

"You are so mean to me and you don't care," "Nobody loves me and I don't care anymore" are typical reposts of kids.

They are so sensitive they become very defensive, and then they are not intimidated by anyone. This escalates to a combination of explosive temper and disregard for authority or the consequences, with repeated violent threats toward parents.

They become totally fearless. They can also experience episodes of rage with great feats of strength and it's the remedy for those who do the impossible, Clint Eastwood, Arnold Schwarzenegger. They are like a grenade waiting to explode, so great is the anger. . . .

Learning to channel this anger is their journey and the purpose of giving the remedy. They can show the opposite face of being easily and deeply upset by discipline, or being told off, or by writing poetry which gives you the clue, the desperately insecure little kid seeking love. . . . They can be so fearful that they can develop varicose veins from holding back, which is what varicose veins are all about.

— PETER CHAPPELL

Agaricus muscarius

Who is this poet of the night?
Ecstasy with inner light
Doesn't like a thunder storm
His nervous system's not quite right
I see him twitching through the day
Ear is itching as from hay
Makes a funny face at me
Frostbite, burning spasming

He seems to be a fearless sort
Doing things with danger fraught
But when he came to tell his tale
He complains, his health does fail
He swears it's cancer on the rise
Every pimple his demise
So disturbed by any sign
I try to tell him it's benign
And then I heard he joined a troop
That helps a rather sickly group
And since that day he seems improved
But don't you go and stimulate
This nervous mushroom into state
Best to let him just refrain
You might confuse this poor guy's brain.
    — SYLVIA CHATROUX, MD

Amanita phalloides

(GREEN DEATH CAP)
A. virosa
A. bisporigera
(DESTROYING ANGEL)
A. ocreata
(WHITE DEATH CAP)

Like Death he stalked the ravished land,
His 'cutting implement' in hand.
Pale Oyster Mushrooms cried in fear:
"The Mad Mycologist draws near!
"His bloodlust will not be abated
"Until we're all decapitated."

He stripped the barren fields and woods
of Chanterelles and Scarlet Hoods.
No Parasol was safe from him.
The Fungus Fiend, the Reaper grim.

Smug Deathcaps smirked: "He won't hurt us
"For we are much too poisonous."

Plump Puffballs pleaded as he passed,
And Weeping Widows wept their last.
The Horns of Plenty blew no more,
As Ceps lay slaughtered by the score.
A small voice cried out: "Please don't eat us!"
The last words of a Bay Boletus.

One day he slew two Agarics
(Defying Bylaw 26)
They gloated: "Ha! We've got him now!"
And hauled him off to court in Slough.
"Off with his head!" the jury cried.
"He's guilty of Mass Fungicide."
The moral of this tragic tale
Is: "Wickedness must not prevail,"
That he who harms a helpless fungus
Is not fit to dwell amungus,
But he shall go Hell to boil
(or lightly fry in olive oil).
    — P. VERSEHOYLE

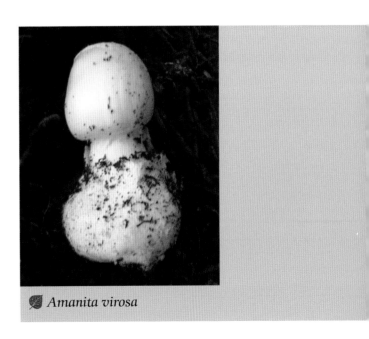

🍂 *Amanita virosa*

49

How sinister this mushroom's deception
Luring with her immaculate
Purity of presence.
Death masquerades as virgin bride with
Remnants of lace upon her cap
And vestiges of veil around her neck.

— Jessie Keiko Saiki, Wisconsin
Mycological Society Newsletter,
Spring 1983

Toxins present in many deadly poisonous *Amanita* species include phalloidin, phalloine, and amanitin. They are collectively know as phallotoxins and amatoxins, and have been found in species of *galerina* and deadly cococybe *(C. filaris).*

Higher concentrations of muscarine are con-tained in both the *inocybe* and *clitocybe* species (3 percent dried) without the other toxins, for a purely cholinergic effect. In the case of ingestion of the related *A. phalloides,* get medical help immediately, and take a glass of salt water every half hour until you reach the hospital. Steyn (1966) found that three hundred milligrams of alpha lipoic acid daily given in the cases of *A. phalloides* and *A. capensis* poisoning as soon as serum transaminase levels were raised restored hepatic and renal function in patients.

Montanini et al. (1999), in a small eleven-patient trial, found acetylcysteine combined with silybin from milk thistle a useful antidote for *A. phalloides* poisoning.

An antiphalloidin serum has been developed at the Institut Pasteur, but must be administered soon after ingestion.

The blusher *(A. rubescens)* is considered edible, but not worth the risk of misidentification.

Ten patients with *Amanita* poisoning who underwent Molecular Adsorbent Recirculating System (MARS) treatment, which helps remove toxins from the blood, were all alive one year later (Kantola et al. 2009).

In a recent case, two people consumed a soup made from *A. phalloides* and showed symptoms of poisoning nine to fifteen hours after ingestion. Intravenous doses of penicillin G, silibinin, and acetylcysteine prevented further damage and both patients were discharged from the hospital eight days later.

A water decoction of *Ganoderma lucidum* was given to twelve patients with acute *Amanita* poisoning and their results were compared to those of patients who were treated with penicillin and reduced glutathione. The researchers found a statistically significant reduction in mortality and recovery rate with reishi treatment (Xiao et al. 2007).

Aucubin, found in herbs like German chamomile, has been found to prevent depression of m-RNA biosynthesis by alpha amanitin intoxication (Chang, I.-M. and Y. Yamaura 1993).

Guang-Sheng Ding and You-Yi Liang (1991) found DMS (dimercaptosuccinic acid) helpful in mushroom poisonings.

Medicinal Use

Phallolysin from *A. phalloides* and rubescens-lysin from *A. rubescens* show in vitro disruption of mast cells in rat mesentery, with 90 percent of cells disrupted within five minutes of ingestion.

Death cap *(A. phalloides)* extracts inhibit the transplantation of Yoshida sarcoma in mice and are believed to provide immune-boosting

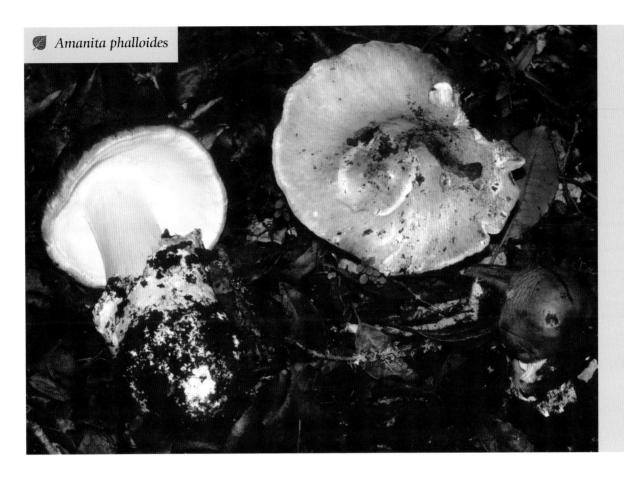

Amanita phalloides

activity. This mushroom is of European origin but is found widely around the San Francisco Bay Area, south to Los Angeles and north to Vancouver (Pringle et al. 2009).

Doljak et al. (2001) found that destroying angel inhibits thrombin by 48 percent, but may be of little use due to its toxicity.

Amanita virosa shows activity against *Pseudomonas aeruginosa* (Damjan et al. 2007)

Homeopathy

Amanita phalloides is used to treat liver damage such as acute yellow atrophy or jaundice. It is also useful in paralysis or conditions with progressive physical deterioration. The rem-

edy may be useful in lower potencies for those conditions, and in higher potency for treating neoplasms, including those with hepatic involvement.

Dose: 6C to 200C. The mother tincture is prepared from the fresh *A. phalloides*. A 2D dilution containing amanitin has been trialed against leukemia, showing stabilization of B-cell chronic lymphatic leukemia. Amanitin stopped the activity of the tumor cells, and then they lyse and migrate. Amanita therapy also showed good results in a variety of other tumors such as colon carcinoma, breast carcinoma, and tongue root tumor.

Antrodia

Antrodia cinnamomea

A. camphorata

(ANTRODIA)

(NIU CHANG CHIH)

A. xantha

Amyloporia xantha

Poria xantha

Daedalea xantha

Chaetoporellus greschikii

(YELLOW PORIA)

A. serialis

Trametes serialis

Coriolellus serialis

D. serialis

P. callosa

Both *Antrodia xantha* and *A. serialis* have been found in parts of the Pacific Northwest. In Finland, the latter is known as *knolticka*.

In Taiwan, cinnamon or camphor *Antrodia* is known as *niu chang* and other variations such as *niu chang ku, niu chang chih,* and *jang-jy*. The wood it grows on has been used traditionally for high-end furniture; it is becoming rare and is now protected. The mushroom is commonly known as ruby mushroom, and is traditionally used by aborigines to treat alcohol abuse and exhaustion.

Fruiting bodies have sold for $15,000 per kilogram due to their rarity.

It is very bitter and smells of camphor.

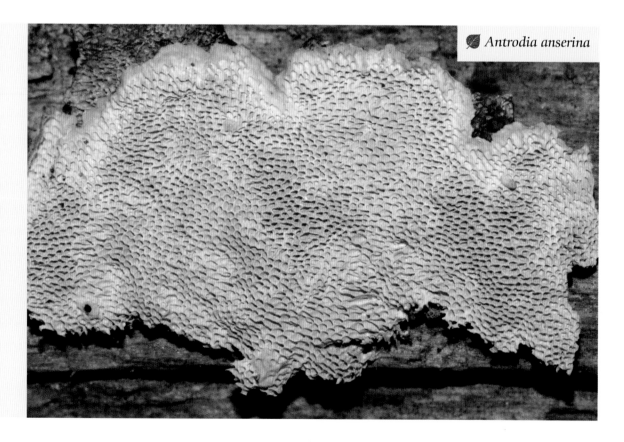

Antrodia anserina

Medicinal Use

Chemical Constituents

- *A. serialis:* **serialynic acid.**
- *A. camphorata:* **antroquinonol.**

Yellow *Poria* has been found to contain serialynic acid, a phenol with an isopentenyne side chain. It shows a weak inhibition of pathogenic fungi, and anti-*Pythium graminicola* activity (Kokubun et al. 2007b).

It shows activity against *Staphylococcus aureus.* Early work by Robbins et al. (1945) found *A. serialis, A. heteromorpha, A. malicola, A. vaillantii,* and *A. rubescens* active against *Staphylococcus aureus* and *E. coli.*

Work by Shih Chung Chen et al. (2005) found extracted polysaccharides of this mushroom to inhibit endothelial tube formation, with fucose, glucose, and mannose the predominant monosaccharides.

In fact, the polysaccharides isolated from *A. xantha* provide greater anti-angiogenesis than those from *Agaricus brasiliensis* and *Antrodia cinnamomea.* It has a mild taste.

The related cinnamon or camphor *Antrodia* from Asia shows anti-hepatitis B virus activity with inhibition of 76 percent at a non-toxic concentration of 100 micromoles per milliliter.

Both the fruiting body and mycelia possess antibacterial, antioxidant, anti-inflammatory, anti-fatigue, and anticancer activity.

They are especially valuable for treating alcohol-induced hepatitis, but also of value in the treatment of diabetes and hypertension, as well leukemia, adenoma, and cancers of the lung, liver, cervix, colon, and breast. One study found a reduction in alcohol-induced

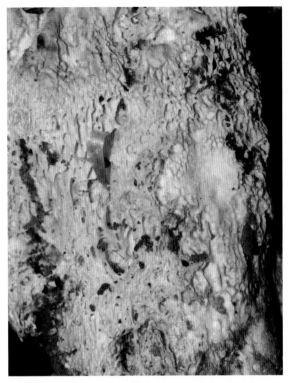

Antrodia radiculosa

fatty liver disease similar to that of silymarin from milk thistle.

Recent research indicates benefit of limiting the growth and proliferation of bladder carcinoma cells (Peng et al. 2007).

Hseu et al. (2006) found inhibition of COX 2 and induction of apoptosis in estrogen nonresponsive breast cancer cells. They later identified pathways of induced apoptosis in human breast cancer cells (Hseu et al. 2008).

Mei-Kuang Lu et al. (2006) found adenosine, a major component, acts through activation of A (2A)-R to prevent serum deprivation-induced PC12 cell apoptosis.

Chia-Yu Chang et al. (2008) found that when combined with antitumor agents it proved to be an effective adjuvant anti-proliferative agent in studies on multi-drug-resistant hepatoma cell lines.

Antroquinonol, isolated from *Antrodia,* has been found to inhibit breast, liver, and prostate cancer cell proliferation at 0.13 to 6.8 micro-moles (Lee, T.-H. et al. 2007).

Methanol extracts show potential anti-inflammatory effects, while both wild and cultivated mycelium show anti-proliferative activity against the Lewis lung carcinoma tumor cell line.

The fruiting body contains new succinic and maleic derivatives that possess anti-inflammatory activity. One compound sig-nificantly increased spontaneous TNF-alpha secretion from un-stimulated RAW264.7 cells, but suppressed IL-6 production in LPS-stimulated cells. This suggests both immune stimulating and anti-inflammatory effects (Chien et al. 2008).

Other work suggests vaso-relaxant proper-ties as well as inhibition of androgen respon-sive prostate cancer cell lines.

Antcin A and B and antrocamphin A have been isolated and found to potently inhibit inflammation. A cytotoxic agent against human leukemia and pancreatic cancer cells, MMH01, was also isolated.

Antrocinnamomin A shows significant inhi-bition of nitric oxide (Wu, M.-D. et al. 2008).

Geethangili et al. (2009) published a review of pharmacological effects and the bioactive compounds online.

Armillaria

Armillaria mellea
Armillariella mellea
A. ostoyae
A. gallica
A. sinapina
A. nabsnona
(HONEY MUSHROOM)
(BOOTLACE FUNGUS)
(SHOESTRING FUNGUS)
(MUSTARD ARMILLARIA)
A. straminea
A. luteovirens
A. floccularia var. americana
Floccularia straminea

Armilla means "a ring" and *mellea* means "honey colored." *Armillaria* is from the Latin meaning "furnished with an armband," in reference to the partial veil. Eastern European settlers to the Canadian prairies, including Poles and Ukrain-ians, know this mushroom as *poppien'ka.*

The honey mushroom grows in clusters at the base of both deciduous and coniferous trees, or on the stumps and dead wood, where they tend to be somewhat larger. The honey mushroom complex, *A. mellea,* has now been split into at least eleven distinct biological spe-cies in North America.

The caps are honey colored, hence their common name. A lemon-yellow color under their ring is an important clue to keep in mind when searching for this mushroom. With age, the mushroom turns a dark brown, but the ring remains distinctively whitish.

It has white spores, often dusted on the cap, and striations around the edge of that cap.

It occurs in large numbers in the late summer and early fall. It can be gathered and dried, but needs to be processed quickly and efficiently. The mushroom is edible when young, but should be cooked before eating. In late August of 2002, and then again, in 2007, I collected baskets of *A. gallica* from the river valley near my home.

They are delicious in stews, or simply fried in butter. The mushroom is great when pickled and used later in salads, cream sauces, and even martinis.

They should be well cooked, for when eaten raw or combined with alcohol, they may cause nausea, vomiting, and diarrhea in some sensitive individuals. The German name for the mushroom, *hallimasch,* is said to be a contraction for "Hölle im Arsch" or "hell in the ass."

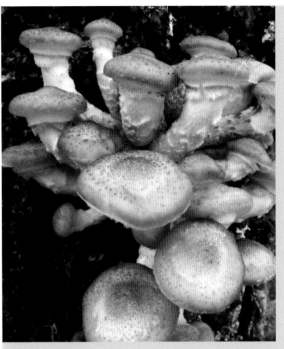

Armillaria mellea

Medicinal Use

Chemical Constituents

- **Sesquiterpene aromatic esters including armillaricin, armillarigin, armillarikin, armillarilin, armillarinin, armillaripin, armillaribin, armillaritin, armillarivin, and armillarizin; Sesquiterpene aryl esters; judeol armillyl everninate; armillol; melleolide; nor-sesquiterpene esters armillasin, armillatin; and AMG-I.**

- *Sporophore:* **E-threitol ($C_4H_{10}O_4$), vitamin A. Polysaccharide content is 1.12 percent in the rhizomorph and 2.27 percent in the fruiting body.**

- *Mycelium extract:* **armillane, volatile organic acids propionic, valeric, isocaproic, and caproic; isobutyric, butyric, isovaleric and hepatonic acids, potassium, iron and manganese, one hundred-sixty micrograms**

per hundred grams, and copper thirty-three micrograms per hundred grams. The protein content is nearly 30 percent, with 384 calories per hundred grams.

In traditional Chinese medicine, the honey mushroom is considered cold and sweet tasting—a good nutritive tonic. It is known as *mi huan ku.*

Honey mushroom tablets are used for the treatment of dizziness, headache, neurasthenia, insomnia, numbness in the limbs, and convulsion in infants.

The fruiting body helps support the intestines and stomach in cases of gastritis and painful digestion, and is used for conditions like poor night vision, weak vision, and dryness of the skin, as well as protection from certain respiratory infections, due in part to its vitamin A content.

Honey mushroom grows in the same areas as the herb *tian ma,* or *Gastrodia elata,* which is valued by practitioners of traditional Chinese medicine. The metabolites of the mushroom are similar to some compounds in the orchid, and may be considered for a substitute. Clinical trials have been completed confirming the use for hypertension, anti-spasmodic, and nerve-relaxing properties.

Calming of liver yang and supporting internal wind is another way of explaining its application. Dizziness, Meniere's disease, tinnitus, vascular headaches, and after-stroke syndromes may benefit from the fermentation liquid of these fungi.

Moody and Weinhold (1972) found rhizomorph production of *A. mellea* stimulated by oils and fatty acids, especially oleic and linoleic acids.

In vitro, honey mushroom has shown antibiotic action against *Staphylococcus aureus, Bacillus cereus,* and *B. subtilis.*

Armillaric acid inhibits both gram-positive bacteria and yeasts. Dervilla M. X. Donnelly et al. (1986) showed significant in vitro antibacterial activity against gram-positive bacteria. Melleolide, isolated from the mycelium, has been found to be antibiotic in nature.

The fruiting body, extracted by five different solvents including ethanol, exhibits activity against *Staphylococcus aureus* (Yamac and Bilgili 2006).

Obuchi et al. (1990) isolated armillaric acid as the antibacterial fraction, and 2-hydroxy-4-meth-oxy-6-methylbenzoic acid, as an antifungal.

Ying et al. demonstrated that a polypeptide dextran exhibited antitumor activity. The inhibition rate against sarcoma 180 is 70 percent, and against Ehrlich carcinoma, 80 percent (Ying et al. 1987).

Animal studies have shown honey mushroom to decrease heart rate, reduce peripheral and coronary vascular resistance, and increase cerebral blood flow. It also exhibits cerebral protective effect with AMG-I (a compound isolated from *A. mellea*) increasing coronary oxygen efficiency without altering blood pressure.

N. Watanabe et al. (1990) isolated AMG-1, an N^6-substituted adenosine with cerebral-protecting properties.

A study on the use of armillaria tablets in forty-three patients with hyperlipidemia conducted at the Central Hospital of Shanghai, Jingan District, found an average of 48 percent serum cholesterol change was found, with an effective rate of 83 percent. In patients with elevated triglycerides, the decline averaged 42 percent, and the effective rate for lowering them was 75 percent. The systolic and/or diastolic pressure of 86 percent of patients

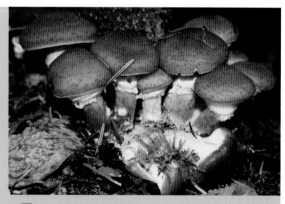

Armillaria mellea

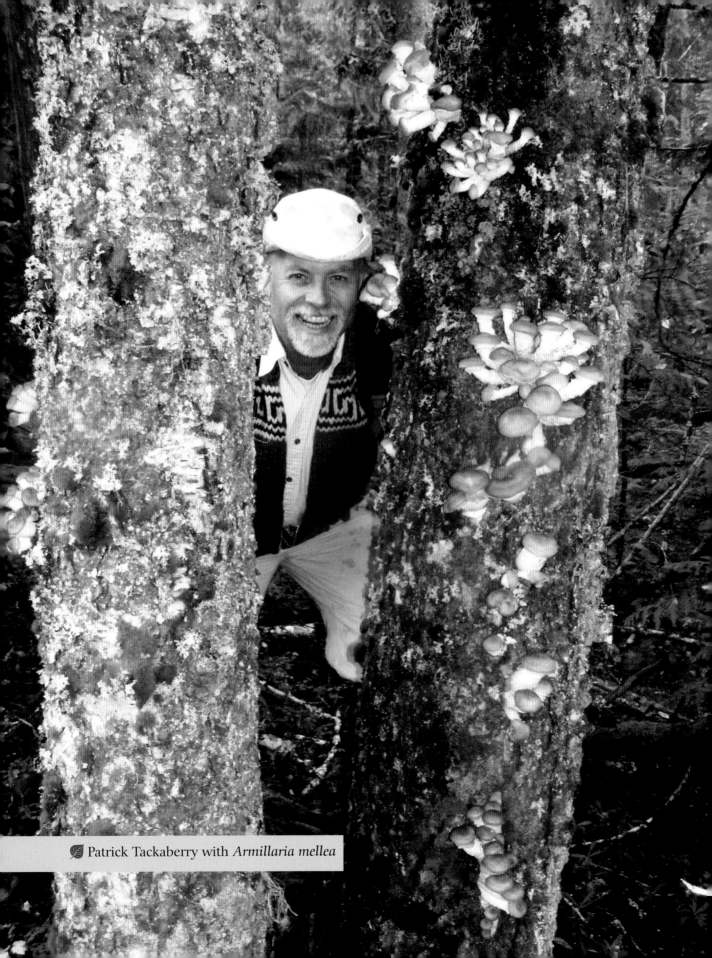

Patrick Tackaberry with *Armillaria mellea*

showed a decline, while symptoms such as dizziness, oppression in chest, nervousness, and other hypertensive symptoms abated.

Polysaccharides have been shown to help protect against the negative side effects of exposure to radiation.

One human clinical trial showed *A. mellea* reduces the symptoms of essential and renal hypertension, as well as neurasthenia, and demonstrated sedative and anti-convulsant activity (Chang, H.-M. and P. P.-H. But 1986).

Studies indicate that honey mushrooms possess antiviral activity when tested against poliomyelitis (Amoros et al. 1997).

Yan-Ping Li et al. (2005) found polysaccharides provide a protective effect caused by cyclophosphamide on mice bone marrow cells.

A fibrinolytic enzyme (metalloprotease) has been identified in the fungi, suggesting a potential use in treating thrombosis.

The mushroom contains significant amounts of copper 330 milligrams per kilogram (Colak et al. 2009).

Shu-Jing Wu et al. (2007) found that ethanol extracts of the mushrooms exhibit significant anti-inflammatory activity by inhibiting NO, iNOS, COX-2, and cytokine production.

It appears that honey mushroom extracts induce maturation of human dendritic cells without inducing cytokine expression (Kim, S. K. et al. 2008). This suggests immune modulation. More recent work found the mushroom induces expression of intracellular adhesion molecule-1 that regulates movement of immune cells to regional inflammatory sites (Kim, Y. S. et al. 2010).

For years, T helper cells were assumed to be either Th1 that remove viruses and bacteria from host cells or Th2 cells that fight parasites, bacteria in blood, and allergens. Then two new Th cells were discovered: regulatory T that dampens the immune system and Th17 that triggers inflammation and autoimmunity. What is interesting is that T helper cells are flexible, and influence from the right molecules can turn off harmful immune responses.

A mycelial tablet, *mi huan jun,* is produced commercially in China and used for the nervous system. It is also said to strengthen the lungs, intestine, and stomach; prevent dry skin; and aid leg and lumbago pain, rickets, and epilepsy.

The closely related *A. tabescens* contains armillarisia A, and has been found to be beneficial for cholecystitis and chronic hepatitis. Inhibition rates of 70 percent have been found for both sarcoma 180 and Ehrlich carcinoma.

It contains a compound, armillarisin B, that when extracted with methanol shows inhibition of *Gibberella zeae* (Shen, J.-W. et al. 2009).

The related yellow-tinged *A. straminea* contains a lectin that inhibits proliferation of MBL2 cells, HeLa cells, and L1210 cells at low doses. It exhibits potent mitogenic activity toward spleen cells and anti-proliferative activity toward tumor cells (Feng et al. 2006).

The use of *Gastrodia* corm extract by intramuscular injection gave results similar to those from a twenty-five milligram tablet of *Armillaria* given orally. In one study of fifty-two cases, the efficacy rates were 83 percent and 81 percent respectively.

Research shows that *Armillaria mellea* possesses anti-epileptic activity and may be more cost-effective and less toxic than standard anti-epileptic drugs (Ojemann et al. 2006).

Fungi Essence

Honey mushroom essence will give you guidance and calmness for group consciousness. It can help you to be as one in a collective space. It is a nutritive tonic, sedative, and good for large intestine and stomach.

— Silvercord

Recipes and Dosage

Dried powder: thirty to ninety grams in tea, capsules, or simply sprinkled on food. Do not consume with alcohol.

Tablets: Three to five 250-milligram tablets or two 400-milligram capsules daily.

Bits and Pieces

Honey mushroom *(A. ostoyae)* can be quite large. In fact, one colony in Oregon's Maleur National Forest is nearly four miles across and covers an area equivalent to more than sixteen hundred football fields, or twenty-four hundred acres. It may be twenty-four hundred years old and still growing.

Another honey mushroom *(A. bulbosa or A. gallica)* mycelium, in the state of Michigan, stretches for some three and a half miles. It has been estimated to weigh more than ninety-one metric tons, covers fifteen hectares, and is estimated to be more than fifteen hundred years old. If you are ever in area, the GPS coordinates are 45° 21' 28" N by 88° 21' 46" W, more or less.

Quite recently, an even larger *A. ostoyae* covering more than eleven thousand acres has been found in Washington state. Paul Stamets

refers to these interlacing mosaics of mycelial colonies as the earth's "natural internet," a kind of neural network of billions of tons of communicating cells.

The Inca discovered and used Quipu recordings as a series of knots and threads. Computations based on weaving are known as topological, as noted by G. P. Collins (2006) in *Scientific American.* Vast looped networks result in topological consciousness.

Dr. Ede Frecska writes, "When we use our topological (direct-intuitive-nonlocal) consciousness that's hidden in the fabric of the sub-cellular matrix, and we liberate it from the suppression of the over dominant perceptual-cognitive-symbolic cognition of ordinary consciousness through the use of particular rituals, we can access the wisdom of the plant kingdom." Fungi, as well! The author contributes three interesting chapters in *Inner Paths to Outer Space,* by Rick Strassman and others. A very good read.

At night, you can see a luminous glow from the wood that contains the mycelium and rhizomorphs of this mushroom. Roger Phillips suggests that the magic wands of folklore may have been inspired by fungal-infected wood. Both Aristotle and Pliny describe this glowing wood. Some even relate it to the perpetual burning bush of Moses, but this is unlikely. Many fairytales and legends do concern shining timber in one form or another. One popular Indian story tells of a Siris tree growing in a cemetery that has lights at the end of each of its branches.

Luminous pieces of tree roots were considered powerful sources of magic, and believed to confer the ability to make gold. It is a sign of vigor, as it is respiring cells that generate the luminescence. The effect can last up to eight weeks if the piece of wood is kept damp.

The glowing roots were used as way markers in the Scandinavian forests during long winter nights. During World War I, troops in the trenches would stick a small piece of infected touchwood on their helmets, to avoid nighttime collisions, especially in areas where naked flames and explosives were not compatible.

Keewaydinoquay, a native herbalist, tells of an Ahnishinauberg shaman who placed two luminescent pillars on each side of her doorway, but removed them for fear of scaring more visitors than they attracted.

Phosphorescence in fungi is due to two substances, luciferin and luciferase, that interact in the presence of oxygen and water. It really should be investigated more thoroughly. The optimal temperature for bioluminescence is seventy-seven degrees Fahrenheit, but light has been noted at just one degree above freezing. Maximum intensity occurs around seven thirty in the evening and minimum the next morning at same time.

The radiation emitted by honey mushrooms will pass through cardboard enclosures and develop photographic plates. Even mushrooms grown on artificial media in laboratories emit a greenish glow.

Auricularia

Auricularia auricula
A. americana
A. auricula-judae
Hirneola auricula-judae
(JEW'S EAR)
(WOOD EAR)
(TREE EAR)
A. polytricha
(CLOUD EAR)
(MU ERH)
(BLACK JELLY FUNGUS)

For the cough take Judas Eare,
With the parynege of a Peare.
And drink them without fear
If you will have remedy.
— UNKNOWN

All the sallets are turned to Jewes-Ears, Mushrooms and Puckfists.
— H. AINSWORTH

This interesting jelly fungus grows on elder, spruce, and other trees, in the shape of a human ear. It is also known appropriately as *Auricularia auricula-judae,* wood ear, or Jew's ear. Another name for it is Judas' ear, from the legend that they grew as a curse on the elder tree where the traitor, Judas Iscariot, hanged himself. Boulet suggests the name *A. americana* is more appropriate as *A. auricula-judae* is a European species. *Hirnea* means "a small jug," hence hirneola.

Cloud ear is named for either its resemblance to the clouds created by the paintbrush in Chinese art, or because dried specimens billow up when soaked in water. The name rat's ear, or *het kanoo,* is used in Thailand. *Polytricha* means "many hairs."

In Japan, cloud ear is highly prized as an edible mushroom, known as *arage kikurage,* meaning "tree jelly fish" or "hairy forest jellyfish."

Wood ear *(A. auricula)* is called *senji,* and more often collected from the wild.

Both wood ear and cloud ear are used in *mu shu* pork, a favorite Chinese dish of both my wife, Laurie, and myself. The latter is known in restaurants as *muk nge.*

Cloud ear mushroom is cultivated in Asia for use in hot-and-sour soups, and can be purchased dried in Asian food stores. It expands five times when soaked in hot water.

Cultivation

One study found that a mixture of sawdust and cornstalk, packed in plastic bags and maintained on ground, led to faster and more abundant cultivation of *A. auricula,* leading to more economical mass production.

Medicinal Use

Chemical Constituents

- *A. polytricha* **contains various polysaccharides, hetero-polysaccharide glucans, and acidic heteroglycans; erogsterol, cephalin, sphingo-myelin.**

The distinct odor is due mainly to dihydro-5-pentyl-2(3H)furanone acid.

Traditional Uses

In traditional Chinese medicine, the cloud ear is considered very beneficial, giving lightness and strength to the body and strengthening the will.

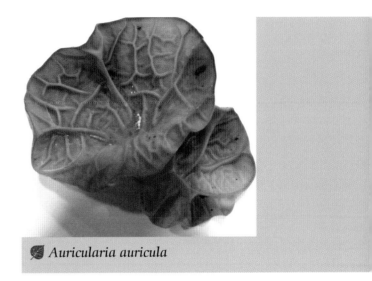

Auricularia auricula

The Chinese consume it for mental and physical energy. It is considered a specific for bleeding, especially from the uterus and hemorrhoids. It nourishes the lungs, replenishes energy after childbirth, and improves blood circulation. It is specifically useful in postpartum thrombo-phlebitis, blood clotting and inflammation of the veins after delivery. It has also been used in China for thousands of years for hemorrhoids and as a stomach tonic. Traditionally, it was boiled in milk or alcohol and used to treat inflammations of the throat. According to Berkeley in 1857, the fungus "owed its reputation in throat cases, probably to the fancied resemblance of its hymenial surface to the fauces." That is, the doctrine of signatures reflects that the hymenium or spore-producing surface of the fungus suggests a resemblance to the throat.

Linnaeus wrote in his *Materia Medica* that wood ear is used in eye complaints, inflammations, and angina. In parts of central Ireland, it was traditionally boiled in milk for treating jaundice, and in the Highlands of Scotland decocted as a gargle for sore throat.

In Germany, the dried fungi are soaked overnight in rose water and applied to styes and infected eyelids (Wells 1994).

The dried wood ear is soaked in vinegar for several hours and then chewed for weakness after childbirth, or cramping and numbness.

For irregular uterine bleeding, the mushroom is stir-fried, and then boiled until soft and served with brown sugar.

This mushroom was used traditionally in folk medicine in Hong Kong to thin blood and reduce clotting problems in postpartum women.

In the early 1970s, wood ear mushroom began to be more widely served in North American Chinese restaurants. Some diners noted blotchy hemorrhages on their face the day after eating them. This became known as the Szechwan *purpura*. This led, in turn, to research and discovery of a new anticoagulant to break up blood clots.

Researchers reported in the journal *Thrombosis and Haemostasis* that even when tree ear mushrooms are chemically treated to remove adenosine, they still inhibit blood clotting in animals.

Auricularia species help achieve a balance in secretions of pancreatic enzymes; and help regulate glycogen production, storage, and breakdown of bioavailable monosaccharides by the liver.

This leads to better control of hypoglycemia and diabetes, keys to maintaining a vigorous immune response.

In clinical studies by Wasser and Weis (1999), anti-tussive effects in wood ear were discovered.

Sang-Chul Jeong et al. (2004) found submerged cultures of *A. auricula-judae* produce an anti-complement exo-polymer with 70 percent activity. Optimal growth and production of the exo-polymer was found at pH 6, twenty-five degrees Celsius and pH5 and twenty-five degrees Celsius respectively.

Acharya et al. (2004) evaluated the antioxidant activity of *A. auricula* and found significant radical scavenging activity as well as significant production of nitric oxide.

Wood ear mycelium extracted with ethanol at two milligrams per milliliter showed an 80.2 percent antioxidant activity (Asatiani et al. 2007).

This species has been shown to lower blood glucose and reduce total cholesterol levels, as well as "bad" cholesterol levels.

The mushroom contains a polysaccharide with activity on blood coagulation, platelet aggregation, and possibly on thrombosis. Seon-Joo Seon-Joo Yoon et al. (2003) found alkali extracts showed significant anticoagulant activity.

The mushroom's anti-platelet activity is similar to that of aspirin, without side effects, such as stomach bleeds. This makes it a good choice for intermittent claudication, where there is leg pain after exercise. It helps blood thinning without the harmful effects on collagen fiber of the blood vessels associated with pharmaceuticals. Recent work suggests the polysaccharide could improve heart function, due in part to strong antioxidant activity (Wu, Q. et al. 2010).

Wood ear shows inhibition of sarcoma 180

from 42 to 60 percent and Ehrlich carcinoma of 80 percent (Ohtsuka et al. 1973).

The constituents of wood ear have stimulated DNA and RNA synthesis by human lymphocytes in vitro, suggesting immune tonic activity. Anti-ulcer, anti-mutagen, and anticoagulant properties also exist. The mushroom helps lower total cholesterol, triglyceride, and lipid levels.

H. P. Zhou et al. (1989) also reported on the anti-hepatitis, anti-mutagenic, and anti-aging effects of wood ear.

Ying et al. (1987) cited anti-hypertensive activity.

They exhibit anti-aging properties, by lowering the lipofuscin content of heart muscles and increasing the SOD activity of the brain and liver. The mushroom is an monoamine oxidase-inhibitor (MAOI), and shows definite activity in cases of chronic bronchitis.

Adenosine has been isolated and reported to inhibit platelet aggregation (Markhija and Bailey 1981). The ingestion of this fungus as food was reported to reduce the chance of heart attack (Hammerschmidt 1980). A combination of this mushroom with hawthorn berry has been developed for its antioxidant and anti-hyperlipidemic properties (Luo, Y. et al. 2009).

Dong Hyun Kim et al. 1996 showed the mushroom exhibits inhibitory effect of Helicobacter pylori urease related to stomach ulcer formation.

Zuomin Yuan et al. (1998) found water-soluble polysaccharides from *A. polytricha* possess hypoglycemic effect. A water-insoluble glucan, similar to beta 1,3 D-glucan and beta 1,6 D-glucan, has been isolated from fruiting bodies.

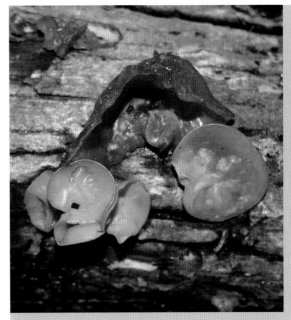

Auricularia auricula

It restricts the growth of *Bacillus cereus, E. coli, Proteus vulgaris,* and *Staphylococcus aureus* (Gbolagade and Fasidi 2005).

Potent activity against sarcoma 180 has also been found (Misaki et al. 1981).

The related *A. mesenterica* inhibits sarcoma 180 and Ehrlich carcinoma cell lines by up to 60 percent, while *A. polytricha* is 90 percent and 80 percent effective respectively.

The related *A. delicata,* a tropical species, is used to enrich blood, lubricate lungs, and stop hemorrhage. It helps to heal hemorrhoids and build up strength.

Recipes and Dosage

Fifteen grams in decoction or powder two times per day. Wood ear inhibits platelet aggregation, with effects lasting for several days. Use cautiously with blood-thinning medications. Women may observe a heavier menstrual bleeding after a meal of these mushrooms. Extracts have been shown to prevent egg implantation in animals, terminating early and mid-pregnancy, suggesting it be avoided by pregnant women or those wishing to conceive.

Bits and Pieces

Mycophagy has been documented for at least twenty-two primates, including gorillas, lemurs, and monkeys. Most spend less than 5 percent of their feeding time on fungi. The Goeldi's Monkey *(Callimico goeldlii)* from South America, however, devotes 63 percent of its time to the consumption of *A. auricula, T. mesenterica,* and other fungi. This small monkey weighs only five hundred grams and yet may consume more than six kilograms of fresh fungi per year. By comparison, humans in North America consume an average of less than two kilograms of fresh mushrooms annually.

An interesting article by Amy Hanson et al. (2003) discusses this interesting phenomenon, made even more so when one considers that these animals are not foregut fermenters and would, therefore, receive very little nutrient from ingestion of these mushrooms.

Terence McKenna suggested that human ancestors first surpassed their monkey cousins when they sought out and ingested hallucinogenic mushrooms—a suggestion not shared by all evolutionary biologists, but interesting nonetheless.

Battarrea

Battarrea stevenii
(DESERT DRUMSTICK)

Battarrea is named after A. S. A. Battarra, the Italian mycologist. *Stevenii* is named for the Finnish botanist Christian Von Steven.

Desert drumstick is a tough and stringy mushroom that releases very sticky spores later in life. It is found in arid and semi-arid regions, and looks like a spiraling tower with a small spore sac on top.

Traditional Uses

When dried under the sun, the peridium of the sporophore can be used to reduce swelling, stop bleeding, and relieve internal heat and fever.

Bjerkandera

Bjerkandera adusta
Gloeoporus adustus
B. fumosa
(SMOKY POLYPORE)

Smoky polypore grows in overlapping, shelf-like ripples on poplar logs and stumps. The small pore surface is gray or black, with whitish margins when young.

The closely related smoky gilled polypore *(B. fumosa)* is widespread throughout North America. In fact, there is some debate whether or not the two are similar enough to be considered variations of the same fungi. *B. fumosa* is larger and thicker, with larger spores, and a stronger anise-like or unpleasant smell. Both are inedible.

Medicinal Use

Chemical Constituents

■ *B. fumosa:* chlorinated p-anisyl metabolites (CAM aldehydes and alcohols), chlorinated 4-hydroxybenzoic acid derivatives, chlorinated hydroquinone derivatives, and veratryl chloride; as well as trametol (also found in *Trametes*), erythro-1 (3',5'-dichloro-4'-methoxy-phenyl), 1,2-propane-diol; and 1-(3'-chloro-4'-methoxyphenyl)-3-hydroxypropan-1-one.

In China, where the fungus is prevalent, it is used for uterine cancer. It contains a lanostane-type triterpene demonstrated to have T-cell-stimulating activity.

Inhibitory, cytostatic, and antifungal activities have been observed for both the dichlorinated aldehyde and alcohols it contains.

Both mycelium and fruiting bodies of the *Bjerkandera* species have been studied for medicinal properties. The fruiting body shows higher proliferation than mycelium on spleen cells, suggesting stimulation of B-lymphocytes.

A stimulating effect on both interleukin-1beta and interleukin-8 (pro-inflammatory cytokines) was found, but no influence on interleukin-2.

Zaidman et al. (2007) found both mycelium and culture broth of *B. adusta* inhibit MCA-kb2 and MCF-7 breast cancer cells, as well as PC-3, DU 145 and LNCaP prostate cancer cells.

Extracts were found to suppress the over-stimulated immune system suggesting a use in allergies and autoimmune disease (Shamtsyan et al. 2005).

Mycoremediation

Jauregui et al. (2003) found *B. adusta* helps transform organo-phosphorus pesticides. Yuxin Wang et al. (2003), from the University of Alberta, found oxidation of polycyclic aromatic hydrocarbons (PAHs) more active in the absence of manganese.

Bjerkandera species have been found to oxidize phenanthrene, suggesting a role in mycoremediation (Terrazas-Siles et al. 2005).

Mineralization of phencyclidine (PCP) has been shown in this species, but it is not as efficient as oyster mushrooms (Ruttimann-Johnson and Lamar 1997).

The *Bjerkandera* spp. strain BOS55 was found to degrade anthracene, benzopyrene, and decolorize Poly R-478 (Field et al. 1992; Kotterman et al. 1998). The anthracene was degraded by 99.2 percent in only twenty-eight days. It degraded 16 PAHs from polluted soil extracted with either 2 percent acetone or ethanol (Field et al. 1996).

The fungi were shown to be the most active degrader of polychlorinated biphenyl (PCB) congeners (Beaudette et al. 1998).

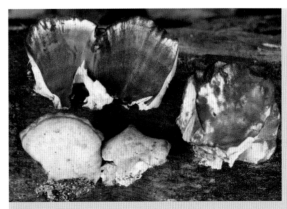

Bjerkandera adusta

Bjerkandera adusta reduced the EC_{20} values from seventy-two to ten after seven days during transformation of HRV5 (Heinfling et al. 1997). They also found it reduced nickel by about 30 percent in an initial HRB thirty-eight concentration of two hundred milligrams per liter. After seven days the EC_{50} value reduced to nine from thirty-seven.

One study demonstrated that after only three days of incubation, *B. adusta* removed 56 percent of fluorene and 38 percent of anthracene.

Three phenylurea-based herbicides were tested for degradation by one hundred fungal strains, and *B. adusta* gave the best results. In two weeks, the fungi depleted 98 percent chlortoluron, 92 percent diuron, and 88 percent isoproturon (Khadrani et al. 1999).

This fungus and oyster mushrooms were found to degrade styrene almost completely within forty-eight hours with the addition of lignocellulosic materials (Braun-Lullemann et al. 1997). The use of white rot fungus mycelium for mycofiltration of polluted air is an exciting prospect.

Kornillowicz-Kowalska et al. (2005) found *B. adusta* strains capable of decolorizing and decomposing the cytostatic xenobiotic from post-production of daunomycin. A related study by Belcarz et al. (2005) found the presence of humic acid from brown coal helped synthesize significant amounts of laccase and lipase. This ability could be useful in constructing new biologically active filters for purification of drinking water contaminated by humic acids.

Markus Thormann (past president of the Alberta Mycological Society) et al. (2002) found a fungus similar to *B. adusta* caused the greatest mass breakdown in spruce wood chips.

Bjerkandera species were tested and found effective in degrading nonylphenol, an endocrine-disrupting compound. Less than 1.3 percent of the chemical remained in the soil after five weeks of incubation.

Work in Portugal suggests that lignin peroxidases of *Bjerkandera* species are closely related to those from *Trametes versicolor*.

Recipes and Dosage

Simmer dried slices of *B. fumosa* in water, using a 1:10 ratio, and drink one cup twice a day after meals. One kilogram (about 2.2 pounds) constitutes a treatment, according to Hobbs and others.

Boletopsis

Boletopsis leucomelaena
Albatrellus leucomelaena
B. subsquamosa
Boletus leucomelas
(KUROKAWA)
(KUROTAKE)
B. grisea
(GRAY POLYPORE)

This variable mushroom has several species names, depending upon the cap color, ranging from gray to blue to black. They are all the same polypore, found mainly under spruce and pine. *Leucos* means "white," *melas* is "black," and *grisea* is "gray."

It is a popular and sought after bitter edible in Japan.

Medicinal Use

The fruiting bodies contain leuco-peracetates of telephoric acid and cycloleucomelone.

Takahashi et al. (1992) isolated a series of terphenyl compounds, B1 I-V, that show inhibition activity of 5-lipoxygenase suggestive of antioxidant activity. Further work concluded these compounds to be a series of cycloleucomelone-leucoacetates.

The mushroom possesses a partial amino acid sequence similar to *Agaricus bisporus* lectin agglutinin. The Kurokawa lectin inhibits proliferation of human monoblastic leukemia U937 cells, due to apoptosis. Yu Koyama et al. (2002) identified this lectin as the first mushroom lectin with apoptosis-inducing activity.

A lectin from *B. leucomelaena* has been found to cause apoptosis in human leukemic U937 cells. More recent work by Yu Koyama et al. (2005) suggests involvement of G2/M cell cycle arrest.

Early work found polysaccharides from the mycelium inhibit growth of sarcoma 180 and Ehrlich carcinoma by 80 percent and 70 percent respectively.

The gray polypore *(Boletopsis grisea)* exhibits free-radical scavenging ability, due in part to p-terphenyl compounds (Liu, J. et al. 2004).

Early work by Robbins et al. (1945) identified pleurotin, also found in oyster mushrooms. It was mildly inhibitory to *S. aureus, Bacillus mycoides, and B. subtilis.*

Boletus

Boletus erythropus
(SLENDER RED PORED BOLETE)
B. regius
(RED CAPPED BUTTER BOLETE)
B. chrysenteron
B. truncatus
Xerocomus chrysenteron
X. truncatus
(RED CRACKED BOLETE)
B. badius
X. badius
(BAY BROWN BOLETE)
B. calopus
(BITTER BOLETE)
Xerocomus rhodoxanthus
Phylloporus rhodoxanthus
(GILLED BOLETE)
B. pulverulentus
X. pulverulentus
(INKSTAIN BOLETE)

Slender red pored bolete *(B. erythropus)* is found under coniferous trees such as spruce and fir. It is considered poisonous and added only for interest regarding its medicinal potential.

Bay bolete is an excellent edible and, for some reason, is often maggot-free. It dries well.

Bitter bolete is common to western North America under mixed forest and conifers at higher elevation.

Gilled bolete has been having a hard time finding its true identity. It looks very much like *B. subtomentosus,* but has bright yellow gills. It is edible, but according to Arora, insipid and slimy, so let's leave it at that.

The eastern *B. speciosus,* or *B. pseudopeckii,* is a good edible.

Medicinal Use

In China, *B. speciosus,* or *B. pseudopeckii,* is used to cure indigestion and abdominal distension by decocting six grams of dried fruiting body and drinking the water twice daily.

Its inhibition rate against both sarcoma 180 and Ehrlich carcinoma is 100 Percent.

Various internet sites report that it contains unidentified hallucinogens and that ingestion of one hundred grams of fresh mushrooms will cause psychotropic effects. I would not recommend it.

Research suggests tryptamine and possibly putrescine content (Smith 1977). The taste and odor are due to piperitone.

The rose-colored *B. regius* is edible, and although not as tasty as king bolete (what is?), has a wonderfully dense flesh. It is more common in British Columbia and south to California, under both hardwoods and conifers.

It has an inhibition rate against sarcoma 180 of 80 percent and against Ehrlich carcinoma of 90 percent.

Red cracked bolete contains five organic acids, including citric, ketoglutaric, succinic, fumaric, and malic. The latter comprises 89 percent of the acids. It is difficult to tell *B. chrysenteron* from *B. truncatus,* unless you look at the spores of the latter that are truncate, or flattened at one end, under a microscope. No asorbic acid is found.

The related *Xerocomus nigromaculatus* naturally contains 1-beta-D-arabinfuranosyl-cytosine, a synthetic cancer drug.

Bay brown bolete may be able to bind radioactive cesium to a pigment called norbadione A. This discovery could lead to mycoremediation of an element with a thirty-year half-life (Garaudee et al. 2002). It also accumulates silver (Komarek et al. 2007).

Bay bolete shows inhibition against sarcoma 180 and Ehrlich carcinoma by 60 percent and 70 percent respectively.

The mushroom exhibits some antioxidant activity and contains L-theanine, a compound extracted from green tea that exhibits mind-relaxing activity. It also contains tryptophan, tryptamine, and serotonin, which may help explain its slumber potential (Muszynska et al. 2009).

Methanol extracts of the fruiting body of the bitter bolete show potent free radical-scavenging activity. Jin Woo Kim et al. (2006) identified the lactone calopin B, in addition to known cyclocalopin A, with IC_{50} values of 1.2 to 5.4 micrograms per milliliter.

Bitter bolete contains cyclopinol, cyclocalopin A, and 0-acetyl cyclocalpin A. Related species such as *B. radicans, B. coniferarum, B. rubripes,* and *B. peckii* also contain this bitter principal (Hellwig et al. 2002).

Gilled bolete shows antitumor activity with 90 percent and 80 percent inhibition of sarcoma 180 and Ehrlich carcinoma cancer cell lines respectively. So does the related *B. pulverulentus.* The widespread *B. rubellus* has similar rates of inhibition.

Boletus edulis

B. edulis var. clavipes
B. clavipes
(KING BOLETE or CEPE)
(PENNY BUN)
(PORCINI)
(CLUB FOOTED BOLETE)

> *My voice*
> *Becomes the wind*
> *Mushroom hunting.*
> — SHIKU

> Some species of fungi appear to have that prize of Fairyland—the Wishing Cap—and by its power be able to take on any form they please. *Boletus edulis* is one of them. Its variableness is puzzling.
> — MCILVAINE

Boletus means "the best kind of mushroom," and *edulis* means "edible." *Boletus* may come from the Greek *bolites*, derived from *bolos* meaning "clod" or "lump," suggesting the shape of the mushroom. Pennybun is named for the cap, which is shaped like a small loaf of bread, and a white bloom that resembles flour dusted on baked goods. The club footed bolete is very similar in appearance.

The name *porcini* has always puzzled me, as in Italian this means "little pig." The *Suillus* genus is from the Roman *suilli* for "hog fungi," which suggests confusion in early times and today.

The Romans prized *boleti*, as they were known, and cooked them in special vessels called *boletaria*. The celebrated poet Martial wrote in the first century AD: "Gold and silver and dresses may be trusted to a messenger, but not boleti."

Boletes are often called squirrel's bread, and tooth marks on the caps are often found. Small, tight, raw specimens add a leafy richness to salads. Larger specimens are best cooked.

In the eighteenth century, the French-born king Karl Johan XIV and other Swedish aristocracy loved to eat boletes. The people named this mushroom *karljohan* in his honor.

Whole, dried cepes, exported from Poland, are considered by many chefs to be the best in quality. Maybe.

King bolete is a good grilling mushroom, but they really shine as a dried and reconstituted elixir. The mushrooms should not be musty, but woodsy with an overtone of leather. The related *Suillus* is sometimes snuck into dried packages from Europe, but adds a slightly acrid odor.

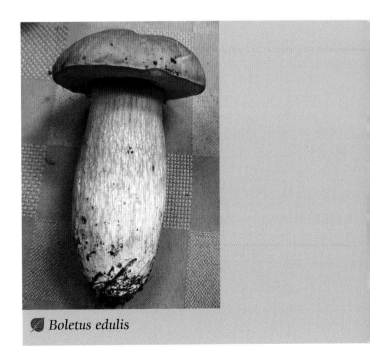
Boletus edulis

Canned cepes can be found in Germany and Switzerland, and frozen versions are sold in Spain. Though many have attempted to cultivate it, the mushroom has refused to cooperate.

Culture and Folklore

Suetonius tells a story that Emperor Tiberius gave Sabinus two hundred thousand sesterces (about five thousand dollars) for making up a conversation between *boleti,* oyster, thrushes, and beccaficos (small birds), as to which of them deserved the title of "best food."

Pliny recorded that "Glaucias thinks *boleti* are good for the stomach." He also wrote that "these are good as a remedy in fluxes from the bowels, which are called rheumatismi, and for fleshy excrescences of the anus, which they diminish and in time remove; they remove freckles and blemishes on women's faces; a healing lotion is also made of them, as of lead, for sore eyes; soaked in water they are applied as a salve to foul ulcers and eruptions of the head and to bites inflicted by dogs."

Juvenal wrote "doubtful fungi shall be served to his clients, the boletus to the lordly patron."

Traditional Uses

Lumberjacks from Bohemia consumed the mushroom believing it protected them against cancer. They were right!

In Latvia, the mushroom is used to treat stomach aches, chilblains, and stenocardia.

It is a part of the Tendon Easing Pills that are used in China to cure lumbago, pain and numbed limbs, discomfort in tendons and bones, tetany, and leucorrhoea.

Medicinal Use

Chemical Constituents

- **Dried boletus contains nearly 52 percent protein, which is high for a mushroom, and nearly 80 percent of this is digestible. Boletus also contains eight essential amino acids.**

Boletus edulis has the highest organic selenium count of any mushroom, perhaps explaining, in part, its antitumor activity. It also contains high levels of organic gold at 235 nanograms per gram.[1]

It accumulates mercury, concentrating this heavy metal by up to two hundred and fifty times, as well as cadmium by ten times, suggesting mycoremediation potential, and also urging caution in where one picks the fruiting bodies.

Studies at the Sloan-Kettering Institute have shown antitumor effect from extracts of *Boletus edulis.* The fruiting body has inhibition rates against sarcoma 180 of 100 percent, and against Ehrlich carcinoma of 90 percent. The water extracts contain four active ingredients, including a peptide.

Back in the 1950s, *B. edulis* advanced to the test phase in the treatment of cancer by natural substances.

Polysaccharides have been shown to produce neutralizing effect on inflammation mediators. In animal studies these caused lymphocyte counts to increase.

Studies from Poland show vaso-protective action by polysaccharides (Grzybek et al. 1992).

The mushroom showed neuronal brain damage inhibition in work by Moldavan et al. (2001).

It contains variegatic and xerocomic acid that has been shown to inhibit cytochrome P450 in a manner similar to erythromycin and cimetidine. This should be considered when concurrently taking drugs with significance to half-life and dosage (Huang, Y.-T. et al. 2009). This relates to the ability of the liver to detoxify.

In king bolete, 66 to 91 percent of the total organic acid content is malic and quinic acid, with minor amounts of succinic, oxalic, and fumaric acids. No ascorbic acid is found in either.

Essential Oil

The edible *Boletus* owes its pleasant smell to a volatile oil. Distillation of the dried fungi yields .056 percent of a dark brown oil that melts at thirty-four degrees Celsius.

Although produced for the culinary market, the oil does present some interesting notes for the aromatherapy, brewing, and perfume industries.

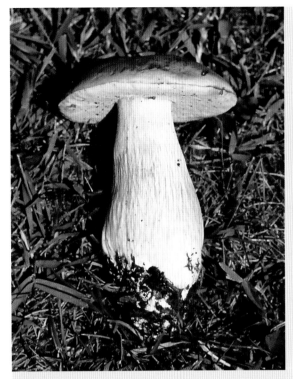

Boletus edulis

Fungi Essence

Penny bun essence is for those on a spiritual quest. It helps one come closer to Mother Earth and her message. It is a good cleanser and immune booster."

— SILVERCORD

King bolete essence helps one develop a firm stand in life. Fixed roots without soil cause a stake in cosmic energy. It helps give solid anchorage and protection."

— MARIANA

Recipe and Dosage

Nine grams three times per day, decocted in water.

Bits and Pieces

Even fungi have fungi, and the king bolete and other *Boletus* are susceptible to attack.

Sepedonium chrysopermum, also called *Hypomyces chrysospermus*, form a mass of yellow powder on the mushroom, which is used to cure external bleeding, by sprinkling and applying it onto cuts and wounds.

Boletus luridus

(PALE YELLOW BOLETE)

(LURID BOLETE)

B. satanus

(SATAN'S BOLETE)

(DEVIL'S BOLETE)

B. pulcherrimus

B. eastwoodiae

(RED PORED BOLETE)

(ALICE EASTWOOD'S BOLETE)

B. piperatus

Chalciporus piperatus

Suillus piperatus

(PEPPERY BOLETE)

B. spadiceus

Xerocomus spadiceus

Boletus luridus and *B. satanus* are poisonous and, after being diluted to homeopathic potencies, are used medicinally. At one time, it was believed that blue-green streaks in boletes indicated a poisonous species, but this is not always true! These two are toxic due to their content of muscarine and, indeed, turn blue-green when cut or bruised.

Steve Trudell, in his excellent book *Mushrooms of the Pacific Northwest,* writes, "the usual advice is that no red-pored, blue-staining boletes should be eaten and, indeed, some are known to be quite poisonous."

The color change is due to boletol (a chromagen) reacting with laccase (an enzyme) in the presence of both moisture and oxygen. That being said, an article on the "Little People" of Yunnan by David Arora (2008) regards the ingestion of undercooked blue-staining boletes in this province of China. He observed nearly twenty species being sold and was told to stir-fry them for ten minutes. When he asked what would happen if he didn't, the vendor said, "Well, then you will see the little people."

Boletus luridus has a similar alcohol-sensitizing action as *Coprinus* species, *Verpa bohemica,* and *Clitocybe clavipes.* It contains muscarine and coprine. *Boletus satanas* contains small amounts of muscarine. It is eaten after cooking in parts of the Czech Republic and Italy.

Red pored bolete, found in the Pacific Northwest, possesses muscarinic effects and should be avoided. In 1994, a couple picked and dined on this mushroom. Both became ill with severe gastrointestinal distress, and the husband died of midgut infarction.

Peppery bolete contains some unusual pulvinic acid dimmers and a yellow-staining chalcitrin. It contains toxins and is too bitter to eat anyway.

Satan's bolete may be psychotropic as it contains indolic and isoxazolic derivatives. It is a gastrointestinal irritant that is not recommended. In the Italian dialect of Trentino, this mushroom is known as *brisa matta,* suggesting the idea of madness.

The related *B. manicus,* from Papua New Guinea, is reportedly psychoactive, as the locals become crazed under the influence, but this may be due to ritualized cultural mania. It looks very similar to *B. satanus,* which is red, has a spongy undersurface, and stains blue when bruised (Heim 1972).

The ammonia scented, blue-staining *B. spadiceus* is inedible, but contains a lectin with hemagglutinating activity was only inhibited by inulin (Liu, Q. et al. 2004).

Homeopathy

Pale yellow bolete is recommended for the treatment of violent pains in the epigastrium (the upper central region of the abdomen) and in urticaria tuberosa (unceasing and itchy swellings).

Satan's bolete is used more often for treating dysentery or vomiting seen along with great debility, cold extremities, or spasms of the extremities and face (Boericke).

Recipe and Dosage

Both used in the first attenuation. The mushrooms are dried and powdered and then diluted with milk sugar powder to the required potency.

Bondarzewia montana

B. mesenterica
(GIANT MOUNTAIN POLYPORE)

This mushroom is named after A. S. Bondartsev, a mycologist who studied polypores. Montana means "of the mountains."

This is an unusual polypore, growing under old conifers, especially fir, or Western red cedars. On a stump, it can form large fruiting bodies for many years. It has a mild anise-like odor and a bitter taste. It is edible and was used traditionally as an antidote for poisonous wild mushrooms.

Medicinal Use

Chemical Constituents

- Montadial A (monoterpenoid).
- Montadial A exhibits cytotoxic effects against lymphocytic leukemia in mice (L1210 tumor cells) as well as promyelocytic human leukemia (HL60 cells) at ten and fifteen micrograms per milliliter, respectively (Sontag et al. 1999).

Bridgeporus

Bridgeporus nobilissimus
Oxyporus nobilissimus
(NOBLE POLYPORE)
(FUZZY SANDOZY)
O. populinus
Polyporus connatus
P. populinus
Fomes connatus
(POPLAR POLYPORE)

The noble polypore is a perennial, native to the old-growth forests of Washington and Oregon, where it is a protected species.

These mushrooms can be massive and at one time were listed in the *Guinness Book of World Records* as the largest mushrooms ever found. One three-by-five-foot specimen, found in 1943, weighed more than three hundred pounds.

Not only is the size remarkable, but so is the fact that they grow exclusively on very large old-growth trees, including fir and western hemlock. It has a soft, spongy surface, and is covered with a hairy, fur-like coat. It is a cause of brown rot, and thus has been moved to its own genus, as *Oxyporus* is a white rot species.

Not much is known of it, but on a recent foray for oyster mushrooms, I found a similar small specimen growing on sanctuary land in western Alberta, Canada. It was, unfortunately, growing on a poplar and thus was probably *O.*

populinus. This is considered an eastern variety growing on maples and other hardwoods. And yet here it was in western Alberta!

The Rainforest Mushroom Genome and Mycodiversity Preservation Project recently awarded Meg Cowden of Oregon State University a research grant to study the former fungi. For more information go to www.mycodiversity .org.

Medicinal Use

The fruiting body has a beta glucan content of 38.5 percent. For comparison, reishi contains only 25 percent.

Perhaps *O. populinus* should be studied for similar beta-glucans. The related *O. corticola* shows antitumor, antifungal, and antibacterial activity, including activity against *Staphylococcus aureus.*

Mycoremediation

Khadrani et al. (1999) found *Oxyporus* species useful in degrading three different phenyl urea-based herbicides.

Calocera viscosa

(STAGHORN JELLY FUNGUS)

Staghorn jelly has bright yellow to orange antler-like rubbery branches. It looks, at first glance, like a *Clavulina.*

Medicinal Use

It contains 5HTP, which is a precursor to serotonin and then to melatonin (Kohlmunzer et al. 2000).

Inhibition of sarcoma 180 and Ehrlich carcinoma cancer cells is 90 percent (Ohtsuka et al. 1973).

Calocybe

Calocybe carnea
Clitocybe socialis
Lyophyllum carneum
Tricholoma carneum
(PINK CALOCYBE)
C. gambosa
(CREAM CALOCYBE)
(ST. GEORGE'S MUSHROOM)

Pink calocybe is a white-spored, pink-capped lawn mushroom found in fairy rings. *Carnea* means "flesh-colored." It is also found among the moss of a spruce bog.

Cream calocybe grows in open woods in the form of roadside fairy rings. It is a fall mushroom with a rich, mealy scent and a nutty flavor when cooked.

It is called St. George's mushroom in England, where it pops up around the time of St. George's Day (April 23). According to some cookbooks, it goes well with chicken.

Medicinal Use

Laboratory testing has shown an inhibition rate against Ehrlich carcinoma of 100 percent and against sarcoma 180 of 90 percent.

The mushroom contains hypoglycemic properties that are worthy of investigation (Brachvogel 1986).

Activity against *Bacillus subtilis* and *E. coli* has been noted (Keller, C. et al. 2002).

Calvatia

Calvatia bovista
C. utriformis
C. caelata
Handkea utriformis
Lycoperdon utriforme
(CHECKERED PUFFBALL)
(MOSAIC PUFFBALL)
C. gigantea
Lycoperdon giganteum
Langermannia gigantea
(GIANT PUFFBALL)
C. booniana
(GIANT WESTERN PUFFBALL)
Lycoperdon umbrium
(AMBER PUFFBALL)
Bovista plumbea
(LEAD COLORED PUFFBALL)
(TUMBLING PUFFBALL)
L. pyriforme
Morganella pyriformis
(PEAR SHAPED PUFFBALL)
L. candidum
L. marginatum
C. candidum
(SNOW WHITE PUFFBALL)
L. perlatum
L. gemmatum
(WARTED/GEM PUFFBALL)
B. dermoxantha
B. pusilla
L. pusillum
L. erictorum
(SMALL TUMBLING PUFFBALL)

L. hiemale
Vascellum pratense
V. depressum
(WESTERN LAWN PUFFBALL)
(MEADOW PUFFBALL)
B. nigrescens
(BLACK PUFFBALL)

I found a giant puffball, weighing twenty pounds
I took it home, sliced it into perfect juicy rounds,
I fried each slice with ginger and spices that I
  knew
Served it up, gulped it down, it tasted like tofu!
  — RDR

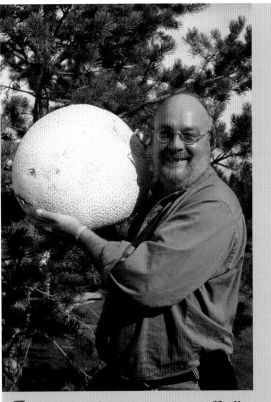

🍃 Author with giant western puffball
(*Calvatia booniana*)

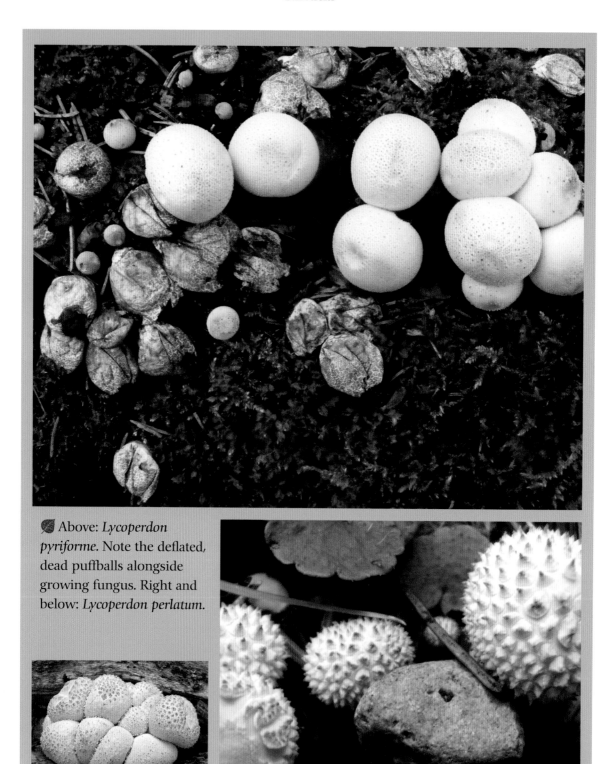

🍃 Above: *Lycoperdon pyriforme.* Note the deflated, dead puffballs alongside growing fungus. Right and below: *Lycoperdon perlatum.*

Bovista is from the Old German *bofist* that was Latinized. *Calvatia* is Latin for "a bald object." *Pyriforme* means "pear shaped." *Utriformis* means "uterine-like." *Plumbea* means "leaden."

Lycoperdon is from the Greek meaning "flatulence of the wolf" or "wolf breaking wind." *Candidum* means "white," while *perlatum* means "widespread," or may be from *perfero,* meaning "to endure."

Puffballs have long been associated with farting. In England they were known as fistballs or bullfists. Theophrastus of ancient Greece called it *pezis* and the Roman Pliny a similar *pezicae.*

In ancient Rome it was *crepitus lupi;* in Spain, *cuesco de lobo;* and in France, *pet de loup,* meaning "fart of the wolf," suggesting the silent but deadly type of wind.

Other names include *puckfist,* which means "fairy fart," from the Gaelic *puca,* or the Welsh *pwca,* meaning "an elf," or "demon or hobgoblin." Puck is a well-known fairy, and the Irish call him *pooka.* He is about at night, causing mischief, sometimes taking the form of a horse and attacking travelers on the road.

Puffballs are commonly found throughout North America. Many years ago, I found a giant western puffball larger than a beach ball. Some are up to five feet across, weigh fifty pounds, and may contain up to seven trillion spores, about three to five microns in size.

The largest recorded giant puffball was found in New York State in 1877 and measured 162.5 centimeters in diameter. From a distance, it was mistaken for a sheep.

In 1987, a specimen of giant puffball measuring more than eight feet across was found in Canada. It was plucked from the ground before it had started to produce spores and weighed more than forty-eight pounds. It was capable of producing more than 10^{25} spores. That is ten followed by twenty-five zeros!

The average giant puffball, weighing two hundred fifty grams, will still produce seven trillion spores. If each were to germinate and grow to the same size, the combined mass would be approximately eight hundred times the size of the planet Earth.

Smaller puffballs, when ripe, will expel one million spores the moment they are struck by a single raindrop. The small aperture through which the spores escape is known as an *ostiole,* meaning "little door."

Bovista fruiting bodies have been found at archeology sites in England, and radiocarbon-dated to before the time of Christ.

When young, they make excellent food. A sliced giant puffball will fill a large frying pan. Jack Czarnecki, in *A Cook's Book of Mushrooms,* shares his tip of using nori seaweed with puffball dishes. He was always distracted by the slightly minty flavor, which nori appears to neutralize.

He suggests tamari, sake, rice vinegar, and other Japanese condiments as the best flavors for puffball cooking. I agree, for as Martin Osis, president of the Alberta Mycological Society often says, if you like tofu, you will like puffballs.

Checkered puffball *(C. bovista)* is known in Malaki as *ngoma wa nyani,* or "the drum of the baboon," and is a prized edible.

Amber puffball *(L. umbrinum)* is found in mixed forests and looks like a smaller brown version of *L. perlatum.* In Mexico, the amber puffball is known as *kapxia,* meaning ball, but in other places it is referred to as *ju'ba'pbich* or "star excrement fungus." It is a popular edible when young.

L. mixtecorum are mushrooms are considered to be the best quality, whereas *L. marginatum* is considered second choice and called *gi i sa wa.*

Small tumbling puffball *(L. pusillum)* is a prized edible in India, and is known as *ghundi,* meaning "nipple-shaped" or "button." To the Santal of India, it is known as *rote putka,* meaning "toad soul plant," and to the Kanaks, "thunder turd." The Buddha is believed to have eaten a piece as a substitute for Soma. It is known as *pûtika.*

Western lawn puffball *(V. pratense)* is believed to contain psychoactive substances.

Black puffball is recorded in the University of Saskatchewan database. It was found in 1972 at Skara Brae in Orkney as a well-preserved specimen carbon-dated to 1750 to 2130 years ago. It was probably gathered for stopping bleeding.

Snow white puffball, according to noted mycologist Schalkwijk-Barendsen, may be hallucinogenic. Edible when young, it may be narcotic in later stages of life.

Culture and Folklore

Throughout the ages, these mushrooms have been associated with the planet Jupiter; and related to wisdom and integrity.

The Santal of India believe that small tumbling puffballs are related to thunder and lightning, that they are animate and have a soul.

Various tribes used puffballs as tinder for starting fires, or dried pieces as incense for holy ceremony to drive away evil spirits. Puffballs were called such names as "no-eyes" and "ghost's makeup."

Puffballs were worn as magic charms, and even filled with seeds or tiny pebbles for use as rattles.

In northern Mexico, a species of fecal-smelling *Lycoperdon (L. marginatum)* known as *Kalamoto* is taken by sorcerers to enable them to approach people without being detected and to make people sick.

Further south, near Oacaxz, the Mixtec use *gi i wa (L. mixtecorum)* to induce a condition of half sleep, during which voices and echoes can be heard.

Traditional Uses

The Alberta Cree call them *pesohkan,* and use the powdery spores on fresh wounds for stopping blood and preventing infection. The soft, dried immature centers are used to remove foreign objects from the eye.

The Blackfoot Nation call them *kakatoosi,* or "fallen stars." They are said to be indicators of supernatural events. The Blackfoot traditionally used the center of dried, unripe puffballs for the same purpose as the Cree and, in fact, so did the ancient Greeks. When available, the dried powder was mixed with spider webs for even more effective clotting of blood.

The Blackfoot drank spore infusions to stop internal bleeding and hemorrhage.

The Blood Nation took pieces of the fruiting body, boiled them in water, and mixed them

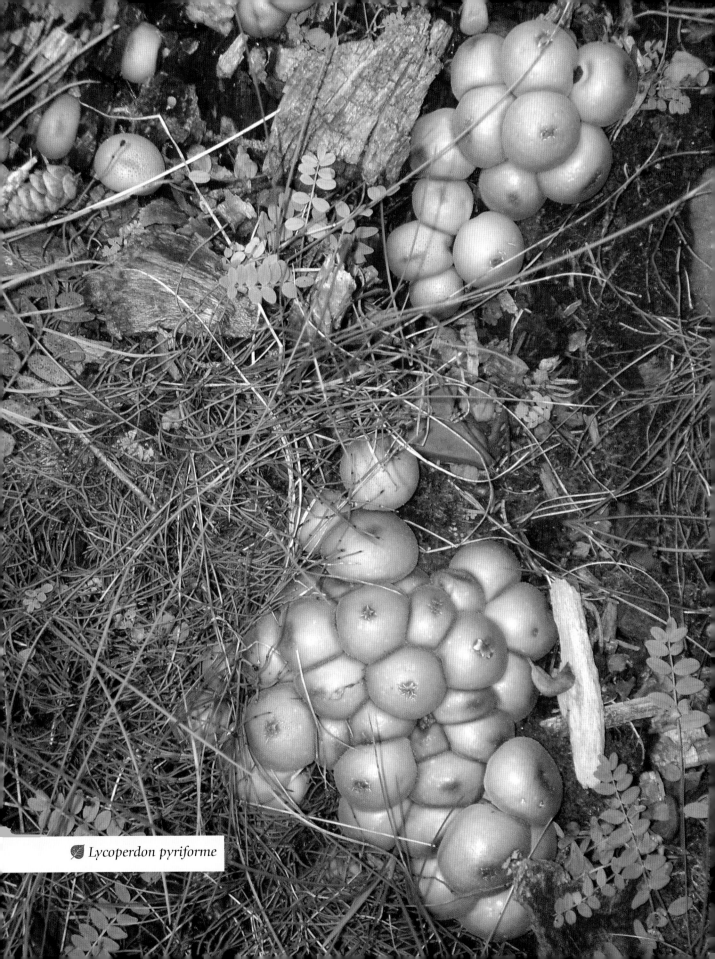

Lycoperdon pyriforme

with grease for ringworm or hemorrhoids. Young puffballs were held against the nose to staunch bleeding.

The Chipewyan, further north, call them *datsa'tsie.* The spores were sometimes used as a baby powder to prevent diaper rash. The Dene call the puffball *wogwichi,* and use the dried spores for staunching bleeding of the nose and skin wounds, as well as to treat skin rashes around the neck.

The larger *C. cretacea,* found in the arctic and subarctic, is known as *atungaujait* by the Inuit of Baffin Island. The dry spores are used for similar hemostatic and disinfecting properties.

Down East, various Iroquois First Nations called the giant puffball by various descriptors. The Mohawk called it devil's bread, the Cayuga knew it as smoke shoots out, and the Onondaga called it either smoking fungus or round fungus.

The Arikara natives made a poultice of spore mass and red baneberry root to treat inflamed or abscessed breasts.

Dried, mature puffballs were used as a remedy for earache and broken eardrum.

Native tribes of British Columbia used the powder for diaper rash, and added alumroot (*Heuchera* spp.) powder if necessary.

The Dakota applied the powder to the cut umbilical cord after childbirth.

Giant puffball is used in Indonesia for swellings. The fungus' flesh is mixed with vinegar and applied to the affected area. It is, of course, a styptic, and the entire fruiting body is mixed with oil as an embrocation. The flesh is often added to ointments for treating hemorrhoids.

In Finland, dried giant puffballs were traditionally fed to calves suffering chronic diarrhea.

Chinese herbalists gather the reddish-brown giant puffball dust in the fall and mix it with honey to treat throat infections, cough, or inflammation including tonsillitis and laryngitis. In tea form, it is used as a menstrual regulator.

The spores are used externally as a reliable hemostat, stopping bleeding effectively, and were used by European surgeons for centuries for the exact same purpose. Topically, a decoction or tincture is used as a mouthwash or gargle for sore throats, and bleeding lips and gums. Whitla remarked that the dried immature flesh is "a soft and comfortable surgical dressing."

Infusions or powder form are useful in the treatment of hemorrhoids, varicose veins, and frostbite.

The related *L. pusillum* showed activity against *Botrytis cinerea* and *Verticillium dahliae.*

Giant puffball tincture has long been used in various nervous affections.

Dried puffball tea is used to treat tonsillitis and swollen, sore throats.

Lead colored puffball (*Bovista plumbea*) is used in traditional Chinese medicine for external application to stop bleeding and swelling. It is used internally to relieve internal heat and fever and as a gargle to cure chronic tonsillitis, as well as sore throat and hoarse voice.

When used externally, it stops bleeding, including nosebleeds, and cures skin ulcers and watery chilblains (acral ulcers, or ulcers affecting the extremities).

Snow white puffball spores were traditionally used to stop nosebleeds.

Medicinal Use

Chemical Constituents

- *C. gigantea:* **burned ash contains about 72 percent sodium phosphate, 16 percent aluminum, 3 percent magnesium, and 0.44 percent organic silicic acid. Gold, in amounts around 160 nanograms per g(-1), has been found in puff balls in unpolluted areas.**

- **The spores contain amino acids, urea, ergosterol, calvacin, gemmatein, polysaccharides, and lipids. The amino acid content is very high, with noteworthy levels of lysine, tyrosine, asparagine, and glutamine.**

- *C. cyathiformis:* **polyhydroxysteroids similar to ecdysteroids, as well as calvasterone, ergosta-4,7,22-trien-3,6-dione; cyathisterone, cyathisterol, ergosta-4,6,8(14),22-tetraen-3-one, and calvasterols A and B.**

- *L. perlatum:* **lycoperdic acid, zinc, copper, lead, and iron.**

Giant puffball *(L. giganteum)* shows activity against *Microsporum boulardii* as well as *Candida albicans* and various *Aspergillus* species (Jonathan et al. 2003).

Lycoperdon species are high in iron and manganese (Colak et al. 2009).

Checkered puffball *(C. bovista/caelata)* has been analyzed and found to contain the protein calcaelin, which has shown antimitogenic activity toward mouse splenocytes and reduced the viability of breast cancer cells (Ng et al. 2003).

Earlier work identified a peptide that potently inhibited proliferation of spleen cells with an IC$_{50}$ of about 100 nanomoles. The viability of breast cancer cells was reduced to half.

Mosaic puffball shows inhibition of a number of bacteria, including *Bacillus subtilis, E. coli, Klebsiella pneumonia, Pseudomonas aeruginosa, Salmonella typhimurium, Staphylococcus aureus, Streptococcus pyogenes,* and *Mycobacterium smegmatis.* A 60 percent methanol extract shows inhibition similar to the antibiotic gentamycin (Dulger 2005).

Studies at the University of Oklahoma have shown giant puffball to possess antitumor properties. Calvacin inhibits the growth of sarcoma 180 in mice. The spores are active, in vitro, against a variety of bacteria including *Staphylococcus aureus, Streptococcus pneumonia, Proteus,* and *Pseudomonas* species. Cancer researchers studied calvacin derived from giant puffball and found that it inhibited sarcoma 180, mammary adenocarcinoma 755, leukemia L-1210, and HeLa cancer cell lines (Lucas et al. 1957).

Giant puffball spores stopped traumatic hemorrhage after operations in nearly 98 percent of 467 patients who were studied in China.

Some molecular weight derivatives from *C. gigantea* are reported effective against poliomyelitis and influenza viruses, according to Cochran in his interesting book *The Biology and Cultivation of Edible Mushrooms.*

Pear shaped puffball *(L. pyriforme)* has been shown to possess anti-carcinogenic effect with a 100 percent inhibition rate against both sarcoma 180 and Ehrlich carcinoma. According to Adrian Morgan, it is also reported to have sleep-inducing effects.

Snow white puffball has been shown to possess antifungal activity against *Candida albicans, C. tropicalis,* and *Aspergillus fumigatus,* as well as *Alternaria solani, Botrytis cinerea,* and *Verticillium dahliae.*

According to traditional Chinese medicine, *C. candida* is good for the throat, relieving heat and fever. The mature spores are styptic.

Warted puffball occurs worldwide, growing in open fields of the woods. It is edible and tasty. The dried sporophores are effective for detumescence, staunching bleeding, and detoxification. In India, it is sold in the markets to "expel cold and bilious humors." Care must to taken, though, as mercury levels as high as 2.94 milligrams per kilogram have been found in specimens.

Calvasterone is a dimeric steroid common to *C. cyathiformis.*

Mycelial culture of a unnamed *Bovista* species (96042) yielded several cytotoxic compounds including illudane psathyrellon B (illudane C3) and protoilludane armillol, 5-desoxyilludosin and 13-hydroxy-5-desoxyilludosin, several new secoprotoilludanes, illudane compound 8 and drimene-2-11-diol, and a novel hexacyclic compound bovistol (Rasser et al. 2002).

Coetzee and van Wyk (2009) have published a good summary of *Calvatia* ethnomycology and biotechnology.

Homeopathy

Giant puffball *(Bovista gigantea)* has a marked effect on the skin, soothing skin rashes brought on by excitement and made worse by bathing. Moist eczema on back of the hands is a symptom of use.

In cases of chronic uticaria, it follows well after Rhus tox, or poison ivy. It is a specific for those suffering from stammering or stuttering.

It is used to treat hemorrhage, cardiac circulatory insufficiency accompanied by hyperemia, anoxemia, gastric pain, and diarrhea.

In female patients, it relieves the diarrhea that comes before or during menses. The menstruation may be heavier at night, or there may be some between-period bleeding.

It may be useful for treating protracted colds with ulcerated nose and lips.

Neuritis, or nerve pain, numbness, and tingling are all improved with puffball. The head may feel enlarged, and there may be an awkwardness or clumsiness with mechanical ability and the hands.

One symptom that may lead one to thinking of this remedy is a toothache ameliorated by fresh air.

Hering suggests that it is an antidote to the ill effects of tar applied externally. Coal tar derivatives are everywhere, including in petroleum jelly and aspirin. This remedy may relieve asthma caused by coal tar ointments used to treat skin eruptions.

Dose: 3C to 6C. The mother tincture is made from the spores of the ripe fungus.

Frans Vermeulen, in his excellent book *Fungi,* suggests that *Bovista* ash is rich in aluminum, and that homeopathic *Bovista* and *Alumina* have nearly one thousand symptoms in common.

Fungi Essence

Puffball spore essence is helpful for those with speech difficulties. The range of helpfulness is from those suffering stage fright at the thought

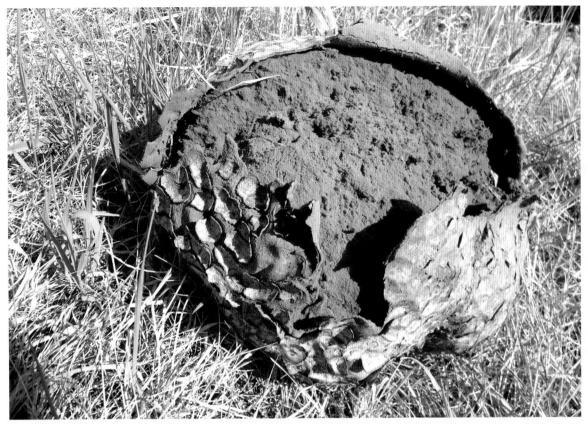

Calvatia booniana; note the billions of spores present.

of performing or having to give a speech to those suffering from chronic or early childhood stuttering.

The essence is much more effective if taken frequently and while the symptoms are manifesting.

— Prairie Deva

Lycoperdon perlatum essence is used when love is the encapsulation of mind. Play the magic wand and illusions disappear.

— Silvercord

Puffball essence is used to help gain insight, perception, and greater awareness. It is for those who hold onto the past. For sore throats, fever, bronchi, and lungs. It has a cleansing and detoxifying action.

— Silvercord

Puffball *(L. perlatum)* essence has a direct effect on the fontanel, opening up the crown chakra and connecting us to higher dimensions. It helps us be aware of the relative importance of different circumstances during difficult times so that we stay focused and centered.

—Korte Phi

Recipes and Dosage

Powder: use one to two grams in honey as needed. The dust is extremely irritating and should be collected wearing a mask over the mouth.

Infusion: two to six grams of dried, immature puffballs in tea. Steep and drink as needed.

Decoction: Hobbs suggests wrapping the dried fruiting body in cheesecloth and decocting for twenty to thirty minutes. Great idea.

Tincture: Five to ten drops as needed. The dried puffball is cut into small pieces and saturated in a 70 percent alcohol solution. Use one part mushroom to five parts solution and soak for two weeks before straining and bottling.

Bits and Pieces

When I raised bees years ago, I used to smolder previously dried puffballs for stupefying the bees during hive inspection or when removing honey. Probably any smoke would do, but I was interested to find out that people in Kenya sold puffballs in the market for the same purpose. The fumes from burning common puffball are narcotic and anesthetic, the gas given off being a derivative of carbonic oxide, or simply carbon dioxide. Smoldering *Piptoporus betulinus* or *Daedalea quercina* will work just as well.

The spores of giant puffball and *Lycopodium,* a clubmoss, were often combined for stage lighting, or to invoke a dramatic flash by blowing it through a flame, in the case of a shamanic ceremony.

Cantharellus

Cantharellus cibarius
(GOLDEN CHANTERELLE)
(GIROLLE)
C. minor
(SMALL CHANTERELLE)
C. tubaeformis
C. infundibuliformis
Craterellus tubaeformis
C. neotubaeformis
Helvella tubaeformis
(TRUMPET CHANTERELLE)
(WINTER CHANTERELLE)
(TUBED CHANTERELLE)
(YELLOW LEGS)
C. cinnabarinus
(RED CHANTERELLE)
C. formosus
(PACIFIC GOLDEN CHANTERELLE)

> I picked a basket of chanterelles
> Avoided the destroying angels
> The ink caps and puffballs
> Gorged all summer on what hadn't made it
>   through.
> "Mushroom," we whispered to each other
> As if the name would kill us.
>   — SHANE RHODES

The boys referred to the "vixens" [Lithuanian for Cantharelle], emblems of maidenhood, uneaten by worms, no insect lights upon their forms.
  — PAN TADEUSZ

Cibarius is Latin meaning "good to eat." Chanterelle is from the Greek *kantharos* for "vase," due to their shape, *formosa* for "finely formed" or "beautiful." Chanterelles symbolize abundance and happiness in the world of mushrooms!

In Russia, the mushroom is called *lisichki* or "little fox."

The Thompson First Nation in British Columbia refer to the golden chanterelle as "little fish-gills." They are often eaten fresh along with salmon and other fish. They were traditionally hung and dried for later use in soup and stews. When plentiful, the mushrooms were roasted over a fire on sticks like marshmallows.

More than two million kilograms are shipped annually in barrels of brine to Germany. Chanterelle is known as *pfifferlinge* there and is highly prized.

Golden chanterelle is orange-yellow and firm overall, with a mild to spicy taste and slight apricot smell. It is scattered amongst reindeer moss (lichen) under jack pine. Very edible and prized by restaurants for serving fresh as well as for canning and drying. The annual harvest in North America is estimated to be worth two billion U.S. dollars.

This is not surprising, as in the Haute Savoie region of France, picking is limited to half a kilogram (just over one pound) per person and one kilogram per vehicle. Washington State has some picking restrictions and without adequate protection, these will soon apply elsewhere. It is very important to avoid damaging mycelium, which take years to recover.

My cousin, Gary Eisnor, often sends me a parcel of *C. lateritius* from near Chester, Nova

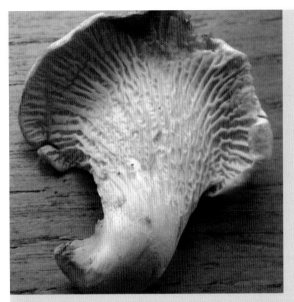

Cantharellus formosus

Scotia. They are smaller and more delicate than those from the Pacific Northwest, with a smoother underside and less distinct gills.

The Pacific golden chanterelle is *C. formosus.* In 1999, it was named the official state mushroom of Oregon.

During a foray to Sicamous in September 2008, which involved picking numerous lobster and honey mushrooms, I also enjoyed a meal of white chanterelles *(C. subalbidus)*. These are a choice edible.

Woolly chanterelle *(Gomphus floccosus)* was found in abundance, but is not recommended. Several novice pickers staying in our motel cooked and ate it, mistaking it for an edible chanterelle. It has a sour taste and causes nausea and diarrhea in some individuals. It contains nor-caperoic acid that has been shown to enlarge rat livers. The rookies felt fine the next morning.

Small or lesser chanterelle *(C. minor)* is also known as rooster mushrooms and is identified by a pink spore print.

Trumpet chanterelle is often found on damp soil from July through September. It is fond of moss and rotten wood, in both solitary and gregarious concentrations. They tend to be waterlogged and quickly lose their shape. Jack Czarnecki calls it "chop suey chanterelle," due to its mushy texture and indistinct flavor. I like them, especially in omelets.

Some consider this a superior culinary mushroom compared to other chanterelles. It forms mycorrhizal relationships with orchids.

Chanterelles have a woodsy, apricot-like scent that is enhanced with dried apricots during cooking. According to expert chef Jack Czarnecki, it is one of the few mushrooms that can be paired with lemon without losing its character. He says that chanterelles are "more like the queen seductress; fruity, peppery, richer, and more difficult to work with from a cooking standpoint, and complex and very singular." Well said.

He pairs them with game or shellfish, or pickles them for later use in salads. A good German white wine like a Riesling is the perfect accompaniment.

The dried mushroom yields very little flavor, but when soaked in vodka for a month, an interesting flavor for sauces develops. Canning is perhaps a better preservation method than freezing, as the raw mushrooms tend to turn mushy when thawed.

I like to fry them gently in butter and then freeze the whole mixture.

According to David Spahr, adding dry powdered chanterelles to Alfredo or béchamel-based sauces is outstanding. He adds that it is not the right mushroom to serve with steak, and I have to agree it is a waste.

Cultivation

In 1997, the first successful inoculation of *C. cibarius* of sixteen-month-old pine seedlings was reported from Sweden.

Traditional Uses

In traditional Chinese medicine, it is prescribed frequently to prevent night blindness and inflammation of the eyes. It also helps to tonify the mucus membranes and may help increase resistance to a variety of infectious respiratory diseases.

In Latvia, a tincture of the fresh or dried fruiting body is used for tonsillitis, furuncles, and abscesses, as well as to delay the growth of tubercular bacillus and promote removal of radioactivity from the body. They are believed to help remove intestinal worms when consumed in large amounts.

Small or lesser chanterelle *(C. minor)* is similar to golden chanterelle in medicinal action. It helps clear the eyes and is beneficial to the liver, intestines, and stomach. It is also used for the treatment of diseases with Vitamin A deficiency such as dry skin, softening cornea, night blindness, and xerophthalmia.

Medicinal Use

Chemical Constituents

- *C. cibarius:* **eight essential amino acids, 21 percent protein, vitamin A and D2, cibaric acid and 10 hydroxy-8-decenoic acid (two**

fatty acids with weak antimicrobial and cytotoxic activity), potassium (507 milligrams per hundred grams), chromium (four micrograms per hundred grams), iron (one milligram per hundred grams), six phenolic compounds (3-, 4-and 5-0-caffeoylquinic acid), caffeic, p-coumaric, citric, ascorbic, malic shikimic tartaric and fumaric acid, hydroxytyrosol, tyrosol, luteolin, apigenin, and very small amounts of amanitine.

Chanterelles contain significant amounts of ergocalciferol, or D2, which regulates calcium transport in humans. It is a rodenticide as it causes accumulation of calcium in mammals, birds, and fish. The presence of D2 in large amounts may explain why insects, slugs, and snails rarely attack this mushroom.

A combination of *Ganoderma, Trametes,* and *Cantharellus* species, as well as *Schizophyllum commune, Phellinus igniarius,* and *Fomes fomentarius* are mixed together in Tanzania to treat HIV, Kaposi's sarcoma, and other health concerns. The combination is known as *gacoca* (Sumba 2005).

The mushroom accumulates radioactive cesium by double, and to a lesser extent, is found in its smaller cousin *(C. minor)* below.

Jeong Ah Kim et al. (2008) identified ergosterol, ergosterol peroxide, and cerevisterol in *C. cibarius.* They also found the mushroom contains potent inhibitors of NFkappaB activation, a finding that requires more intense study.

Yagi et al. (2000) found a human blood type A hemagglutinate.

Extracts of the sporophores show inhibition of certain species of bacteria (Robbins et al. 1945).

Outila et al. (1999) conducted a human bioassay on the bioavailability of vitamin D in this species and others.

The related *C. xanthopus (C. lutescens)* exhibits 36 percent thrombin inhibitor activity (Doljak et al. 2001).

Fungi Essence

Chanterelle essence invites one to drink from my endless well of knowledge that I can transmute your dreams into reality. It is used for skin problems and will tone up mucus membranes, eyes, and bronchi.

—SILVERCORD

Cosmetics

Canthaxanthin, a carotenoid from the red cap, is used as a color additive in suntanning agents. It is present in various marine crustaceans and believed to give pink flamingos their beautiful coloration.

Catathelasma

Catathelasma imperialis
C. imperiale
(IMPERIAL MUSHROOM)
C. ventricosa
(SWOLLEN STALKED CAT)

Several years ago, a member of our Mycological Society returned from a camping trip to the Rocky Mountains with a humongous fungus that was later identified as the imperial mushroom. It is known as potato mushroom in Alaska, due to its firm flesh.

A smaller relative, *C. ventricosa* also grows under spruce and fir in the same region, so it may have been this species. It has a paler cap and is sometimes mistaken for the pine matsutake, but has a mild cucumber scent and no cinnamon odor. Both are firm and edible. It is known in Japan as *momitake,* or "mock matsutake."

Medicinal Use

The latter fungus contains three glycosphingo-lipids with a cis-Δ^{17}-fatty acyl moiety, specifically catacerebrosides A-C (Zhan and Yue 2003).

These compounds are not well studied, but cerebrosides in general are nerve cell membrane activators, and play a role in antitumor and immune stimulation.

The polysaccharides from the mycelium have been found to inhibit both sarcoma 180 and Ehrlich carcinoma cancer cell lines by 90 percent.

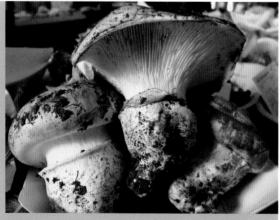

🍃 *Catathelasma ventricosa*

Ceratocystis

Ceratocystis populina
C. fimbriata

Ceratocystis populina is an ascomycete that grows on the Aspen poplar. It is a blue-staining fungus that causes cankers in poplar species.

Essential Oil

When steam distilled, it produces a pleasant fruit-like essential oil that includes various fruit esters, acyclic mono- and sesquiterpenes, terpenoids, and 2-phenyl-ethyl acetate.

Stefer et al. (2003) found a mixture of esters and alcohols produced by the fungus that can be defined as natural.

The related *C. piceae,* found on pine and other conifers, contains 6-protoilludene as the major volatile metabolite. It is related to *C. ulmi,* the dimorphic fungus implicated in Dutch elm disease.

Ceriporiopsis

This common yet easy to miss fungus contains novel enzymes that help break down wood chip lignins prior to mechanical application, resulting in energy savings of 30 to 40 percent.

Medicinal Use

Yaghoubi et al. (2008) found fungal enzymes reduce wheat and barley biomass by 21 percent and 19 percent respectively.

Akin et al. (1993) found the mushroom helps improve in vitro digestion and volatile fatty acid production by ruminal organisms by 80 percent. This suggests application for feedlot and beef producers.

Other Uses

It is a good biological devulcanizer of rubber (Sato, S. et al. 2004).

Cerrena

Cerrena unicolor
Coriolus unicolor
Polystictus unicolor
Daedalea unicolor
Trametes unicolor
(GRAY POLYPORE)
(MOSSY MAZE POLYPORE)

Cerrena is Greek meaning "like a shield" and *unicolor* from the Latin meaning "of one color," in this case gray.

This is a widespread and cosmopolitan mushroom, living as a wound parasite on deciduous trees like poplar. It grows along the grooves of the bark on horizontal logs, but on standing trees takes the form of one large gray, brown-edged fungus covered with green algae.

Medicinal Use

Research shows that the mushroom has an affinity for fibrin and has a direct and stable influence on new thrombosis. More research would be welcomed, as it is plentiful.

It contains anti-carcinogenic substances that inhibit Ehrlich carcinoma in mice studies (Shibata, K. et al. 1969).

Early work by Hervey, found activity against *Staphylococcus aureus* (Hervey 1947).

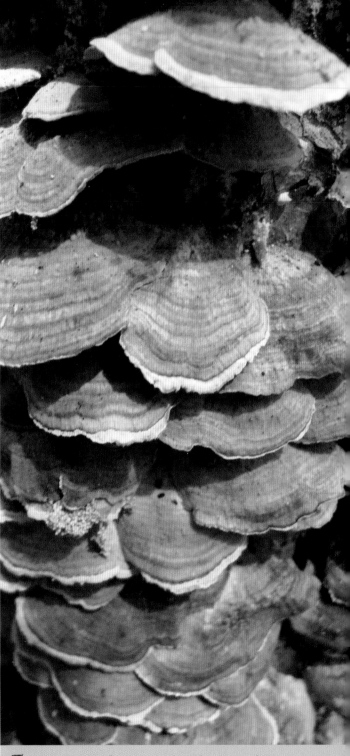

Cerrena unicolor, covered with green algae

89

Mycoremediation

Michniewicz et al. (2005) found laccase levels as high as 22 percent obtained with the fungus grown in tomato juice. Two isoforms were produced and remained stable at pH 7 and 10, with optimal performance at sixty degrees Celsius. These laccases are composed of glycoproteins including mannose, galactose, and N-acetylglucosamine.

Gray polypore on wheat bran substrate produces high levels of manganese peroxidase (6.3 international units per liter) by day eleven. Ethanol production wastes also provided high laccase levels. At a pH of 5.5, laccase appeared on the second day and peaked on the eleventh day at 233 international units per liter (Rebhun et al. 2005).

Cellobiose, instead of avicel as a carbon source, results in a twenty-fold increase in laccase activity.

Wheat straw is useful for the hemagglutinating activity accumulation by this mushroom (Davitashvili et al. 2008).

High laccase levels were identified in *Cerrena* species by Elisashvili et al. (2002b).

The related *C. maxima,* also an active laccase producer, consumed up to 50 percent atrazine in a five-day cultivation, and 80 to 90 percent in forty days.

Chlorophyllum

Chlorophyllum molybdites
Lepiota morgani
L. molybdites
C. rachodes var. hortensis
(GREEN SPORED PARASOL)
C. rachodes
Lepiota rachodes
Macrolepiota rachodes
Leucoagaricus rachodes
(SHAGGY PARASOL)

Rachodes is Greek meaning "ragged or tattered garment." This handsome mushroom is common to the western side of North America and is often found growing on lawns.

Green spored parasol is responsible for more poisonings than any other mushroom in North America.

In Fresno County, California, nineteen cases of mushroom poisoning were reported by local hospitals in one seventeen-day period, all caused by this specific mushroom. It resembles edible mushrooms like the shaggy mane or shaggy parasol, forming fairy rings on lawns.

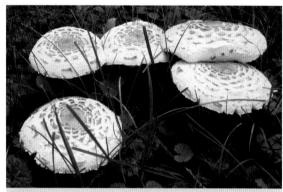

🌿 *Macrolepiota rachodes*

90

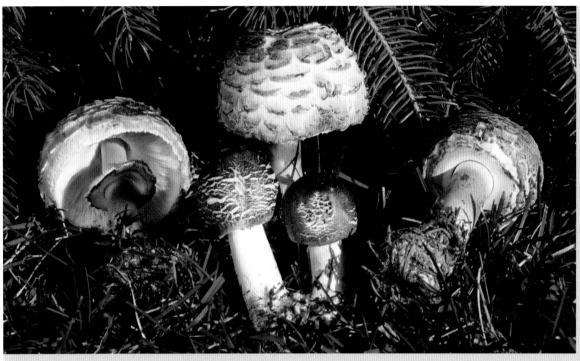

🍃 Shaggy parasol (*Macrolepiota rachodes*)

Fortunately, although it can cause severe gastrointestinal distress, people do not die, and the symptoms pass in a few days.

Shaggy parasol *(C. rachodes)* is a smaller version of the parasol mushroom *(Macrolepiota procera)*. It has white spores and is a great edible. To be sure, take a spore print!

This mushroom was transferred to the *Chlorophyllum* genus in 2003, based on DNA markers. *Chlorophyllum* means "green leaves," but refers to the color of the mature gills.

Medicinal Use

Suay et al. (2000) showed moderate activity against *Staphylococcus aureus* bacteria.

The green-spored parasol has tested positive against the poliomyelitis virus.

One compound was found to exhibit cytotoxicity against Kato III cells related to gastric cancer cells (Yoshikawa, K. et al. 2001).

Mycoremediation

It myco-accumulates arsenic, lead, mercury, and copper, but no definitive studies have found the degree of concentration.

Bits and Pieces

Paul Stamets cloned the shaggy parasol *(C. rachodes)* mushroom and, based on his observations that it grows in grass clippings, he spread a bag of spawn over two inches of raked clippings. He covered this with another two to four inches of grass clippings and left it alone. Six months later, the fruiting bodies

91

appeared. They continued to reappear for the next four years.

It is an excellent recycler of garden debris and, according to Stamets, the mycelium may produce antibiotics that protect ant colonies from parasitic disease.

Chondrostereum

Chondrostereum purpureum
Stereum purpureum
(VIOLET TOOTH)
(SILVER LEAF FUNGUS)

This small silvery-violet-colored, pored fungus is a decayer of cherry, maple, birch, and poplar.

This fungus causes "silver leaf" on apple and plum trees, as well as other hardwoods.

Bits and Pieces

Dr. Jean Barry (1968) of Bordeaux, France, published a study on inhibiting the growth of the violet tooth by mental concentration. The fungus was cultivated in Petri dishes under optimal lab conditions and controls. Nine sessions were completed with ten subjects, and the number of "thinkers" in each session varied from three to six. Each was assigned ten dishes of cultivated fungi. In a total of 195 dishes, 194 showed a difference and 151 showed inhibition of growth! Imagine. Mediums affecting mediums!

Medicinal Use

This fungus has been shown to inhibit HIV-1 reverse transcriptase by 62 to 64 percent in a dose-dependent manner (Mlinaric et al. 2005).

Agroforesting

Wall (1990) found the mushroom extract works as a sylvicide to control stump sprouting in hardwood trees.

Vartiamäki et al. (2009) found application to birch stumps in May and June reduced growth to 12.5 percent compared to 74 percent reduction on control stumps over two years.

Various sesquiterpenes and sterpurene, which has been formed by chemical process in labs, have been identified.

Myco-Tech™ Paste, isolated from a HQ1 strain, is a commercial product that is applied to deciduous trees within thirty minutes of cutting for inhibition of sprouting and regrowth. It is also used in conifer forest management, where poplar suckers can crowd out seedlings.

Chroogomphus

Chroogomphus rutilus
C. viscidus
(PEG TOP)

Chroogomphus is from the Greek meaning "skin-colored peg" and *rutilus* is Latin for "red-gold."

This mushroom is common among conifers. It is edible but not choice, and turns black when cooked or pickled.

Medicinal Use

Yamac and Bilgili (2006) found different solvents gave the fruiting body activity against various bacteria.

Acetone extracts showed activity against *E. coli, Enterobacter aerogenes, Salmonella typhi-*

murium, Pseudomonas aeruginosa, Staphylococcus aureus, and *Bacillus subtilis.* Ethanol extracts were effective in most of these cases.

It contains a water-soluble polysaccharide with antioxidant activity (Sun, Y. et al. 2010b).

Clavaria

Clavaria zollingeri
C. lavendula
(PURPLISH CLAVARIA)
(MAGENTA CORAL)
C. viscosa
Calocera viscosa
(STAGHORN JELLY)
Clavulina cinerea
(GRAY CORAL)
Clavariadelphus truncatus
(TRUNCATE CLUB CORAL)
(FLAT TOPPED CORAL)
C. ligula
(STRAP CORAL)
C. pistillaris
(PESTLE SHAPED CORAL)
C. fusiformis
C. ceranoides
Clavulinopsis fusiformis
(YELLOW SPINDLE CORAL)
(GOLDEN FAIRY SPINDLE)
C. purpurea
Alloclavaria purpurea
(PURPLE FAIRY CLUB)
(PURPLE CORAL)

Zollingeri is named after the Swiss mycologist Heinrich Zollinger. *Clavaria* means "small club." *Clavulina* is Latin for "little nail." *Clava-riadelphus* means "brother of Clavaria," suggesting their close relationship. *Clavulinopsis* is "little *Clavaria.*" *Pistillum* is Latin for "pestle."

This mushroom is small and elegant, looking like elk antlers, and often found on poor soil. The flesh is quite brittle, mild, odorless, and yet very tasty.

The fermentation of purplish clavaria yields a liquid exhibiting antibiotic activity on the bacillus tubercle (tuberculosis).

Gray coral is in a genus related to *Clavaria.* It is a gray-purple branched fruiting body with white spores.

Pestle shaped coral is common amongst mixed hardwood and conifer forests in Pacific Northwest. It is edible but slightly bitter.

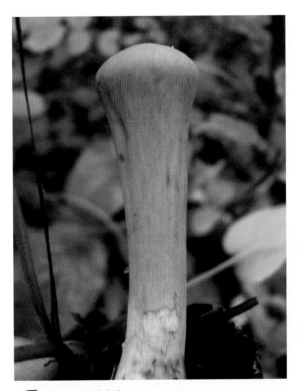

🌿 *Clavariadelphus truncatus*

93

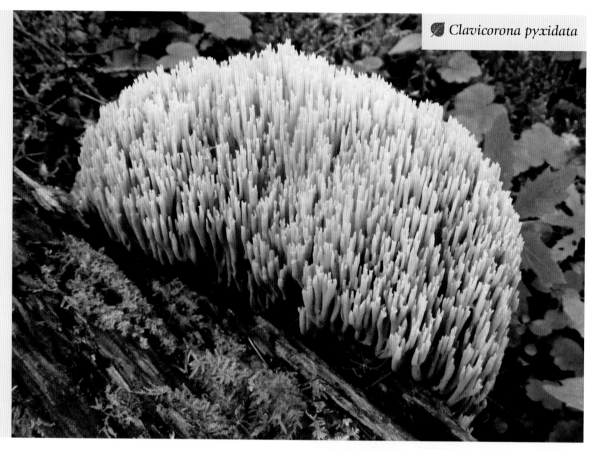

Clavicorona pyxidata

Staghorn jelly fungus looks like a yellow coral mushroom but is not. It is placed here for convenience as much as anything. The rubbery texture makes them more related to wood ear (*Auricularia* species).

Medicinal Use

Clavaric acid, a triterpenoid found in *C. truncatus* and possibly other members of this extended family, is a compound that inhibits farnesyl-protein transferase (FPTase) with a low IC_{50} value of 1.3 nanomoles. Inhibition of FPTase activity has been shown to reduce tumor development in mice challenged with oncogenic forms or ras, which plays a role in cancer signal

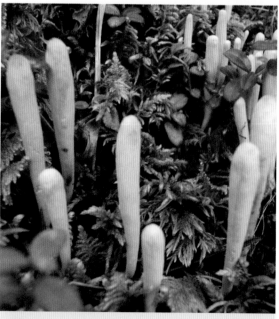

Clavariadelphus ligula

transduction and is found in one-third of all human cancers (Jayasuriya et al. 1998).

It inhibits FPTase with an IC_{50} value of 1.3 micromoles without interfering with geranyl-geranyl-protein transferase-I or squalene synthase activity. It is competitive to ras and is a reversible inhibitor of FPTase.

Pancreatic, colon and lymphatic cancers may be a target of this FPTase enzyme (Lingham et al. 1998).

Yamac and Bilgili (2006) found *C. truncatus* mycelium extracts possess some antibacterial activity. *Staphylococcus aureus* and *Bacillus subtilis* showed sensitivity similar to ceftriaxone, while weak activity was shown against *E. coli, Enterobacter aerogenes,* and *Salmonella typhimurium.*

Ohtsuka et al. (1973) identified four *Clavaria* species, one *Clavina* species, and two *Clavariadelphus* species with activity against sarcoma 180 from 60 to 90 percent and against Ehrlich carcinoma from 60 to 100 percent.

The cultivated mycelium of staghorn jelly contains 5-HTP, or 5-hydroxytryptophan (Kohlmunzer et al. 2000).

The mycelia show inhibition of sarcoma 180 of 70 to 90 percent, whereas the fruiting body is 60 percent effective against both sarcoma 180 and Ehrlich carcinoma cancer cell lines.

Golden fairy spindle exhibits 80 percent inhibition of both sarcoma 180 and Ehrlich carcinoma cell lines; *A. purpurea* shows inhibition of 80 percent and 70 percent respectively.

The related *C. vermicularis* inhibits both by 90 percent (Ohtsuka et al. 1973).

Fungi Essence

Gray coral fungus strongly stimulates all types of mental activity by directly affecting the nervous system. Helps harmonize intellect and intuition by opening us to higher perceptions and thought processes.

— KORTE PHI

Clavariadelphus pistillaris essence connects us to our higher-level chakras, starting with the eighth chakra (above the crown). Through this contact, we recognize clearly what is right and important at every moment so we can direct our energies accurately.

— KORTE PHI

Claviceps purpurea

(RYE ERGOT)
C. paspali
(BARLEY ERGOT)

Look how Mother Clio-Erato smokes her *Claviceps,* a fungus, called "cock's spur," not yet in the field guides, those passive paradigms in our shaking hands.

— GEORGE QUASHA

Claviceps purpurea (Secale cornutum) is an ergot found on both wild and domesticated rye.

Acute poisoning from large amounts of ergot rye results in headaches, hallucinations with enlarged pupils, abdominal pain, depressed pulse, nausea, retching, vomiting, a sensation of increased warmth in the stomach, and salivation.

The related *C. paspali* is an ergot on related grasses, including barley, but does not cause the same powerful effects.

Medicinal Use

Chemical Constituents

- **Cornutum, ergotine, secalonic acid, sphacelinic acid, ergotinic acid, ergotamine, ergocryptine, ergosine, ergocristine, ergonovine, ergocornine, isoergine (lysergic acid amine), sphacelotoxin, picroscleratine, secaline, ergochrysine, chrysotoxin, secaltoxin, clavine, as well as fatty oils, phosphates, potassium, magnesium, calcium, and sodium.**

The dextrorotary "-inine" alkaloids are considerably less active than the laevorotary "-ine" alkaloids.

The insoluble polypeptide alkaloids are stimulants of smooth fiber, especially uterine and vascular, and affect the sympathetic nervous system, counteracting the effect of adrenaline.

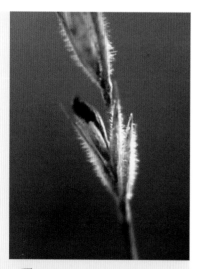

Claviceps purpurea

Ergotamine is the most active and the least toxic. Ergometrine is only oxytocic and constricts the unstriped muscles of the vessels.

Ergotine is used in allopathic medicine as a constrictor of blood vessels, to encourage homeostasis, and in uterine hemorrhages.

The half-life of rye ergot is two hours, as it is metabolized by the liver and 90 percent of it is excreted in bile.

Numerous and interesting medicines have been derived by studying the ergot molecule.

One extract of ergot, produced by Sandoz Pharmaceuticals, is hydergine, approved by the FDA in the United States for the treatment of age-related mental incapacities.

An employee of Sandoz, Albert Hoffmann, was working on ergot extracts in 1943. By accidentally ingesting a sample, he discovered the effects of LSD, a potent hallucinogen. It is recorded that his bicycle ride home was hair-raising, to say the least.

Studies have shown that hydergine causes an increase in the brain of superoxide dismutase (SOD) and, the body's natural antioxidants and among our most effective free radical scavengers.

It appears to safely inhibit toxic monoamine oxidase (MAO) levels. Elevated levels can damage brain cells and cause pathological disorders such as Parkinson's disease. Age-related depression is linked to excess as well and drugs that inhibit MAO are widely used for treating depression.

Other studies have shown hydergine to improve blood and oxygen supply to the brain; increase intelligence, memory, learning, and recall; lower the deposit of lipofuscin (age pigment) in the brain; enhance the use of glucose by brain cells; increase ATP levels in the brain; and raise the brain levels of serotonin.

Another drug derived from ergot, bromo-criptine, is used to treat Parkinson's disease, as it stimulates dopamine receptors in the brain. It also acts on the pituitary, discouraging it from releasing prolactin and growth hormone.

This hormonal action has been used with success to treat prostate problems, reduce excessive lactation in women, and treat acromegaly, a disorder in which the hands, feet, and head grow too large.

Homeopathy

Secale cornutum (Claviceps purpurea) ergot is used when these symptoms appear: sensation of numbness, cramps, and paralysis of the extremities; gangrene; intermittent claudication or varicose ulcers, sometimes called smoker's leg; stomach cramps, exhausting and involuntary diarrhea, and paralysis of the anal sphincter; and copious menses, as well as seeping hemorrhage from an insufficiently contracted uterus postpartum.

When giving doses of fluid extract, observe Paget's rule: so long as anything remains in the uterus—child, placenta, afterbirth—do not give *Secale!*

Secale has a typical craving for the cold and sometimes, an unquenchable thirst. Great objective coldness of body surface is felt and yet the patient cannot bear to be covered up. There is burning in all parts of the body, as if sparks had fallen on them. This is found in both cholera and gangrene.

Dose: 1C to 30C. Use one-half to one dram of mother tincture when there is hemorrhage during puerperium, or secondary bleeding when the uterus does not completely restore shape.

The mother tincture is prepared from the dried ergot (Boericke).

Ergotin (from *Secale*) is used when beginning arteriosclerosis is progressing rapidly. There may be increased blood pressure. Use the 2C dose in this case.

Edema, gangrene, and purpurea hemorrhagia can all be treated with *Secale*. If it fails, use ergotin.

Ergotinum is primarily a female remedy, especially indicated in cases of short loss of consciousness or for migraines that occur shortly before menstruation.

Menorrhagia due to infections, seen in young women due to hyperfunctioning of the pituitary and ovaries, may be relieved, as well as vaginal itching and congestion, when no infection is present.

It can be used to treat lack of bladder control in both sexes, when no anatomical lesions exist.

It may help various forms of alopecia.

Dose: 6C or 9C, usually in suppository form for more certain action.

Bits and Pieces

Years ago, ergotism (ergot poisoning) was not recognized as a disease, but was thought to be caused by possession by demons. The Order of St. Anthony was founded to care for those afflicted. Convulsive ergotism was known as

"St. Anthony's fire" or "holy fire," named after a hermit who lived in the North African desert in the fourth century A.D.

In 1951, a case broke out in a small French village, where a baker unknowingly used contaminated flour, and nearly the entire populace died. One young girl who survived believed she saw geraniums growing out of her arms.

It is speculated that the related species *C. paspali* played a role in the *kykaeon,* a type of porridge used in celebration at the mysteries of Eleusis in ancient Greece. It has a higher proportion of psychoactive compounds, but less toxic simple ergot and peptide ergot alkaloids. Wasson and Hoffmann, in the *Road to Eleusis,* suggest that macerating the ergoty grain in water helps separate the water-soluble desired alkaloids from the fat-soluble toxic alkaloids (Wasson et al. 2008).

It is likely that the ergoty barley was brewed as a beer. Wasson wrote:

"Clearly ergot of barley is the likely psychotropic ingredient in the Eleusinian potion. Its seeming symbiotic relationship to the barley signified an appropriate expropriation and transmutation of the Dionysian spirit to which the grain, Demeter's daughter, was lost in the nuptial embrace with Earth. Grain and ergot together, moreover, were joined in a bisexual union as siblings, bearing at the time of the maiden's loss already the potential for her own return and for the birth of the phalloid son [the mushroom] that would grow from her body."

The purple robe of Demeter may be related to the purple sclerotia, according to Terence McKenna in *Food of the Gods.*

The Eleusianian mysteries may never be solved. Whatever occurred was significant. As the Greek scholar Pindar wrote, "Happy is he who, having seen these rites, goes below the hollow earth; for he knows the end of life and he knows its god-sent beginning."

Climacodon

Climacodon septentrionalis
Steccherinum septentrionale
(SHELVING TOOTH)
(NORTHERN TOOTH)

Shelving tooth fruits in tight layers that are yellow-white and turn tan with age. It is widespread, though not common, and is found on various hardwoods, particularly maple, but also poplar.

It looks like a polypore, but has spines instead of pores. The odor is said to resemble ham.

It is interesting that we have so many mushrooms associated with or named after animal foods, such as turkey tail, chicken of the woods, beefsteak, and pig's ear.

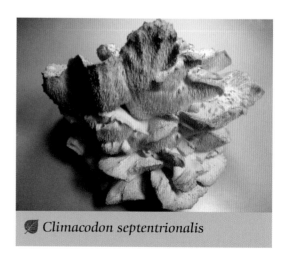

Climacodon septentrionalis

Medicinal Use

In 1945, Robbins et al. found moderate activity against *Staphylococcus aureus* and *E. coli* bacterium.

Clitocybe

Clitocybe candicans
Leucopaxillus candidus
C. candicans var. dryadicola
(MOUNTAIN AVENS CLITOCYBE)
C. nebularis
Lepista nebularis
(CLOUDY CLITOCYBE)
(CLOUDED AGARIC)
C. odora var. alba
(WHITE ANISEED CLITOCYBE)
C. odora var. odora
(GREEN ANISE SCENTED FUNNEL
   MUSHROOM)
C. fragrans
(SLIM ANISE MUSHROOM)
C. geotropa
(TRUMPET MUSHROOM)
(TRUMPET FUNNEL CAP)
(MONK'S HEAD)
C. gibba
C. infundibuliformis
(SLIM FUNNEL MUSHROOM)
C. inversa
C. flaccida var. inversa
(TAWNY FUNNEL CAP)
(ORANGE FUNNEL CAP)
(INSIDE OUT AGARIC)
C. clavipes
Ampulloclitocybe clavipes
(CLUB FOOT)
C. robusta
C. alba
(STURDY CLITOCYBE)
C. nudu (see *Lepista nuda*)
C. multiceps (see *Lyophyllum decastes*)
C. gigantea (see *Leucopaxillus giganteus*)
C. socialis (see *Calocybe carnea*)
C. maxima
(LARGE FUNNEL CAP)

Clitocybe means "sloping head," referring to the funnel-shaped cap. *Geotropa* is Greek for "turn the earth." *Fragrans* means "fragrant or odorous." *Odora* means "perfumed." *Gibba* means "humped." *Nebularis* is from *nebula* meaning "a cloud. *Clavipes* means "clubfoot."

Mountain avens *Clitocybe* is usually found in the fall on the floor of spruce forests. It is edible.

Cloudy *Clitocybe* is a smoky-colored forest floor mushroom. Found during the summer and early autumn, it is somewhat edible, but not recommended. The odor is unpleasant, like a dirty mouse cage or skunk cabbage. Young specimens can be dried for flavoring winter meals.

Clitocybe odora, as the name suggests, has a strong anise odor that is not destroyed by cooking. The dried mushroom is powdered and added to sweet and savory dishes.

Trumpet mushroom grows in rings, similar to *Marasmius,* that can be quite large. One ring in France is more than half a mile in diameter and is estimated to be more than seven hundred years old. It is easily identified by its distinct lavender scent, with peach and bitter almond undertones. It is a very pleasant and edible mushroom when young.

Giant funnel cap *(C. maxima)* is undergoing research into its viability as a commercially cultivated mushroom.

Clitocybe inversa, also known as *Lepista inversa,* is widespread from Alaska to California and found mostly in wooded areas. It is considered a good edible by some, though others find it to be bitter. It has a mild peach odor. It is best when young. It myco-accumulates arsenic and cadmium, so caution is advised when picking.

Clitocybe inversa and *C. flaccida* are closely related and may or may not be the same mushroom. Work by Boustie (2005) suggests the former may have chlorinated compounds not present in the latter.

Clubfoot *(C. clavipes)* contains toxins that are not compatible with alcohol, leading to similar unpleasant symptoms as smooth inky cap *(Coprinus).* Otherwise it is considered edible.

Medicinal Use
Chemical Constituents

- *C. candicans:* **clitocybin.**
- *C. nebularis:* **nebularine or 9-(beta-D-riboufruanosyl)purine.**
- *C. inversa:* **clitocine.**
- *C. flaccida:* **clitolactone or 5-[chloromethyl]-3-methyl-2 [5H]-furanone.**
- *C. nivalis:* **strobilurins and oudemansin A.**

Mountain avens *Clitocybe* contains clitocybin that may be effective in resisting pulmonary tuberculosis, and has been shown in studies to be effective against both gram-positive and gram-negative bacteria.

Research conducted shortly after World War II showed promise for curing tuberculosis, as clitocybin inhibits the growth of Koch's bacillus. When streptomycin was discovered, the research was abandoned.

Cloudy *Clitocybe* produces nebularine 9-(beta-D-riboufruanosyl)purine, which moderately inhibits the growth of sarcoma 180 in white mice. Studies indicate nebularine is bacteriostatic. What is interesting is that a water concentration of one in three hundred thousand is active against mycobacterium but shows no activity against *E. coli.* Considerable dilution also shows preferential activity against cancer cells, including sarcoma 180.

Earlier research found that the fresh-pressed juice possessed antibiotic activity (Ehrenberg et al. 1946).

Ehrenberg's colleague Lofgren wrote in a private communication in 1947 that the substance, though still impure, inhibited tubercle bacilli at a dilution of one in two million.

C. nebularis has been found active against five bacteria: *Bacillus cereus, B. subtilis, Streptococcus aureus, E. coli,* and *Salmonella typhimurium.*

Work by Milton et al. (1992) at the University College of Swansea examined the culture of the fungi for production of nebularine. Growth was better in dark conditions at twenty-one degrees Celsius.

Extracts contain aspartic proteases, which have biotechnology application and use in drug design (Sabotic et al. 2009).

A lectin has been found to bind to carbohydrate receptors on human leukemic T-cells, suggesting anti-proliferative activity (Pohleven et al. 2009).

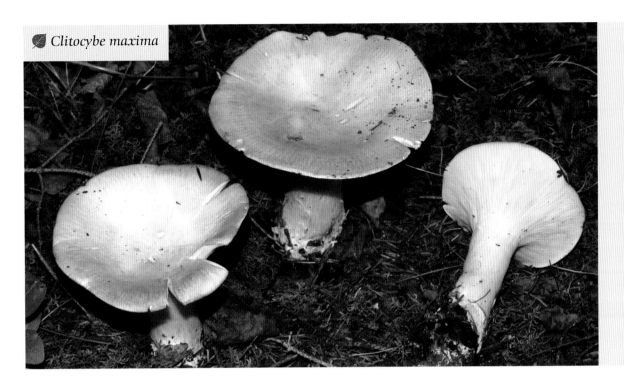

Clitocybe maxima

The related slim anise *(C. fragrans)*, trumpet mushroom *(C. geotropa)*, and slim funnel *(C. gibba)* showed inhibition rates of 70 to 80 percent against sarcoma 180 and Ehrlich carcinoma.

The anise funnel showed inhibition of 70 percent and 60 percent respectively.

Activity against *Staphylococcus aureus, Bacillus subtilis,* and *Saccharomyces cerevisiae* by trumpet mushroom was found (Yamac and Bilgili 2006).

The related *C. suaveolens* or *C. deceptiva* is edible but has an anise odor, due to the presence of N-methyl nitro aminobenzaldehyde.

Clitocybe veneriata contains antibiotic substances.

Both the white and green anise *Clitocybes* contain one milligram per kilogram of vanadium. This mineral plays a key and vital role in the production of insulin by the pancreas.

Potential for commercial production of organic vanadium could be explored.

Research in Norway found that radioactive cesium released from Chernobyl began showing up in domesticated animals. The vascular plants and soil were quite stable, and this led researchers to fungi. The levels were ten to one hundred fifty times higher than in adjacent plants, with one particular *Clitocybe* containing 270 times the cesium than the surrounding soil and plants.

Slim funnel *Clitocybe* releases hydrogen cyanide (HCN) gas into the air, but this dissipates upon heating. The mushroom inhibits thrombin, which is a key serine proteinase of the coagulation cascade. *C. gibba* has been shown to inhibit thrombin by 49 percent, suggesting a model for further research into blood coagulation and safer thrombin inhibitors (Doljak et al. 2001).

Extracts of *C. infunibuliformis* have been found

active against *Bacillus cereus* and *B. subtilis*. Inhibition rates against sarcoma 180 and Ehrlich carcinoma are 70 to 80 percent.

It is noted for its antitumor activity. Its extract has been shown to be effective against transplanted lymphatic leukemia in mice (Bezivin et al. 2003b).

It has also been shown to be active against both lymphocytic leukemia and Lewis lung carcinoma cell lines (Bezivin et al. 2002). Methanol extract from the fruiting body showed significant activity against the human cancer cell lines K562, U251, DU145, and MCF7 greater or equal to the bark extracts of *Taxus baccata*. This genus led to the production of taxol and tamoxifen. Clitocine is the major compound responsible, and may work via induction of apoptosis, or programmed cell death.

Early work identified antibacterial activity against *Bacillus cereus* and *Staphylococcus aureus*.

It has been shown to be active against herpes simplex virus 1 and 2, as well as poliovirus and vesicular stomatitis virus (VSV). Follow-up research found this mushroom rated the highest antiviral activity of 121 species tested. It showed low toxicity against Vero cell line (that's good), as well as high activity against poliovirus and VSV (Amoros et al. 1997).

Tawny funnel cap *(C. flaccida)* contains a compound, clitolactone or 5-[chloromethyl]-3-methyl-2 [5H]-furanone, a natural chlorinated compound that exhibits anti-feeding activity against slugs (Wood et al. 2004).

The related *C. nivalis* produces the antibiotic metabolites strobulurins and oudemansin A on natural substrates.

Both *C. robusta* and *C. obsoleta* exhibit activity against *Staphylococcus aureus* (Hervey 1947).

Clubfoot mushroom *(C. clavipes)* contains fatty acids that are antibacterial against *Bacillus subtilis, B. cereus,* and *Sarcina lutea;* as well as antifungal activity (Arnone et al. 1994). It contains a novel tyrosine kinase inhibitor that may find use as an antitumor agent (Cassinelli et al. 2000).

Essential Oil

The hydrodistilled *C. odora* essential oil is 81.4 percent p-anisaldehyde, 8 percent benzaldehyde, and minor amounts of 1-Octen-3-one, 1-Octen-3-ol, 3-Octanone, limonene, 2-phenylethanal, and linalool (Rapior et al. 2002).

Fungi Essence

Trumpet funnel cap *(C. geotropa)* essence frees energy blockages and disturbances from the first and second charkas, thereby strengthening our basic vitality. It also draws out poison residues at an energy level in the cause of fungus-related diseases.

— KORTE PHI

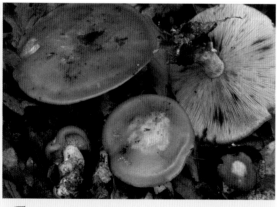

Clitocybe nuda

Clitocybe dealbata

C. dealbata var. sudorifera
(SWEATING MUSHROOM)
(IVORY CLITOCYBE)
(SUDORIFIC CLITOCYBE)
C. rivulosa
(DEADLY CLITOCYBE)
C. cerussata
(LEAD WHITE CLITOCYBE)
C. illudens (see *Omphalotus olearius*)

> Nicely groomed, like a mushroom
>> Standing there so sleek and erect and eyeable
>> And like a fungus, living on the remains of
> bygone life, sucking his life out of the dead
> leaves of greater life than his own.
>> And even so, he's stale, he's been here too
> long, touch him, and you'll find he's all gone
> inside just like an old mushroom, all wormy
> inside, and hollow under a smooth skin and an
> upright appearance.
>> — D.H. Lawrence

I have grouped these *Clitocybes* in a separate category, as they are often considered poisonous, toxic, or deadly. And because they are often found in fairy rings (see *Marasmius* below), they should be discussed.

Dealbata is from *dealbo* meaning "to whitewash," due to its ivory-white top.

The sweater *(C. dealbata)* is representative of the group, as they all contain muscarine. This is the same toxin present in small amounts in *Amantia muscaria,* stimulating the parasympathetic nerve endings of the autonomic nervous system. It causes profuse glandular secretions that can result in sweating, salivation, and tears, as well as muscle spasms, slowed heartbeat, and pinpoint pupils. This toxin is treated with atropine, the most commonly used antidote in mushroom poisoning, but it usually has little effect and may even exacerbate the condition. It is worth noting that muscarine poisoning responds well to calm, quiet, and the knowledge that it will wear off in about six hours. In some cases, atropine can serve as an antidote for muscarine poisoning, as the toxic effects are the result of stimulation of parasympathetic effector organs that are antagonized by the peripheral action of atropine.

Some authors consider *C. rivulosa* a synonym, while others think it is a separate species. *C. dilatata* and *C. morbifera* are others in this group that you should avoid ingesting.

Homeopathy

The related *C. acromelalga* contains acromelic acid, which is closely related to L-kainic acid and similar to domoic acid, found in some shellfish.

It has a structural relationship to the neurotransmitter glutamate and has been shown to be a powerful agonist in neuro-muscular junctions.

Ingestion of this mushroom produces sharp pains with marked, reddish swelling of the hands and feet (erythro-melalgia) about seven days later. This painful condition can last for months. In rat studies, it appears the mushroom increases conversion of tryptophan to niacin. Perhaps an eager homeopath would consider a studying this mushroom as a remedy for these symptoms in gout, erythema, and various painful neuro-muscular diseases.

Coltricia cinnamomea

(FAIRY STOOL)

C. perennis

(TIGER'S EYE)

Both of these mushrooms are widely distributed in North America. They dry nicely for use in flower arrangements.

Medicinal Use

The inhibition rate against sarcoma 180 and Ehrlich carcinoma is 90 percent and 100 percent for the former and 100 percent and 90 percent for the latter (Ohtsuka et al. 1973).

Other Uses

Tiger's Eye shows significant production of hydrolytic enzymes including protease, amylase, carboxyl esterase and lipase (Goud et al. 2009). These are all significant to various industries, including food, paper, textile, alcohol, and biodiesel.

Conocybe siliginea

C. siligineoides

(SLIM CONOCYBE)

Siliginea is from the Latin meaning "looking like wheat kernels." *Conocybe* is from the Greek meaning "conical head or cap."

A cult based around *Tamu*, a *Conocybe* species, known as the mushroom of knowledge, was discovered in the Ivory Coast (Samorini 1995). Maybe this is where the term "conehead" comes from!

Slim *Conocybe* has a small cone-shaped cap and tall thin stalk; both tan-brown. It is found on lawns, and may be prevalent at times. In culture work, the compounds conocenol A-D, conocenolide A and B, tremulenediol A, 5 tremulane-type sesquiterpenes, and three new aliphatic diketones have been identified.

The first tremulanes were found in *Phellinus tremulae* on aspen poplar. The biological activity is as yet unknown.

Some members of the genus, such as *C. filaris,* contain amatoxins that destroy the production of specific proteins in the liver and kidneys, leading to failure and death. This species and other related mushrooms have a membrane ring on the stalk that may fall off. Hence, identification is essential. Twenty to thirty caps are the equivalent of one half cap of *Amanita phalloides!*

The related *C. tenera,* or brown dunce cap, also found on lawns and gardens, is too similar to *C. filaris* to chance edibility. White dunce cap (*C. lactea*) is a soft, white, so-called edible found on lawns, but caution is advised. Hallen et al. (2003) have detected minor amounts of phallotoxins. I wouldn't eat either.

Hutchison et al. (1996) found appendages, similar to those of oyster mushroom, that paralyze and kill nematodes. Unlike the oyster mushroom, this mushroom does not use the nematodes for food, thus the appendages are more likely simply a defense mechanism.

The related *C. siligineoides* was collected by Dr. Wasson in Mexico in 1955, and determined to be one of the hallucinogenic mushrooms. It is found growing on pieces of decayed wood.

104

Other "pupil dilating" species, as David Arora calls them, are *C. smithii* and *C. cyanopus*. The former are found in bogs, the latter on lawns or moss.

It contains 0.93 percent psilocybin by dry weight and some baeocystin. The whitish stem is blue-green at base and turns blue when squeezed.

Care must be taken to ensure it is not ringed cone head *(C. filaris),* which contains deadly amanatoxins.

The related Kuhner's *Concybe (C. kuehneriana)* also contains psilocybin. It looks similar to the poisonous *C. filaris,* but has a reddish-brown spore print. Caution is advised.

Coprinopsis atramentaria

Coprinus atramentarius
Agaricus atramentarius
(SMOOTH INKY CAP)
C. plicatilis
Parasola plicatilis
(JAPANESE UMBRELLA)
(JAPANESE PARASOL)
C. micaceus
Coprinellus micaceus
(GLISTENING INKY CAP)
(MICA CAP)
C. domesticus
(DOMESTIC INKY CAP)
(RETRO INKY)
Coprinopsis lagopus
(HARE'S FOOT INKCAP)
(WOOLLY INKCAP)
C. nivea

Have you not seen in the woods, in a late autumn morning, a poor fungus or mushroom—a plant without any solidity, nay, that seemed nothing but a soft mush or jelly—by its constant, total, and inconceivably gentle pushing, manage to break its way up through the frosty ground, and actually lift a hard crust on its head? It is the symbol of the power of kindness.

— RALPH W. EMERSON

Coprinus may be from the Greek *kopros* meaning "dung." *Atra* means "blackened," and *atramentum* means "ink." *Comatus* means "covered with hair." *Micaceus* is from the Latin *mica* meaning "crumb, grain or granular." *Plicatilis* is from the Latin meaning "with fine folds." *Domesticus* is also Latin, meaning "domestic," while *atramentarius* means "ink." *Lagopus* is Greek for "hare" and "root."

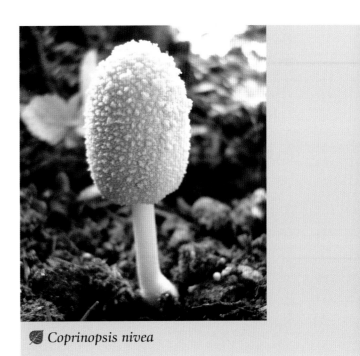

🍃 *Coprinopsis nivea*

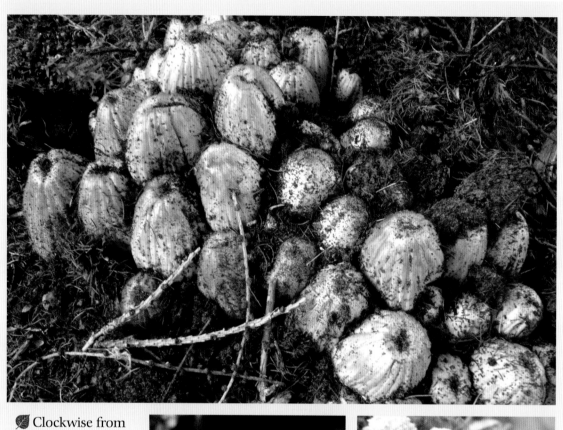

Clockwise from above: *Coprinopsis atramentaria; Coprinopsis nivea; Coprinus plicatilis (Parasola plicatilis); Coprinopsis nivea.*

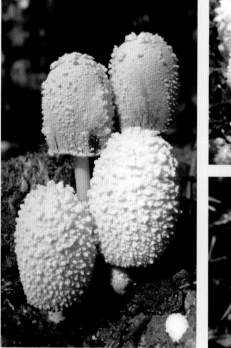

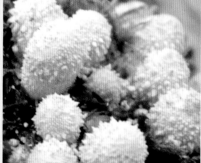

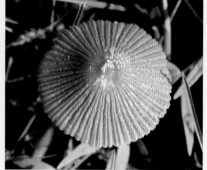

Smooth inky cap is common to roadsides, where it very quickly turns black and inky as the name suggests. It is most edible in its younger stage, when it consists of 21 percent protein and 5.7 percent fat and contains illudins.

C. atramentarius, C. micaceus, and *C. comatus* have been shown to contain tryptophan and tryptamine.

It should not be consumed with alcohol, as this may cause mild poisoning with accompanying rapid heartbeat, tinnitus, or ringing in ears, collapse, and creeping chill or agitation. It contains significantly greater amounts of coprine than its cousin, the shaggy mane.

C. plicatilis, or Japanese umbrella, grows in old leaves and other wood debris. A small version is sometimes found in potted houseplants. It is a very fragile species, fruiting in spring.

Glistening inky cap, or mica cap, is often found near old rotten stumps, growing in bunches. They are edible and tasty in omelets.

The whole genus contains coprine, a water-soluble substance whose action inhibits the liver enzyme acetylaldehyde dehydrogenase. If even small amounts of alcohol are combined with several days of eating the mushrooms, acetylaldehyde accumulates in the liver, creating toxicity. Normally, the enzyme catalyzes the conversion of acetylaldehyde to acetic acid (vinegar), which can easily be broken down to carbon dioxide and water. To be effective the enzyme requires molybdenum and a substance in the mushroom binds this element.

Coprine is similar to disulfiram (Antabuse), a prescription drug that interferes with the metabolism of alcohol.

Symptoms of poisoning include low blood pressure and cardiovascular collapse and last several hours. There is no antidote, but symptoms usually fade within few hours.

It may be used externally to cure sores or eaten to improve digestion and reduce phlegm.

Culture and Folklore

Grandfather dug the serving fork into the platter of *Coprinus* crispies (French-fried *C. atramentarius*) . . . and poured himself half a water glass of elderberry wine . . . [Dinner] was usually fun, but that day it was an unhappy meal. By the time Grandmother stood up to bring in the dessert, Grandfather Sauganash began to turn red, blue, purple, and white, and made strange growling noises deep in his throat. My mother whisked me upstairs to the bedroom and locked me in. Of course I didn't stay there.

It took me a little while to figure out how to unlock the door. I crept down to the stair landing in my bare feet, and an utterly weird sight met my eyes. Dignified Grandfather Sauganash was dancing on the dinner table, shouting some strange song in a foreign tongue, throwing dinner knives through the window and door panes, and laughing uproariously as they shattered. . . .

Mother did what she usually did when there was trouble—ran for father . . . Father hesitated, and while he did so, a gravy boat caught him on the jaw and splattered brown ooze down the front of his only white linen shirt. Once my father decided, it was all over in a split second. Grandfather Sauganash lay on the floor smiling like a baby in his sleep. . . .

When Grandfather awoke early the next morning . . . he looked around at us all, and he chuckled. Then he laughed... "Ho, ho, ho ... out like a light, eh Margaret?" I ask for forgiveness for doubting your word. I should have known better by this time.

— Keewaydinoquay Peschel

Several species, including *C. narcoticus, C. radicans,* and *C. niveus (Coprinopsis nivea),* are said to have psychoactive properties when eaten fresh. The latter is very white and grows on horse or cattle dung. It is quite beautiful.

Traditional Uses

In Sweden, smooth inky cap is applied to sores caused by burns.

In traditional Chinese medicine, the mushroom is used as an anti-inflammatory and applied externally to dermatitis, furuncles, and sores. It is considered cold and sweet, and taken internally for improving digestion and reducing phlegm.

The black ink has been used in the past for writing, and, when boiled with cloves or avens root, produces a good quality calligraphy ink. Iron filings are also used as a fixative for the ink.

Medicinal Use

Smooth inky caps' inhibition rate against sarcoma 180 and Ehrlich carcinoma is 100 percent. Studies have shown it contains high levels of ergosterols.

Studies have shown *C. plicatilis* has inhibition rates against sarcoma 180 of 100 percent, and against Ehrlich carcinoma of 90 percent (Ohtsuka et al. 1973).

It exhibits activity against *Bacillus cereus* and *B. subtilis* (Bianco and Giardino 1996).

Glistening inky caps have been shown in clinical trials to inhibit sarcoma 180 by 70 percent and Ehrlich carcinoma 80 percent (Ohtsuka et al. 1973).

Studies indicate that *C. micaceus* possesses antiviral properties when tested against poliomyelitis.

Work by researchers at the University of Winnipeg identified two natural compounds from this species on the prairies.

Micaceol, a sterol, shows antibacterial activity against *Corynebacterium xerosis* and *Staphylococcus aureus.*

The other compound, (Z,Z)-4-oxo-2, 5-hetpadienedioic acid exhibits inhibition of glutathione S-transferase.

Domestic inky cap is closely related to mica cap, and is found in the woods, gardens, parks, and even coal mines. It is characterized by a distinct orange, straw-like mycelium.

Clinical work shows that the mushroom has a large affinity for fibrin and can cause fibrinolysis. It appears to have a direct and stable effect, especially on fresh thrombosis.

The same researchers also found, in rat and guinea pig experiments, that *C. domesticus* reduced total cholesterol, increased HDL, and lowered LDL, in serum blood and liver.

Woolly ink cap is a non-poisonous but inedible mushroom that is quite short-lived. Early work found it active against sarcoma 180 and Ehrlich carcinoma with inhibition rates of 100 percent and 90 percent respectively (Ohtsuka et al. 1973).

Lagopodins A and B show activity against gram-positive bacteria (Bu'locn and Darbyshire 1976).

The mycelium has been shown to be active against both gram-positive and gram-negative bacteria.

The related magpie mushroom *(C. picaceus)* contains picacic acid with weak activity against *Staphylococcus aureus, S. typhi,* and *Streptococcus pyogenes.*

Coprinol, a cuparane isolated from the wood-loving *Coprinus* species, shows activity against grams positive bacteria strains, including penicillin-resistant *pneumococci,* methicillin- and quinolone-resistant *staphylococci,* vanomycin-resistant *enterococci,* and *staphylococci* (Johansson et al. 2001).

The related little helmet, *Coprinellus disseminatus,* inhibits proliferation and induces apoptosis in human cervical carcinoma cells by activation of caspase (Han, B. et al. 1999).

Early work showed inhibition of sarcoma 180 and Ehrlich carcinoma by 100 percent and 90 percent respectively. The mushroom does not deliquesce leading to the alternate name *Pseudocoprinus disseminatus.*

Fungi Essences

Cap essence is for those who doubt their own beliefs, need to express and communicate oneself. For fears and a need for extra emotional protection. It helps skin conditions, dermatitis and burns.

— Silvercord

Japanese umbrella essence will encourage self-control, promoting strength of convictions to become more disciplined and self-sufficient. For those sensitive to environment and to help boost the immune system.

—Silvercord

Mycoremediation

Several *Coprinus* species were investigated and evaluated as cost-effective alternatives to horseradish peroxidase for aqueous phenol treatment. Removal efficacy was similar, with a broader range of pH activity than other plant peroxidases. Ikehata et al. (2005) found that it may be useful in treating industrial wastewater.

Earlier work by this same team at the U. of Alberta found optimal glucose and peptide concentrations required for maximum peroxidase activity (Ikehata et al. 2004).

Personality Traits

Mushrooms have strange and unique qualities. Take the inky cap mushroom that grows in grass or on decaying wood. It is a charming little fungus with a gray-brown cap, resembling a partly closed umbrella. As the mushroom matures, the cap turns inky black, hence its name. But that's not the strange part.

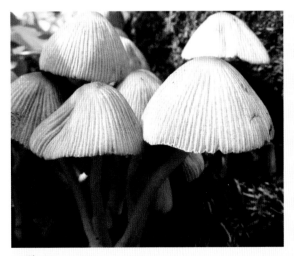

Coprinellus micaceus

The inky cap is an edible mushroom that is normally quite harmless—unless you make the mistake of drinking alcohol with it. Some species of this group contain the chemical coprine, which disrupts the normal metabolism of alcohol in your body, even up to several days after eating the mushrooms. The result can be a rapid buildup of toxins, producing stomach upset, facial flushing, nausea, heart palpitations, and other disturbances.

Unhealthy combinations are always best avoided—whether it be mushrooms and alcohol, or people and situations. For example, some personalities are better suited to certain kinds of livelihoods than others. The methodical, unhurried thinker should not pursue a fast-paced, on-the-edge career. Conversely, the high-energy, lightning-speed, problem-solver would shrivel in a sedate job. Your livelihood should not clash with your disposition. It's just not healthy.

— GINA MOHAMMED

Inky caps are pioneers, and are self destructive for the purpose of reproduction. They are fragile and short lived, yet pushy and pressing ahead. They pop up massively, seize control, overrun others and monopolize. They are the soldier among mushrooms; Attila the Hun.

— VERMEULEN

Fungal Signature

Disturbed ground, self-destruction, dissolution, perfect timing, delicate yet strong, soldier, intruder, control, suppression, benefit of cooperation, black.

— VERMEULEN

Coprinus comatus

(SHAGGY MANE)
(LAWYER'S WIG)
(INKY CAP)

One fine day, I spied, projecting from its lawn, what seemed to be the five fat fingers of a buried hand! Gloved, moreover, in shag! The fact that shag-gloved gestures from the grave came to mind rather than the immediate recognition of young shaggy mane mushrooms . . . indicates the extent of my then fashion orientation and the totality of my mycological ignorance. . . . On cutting them open in culinary preparation, I experienced an epiphany!

Never had I seen anything more beautiful, their baby gills were pink as a peony petal, lustrous as the interior of a shell, they demanded to be painted, not cooked! Later, on being refrigerated for further observation, these angelic apparitions vanished overnight, leaving behind nothing but blobs of black ink.

— WILLIAMSON

Coprinus is from the Greek *kopros,* meaning "dung." *Comatus* is from the Latin *coma,* meaning "shaggy" or "adorned with hair tufts." This is the fungi *candidi* of the Romans and *Velut apice Flaminis insignibus pediculis* of Pliny.

The Thompson of British Columbia named the mushroom "thunderstorm head," coming up in clumps after a heavy rain. Others believe the true thunderstorm head comes in spring, and may be *Tricholoma gambosum.*

Shaggy mane has long been a favorite of mushroom hunters throughout Europe and North America. It is easy to identify and difficult to confuse with anything poisonous. It

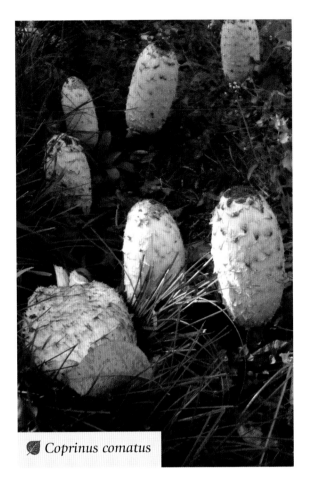

Coprinus comatus

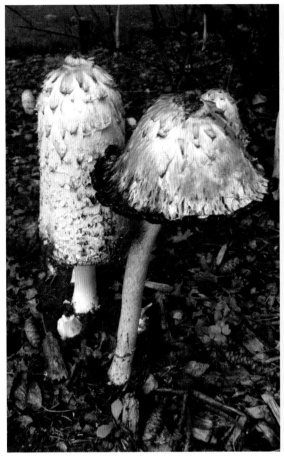

is able to push up through asphalt, which is amazing considering their fragile appearance. It often appears after disturbance, frequently found near highways. They are prolific spore producers. According to one expert, it can eject 1,660,000 spores a minute to a total of 5.25 billion spores before its life is over.

When young, this mushroom contains more than 25 percent protein, while later in life it turns inky black like its cousin. If the freshly picked mushrooms are quickly put in water, they will last several days.

The flavor is mild but delicious. When I lived on a hippie commune in the mid-1970s, this was my favorite omelet mushroom for fall, while the morel mushroom was for spring-time meals.

It has lots of flavor, due to presence of 3-octanone, 3-octanol, 1-octen-3-ol, 1-octanol, l-dodecanol, caprylic acid, as well as n-butyric and isobutyric acids.

It contains a lot of 1,3 beta-glucans, compared to eighteen other medicinal and culinary species.

Cultivation

In commercial cropping, it yields two to three pounds per square foot over the course of a month. Most, however, are picked wild. Shaggy mane is easy to clone and cultivate. Before it can be commercialized, it will be necessary to cultivate a spore-less strain. Maturing spores, as noted above, trigger deliquescence, or disintegration into a black, spore-enriched liquid.

Freeze-drying and nitrogen packing are two options that may lead to more commercial cultivation. It appears to grow better in soil rich in magnesium.

Medicinal Use

The Chinese know this mushroom as *maotouguisan* and use it to help improve digestion and treat hemorrhoids.

Inhibition of sarcoma 180 and Ehrlich carcinoma cancer cell lines is 100 percent and 90 percent respectively (Ohtsuka et al. 1973). Extracts from fresh specimens have been shown to have antibiotic properties.

Water extracts have been found to contain compounds that are active against breast cancer and it has been found to inhibit the growth of both ER+ and ER– breast cancer cells, inducing them both to die via apoptosis, and inhibit the formation of tumors in vitro (Gu and Leonard 2006).

Liping Wu et al. (2003) identified an alkaline protein, y3, that inhibits gastric cancer cell lines with an IC50 of twelve milligrams per milliliter.

Ethyl acetate extracts inhibit human ovarian cancer cell lines at low doses (Rouhana-Toubi et al. 2009).

Early studies indictate that *C. comatus* contains pronounced antifungal activity. Coprinin is a natural antibiotic, with activity against *Aspergillis niger, Candida albicans, E. coli, Pseu-domonas aeruginosa, Staphylococcus aureus,* and various *Bacillus* species.

Coprinol, obtained by fermentation process, has been found active against a variety of multi-drug-resistant gram-positive bacteria (Johansson et al. 2001).

Pseudomonas aeruginosa, for example, is responsible for minor irritations such as urinary tract and otitis externa infections, as well as more serious conditions associated with diabetic complications and progressive lung disease.

The bacteria are responsible for one in ten hospital-acquired infections, attacking those with already weakened immune systems. Paul H. McCay et al. (2010), professors at the National University of Ireland in Galway, performed a study in 2009 showing how the bug mutates and builds resistance to disinfectants such as BSK, or benzalkonium chloride, used in many cleaning products. The DNA-altered bacteria can withstand BSK up to four hundred times greater than non-mutated strains, and more worrisome is that they are up to ten times more resistant to ciprofloxacin, a front-line drug.

Cystic fibrosis patients have a thick mucus secretion that clogs the bronchial tubes and the passages of the pancreas and intestine. They are prone to this bacterial infection, as are diabetic patients with leg ulcers and burn victims.

Serum lysozyme activity is an indicator of immune strength as it breaks down polysaccharides on bacteria cell walls and binds to their surface, making it easier for white blood cells to ingest them. One study found polysaccharides from this mushroom increase serum lysozyme activity.

The bacterium *E. coli* has also developed multi-drug-resistant strains, causing urinary and bloodstream infections that are very difficult to treat.

Potron et al. (1956) found it to be one mushroom capable of lowering blood sugar levels in diabetics. *Amanita virosa and A. verna* were mentioned in same study but are highly toxic.

More recent work by Kronberger et al. (1964) has confirmed this property.

A more recent study by Bailey et al. (1984) reported lower blood glucose levels in mice after feeding dried powder of the fruiting body.

Fermented mushrooms rich in vanadium also inhibit high blood sugar (Han, C. et al. 2003). Further work found lower levels of blood glucose induced by adrenalin, lower levels of glycosylated hemoglobin, and even normal mice improved their tolerance to sugar. Lower doses of vanadium with mushroom extract significantly decreased blood glucose and glycosolated levels in diabetic mice (Han, C. et al. 2006).

Comatin improved glucose tolerance and lowered blood cholesterol and triglycerides in diabetic rats (Ding, Z. et al. 2010).

Ethanol extracts from this mushroom have been found to show anti-androgenic activity, selectively inhibiting LNCaP cell proliferation. This may lead to products useful for preventing or treating prostate enlargement or cancers (Zaidman and Mahajna 2005).

More recent work found ethanol and ethyl acetate extracts of both *C. comatus* and *Ganoderma lucidum* possess anti-androgenic activity with G1 phase arrest in androgenic dependent LNCaP cells, decreased levels of AR regulated PSA levels, and decrease in AR protein in both prostate and breast cancer cell lines (Zaidman et al. 2008).

Coprinus cinereus contains coprinastatin 1, found to inhibit growth of murine P388 lymphatic leukemia cell lines and the bacterium responsible for gonorrhea, *Neisseria gonorrheae* (Pettit et al. 2010).

Zenkova et al. (2003) looked at the antimicrobial activity of *Coprinus* species, including *C. comatus, C. micaceus,* and *C. radiatus.* There was variation in activity from species to species, as regards gram-positive and gram-negative bacteria, as well as Candida albicans.

Inhibition of sarcoma 180 is 70 percent and Ehrlich carcinoma is 80 percent for both *C. micaceus* and *C. radians.*

Inhibition rates for the related *C. plicatilis,* or pleated inky cap, are 100 percent and 90 percent respectively.

Early work by Hervey (1947) showed activity against *Staphylococcus aureus.*

The related *C. sterquilinus,* found on compost or dung, is used in traditional Chinese medicine to aid digestion and reduce phlegm. The dried powder is combined with vinegar into a paste for skin sores, boils, and other external application. Its inhibition rate against both sarcoma 180 and Ehrlich carcinoma is 60 percent.

Kyung-Ae Lee et al. (2005) found rats given carbon tetrachloride and an extract of *C. comatus* grown on brown rice showed diminished lipid degeneration and infiltration of local inflammation was alleviated, suggesting liver protecting mechanisms.

Submerged fermentation of mycelia gives a culture in five days, and subsequent purification yields polysaccharides.

Water extracts of mycelium show significant antioxidant activity at over 85 percent when using two milligrams per milliliter (Asatiani et al. 2007).

It contains ergothioneine, a substance with superior antioxidant activity (List et al. 1957; Badalyan et al. 2003).

Fungi Essences

Little inky cap *(Coprinus species)* is a little mushroom essence which helps letting go of emotions; when you feel vulnerable this essence will bring emotional strength and give universal trust. Little inky cap helps you rise above emotions and promotes the letting go of old anger and emotions quickly and easily.

— BLOESEM

Inky cap essence is for those who doubt their own beliefs, and need to express and communicate one self. For fears and need for extra emotional protection. Also for skin conditions, dermatitis, and burns.

— SILVERCORD

Inky cap *(C. comatus)* essence is for those who have any difficulty with any aspect of communication or who over do it.

— BRYNAHERB

Mycoremediation

The closely related *C. cinereus* contains an iron peroxidase. Dr. Joel Cherry, working at a Novo Nordisk Lab, in Davis, California, discovered that enzymes from this mushroom may be a solution to neutralizing white clothes that become tinted by others in a washing machine.

The enzyme catalyzes a peroxide reaction that removes the color from dyes. But it only works on dyes that have leached into the wash water; the fabrics themselves are left alone. That is, the color from an errant bright red sock would not harm the rest of the load.

His team has modified the enzyme to tolerate high temperatures and the alkaline and oxidative environment of detergents. Through random and directed mutation, this led to the creation of an enzyme with 174 times the thermal stability and one hundred times the oxidative stability of wild *Coprinus cinereus.*

Auer et al. (2005) found *C. cinereus* caused a 37 percent decrease of nitrocellulose in liquid cultures.

Peroxidase from *C. cinereus* is as effective at quenching free radical activity as lipoxidase from soybean (Budde et al. 2001). This may have application for the degradation of phenols.

The related *C. macrorhizus* contains peroxidase that can help remove phenols in continuous batch reactors (Al-Kassim et al. 1994).

The mushroom is a myco-accumulator of heavy metals including mercury by twenty-seven times, arsenic by twenty-one times, and cadmium by eight times, suggesting a big role in mycoremediation.

Insecticide

Like many other mushrooms, shaggy mane kills nematodes by producing penetration pegs with which hyphae colonize the bodies. Unlike oyster mushrooms that paralyze with toxic droplets, this fungus has an unusual spiny ball that helps kill, digest, and consume nematodes within a few days, with the hyphae growing out of the carcass (Luo, H. et al. 2004).

Coriolus versicolor

(see *Trametes versicolor*)

Cordyceps

Cordyceps militaris
(CATERPILLAR FUNGUS)
(TROOPING CORDYCEPS)
(SCARLET CATERPILLAR CLUB)
C. ophioglossoides
(ADDER'S TONGUE)
C. capitata
(TRUFFLE EATER)
(ROUND HEADED CORDYCEPS)
C. myrmecophila
(ANT FUNGUS)
C. canadensis
C. longisegmentis
(CANADIAN TRUFFLE EATER)
(CANADIAN ROUND HEADED
  CORDYCEPS)
C. sinensis
Sphaeria sinensis
Ophiocordyceps sinensis
(CHINESE CORDYCEPS)
(CHINESE CATERPILLAR FUNGUS)

The caterpillar fungus is a fascinating tale
Ingested by its host, the spores start to exhale
Control both direction and when it finally dies
Helps the fruiting body pop up between
  the eyes.
To some it seems incredible
That such a gruesome fate,
Can help improve your sex life
Immunity and weight.

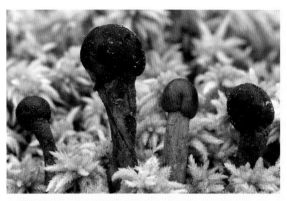

🍃 *Cordyceps capitata*

What existential twist can be so profound
As a moth consumed by mushrooms, instead of
  the other way around?
  —RDR

Cordyceps is from the Greek *kordyle* meaning "club" and *ceps* for "head." *Sinensis* means "from China" and *canadensis* means "from Canada." *Orphioglossoides* is from *ophi* meaning "snake" and *gloss* for "tongue." *Militaris* may relate to the growth pattern that looks like a regiment of toy soldiers.

Chinese caterpillar mushroom *(C. sinensis)* is known in Japan as *tochukaso*, in Tibet as *aweto*, and variously in Mandarin as *dong cao, chong cao,* or *dong chong xia cao*.

It is sometimes called "winter worm, summer grass" as the ancient Chinese believed this fungus to be a vegetable in summer and an animal in winter.

Cordyceps is the fruiting body of fungi parasitizing other fungi, such as the deer truffle *(Elaphomyces* spp.), or insects, such as caterpillars of moths, ants, and beetles. It grows inside the caterpillars and other insects to produce

115

hyphae. When they die, the fungus produces a fruiting body that sporulates into the wind to infect another generation. According to Bryce Kendrick, a single stroma will produce an estimated sixty-four million spores. And so it goes!

One ant fungus (*C. curculionum*) begins as a spore that attaches to its host, germinates, and then begins to feed on the inside. The ant goes about normal activity until one day it suddenly decides to climb to the top of a tree. It reaches a desired height and then chomps down on a leaf and remains there until it dies, releasing spores from the forest canopy.

With the exception of the Chinese species, the others listed may be found throughout North America. None of them are common, or at least they are not frequently identified by the amateur mycologist.

Cordyceps sinensis is the most well known, but the genus can claim several other medicinal stars. It parasitizes the larvae of a bat moth.

It is estimated that over 680 varieties of *Cordyceps* have been discovered and named, and more than thirty are common in alpine terrain.

I lived in Peru in the early 1980s and recently read that two hundred fifty new species of *Cordyceps* discovered there have yet to even be named!

The growth of the fungus on insects lead to the early belief in Tibet that it imparted immortality, with stone effigies placed in burial grounds with the dead.

The high mountain grasses of Tibet and Nepal are used for springtime grazing of domestic yaks. They dig their hoofs into the recently frozen soil and dig up *Cordyceps*. Soon after, the rutting season begins. This was observed by astute herdsmen who tried the mushroom themselves and passed the information on to monks. The Mykot of the region still make a yak yogurt by soaking the dried *Cordyceps* in milk overnight.

In ancient times, its use was restricted to the Emperor's Palace, and baked in duck as a tonic similar to Ginseng. It sold at one time for four times its weight in silver. Today, you will pay considerably more for good quality wild-crafted product!

It has a spicy, cinnamon fragrance that lends itself to soups and broths.

Cultivation

Although the use of wild fungi for medicinal purposes is appealing, the fermentation of mycelium on wheat and other grains produces a safer and more consistent product. Various studies indicate similar antioxidant properties between wild and cultivated strains. Another advantage of the fermented product is that it is 100 percent vegetarian. Various substrates have been used including wheat, rice, sorghum, and even organic purple corn.

Phillip Cleaver et al. (2005) isolated a new *C. sinensis* anamorph with potential to improve cultivated lines.

Aloha Medicinals produce 175,000 kilograms per month of cultured *Cordyceps* that are bio-identical, and perhaps superior in activity to those found in the wild.

Traditional Uses

Adder's tongue is mild, slightly acrid, and used in traditional Chinese medicine as a lung and

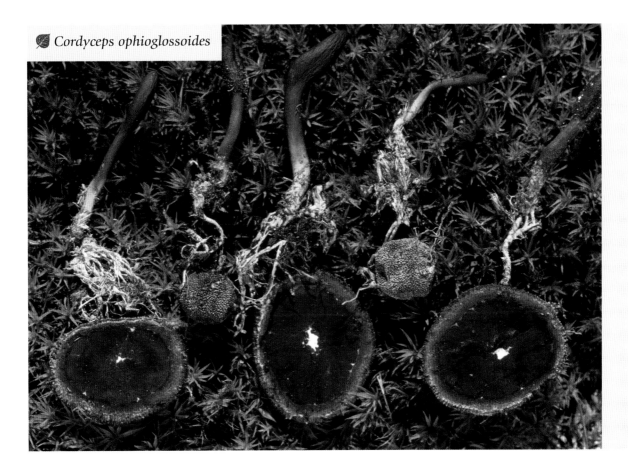

Cordyceps ophioglossoides

kidney tonic. It increases production of red blood cells, increases sperm production, and strengthens *qi*. It was traditionally stuffed into a duck after boiling the cleaned animal in hot water. This makes a pleasant and sweet broth that helps alleviate colds, coughs, anemia, and joint pain. The related *C. sinensis* is used in a similar manner.

It regulates menstruation, and is used to treat metrorrhagia, in-between-period bleeding, as well as abnormal or excessive bleeding associated with perimenopause or fibroids.

It combines well with Garden Burnet *(Sanquisorba officinalis)* root for menorrhagia and irregular menstrual cycles. This is probably due to two compounds isolated from the mycelium that possess estrogenic activity (Kawagishi et al. 2004b).

In Japan, the species *C. sabolitera,* known as *semitake,* is used both to treat postpartum exhaustion and as an antibiotic.

Chinese caterpillar mushroom *(C. sinensis)* has been used as an aphrodisiac for nearly two thousand years, with the first written record in the Classic *Herbal of the Divine Plowman* from 200 AD.

Cordyceps strengthen both the mind and body at a very basic level, replenishing *yin jing* and restoring the deep energy depleted by excessive stress.

It is mainly a restorative to the lungs and a metabolic enhancer and balancer to the entire hypothalmic pituitary adrenal axis.

In traditional Chinese medicine, the mushroom is used for fatigue, wheezing, shallow breathing, and loss of stamina associated with kidney and lung *yang* deficiency.

The lungs rule *qi* and the flow of air, so nose and throat disorders are helped by *Cordyceps*. The kidneys store *jing,* the source of regeneration in the body.

Because it tonifies both *yin* and *yang,* it can be used safely in nearly any endocrine condition to help relieve fatigue and calm the nervous system. To be more exact, *Cordyceps* is both *yin*-nourishing and *yang*-invigorating.

Medicinal Use

Chemical Constituents

- *C. sinensis:* **various sterols, polysaccharides, galactomannans, cordycepic acid 7 percent, 25 percent protein, adenine, adenosine, uridine, uracil, cordycepin, mannitol 9.5 percent, eighteen amino acids, ergosterol, vitamin B12, trace elements, and saturated and unsaturated fatty acids.**

- *C. ophioglossoides:* **ophiocordin and three galactosaminoglycans.**

- *Mycelium:* **ethyl (E)-8-oxo-9-oactadecenoate and 4-(2-hydroxyethyl) phenol.**

- *C. militaris:* **cordycepin, ergosterol, beta sitosterol, adenosine, adenine, and D-mannitol.**

- *C. capitata:* **indole alkaloids.**

In 1996, *Cordyceps subsessilus* was discovered to be the anamorph of *Tolyopcladium inflatum,* the white mold used for the blueprint of cyclosporine. Cyclosporine A is used to prevent the rejection of organ transplants as well as to treat severe urticaria, diabetes, and angioedema. *Cordyceps subsessilus* is found in Europe and North America but is somewhat rare. It parasitizes scarab beetle larvae.

Adder's tongue contains amino acids that regulate moisture to the surface of the skin. The compound ophiocordin possesses antiphlogistic and antibacterial properties, and the polysaccharide CO-1 stimulates peripheral blood flow.

Adder's tongue contains ophiocordin, with antibiotic properties (Furuya et al. 1983). This compound possesses antifungal activity, and is immune-stimulating and anti-fighting in animal trials (Kneifel et al. 1977). Activation of macrophages appears to be part of the picture.

It contains CO-N, SN-C and CO-1, three compounds that possess antitumor activity (Ohmori et al. 1988a, 1988b, 1989).

CO-N, for example, is a water-insoluble glycan that is highly active against sarcoma 180, showing inhibition of 98.7 percent. SN-C shows a broader range of activity against tumors than isolates from shiitake (lentinan) or *Trametes versicolor* (PSK). SN-C is cytotoxic and immune-stimulating.

CO-1 is the primary polysaccharide in SN-C and is very similar to lentinan in structure. It is not soluble in water but reacts favorably in citric, acetic (vinegar), or lactic acid. This compound shows strong inhibition of sarcoma 180 (Yamada et al. 1984).

C. militaris contains cordycepin that shows reverse transcriptase inhibition (Penman et al. 1970). According to Christopher Hobbs, in his inspiring book *Medicinal Mushrooms*, cordycepin (3'-deoxyadenosine) was dropped as a clinical isolate for cancer due to its toxic side effects.

Hui Mei Yu et al. (2006) compared the oxidative damage protection of *C. militaris* and *C. sinensis*. The content of adenosine and cordycepin is higher in the former and both show antioxidant protection.

Guoking Zhang et al. (2006) found *C. militaris* more hypoglycemic in activity than in *C. sinensis.* Rukachaisirikul et al. (2004) identified cordycepin, pyridine-2,6-dicarboxylic acid, and cepharsparoides C, E, and F in this species.

Work by Wen-Hung Lin et al. (2007) on sub-fertile boars found both the quality and quantity of sperm increased by supplementation with *C. militaris* powder.

Water extracts of *C. militaris* have been found to induce apoptosis and growth inhibition of U937 leukemia cells. The regulation of several major growth gene products such as Bcl-2 family expression and caspase protease activity suggests therapeutic potential for human leukemia (Park, C. et al. 2005).

The fungi induced IL-18 and acted on IFN-y production (Kim, C. S. et al. 2008).

Cordycepin suppresses TNF-alpha gene expression, 1kBalpha phosphorylation and nuclear translocation of p65. It also decreases the expression of COX-2 and iNOS due to the down regulation of NFkappaB activation, Ak1 and p38 phosphorylation (Kim, H. G. et al. 2006).

At low doses, cordycepin inhibits the growth and division of cancer cells, while at high doses

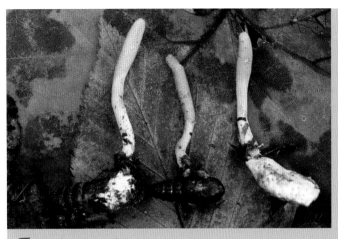

🍂 *Cordyceps militaris*

it stops cells from sticking together. The effects on translation and mTOR are similar to Metformin, and as an inhibitor of Akt and activation of AMPK, cordycepin may be useful in type 2 diabetes, inflammatory conditions, and as a putative cancer drug.

Extracts of *C. militaris* have been found to exhibit anti-angiogenetic properties and repress growth of B16-F10 melanoma cells in mice compared to controls (Yoo et al. 2004).

Haemi Lee et al. (2006) found a hot-water extract of *C. militaris* inhibited cancer cell proliferation by inducing cell apoptosis through the activation of caspase-3, and that the extract may have potential in human leukemia.

A polysaccharide isolated from culture, CPS-1 has been shown to possess significant anti-inflammatory activity and suppressed the humoral immunity in mice, but no significant effect on cellular and non-specific immunity has been found (Yu, R. et al. 2004).

Cordlan, a polysaccharide isolated from this species, increases dendritic cell maturation through TLR4-signaling pathways (Kim, H. S. et al. 2010).

This species induces apoptosis of lung carcinoma cells A549 via diminished telomerase activity (Park, S. E. et al. 2009).

It appears to up-regulate the dopaminergic system and may provide neuroprotection (Sapkota et al. 2010).

Cordycepin can be produced in large amounts in a two-stage process in bioreactors. Work by Xian-Bing Mao and Jian-Jiang Zhong (2004) gives great direction for further commercialization.

Ji et al. (2010) identified anti-aging potential.

Siu et al. (2004) found immune-potentiating effect from an increase in interleukin 11 production, as well stimulation of myocardial ATP generation and enhancement in mitochondrial electron transport. It is rare to find this combination.

X. X. Lin et al. (2001) found fermented Cordyceps powder may be useful for the prevention and cure of asthma.

It is relaxing and restoring to the nervous system, especially when associated with irritability, anxiety, and hypertension.

As an adrenal restorative, it helps premature aging, menopause, impotence, chronic kidney conditions, and seminal incontinence with spermatorrhea. It reduces blood cholesterol and is hemostatic, when needed. Kidneys control the bones and health of bone marrow, according to traditional Chinese medicine.

Xia Zhang et al. (2004) found Cordyceps sinensis inhibits liver cirrhosis induced in rats. It decreased damage to hepatocytes by CCl4 and inhibited hepatic fibrosis. Six weeks after drug administration, the activity of hepatic insulinase began decreasing, but Cordyceps could not inhibit the decrease of activity of hepatic insulinase.

It appears that Cordyceps boosts depressed immune system function, but does not stimulate normal functioning systems. As with many immune stimulants, it is immuno-suppressive in large amounts in a manner comparable to cyclosporine.

As mentioned above, cyclosporine A was derived from an anamorph of Cordyceps species. Although it helps save lives, the drug possesses kidney toxicity. In one small study of seven kidney transplant patients taking azathipirine, cyclosporine, and prednisone, Cordyceps was substituted for the first drug and showed equal results with no inhibition of leukocytes. A larger study on cyclosporine at Nanfang Hospital and Taizhou Medical School in China involving thirty-nine control patients and thirty taking Cordyceps showed reduced kidney toxicity in the latter group.

Cordyceps stimulates in vivo corticosterone production in mice, but does not show constant stimulatory or inhibitory effects on the weights of the body and adrenal glands (Leu et al. 2005).

Lupus nephritis, resulting from an autoimmune condition, responds favorably to a combination of Cordyceps powder before meals and artemisinin after meals. The combination has been shown to prevent recurrence of Lupus nephritis and protect kidney function in a five-year study (Lu, L. 2002). The treatment was markedly effective in 83.9 percent, effective in 12.99 percent, and ineffective in only 3.2 percent of the thirty-one treated patients.

Jiun-Lang Chen et al. (2009) found benefit treating lupus in mice studies.

It shows antitumor activity against lung cancer in humans.

The mycelium increases production of 17 beta-estradiol, due, at least in part, to increased StAR and aromatase expression. This suggests a role for *Cordyceps* in fertility issues where the quality of maturing oocytes is of concern (Huang, B.-M. et al. 2004). It is not recommended during pregnancy or breastfeeding.

In one clinical study of breast and lung cancer patients, the mushroom helped restore immune function (Zhou, D. H. and L. Z. Lin 1995).

Breast tissue cells have an average lifespan of ten days, and then they divide and form new cells. Breast cancer cells divide every twenty minutes, or seven hundred fifty times faster. Cordycepin, if equally toxic to both, would kill off cancer cells seven hundred fifty times more quickly, but cordycepin does not interfere with healthy cell replication and thus only attacks abnormal cells.

On the other hand, water extracts induced apoptosis of B16 melanoma cells in vitro. When combined with methotrexate in vivo, it appeared to extend survival time, and may be of benefit as an adjuvant therapy in the prevention of tumor metastasis in cancer chemotherapy (Nakamura et al. 2003).

Additional work by Jian Yong Wu et al. (2007) found *Cordyceps* mycelium inhibits a variety of cancer cells in culture and B16 melanoma in mice, with a 60 percent decrease in twenty-seven days.

Yu-Jen Chen et al. (1997) found *Cordyceps* inhibits the proliferation of human leukemia cells. This may be due to targeting of terminal deoxynucleotidyl transferase positive cells, and enhanced in the presence of an adenosine deaminase inhibitor (Kodama, E. N. et al. 2000).

Mice inoculated with sarcoma 180 tumor cells, showed significant increases in life span and decreases in tumor weights and volumes when administered ethanol extracts of the fungus (Shin, K. H. et al. 2003).

The mechanism is not exactly known, as compounds other than cordycepin and polysaccharides exhibit tumor inhibition (Kuo, Y.-C. et al. 1994). Earlier work by the author found water extracts of the mycelium doubled production of macrophages.

An exopolysaccharide extract was shown to exhibit immune modulation and antitumor activity by Weiyun Zhang (2005). Metastasis to lungs and liver was significantly inhibited, and levels of Bcl-2 decreased.

The same researchers later found exopolysaccharides significantly elevate immunocyte activity in tumor-bearing mice (Zhang, W. et al. 2008).

Water extracts modulate immune parameters through immunoglobulin production; this results from decreased T lymphocyte helper 2 cytokine secretion and reduced cytokine secretion in mesenteric lymph node lymphocytes (Park, D. K. et al. 2008).

Cordycepin, found in water extracts, was tested on mice inoculated with B16 melanoma cells. Taken orally for two weeks, the compound reduced the primary tumor lump by 36

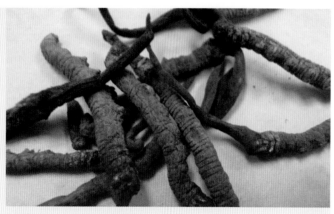

Ophiocordyceps sinensis

percent compared to control mice (Yoshikawa, N. et al. 2004).

Cordycepin (3'-deoxyadenosine) is nearly identical to adenosine except it is lacking an oxygen on the ribose part of the molecule at the three position. This may be important, as the structure of DNA depends upon oxygen to bond adjacent nucleosides between the three and five positions, helping form the ladder of DNA.

When a cell divides, the first step is separation of DNA molecules and insertion on new complement nucleosides, which form hydrogen bonds. The original strand of DNA is copied twice, each a genetic code for new cells. When cordycepin is available, there is no oxygen available to form the three-to-five bond and replication stops. This is not critical to healthy cells as they have an inherent repair mechanism, but cancer cells have lost their self-repair mechanism and cannot duplicate. Many bacteria and viruses also lack this self-repair mechanism.

Cordyceps shows both in vitro and in vivo stimulation of testosterone levels in lab studies (Hsu, C.-C. et al. 2003). This is no great surprise, as athletes taking *Cordyceps* extract shattered nine world records at the Chinese National Games in 1993. In the ten thousand meter run, for example, the world record was broken by forty-two seconds (Steinkraus and Whitfield 1994).

The potential for helping insufficient testosterone production in the aging male should not be ignored. One clinical study on sexual dysfunction in men showed a 64 percent improvement (in 183 of 286 patients) after ingesting one gram three times per day for forty days. Although not as quick-acting as elk antler, it gives long-term restoration in cases of impotence, frigidity, and sexual malaise. Mark Plotkin, noted ethnobotanist, calls it "fungal Viagra."

It could be useful for patients recovering from operations, or following a debilitating illness. It is frequently recommended to patients suffering fibromyalgia or exhaustion from Lyme disease.

A study by Hiyoshi et al. (1996) looked at the effect on long-distance runners. Significant improvement was found in 71 percent of runners, due to increased respiratory effect and removal of lactic acid. *Cordyceps* helps restore skeletal structure, and is useful in treating pain in the lower back, knees, and ankles.

Yue et al. (2008) found both *C. sinensis* and *C. militaris* may affect the anion movement from the basolateral to apical compartments in lung epithelia. This could have some significance in cystic fibrosis, if my science is up to snuff.

Cordyceps increases ATP (adenosine triphosphate) levels by nearly 28 percent. Imagine giving your body 28 percent more energy supply, as ATP is required for nearly all enzyme systems.

Cholesterol levels are also reduced. Yamaguchi et al. (2000) found inhibition of cholesterol deposition in the aorta of the heart by inhibiting LDL oxidation. Other work shows that water extracts dilate the aorta by 40 percent under stress, suggesting a possible mechanism for athletes (Naoki et al. 1994).

In another study, heart disease patients were given three grams of *Cordyceps* daily for twelve weeks. Blood viscosity dropped, as did blood cholesterol, by 21 percent.

In a large two-month trial of 273 patients receiving one gram three times per day, cholesterol levels dropped an average of 17 percent.

More than 80 percent of patients taking fifteen hundred milligrams of cordyceps daily for two weeks showed improvement in ventricular arrhythmia. Other studies appear to confirm this benefit, which seems to improve with continuity of supplementation.

Alcohol extracts appear to show activity against Coxsackie virus B3 associated with viral myocarditis. Induction of IFN gamma and regulation of T-lymphocytes are involved.

In patients aged sixty to eighty-four years, a placebo-controlled trial found levels of SOD (superoxide dismutase) rose to levels usually associated with people aged seventeen to twenty-one years.

In a clinical study of 256 patients with chronic viral hepatitis, the mushroom helped 80 percent. It is believed that 350 million peo-ple suffer from this disease worldwide, with a million dying each year. In another study, eighty-three virus-carrying but symptom-free patients aged two to fifteen years were given *Cordyceps* for three months, after which thirty-three showing the virus were no longer contagious. This is highly significant as 95 percent of infected newborns become chronic carriers, and in children under the age of six, about 30 percent become chronic.

A study of thirty-two hepatitis B patients given 3,750 milligrams per day for thirty days showed liver function improvement in twenty-three patients. Another study of twenty-two patients with post-hepatitis cirrhosis found that by giving six to nine grams daily for three months, all of the patients' symptoms improved. Cirrhotic cells disappeared in fifteen patients and decreased significantly in another six.

It helps prevent kidney disease in elderly patients, by ameliorating aminoglycoside toxicity (Li, L. S. et al. 1996).

Cordyceps may be useful in the regulation of blood sugar levels. In a clinical trial of forty-two diabetic patients, half received an herbal formula including cordyceps, and half just the herbs. Fifty-five percent of the patients in the latter group showed improvement of blood sugar levels after thirty days, while 95 percent of those taking the formula including the mushroom showed improvement. This may be due to CS-F30, a polysaccharide composed of galactose, glucose, and mannose.

Recent work evaluated the efficacy of *Cordyceps sinensis,* combined with low doses of cyclosporine A, on long-term treatment of kidney transplant patients. The combination had less complications with significantly lower serum levels of the drugs.

Rat trials found fruiting bodies attenuated diabetes-induced weight loss, polydipsia, and hyperglycemia (Lo, H.-C. et al. 2004).

In vitro tests show inhibition of *Streptococcus, Bacterium mallei, Bacillus anthracis, Pasteurella suiseptica,* and *Staphylococcus* species, as well as *Microsporum gypseum* and *M. lanosum.*

The related *C. brunnearubra* contains cordyformamide, a compound with activity against the life form associated with malaria (Isaka et al. 2007).

Work by Dong and Yao (2005) gives some excellent suggestions for submerged culture in mass production.

A strain of *C. sinensis* shows a new degradation pathway for dioxins (Nakamiya et al. 2005).

A thorough review of medicinal uses of *C. militaris* has recently been published (Das 2010).

Fungi Essence

Cordyceps essence strengthens and heals the second chakra. It also assists the kidneys. Its effect is very deep as it helps eliminate the emotional poisons that have gotten a foothold in our body.

— Korte Phi

Agriculture

Chickens fed *Cordyceps* have been shown to produce eggs containing cordycepin, which has proven medicinal benefits. Collaboration in Singapore between Chew's Agriculture and AP Nutripharm led to this idea, while seeking alternatives to antibiotics in animal feed.

The eggs are 30 percent lower in cholesterol and have a sweeter yolk than those from chickens not fed the mushrooms. They also sell for twice the regular price, another example of innovative functional food.

Cosmetics

Cosmetic applications that cool and sooth, such as refreshing facial lotions, moisturizing creams, and after-bath skin-care products come to mind.

Recipes and Dosage

Powder: two grams two to three times per day.

Tincture: make at a one-to-five ratio and 40 percent alcohol. Ten to fifteen drops two to three times per day.

Do not use during fever. Combining with vitamin C is said to improve its benefit. Much of the *Cordyceps* used today is grown as fermentation cultured mycelium.

Cortinarius sanguineus

(BLOOD RED CORTINARIUS)
C. cinnamoneus
(YELLOW CORTINARIUS)
C. collinitus
C. muscigenus
(MOSS CORTINARIUS)
(BELTED SLIMY CORT)
C. violaceus
(PURPLE CORT)
C. purpurascens
Phlagmacium purpurascens
(PURPLE STAINING CORT)

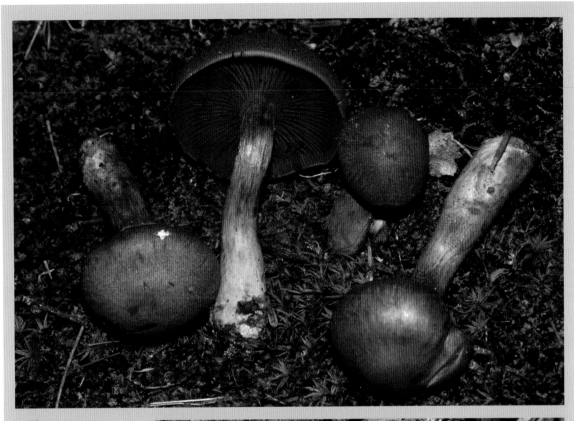

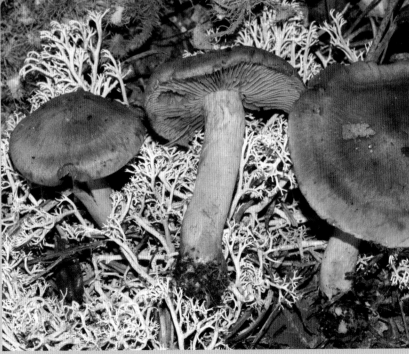

Above: *Cortinarius sanguineus*. Below: *Cortinarius huronensis*.

C. flexipes
C. paleaceus
(PIXIE WEBCAP)
(PELARGONIUM WEBCAP)
C. brunneus
(BROWN CORT)
C. infractus
(SOOTY OLIVE CORT)
C. huronensis var. huronensis
(HURON CORT)

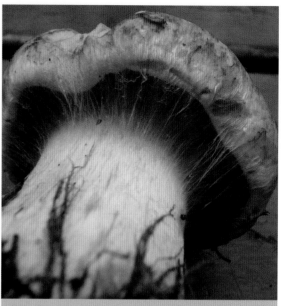

Note the *cortina,* or "little curtain," which identifies the Cortinarius genus.

Cortinarius means "a cobwebbed veil." This is a major identifier of this huge genus.

Sanguineus means "bloody" or "red," while *purpurascens* means "purple." *Collinitus* means "viscous" or "sticky." It may be from *collino* meaning "to besmear."

Blood red *Cortinarius* is a common mushroom found growing in groups among forest moss. It is edible despite a bright red color. Purple *Cortinarius* is also edible, although of poor quality. The yellow is not really recommended for eating, but it is not at all poisonous.

Purple staining *Cortinarius* is often found growing among willow and poplar with wet feet. It has a pleasant sweet, cocoa-like, and fruity odor that has scored high on organoleptic tests for pleasant scents. It has no great texture or taste, but is edible.

Purple cort has a cedarwood-like smell that is most attractive, but the taste is insipid.

C. collinitus is widespread and common, with rusty patches on the base and a slimy texture. It is edible.

Pixie webcap is found in mossy bogs under spruce. It has a distinct geranium-like scent.

Sooty olive *Cortinarius (C. infractus),* from the West coast, is bitter and not considered a choice edible.

The related *C. suaveolens* is an aromatic fungi discovered in the woods of Fontainebleau. It has a strong odor of orange blossom that remains while the fruiting body is fresh.

Brown corts *(C. brunneus)* are red-brown, sometimes with blue tones, common to Sitka spruce forests of the Pacific Northwest.

Many members of this family are deadly poisonous. Be very careful with identification as many contain orellanin, which destroys both liver and kidneys.

An outbreak of poisoning from consuming *C. orellanus* occurred in Poland in 1952. Several people died died, 11 percent of 132 poisonings. The toxin responsible was never identified, but it was probably orellanine, which is toxic to the kidneys. Symptoms are delayed from three to fourteen days.

Michael Beug is head of the NAMA committee recording poisonings. In nearly forty years, he has not encountered significant poisoning from the more than eight hundred *Cortinarius* species in North America. Still, be careful.

Medicinal Use

Chemical Constituents

- *C. sanguineus*: **dermocybin, dermoglaucin, physicon, emodin, and four anthraquinone carboxylic acids.**

Brown corts contain brunneins A-C, with the former a low cholinesterase inhibitor with no cytotoxicity (Teichert et al. 2007).

C. sanguineus has shown inhibition rates against both Ehrlich and sarcoma tumors of 60 percent, while the Purple cort shows 100 percent inhibition. The yellow cort shows an inhibition rate against sarcoma 180 of 80 percent and against Ehrlich carcinoma of 90 percent.

C. collinitus has a rate of inhibition against sarcoma 180 of 80 percent, and against Ehrlich carcinoma of 90 percent. *C. elatior* has rates of inhibition of 70 and 80 percent respectively and *C. turmalis,* 70 and 60 percent. *C. latus* shows 100 percent inhibition for both, *C. salor* 80 and 90 percent respectively, and *C. hemitrichus* 80 and 70 percent respectively.

Purple *Cortinarius* shows 100 percent inhibition of the two cancer cell lines above.

Early work by Ohtsuka et al. (1973) found pixie webcap inhibits sarcoma 180 by 80 percent and Ehrlich carcinoma cells by 70 percent.

Sooty olive *Cortinarius (C. infractus)* contains infractine (beta carboline, 1-proponic acid methyl ester), and eudistomin M, which requires further study. It contains infractine (above), 6-hydroxyinfractine, and infractopicrine, responsible for the bitter taste. These compounds have a chemical structure similar to harmaline, which is an MAO inhibitor, suggesting some hallucinogenic effect, but toxic compounds similar to orellanine are present in small amounts, suggesting it is better to pass it by.

Infractopicrin and 10-hydroxyinfractopicrin inhibit acetylcholinesterase with higher selectivity than galanthamine found in snowdrop (Geissler et al. 2010).

Cortinarius umidicola contains rare C_{17}-phytosphingosine and cerebroside B and D, and again, more research would be welcomed.

Bitter *Cortinarius (C. vibratilis)* contains vibratilicin with a glycerol and hydroxyamic acid moiety. It is a derivative of neoengleromycin from the fungus *Engleromyces goetzii* (Liu, Yu et al. 2002).

Various constituents from *Cortinarius* species exhibit anti-malarial effect. Phlegmacin B1, rufoolivacin, and other isolates show effect against *Plasmodium falciparum* in vitro (Francois et al. 1999).

Cortamidine oxide has been isolated from *Cortinarius* species and exhibits both antimicrobial and cytotoxic activity. It is an asymmetrical disulphide metabolite (Nicholas et al. 2001).

Caesium and aluminum are accumulated by various *Cortinarius* species.

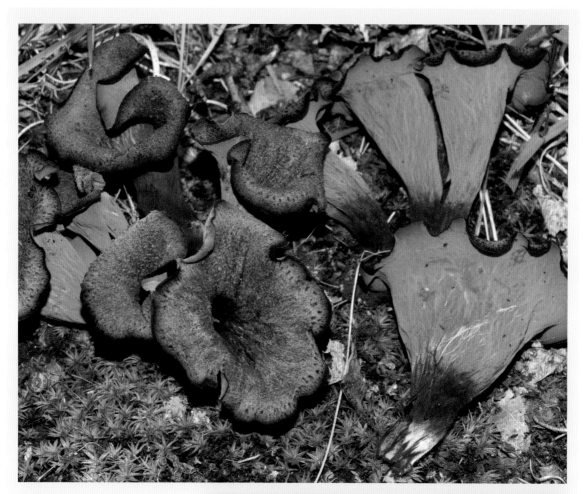

🍂 Above and right:
Craterellus cornucopioides.
Below: *Craterellus fallax.*

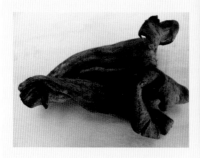

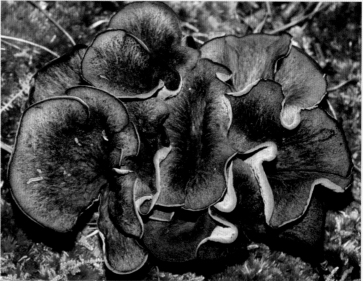

Craterellus

C. cornucopioides
(HORN OF PLENTY)
(FALSE TRUFFLE)
C. fallax
(DECEPTIVE HORN)
(BLACK TRUMPET)
C. tubaeformis (see *Cantharellus*)

Craterellus is Latin for "a small mixing cup." *Cornucopioides,* of course, is from *cornucopia,* "the horn of plenty." *Fallax* is Latin meaning "deceptive." Recent DNA suggests these may be the same mushroom despite slightly different looks and spore print colors.

False truffle refers to using specks of the dark mushrooms in dishes to resemble the real, and very expensive, true truffle.

The horn of plenty is named because of its shape. In France it is often called the *trompet de mort* or "trumpet of death," unusual considering it is an excellent, edible mushroom. Delicatessens in that country may advertise "truffled" cooked meats actually stuffed with horn of plenty.

It is smoky brown on top, with a brownish-purple stem. It has a buttery, woodsy flavor when fresh, and when dried and reconstituted, produces a dark, rich liquid that is perfect for fish sauces. A crock pot of pork and Jerusalem artichokes with a puree of green olives is enriched with this reconstituted sauce.

It is good in egg dishes and pâté, and may be best when simmered in cream.

David Spahr suggests combining it with "foods associated with white wine, such as sea-food, chicken, veal, pork, rice, pasta, cheese, and certain sauces."

When dried, it is more than 50 percent protein (Colak et al. 2009).

Medicinal Use

Investigation by Gruter et al. (1990) has shown that ethanol extracts of this mushroom are anti-mutagenic in vitro. The interesting part is that the activity is heat stable. The agent appears to inhibit the development of tumors provoked by aflatoxins and benzopyrene.

The fruiting bodies inhibit sarcoma 180 and Ehrlich carcinoma by 60 and 70 percent respectively (Ohtsuka et al. 1973).

Tryptophol esters are compounds related to plant hormones and formed in large amounts in this fungus. These are suitable for transport through lipid membranes and storage in lipophilic cell compartments (Magnus et al. 1989). Interesting!

Fungi Essence

Mushroom essence integrates us with our shadow side, grounds us, and releases hidden blockages. Intensely connects us with the Earth, with our darker, deep and physical nature. Through this funnel the Earth inhales and exhales. This essence raises our energies up from a purely physical level through an "in and out" movement similar to breathing. It stimulates the first (root) chakra, liberating our vital life energies.

— KORTE PHI

Mycoremediation

Horn of plenty produces a number of hydrolytic enzymes with commercial application. Work by Goud et al. (2009) found protease, amylase, phytase, carboxyl esterase, and lipase activity. In their study of fifty basidiomycetes for production of enzymes, only four were positive for all five enzymes. More research is needed.

Creolophus cirrhatus

Hydnum cirrhatum
(SPINE FACE)

This relatively rare hardwood stump bracket fungus has rather long spines under its cap.

Work in France found fermentations from the fruiting body produced five new norhirsutanes with fourteen carbon atoms (hirsutanes have fifteen). Creolophins A-E and known complicatic acid were found.

Creolophin E and its dimmer neocreolophin show antibacterial and cytotoxic activity (Opatz et al. 2007; Birnbacher et al. 2008).

Crepidotus mollis

(SOFT CREPIDOTUS)
(SOFT SLIPPER TOADSTOOL)

Crepidotus is Greek meaning "base like an ear" or "shaped like a crepe/pancake." *Mollis* is Latin for "soft."

Soft *Crepidotus* is a small, inconspicuous recycler of wood.

Medicinal Use

Chemical Constituents

■ **CPS (beta-glucan).**

Early work by Ohtsuka et al. (1973) identified three *Crepitodotus* species active against sarcoma 180 from 60 to 100 percent and against Ehrlich carcinoma from 90 to 100 percent.

Even earlier work by Hervey (1947) found activity against both *E. coli* and *Staphylococcus aureus.*

Cryptoporus volvatus

Polyporus volvatus
(POUCH FUNGUS)
(CONCEALED POLYPORUS)

Crytoporous is from the Greek *krypto* meaning "hidden" or "concealed." *Volvatus* means "possessing a volva."

This interesting mushroom has an annual, leathery, pouch-like structure about four-by-five centimeters in size. They are found by the hundreds on spruce and fir, usually the year after the death of the host due to fire or old age.

In Tibet, the polypore is known as *songganian.*

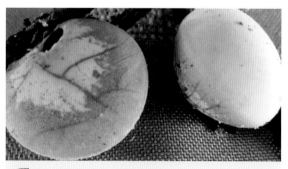

🍃 *Cryptoporus volvatus*

Traditional Uses

The pouch fungus is white to yellowish-brown with age. The whole fruiting body is very fragrant when sucked on, after starting out with a bitter taste. For sore throat, five to eight pieces previously simmered in water are held in the mouth without chewing (Zang et al. 1984).

It is used in traditional Chinese medicine to stop bleeding in the intestines; to treat hemorrhoids, carbuncles, furuncles, and toothaches; and, decocted, as an anti-inflammatory for asthma and bronchial conditions.

Mothers give small ones to their infants to be used like pacifiers as an aid in weaning.

Medicinal Use

They contain various constituents of interest, including ergosta-7,22-dien-3b-ol and fungisterol.

The branched 1,3 beta D glucans from the fruiting bodies were investigated by Kitamura et al. (1994) and showed antitumor activity against sarcoma 180 cancer cell lines.

S. H. Jin et al. (2003) found the polypore capable of leukotriene production.

Cryptoporic acid E, a sesquiterpenoid isolated from the fungus, was shown to inhibit colon cancer development in rat and mice studies (Narisawa et al. 1992).

The sesquiterpenoid cryptoporic acids A-G inhibit tumor promotion, due to their strong free radical scavenging activity (Hashimoto and Asakawa 1998).

G. Ren et al. (2006) found ether and ethyl acetate extracts exhibit cytotoxic effects against human cervix and hepatoma cell lines.

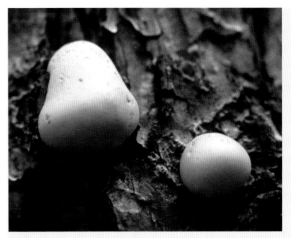

Cryptoporus volvatus

Qiang-Min Xie et al. (2006) found polysaccharides from water extracts useful in allergic rhinitis and to inhibit eotaxin in mRNA expression.

Work has been continuing on this interesting fungus. S. H. Jin et al. (2003) found inhibition of leukotriene B4 suggesting use in reducing inflammation in asthma conditions.

Xiao-Yan Zhao et al. (2004) found *Cryptoporus* polysaccharides protect the lungs in guinea pig studies. Inhibition of airway constriction, eosinophil release and chemotaxis were all noted, suggesting a novel anti-inflammatory agent for treating asthma and allergic conditions.

A U.S. patent has been filed for the use of fruiting body cryptoporic acids for antifungal activity against *Candida albicans*, *Cryptococcus neoformans*, and *Aspergillus* species.

Another patent, granted to Guo et al. in 2004, is for a fermentation technique for a product that prevents and treats irritability diseases, including allergic rhinitis, bronchial asthma, allergic gastroenteritis, and ophthalmology concerns related to pollen and such.

This follows work by Asakawa et al. (1992) on cryptoporic acids.

Work by Hua et al. (1991) at Zhejiang Medical University shows that commercial culture mediums require a carbon to nitrogen ratio of twenty to twenty-five, an optimal pH of 5.5 to 6.5, and a temperature of twenty-five to thirty degrees Celsius.

Cosmetics

Hang Zhao and Wenquan Liang (2004) looked at the best method to extract oil from *C. volvatus*. Soaking the fungus for one hour, and decocting for eight hours in ten times the amount of water was simple and easy. The oil simply floats to the top. This may be an interesting odor for perfume work.

Crucibulum laeve

(WHITE EGG BIRD'S NEST)
C. vulgare
(YELLOW BIRD'S NEST)

Crucibulum means "lamp" and *laevis* means "light" or "soft." This genus is part of the Nidulariaceae, or Bird's Nests, and closely related to *Cyathus* below.

This fungus can be found far north into the Arctic.

Medicinal Use

A fermentation broth of *Crucibulum* species yields a range of salfredins, which possess aldose reductase inhibition. Further research may identify a role in eye health, including prevention of glaucoma or cataract formation associated with blood sugar regulation.

Cyathus striatus

Nidularia striata
Peziza striata
(RIBBED SPLASHCUP)
(STRIATE BIRD'S NEST)
(FLUTED BIRD'S NEST)
C. stercoreus
N. stercoreus
(DUNG LOVING BIRD'S NEST)
Nidula candida
(JELLIED BIRD'S NEST)

As the name suggests, this brown mushroom is shaped like a bird's nest. It is found in rotten wood on the grounds of birch and poplar forests during summer and fall. *Cyathus* means "cup" and *striatus* means "ribbed" or "fluted."

The related dung loving bird's nest, *C. stercoreus,* is ground up in water, filtered, and used as eye drops for conjunctivitis, redness, and swelling. It is also used to stop stomachache, by decocting nine to sixteen grams of powder with boiling water.

It is a very interesting looking mushroom, woolly on the outside, and containing small round blue-black flat and smooth "eggs."

Medicinal Use

Ribbed splashcup is used to treat gastralgia in China.

Ribbed splashcup contains cyathin, a compound that significantly inhibits *Staphylococcus aureus.*

Early work by Anke and Oberwinkler (1977) isolated striatins isolated from the mycelium showing activity against both gram-negative and gram-positive bacteria. Studies indicate *C. striatus* possesses antibiotic activity against both *Bacillus cereus* and *B. subtilis.*

Diterpenes with a cyathane skeleton are typical for this species (Ayer and Taube 1973).

Recent work by Petrova et al. (2007) identified significant inhibitory effect on NFkappaB, a protein complex that regulates the immune system. In some forms of cancer, including MCF7 breast cancer lines, this pathway is always turned on with significant damage and cells running wild.

Twelve different *Cyathus* species were tested for antimicrobial and antifungal activity. Inhibition of human pathogenic fungi including *Aspergillus fumigatus, Candida albicans,* and *Cryptococcus neoformans* was noted (Liu, Y.-J. and K.-Q. Zhang 2004).

Striatins A and B show in vitro activity against *Leishmania* species and *Trypanosoma cruzi* at very low doses. In vivo studies on mice suggest striatin A may have some application in *L. amazonensis* with a decrease in parasite burden only 25 percent of that of the reference drug, N-methylglucamine antimonite (Inchausti et al. 1997).

Dung loving bird's nest contains cyanthusals A-C and pulvinatol, both of which possess antioxidant activity (Kang, H.-S. et al. 2007).

Jellied bird's nest contains nidulal and niduloic acid that possess antibiotic and cytotoxic activity. The former compound induces differentiation of leukemia cells (Erkel et al. 1996).

Mycoremediation

This same species showed a three- to five-fold improvement in enzymatic cellulose digestibility of corn stover after pretreatment (Keller, F. A. et al. 2003). Earlier work studied the production of ligninolytic enzymes and synthetic lignin mineralization relevant to myco-pulping and myco-bleaching methods.

C. stercoreus was found to be the quickest of four species to degrade and detoxify TNT.

Bits and Pieces

The related *N. niveo-tomentosa,* common to the Pacific Northwest, produces raspberry lactones in submerged culture (Böker et al. 2001). Production increases in presence of UV-A light (Taupp et al. 2008). Clouds of raspberry lactones have been found in Saggitarius B, near the center of the Milky Way. Is it really an aromatic universe?

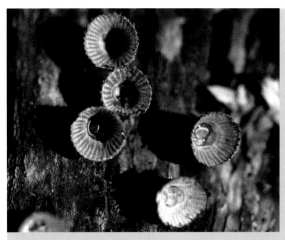

Cyathus striatus

133

Daedaleopsis confragosa

Daedalea confragosa
Trametes confragosa
Daedalea confragosa
Cellularia cookii
Lenzites cookii
Ischnoderma confragosum
(THIN WALLED MAZE POLYPORE)
(BLUSHING BRACKET)

Daedaleopsis is derived from Daedalea, of Greek mythology.

The common name comes from the maze-like (Daedaloid) pattern of the pores, which range from round to elongated.

Thin walled maze polypore is found mainly on willow. It likes birch but is rarely found on conifers.

The closely related thick walled maze polypore *(Daedalea quercina)* emits an apple-like fragrance. This may be due in part to carboxyacetylquercinic acid. Found on hardwoods like oak, it was used for tinder, and sometimes used to rub down horses in the manner of a currycomb, and by humans to brush hair.

The related *D. biennis,* also known as *Heteroporus biennis, Abortiporus biennis,* and *Polyporus biennis,* is found under oak and sometimes pine trees. David Arora calls it an "unimposing, profoundly forgettable, pitiful excuse for a polypore."

Culture and Folklore

Daedalus was a member of the Athenian royal household and renowned craftsman, painter, and inventor. Daedalus attempted to kill his nephew, Pedrix, who had invented the saw, by throwing him over a cliff, but the gods changed Pedrix into a partridge. Daedalus fled to Crete, where he entered the service of King Minos and his queen Pasiphae. She ordered him to build a life sized, hollow heifer in which she could hide to have sex with a bull. As a result, she conceived and gave birth to Minotaur, half man and half bull. The outraged Minos ordered Daedalus to construct a Labyrinth to hold the creature prisoner. Later, Daedalus gave King Minos' daughter Ariadne a ball of twine so that the hero Theseus could navigate the labyrinth and slay the minotaur. Minos became so upset that he locked Daedalus in the labyrinth maze with his young son Icarus. To escape, Daedalus made two pairs of wings from wax and feathers, warning Icarus not to fly too close to the sun or his wings would melt. He didn't listen, of course, and fell to his death. Daedalus made his way to Sicily, where he lived out his years. Probably eating mushrooms.

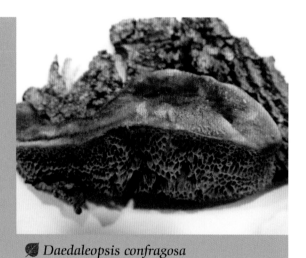
Daedaleopsis confragosa

134

Medicinal Use

Chemical Constituents

- **3alpha carboxy-acetoxy-quercinic acid, 3 alpha carboxyacetoxy-24-methy-lene-23-oxolanost-8-en-2 6-oic acid, 5alpha,8alpha epidioxyergosta-6,22-dien-3beta ol; various sterols and fatty acids.**

Its close relative *D. flavida* (snuff fungus) has been used in India for the treatment of jaundice. Some five grams of the dried powder are snorted throughout the day for three days, dramatically reducing bilirubin and other enzymes indicative of jaundice. If the condition is chronic, a repeat three-day treatment follows after a two-day break.

Melzig et al. (1996) screened thin walled polypore, as well as *P. betulinus, G. applanatum, H. annosum,* and *Fomitopsis pinicola* for pain-relieving compounds. All showed inhibition of neutral endopeptidase (enkephalinase) with IC 50 values between forty and fifty-five micrograms. It is believed that selective inhibitors of this metallo-endopeptidase may be useful in the treatment of pain in a manner similar to opioids.

The related *D. tricolor* shows tumor inhibition (Ikekawa et al. 1969). An extract of the cultured mycelium shows 90 percent inhibition of sarcoma 180 cancer in mice.

The dry, fruiting body contains 20(29)-lupen-3-one. E. M. Kim et al. (2001) showed the compound to possess antibacterial activity against *E. coli, Proteus vulgaris, Pseudomonas pyocyanea, Bacillus subtilis,* and *Staphylococcus aureus.* It possesses antioxidant activity similar to alpha tocopherol.

The conk shows inhibition of ACE or angiotensin converting enzyme and neutral endopeptidase, suggesting pain relief and blood pressure regulation (Melzig et al. 1996).

Hervey (1947) found activity against both *E. coli* and *Staphylococcus aureus.*

The related *D. heteromorpha* and *D. juniperina* showed activity against both bacteria in same journal (Robbins et al. 1945).

Gregory et al. (1966) found inhibition of sarcoma 180 cancer cell lines.

The related *D. gibbosa* mycelium has selective anti-proliferative and apoptosis inducing activity against K562 cells line, a lab model for human chronic myelogenous leukemia. An active fraction, F6 inhibits kinase activity of native and T3151 mutated Bcr-Abl, suggesting great potential in cancer therapeutics (Yassin et al. 2008).

Bits and Pieces

Seven-thousand-year-old fragments of this polypore were found in ruins of ancient Rome (Bernicchia et al. 2006).

Mycoremediation

Sasek et al. (1998) identified the fungus as a myco-degrader and decolorizer of synthetic dyes.

Daldinia concentrica

(CARBON BALLS)
(KING ALFRED'S CAKES)
(CRAMP BALLS)

Daldinia is Greek meaning "round charcoal." *Concentrica* means "concentric" or "round," from the Latin.

King Alfred's cakes are named for their resemblance to cakes burned by King Alfred. You probably had to be there to get the joke.

Cramp ball is related to the ancient belief that carrying them helps ward off cramps.

Carbon balls are hard, small balls that grow in groups on the stumps of deciduous trees or in the wounds of living poplar, birch, and alders of Alberta's Parkland region.

When young, they are reddish brown, later turning shiny and black. When ripe, the fungi release up to two billion spores from ten o'clock in the evening to five o'clock in the morning, peaking at eleven o'clock in the evening. Even under laboratory-controlled conditions, this timed pattern does not change.

Traditional Uses

Carbon ball can be dried and ground into a powder for relieving cramps.

In India, the mushroom is called *kala pihiri,* meaning "black mushroom." It is used for chronic coughs, by taking the dried fruit bodies and a piece of old earthen vessel and powdering separately. This is then mixed with equal parts of honey and given at a dose of one teaspoon twice daily.

The Igbo of Nigeria use this fungus for medicinal purpose. In that country, eight to twelve different mushrooms are consumed, with over one-third of the population using some mushrooms for medicinal purposes.

The fungus is used in Chinese medicine for treating cramps and other spasmodic conditions.

Medicinal Use

Chemical Constituents

- **5-hydroxy-2-methyl chromone; 2-6-dihydroxybutyrophenone; 2,6-dihydroacetophenone; 4, 9, di-hydroxyperylene-3-10 quionone; 8-methoxy-1-naphthol di-methoxy naphthalene; 4,5,4',5'-tetra hydroxydi-naphthyl; 5-hydroxy-2-methyl chroma-none; at least seventeen 10-phenyl (11)-cytochalasans; 1,8-dihydroxy-naphthalene; concentricolide, friedelin, ccytochalasin L-696,474, armillaramide, russulamide; two aromatic steroids with unusual methyl group positions; daldinone A and B; daldiniapyrone; daldinialanone, (+) orthosporin; curuilignan D; concentricols B-D (squalene type triterpenoids); phenochalasin B; 3.4.5-trihydroxy-1-tetralone; and (22E)-cholesta-4,6,8(14),22-tetraen-3-one.**

Concentricolide inhibits HIV-1-induced cytopathic effect with an EC_{50} value of 0.31 micrograms per milliliter, and therapeutic index of 247. The compound exhibited blockage on syncytium formation between HIV-1-infected and normal cells (Qin et al. 2006).

Cytochalasins are a group of fungal secondary metabolites with a wide range of biological activity. They are best known for their various effects on mammalian cells. The most unusual of their properties is their ability to cause cells

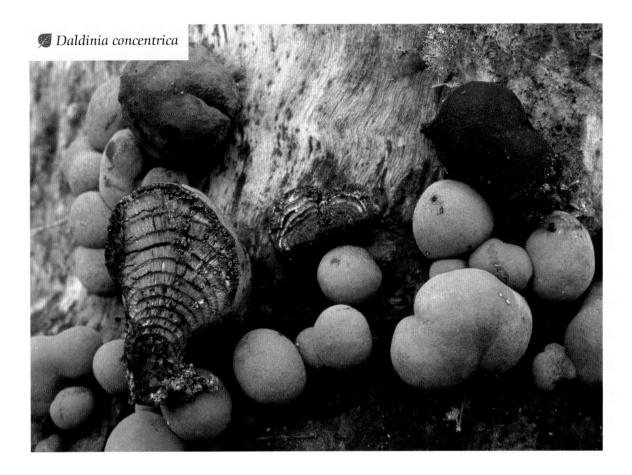

Daldinia concentrica

to extrude their nuclei, leading to the formation of nuclei-free cells. At low concentrations they interfere with cell division by preventing cytoplasmic division, leading to binuclear or polynuclear cells. They also inhibit cell movement.

A recent study found an extract of the fruiting body induces estrogen-like effects on ER positive cell lines, but has no influence on ER negative or androgen cells (Benie et al. 2008).

Work by Qin and Liu (2004) suggests the aromatic steroids could be the long-sought biological precursor steroids for organic matter in Earth's subsurface.

Buchanan et al. (1995, 1996a, 1996b) identified seventeen new cytochalasins.

Inhibition against *Bacillus cereus, E. coli,* and *S. aureus,* and to a lesser extent, *Klebsiella pneumoniae* and *Proteus vulgaris,* was found (Gbolagade and Fasidi 2005).

Anke et al. (1995) identified two naphthalenes derived from the melanin biosynthetic pathway in this fungus.

The related *D. childiae* contains daldinal B that inhibits iNOS mRNA synthesis (Quang et al. 2006).

Other Uses

Cramp balls have been used as a smoldering fruit body to smoke and calm bees, in the manner of puffballs.

137

Echinodontium tinctorium

(INDIAN PAINT FUNGUS)
(TOOTHED CONK)

Indian paint fungus is common in the Pacific Northwest, associated with balsam fir, douglas fir, and western hemlock.

It looks like a conk, but has long teeth on the underside. The bright reddish-orange flesh is distinctive, and was used at one time as a red dye. The common name is related to the use of this dye for ceremonial and war paint.

Traditional Uses

The Eastern Cree call it *meah kis igum*. They used the dried fungus as a styptic and the moistened powder as a poultice. When steeped, the powdered fungus was used as an emetic.

It was widely used by First Nations of British Columbia, mainly for face paint or tattoos as well as to protect the skin from insects and

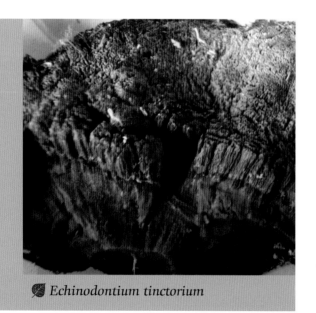

Echinodontium tinctorium

sunburn. The Thompson called it "owl wood of hemlock." They combined the dried powdered fungus with deer grease and then subjected this to heat.

It was often applied under the eyes, like bloodroot, to reduce chances of snow blindness during the bright winter days. The paint was prepared by heating the fungus over a fire and adding the crushed powder to melted fat.

Some First Nations people, including the Kwakwaka'wakw, mixed the red powder with western hemlock gum resin for face paint. They produced paint by placing the fungi on hot rocks, which were then covered with lady fern and left until a red powder appeared.

Medicinal Use

It contains echinodol. Echinolactones (Illudalane sesquiterpenoids) have been isolated from the related *E. japonicum*.

Ohtsuka et al. (1973) identified two *Echinodontium* species with activity against sarcoma 180 of 70 to 90 percent and against Ehrlich carcinoma of 60 to 80 percent.

Hervey (1947) showed activity against *Staphylococcus aureus*.

Textile Industry

It is used in fungal dyes and pigments. Miriam Rice and Dorothy Beebee have published a book on using mushrooms for dyes, pigments, and paper. One unusual application to this beautiful art is Myco-stix™, which combines the pigment with beeswax or *Pseudohydum gelatinosum* as a binder.

Elaphomyces granulatus
(COMMON DEER TRUFFLE)

This is a small, rarely found mushroom, and yet it is very common. It grows underground, near conifers.

It is sometimes parasitized by species of *Cordyceps,* which will help the mushroom seeker find where it grows. It is not edible. See *Cordyceps.*

Alexander Smith called it the most common underground fungus in North America. It was associated with the witches of Germany and Austria, and believed to derive from sorceress' spit, giving rise to the popular name of witches' saliva, or *hexenpizet.*

Medicinal Use

Dr. King, one of the great Eclectic physicians of the nineteenth century, recommended the fungi for its stimulating effects.

Stanikunaite et al. (2007) looked at this species and various *Rhizopogon* species for antioxidant, anti-inflammatory, anticancer, and anti-tuberculin activity.

Mycoremediation

This fungus concentrates cesium at 25,600 becquerels per kilogram. This suggests a use in monitoring nuclear plants or cleaning up contaminated sites.

Bits and Pieces

Resembling an earthball, it was said to have arisen from the spilled semen of copulating deer. Deer truffle was formerly regarded, therefore, as an aphrodisiac, and known as *fungi cervini.* It was used in the preparation of love potions according to J. Bauhin's *Historia 1651.*

Entoloma abortivum

Fibropilus abortivus
Clitopilus abortivus
Rhodophyllus abortivus
(ABORTED ENTOLOMA)
E. nitidum
(STEEL BLUE ENTOLOMA)

Aborted *Entoloma* is a pink-spored edible mushroom that is both widespread and common. *Entoloma* is Greek for "inrolled margin," one of the identifying markers. Many of the genus are poisonous, but this one is not!

The fungus attacks Armillaria species, causing them to look like fur-covered balls. Early books had it the other way around, but we now know that *Entoloma* is the attacker. Tom Volk, renowned mycologist, suggests they should be called aborted *Armillaria*. This fungi represents a potential myco-control of the destructive honey mushroom (Czederpiltz et al. 2001).

They possess a nutty flavor that is best brought out by sautéing. Do not eat the gilled versions, as they may be poisonous.

Medicinal Use

The inhibition rate of aborted *Entoloma* against sarcoma 180 and Ehrlich carcinoma is 90 percent.

The related but poisonous *E. clypeatum (R. clypeatus)* and *E. lividum (E. sinuatum)* show

139

inhibition of 100 percent against various cancer cell lines.

The rare alpine species *E. nitidum* shows activity against sarcoma 180 and Ehrlich carcinoma cancer cells lines by 60 percent and 70 percent respectively (Ohtsuka et al. 1973).

Favolus alveolaris

Polyporus mori
P. alveolaris
(SMALL BRACKET POLYPORE)
(HEXAGON PORED POLYPORE)
F. apiahynus
P. brumalis
(WINTER POLYPORE)

Small bracket polypore is a soft-fleshed mushroom growing on dead broadleaf trees, east of the Rockies. It smells of apricots and has unusual comb-like or diamond-shaped spore openings. The conk was formerly used in Italy for dyeing various fabrics and, depending upon the strength and length of submersion, various shades of yellow green such as *jaune chamois* and *jonquille* were obtained.

Medicinal Use

The mushroom has been shown in both ethanol and hot-water extracts to inhibit the growth of sarcoma 180 cancer cell lines by up to 71.9 percent (Ohtsuka et al. 1973).

The cultured mycelium inhibited sarcoma 180 cancer cell lines by 90 percent in early studies.

Other Uses

Winter polypore has been used in a number of experiments to determine the effects of zero gravity on fungal growth (Kasatkina et al. 1980).

Fistulina hepatica

(BEEFSTEAK FUNGUS)
(POOR MAN'S BEEFSTEAK)
(THE JELLY TONGUE)

Before reclassification by Linnaeus, this mushroom was known as *fungus cariaceus quercinus haematodes*. *Hepatica* refers to the shape, and texture that resembles the liver. *Fistulina* may be from the Old or Middle English *fyst* meaning "fist" and, in turn, from the Greek *faust* or *fust* meaning "five," as in "five clenched fingers," and hence little fist. Some authors believe it means "a pipe." *Hepatica* is Greek for "resembling the liver."

Beefsteak is named for its texture and oozing red juice. It is a delicious, but strong, sour edible that initially appears to be a polypore on oak and other hardwoods. It does have dis-

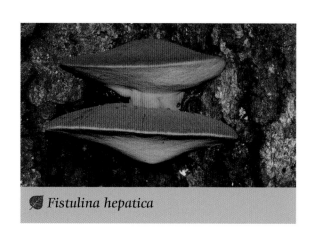

Fistulina hepatica

tinct tubes and is rarely attacked by insects.

The dark discoloration it gives to wood, known as brown oak, is prized by cabinet-makers for furniture.

It is a prized edible when young. It can be sliced and eaten raw in salads, and when cooked begins to resemble liver, hence the common name.

Most mushrooms, like meat, are deficient in vitamin C. This particular fungi, however, contains up to a hundred and fifty milligrams of ascorbic acid per hundred grams—or about five times our daily requirement. This is the source of the sourness. David Arora mentions that he likes to marinate thin raw slices in vinegar and olive oil. It is presently being explored for commercial production in China.

In ancient Ireland, it was laid on old indolent skin ulcers to promote healing.

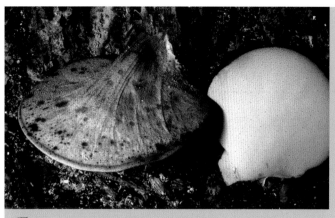

Fistulina hepatica

Medicinal Use

A gray-white powder may be made from a hot-water extract with a melting point of 230 to 260 degrees Celsius. It contains gelatose, xylose, and arabinose. The water extract exhibits inhibition of sarcoma 180 by 95 percent and Ehrlich carcinoma by 90 percent (Kameda et al. 1978).

Cinnatriacetins A and B are two antibacterial triacetylene derivatives identified in the fungus. Coletto et al. (1981) found the mycelium active against *E. coli, Staphylococcus aureus,* and *Bacillus subtilis.*

The fruiting body also showed some inhibition of *S. aureus* in early studies (Robbins et al. 1945).

Coletto et al. (1992) found activity against *Klebsiella pneumoniae.*

Farrell et al. (1973) found a natural acetylene with antibacterial activity similar to cephalosporin C against *S. aureus,* and *Salmonella typhi.*

The fungus contains 49.7 percent ellagic acid of the five phenolic compounds identified, and nearly 58 percent malic acid of the six organic acids (Ribeiro et al. 2007). Strong antioxidant activity and xanthine oxidase inhibition, as well as weak protective effect against hypochlorous acid were also found. Inhibition of xanthine oxidase suggests that it may be useful in treating gout and gouty arthritis.

Essential Oil

This mushroom contains a number of volatile compounds that contribute to its flavor and sweet, wildflower scent. These include 1-octen-3-one, 1-octen-3-ol, linalool, phenyl-acetaldehyde, butanoic acid, (E)-2-methyl-2-butenoic acid, (E)-methyl cinnamate, (Z)-9-hexadecenoic acid, methyl ester, bisabolol oxide B, phenylacetic acid (Wu, S. et al. 2005b).

141

Flammulina velutipes

Collybia velutipes
(VELVET FOOT)
(VELVET STEM)
(FURRY FOOT COLLYBIA)
(WINTER MUSHROOM)
(ENOKI)

Flammulina is derived from the Latin *flammeus* for "a small flame," referring to the yellowish-orange to reddish-orange color of the cap. Velutipes is the conjuction of two Latin words: *velutinus,* meaning "covered with fine hairs," and the noun *pes,* or "foot," hence "velvet foot."

Enokitake is Japanese for "the snow peak mushroom," while the enoki tree is the Chinese hackberry tree on which the wild mushroom grows. In Thailand, it is called the golden mushroom, and in Germany, *Samtfußrübling,* due to its brown, furry stem.

There is some controversy over whether this mushroom is the same as the famous enokitake mushroom of Japan. Both have yellow-brown caps with rusty-brown velvety stems. They grow all summer in clusters on buried roots and rotting poplar logs. They are edible and delicious. The closely related *F. fennae* or *F. populicola* may be our North American species.

In Japan, a tender white cultivated version called *enoki* is readily available in North American supermarkets. Two of the popular commercial strains in Japan are maruei and ebios. These are widely available and add a flavor reminiscent of white pepper and lemon to salads or light soup broths. They are good in fish dishes, stir-fries, or as a stuffing for chicken, when finely chopped and combined with summer savory. My local Chinese hot pot restaurant serves them with beef, ginger, and green onion. This dish is one of my favorite winter lunches.

Cultivation

The small cap and long stem of commercial strains are achieved by elevating carbon dioxide levels and limiting light levels. White fir wood that has been sterilized is a good medium, according to Paul Stamets. The mushroom can withstand cold temperatures and may have a role in mycoremediation of areas with repeated freezing. It is circumpolar in distribution. Wheat bran added to sawdust medium caused increased biological efficiency and quicker spawn running than control (Sharma et al. 2008).

Medicinal Use

Chemical Constituents

- **Valine, lysine, and various polysaccharides including PA3DE. Also contains ergosta-5,8,22-trien-3-beta-ol; enokipodins A-D, and FIP-fve, cerevisterol, and its 22(23)-dihydroxy derivative, flammulin, and tetraol. They contain 31 percent crude protein, various B vitamins, and vitamin C. Niacin content is 107 milligrams per hundred grams of dry weight.**

- **Mycelium: fermented ergosterol, ergosta-3-0-glucopyranoside, ergosta-7,22-dien-5,5-epoxy-3-ol, 5-alpha-stigmastan-3,6-dione, (24R)-stigmast-4-ene-3-one, genistein, adenosine, and cinnamic acid.**

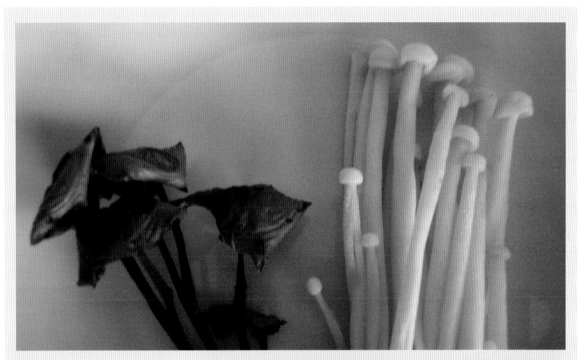

Above: Dried *Flammulina populicola* (left) and commercial enoki (right). Below left: *Flammulina velutipes*. Below right: *Flammulina populicola*.

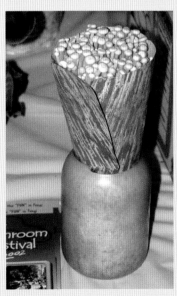

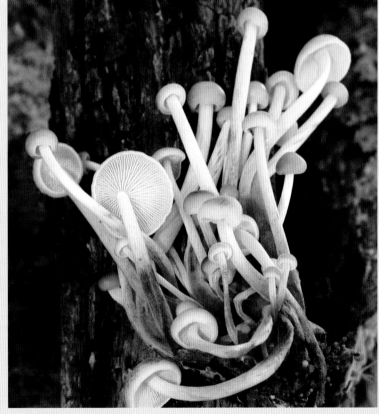

The polysaccharide PA3DE from velvet foot has a molecular weight of 5.4 times ten to the sixth. It contains D-glucose, D-mannose, and L-fucose in the molar ratio of 22.31:1; 46:1; and had beta-glycosidic linkage; a new antitumor glyco-protein proflamin, fucose, and arabinose.

Taken on a regular basis, it is said to cure stomach ulcers and liver disease.

An epidemiological study in Japan, found that enoki growers near the city of Nagano had unusually low cancer rates. Frequent consumption was considered to be the main difference.

The raw mushroom contains a cardiotoxin protein (flammutoxin) that is destroyed when heated to one hundred degrees Celsius for twenty minutes. This same protein has been shown to cause swelling and respiratory inhibition of Ehrlich ascites tumor cells.

In 1968, Ikekawa et al. reported that the mushroom's extracts possess anticancer activity. Earlier work by Komatsu et al. (1963) first identified flammulin and its antitumor activity.

Flammulin, a water-soluble polysaccharide, has been shown to be 80 to 100 percent effective against sarcoma 180 and Ehrlich carcinoma.

A recent study, conducted at Tokyo Pharmacology Institute, on guinea pigs given 30 milligrams daily, found a prevention rate of sarcoma 180 of 81.1 percent.

More recent work from Korea by D. H. Kim et al. (1996) confirms traditional use of this mushroom for ulcers. In studies involving *Helicobacter pylori,* the fungus was found to inhibit the HP urease. Nitric oxide synthase was identified (Song, N.-K. et al. 2000).

Mannick et al. (1996) found *H. pylori* expressed NOS immunoreactivity that was inducible in vivo and in vitro from duodenal ulcer patients. This may also be part of the connection. It has also been determined that the polysaccharides promoted the transformation of lymphocytes.

A new fungal immunomodulatory protein, FIP-fve has been isolated from *F. velutipes* (Ko, J.-L. et al. 1995). It consists of 114 amino acid residues with an acetylated amino acid end that lacks methionine, with half cystine and histidine residues.

The protein is able to hemagglutinate human red blood cells. The immunomodulatory activity of FIP-fve was demonstrated by its stimulatory activity toward human peripheral blood lymphocytes and its suppression of systemic anaphylaxis reactions and local swelling of mouse footpads. FIP-fve was found to enhance the transcriptional expression of interleukin-2 and interferon-gamma.

The protein shows activity against HeLa cervical cancer cell lines (Lee, S. L. et al. 2010).

Ng et al. (2006) found hemagglutinin inhibits the proliferation of leukemia L1210 cells.

Velutin is a ribosome inactivating protein that inhibits HIV-1 reverse transcriptase (Wang, H. and T. B. Ng 2001).

One study found that mycelia reduced the total cholesterol, increased HDL and reduced LDL in experiments on rats and guinea pigs.

Enoki contains a polysaccharide called EA3 and a second of higher molecular weight called EA501, which do not directly affect cancer tumors, but appear to support the immune system in a manner not fully understood.

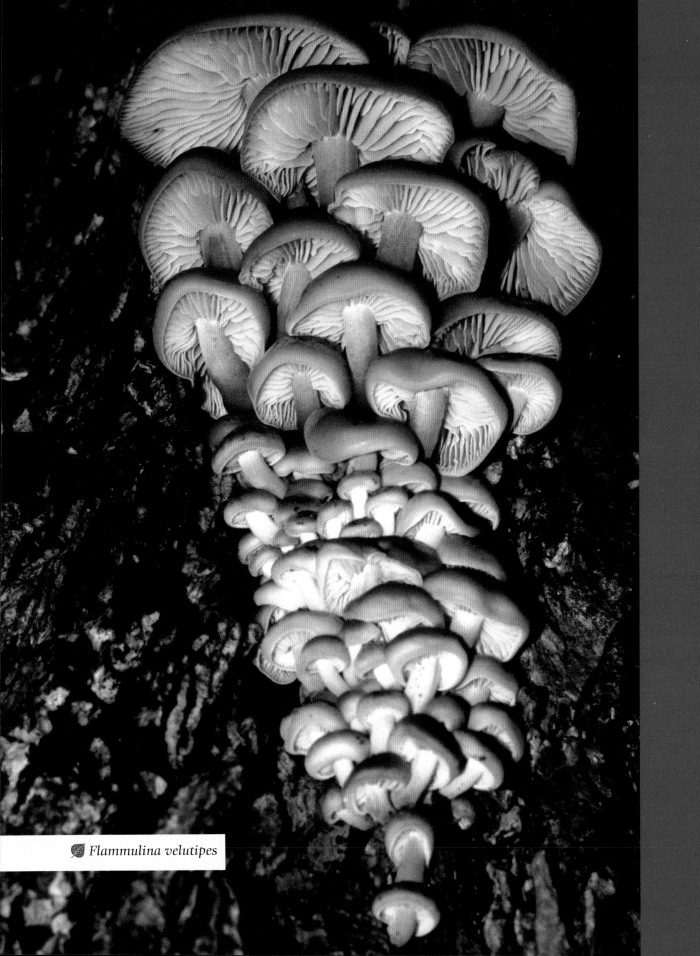

Flammulina velutipes

Another protein-bound polysaccharide, EA6, was studied by Maruyama and Ikekawa (2005). They found that administered alone, the EA6 exhibited inhibitory effect on Meth-A fibrosarcoma tumor cells in combination with surgical excision, in a manner mediated by CD4 positive T-cells. Oral administration also increased the lifespan of mice with Lewis lung carcinoma and B-16 melanoma.

Enokipodins A-D have been found active against *Bacillus subtilis* and *Staphylococcus aureus;* and antifungal against *Cladosporium herbarum* (Ishikawa et al. 2001).

Paul Stamets, in *Mycelium Running,* suggests it exhibits activity against prostate cancer.

Proflamin, a glycoprotein produced from cultured medium, is 90 percent protein and 10 percent saccharide. It shows activity against allogeneic and syngeneic tumors.

Po-Hui Wang et al. (2004) isolated an immune modulating protein similar in structure to human immunoglobulin. It appears to have an immune-modulating response similar to reishi, and may provide another tool in treating hyper-allergenic conditions.

The mushroom appears to reduce allergic immune response in the case of food allergies (Hsieh, K.-Y. et al. 2003).

In summary, *F. velutipes* is antibacterial, antifungal, antiviral, anti-lipemic, antitumor, antiinflammatory, anti-allergenic, and immune modulating.

Fungi Essence

Velvet shank *(F. velutipes)* essence opens us to new and lighter thought patterns. It helps us let go of old, worn-out ways of thinking by opening our mind to the winds of change. The effects can be invigorating and tingling.

— Korte Phi

Fomes fomentarius

Polyporus fomentarius
Pyropolyporus fomentarius
Ungulina fomentaria
(TINDER FUNGUS)
(AMADOU)
(GERMAN TINDER)
(SURGEON'S AGARIC)

Fomes means "tinder," "to burn," or "heat up," as in "foment." *Amadou* is derived from a northern French dialect, meaning "amorous" or "inflames life," from the Latin *amare,* and, in turn, French for "punk." The term "punk" traditionally meant a harlot who sparked her lover into flame. Spark and spunk (semen) are

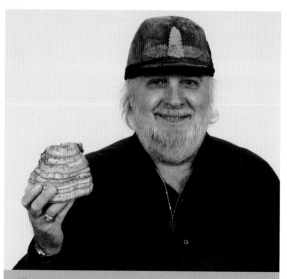

Author, with hat made from *Fomes fomentarius* (polypore in hand).

related derivatives. Pliny the Elder called this mushroom *Aridus fomes fungorum.*

Mors Kochanski, a friend and survival expert I much admire, calls it false tinder conk because it requires preparation to act as tinder. Makes sense to me. He calls chaga *(Inonotus obliquus)* the true tinder conk, due to its use in both igniting and maintaining fires.

False tinder fungus is a hoof-shaped, hard-crusted fungus found on birch. The designation of false tinder conk is sometimes given to the aspen conk *(Phellinus tremulae)* as well as this polypore.

Culture and Folklore

The Khanty tribe of Siberia combined the fungus with silver fir bark as ritual incense used in the house of a deceased person until the body could be removed. "The aim of the procedure was not to let the dead or supernatural being have any influence on the living" (Saar et al. 1991).

Similar rituals were held by the Ainu of northern Japan to banish bad spirits in times of epidemics.

The fungus is depicted in a scene of the temptation of Saint Anthony on Matthias Grunewald's Isenheim Altar as a symbol of the transitory nature of life.

Traditional Uses

Discovery of mushroom remnants dating back to Mesolithic campsites (8,000 B.C.) indicate it may be one of the earliest fungi used by mankind.

This is the Mukes of Hippocrates (400 BC) used for cauterizing wound and treating external inflammation. Cauterizing involved lighting the tinder conk and applying the smoldering mass to the skin on the outside of the affected organ. Laplanders were reported to use pieces of the dried fungus for a similar purpose.

The fungus was powdered by the Cree and applied to the skin as a treatment for frostbite. It was used to treat arthritis by being cut into strips and burned on the skin in the manner of moxibustion to bring blood to the area.

Oetzi, the famous Ice Man found on the slopes of the Alps in 1991, carried whole fruit bodies of *Piptoporus betulinus* and the dissociated context hyphae of *F. fomentarius,* the latter for fire starter and the former to treat intestinal parasites.

In Europe, it was used to treat ingrown toenails, by inserting a strip between the nail and flesh. Pharmacist's polypore, as it was called, was used in European folk medicine as tea taken internally for bladder complaints. Other traditional uses are as a styptic; to cauterize wounds; to treat bladder infections; treat cancer of the stomach, uterus, or esophagus; or smoked with tobacco.

Killermann (1938) reported its use as a remedy for dysmenorrhea, hemorrhoids, and bladder disorders, the active substance being called "fomitin."

Bracket fungus was used by the Okanagan-Colville of British Columbia to cure rheumatism. The fungus was pounded and softened and put over the affected area and ignited, or simply used as a poultice for pain and prevent infection.

The fungi is burned and used as a substi-

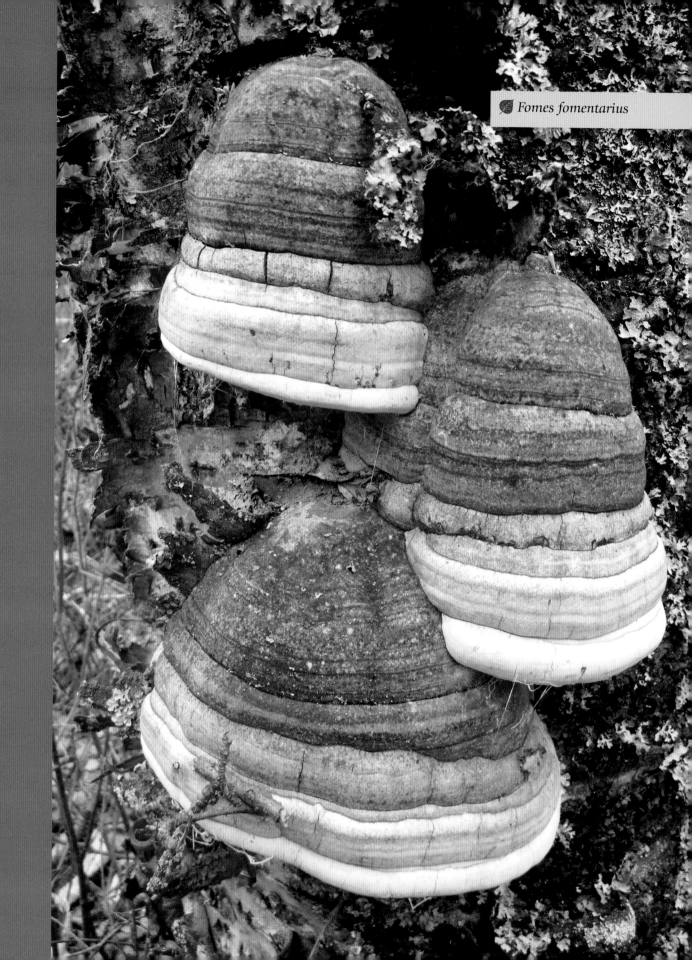

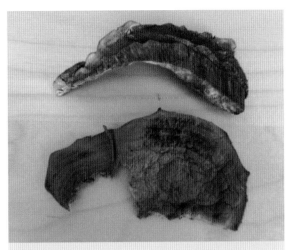

🍃 Context fiber carved from *Fomes fomentarius* as a fire starter (and to make hats).

tute for *Phellinus igniarius* ash with tobacco in Alaska and the Yukon, as well as amongst the Ostiaks of Siberia and other Inuit across northern Canada.

Surgeons have used it to absorb blood and stop bleeding. Dentists have used it instead of cotton wool for drying teeth cavities. It was known formally as "agaric of the chirurges" or "surgeon's agaric."

In traditional Chinese medicine, this fungus warms the lungs, removes lumps from the abdomen, soothes vital energy, and reduces asthma and edema. It is mild in nature, slightly bitter to taste, and is used to resolve indigestion and reduce stasis.

In Japan, where it is known as *tsuriganetake,* it has been used traditionally as a dressing to staunch blood from deep wounds and in the form of a tea for colds, flu, bronchitis, and general debility.

In India, it was known as Gharikum or Chattri-Kiain, and used as a diuretic, laxative, or

nerve tonic. It was also used externally as an absorbing dressing for wounds and burns.

The mycelium has been shown to have an appetite for *E. coli* and other coliformis. Paul Stamets suggests this antimicrobial activity may have been used in ancient times to prevent spoilage in soups and stews.

Because the mycelium can be grown on grains, it could be more commercially available in the future. The wild harvested conks are plentiful in northern boreal forests.

Medicinal Use

Chemical Constituents

■ **Ergosta-7,22-diene-3-one; fungisterol; ergost-7en-3-one; ergosterol; peroxide; three linoleic acid steryl esters; 15 percent protein, 3.5 percent fat, 70 percent complex carbohydrates, 66 international units vitamin D per hundred grams, and 760 milligrams potassium per hundred grams; traces of niacin, copper, iron, selenium, and vitamin B5; benzotropolones including anhydrodehydrofomentariol, anhydrofomentariol, fomentaric acid, glucose oxidase enzymes, polyporic acid C, and ugulinic acid, a lectin that is N-acetylgalactosamine-specific, and B-type erythrocytes specific with molecular weight of seventy kDa with high sugar content (25 percent) and extreme viscosity.**

In China, it is used to treat esophageal cancer and gastric and uterine carcinoma. It has been decocted with red rock lichen to relieve indigestion and reduce stasis.

A lignin from *F. fomentarius* completely inhibits *herpes simplex* virus, in vivo.

Aoki et al. (1993) showed *F. fomentarius* to

possess antiviral substance with systemic effect. The most active compound was identified by Lindequist et al. (1989) as ergosterol peroxide.

Methanol extracts of the conk inhibit nitric oxide synthase (iNOS) and COX expression via down-regulation of the NF-kB, or nuclear transcription factor binding activity to DNA. This suggests both anti-inflammatory and anticancer possibilities (Park, Y.-M. et al. 2004).

Suay et al. (2000) found tinder conk to inhibit the growth of *Pseudomonas aeruginosa* and *Serratia marcescens*. The former is a potentially deadly bacterium that is showing increasing resistance to antibiotics and the leading cause of hospital-acquired infections in the United States.

Serratia causes septicemia and pulmonary disease in immune-compromised patients, and is a most serious bacterium.

Ito et al. (1976) showed that isolated polysaccharides from this mushroom are tumor inhibiting in mice. Rate of inhibition against sarcoma 180 is 80 percent.

Rosecke et al. (2000) found novel ergosterol peroxides in the polypore.

Exopolysaccharides from the fungi have direct anti-proliferative effects on human gastric cancer cells. The sugar complex sensitized the drug doxorubicin, which in turn also inhibited cancer cell growth (Chen, N.-Y. et al. 2008).

Work by Peintner et al. (1998) found antibacterial properties in the fungus.

The conk contains polyporic acid C with antibacterial activity, and ugulinic acid of unknown benefit.

In vitro studies from mushrooms provided by Paul Stamets, found tinder fungus completely inhibited *E. coli* by stopping the bacterial growth ahead of the creeping mycelia. This suggests the possibility of an extracellular antibiotic.

Volc et al. (1985) examined forty species of fungi and found this species and turkey tail *(Trametes versicolor)* contain the highest enzyme activity converting D-glucose into dicarbonyl sugars, useful in fermentation manufacture.

A lectin with an unusually high sugar content (25 percent) and extreme viscosity is B type erythrocytes and N-acetylgalactosamine-specific.

Davitashvili et al. (2008) found wine bagasse gave the highest specific hemagglutinating activity for this polypore.

Essential Oil

Fomes fomentarius has been analyzed for essential oil content and found to contain more than ten sesquiterpenes including octen-3-one, cis-furanoid linalool oxide, (R)-and (S)-oct-1-en-3-ol, beta phellandrene, beta-mycrene, and beta-barbatene.

Fomotopsis pinicola shows a similar composition of volatiles.

Cosmetics

The conk has application in cosmetic preparations for the treatment and repair of signs of skin aging. Various mucopolysaccharides and flavonoids are free radical scavengers, while various saponins exhibit anti-phlogistic action. Cyclic adenosine monophosphate is also present, and shows effectiveness in preventing skin cell aging. It may act as a secondary messenger for metabolic processes in the deeper dermal levels to prevent cellular change and retard skin breakdown. Extracts may be used in after-sun preparations, facial lotions, hair care products, creams and lotions for rough and irritated skin, and moisturizing preparations.

Its distinct odor is due mainly to content of beta phellandrane and beta mycrene.

Textile Industry

Although flammable, it has been woven into clothing and blankets, due to its warm, insulating power. In Romania, Hungary, and other parts of Europe, the pliable "felt" is used to manufacture hats, purses, and other clothing. The tougher parts are soaked in hot water with ashes, and then beaten with a wooden object. It was then stretched to ten times its original size. It is sometimes referred to as German felt.

Dr. Solomon Wasser, a leading authority on medicinal mushrooms, kindly sent me a hat made from this polypore that I highly prize.

In parts of Germany and former Bohemia, the fruiting bodies were hollowed out as flowerpots.

The context material is also used for mounting flies and mosquitoes for entomological collections.

It is used as a pincushion that prevents needles from rusting.

A patent for the use of the fruiting body as a tobacco filter has been filed (U.S. Patent 59122092 1984.)

Insecticide

Paul Stamets suggests that it may be an endophyte, infecting trees and helping prevent disease from other fungi, bolstering the tree's defenses especially in forests subject to pollution and other stressors. This could be accurate, as *Phellinus tremulae* appears to prevent other fungal growths on Aspen poplar trees.

The mushroom contains rac-oct-1-en-3-ol, which is an attractant to various wood-living beetles such as *Malthodes fuscus, Anaspis marginicollis,* and *A. rufilabrus.* The fungi is used as a field attractant for saproxylic beetles. Work in Norway may help explain the role played by beetles in transmitting fungus spores throughout the forest (Olberg and Andersen 1999).

Other Uses

Wood impregnated with the mycelium is known as punkwood and makes excellent tinder. It was widely used by the Cree of Alberta, who called it *wasaskwitoy* or *wa-patos,* for carrying fire from site to site. The tinder fungus was dried, and hollowed out, and then filled with hot embers and repacked with the hard shell covering. This could be carried for days, slowly smoldering. At the new site, it was unwrapped and the embers flamed into fire. It was commonly put on fires at night to glow and smolder and to keep wild animals at bay.

Another use of tinder conk involves pounding the moistened fungus with a rock so that the coating is broken down. It can also be cut into strips, soaked again in saltpeter, and dried for use as tinder. The smallest spark from flint and steel will catch fire and glow for a long time. Before saltpeter, the strips were soaked in dung water.

Sand was sometimes added to the soft fruit body for sharpening razors. The leftover woolly mass can easily be ignited with friction fire after cooking for two hours in a potash lye solution or dung water and then dried.

In the past, it was mixed with saltpeter and used in the musketeer's tinderbox. A spark to the gun's hammer striking the flint ignited it. This lit the wick that then set off the main charge for firing the shot.

In Germany, a Good Friday custom called *weihfeuertragen* involves carrying holy fire in partly hollowed conks.

Fungi Essence

> *Fomes fomentarius* essence helps the artist find new approaches and promotes creativity. It is for burned out artists to help spontaneity.
> — MARIANA

Recipe and Dosage

Fifteen to twenty grams of dried fungus twice daily as water decoction for cancer of the esophagus, stomach, or uterus. Prepare tincture at 1:10 ration. See *Ganoderma applanatum* for directions.

Bits and Pieces

It has been estimated that one average sized polypore releases more than a trillion spores per season, or more than its own weight in spores.

Fomitiporia punctata

Poria punctata
Fuscoporia punctata
Phellinus punctatus
(POLYPORE PONCTUÉ)

This polypore is a flat sporophore with a thickness no greater than fifteen millimeters. It is usually found on hardwood trees.

Traditional Use

The dried fungus is used in China to treat coronary heart disease.

Fomitopsis cajanderi

Fomes cajanderi
F. subroseus
(ROSY CONK)
Fomitopsis rosea
Rhodoformes roseus
(PINK POLYPORE)

Rosy conk is found on dead conifers, as well as fruit trees.

Pink polypore looks similar but paler and also enjoys eating dead conifers.

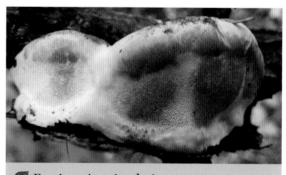
🍃 *Fomitopsis cajanderi*

Medicinal Use

Rosy conk contains anti-carcinogenic substances and has an inhibition rate against sarcoma 180 of 70 percent (Ohtsuka et al. 1973).

Jian He et al. (2003) identified fomlactones A-C. Other compounds include ergosterol, ergosterol peroxide, and various methyl esters.

Early work by Hervey (1947) found activity against both *Staphylococcus aureus* and *E. coli*.

Popova et al. (2009) confirmed triterpenes activity against *S. aureus*.

The related pink polypore, or *F. rosea,* shows inhibition rates of 70 percent against sarcoma 180 in mice studies (Ohtsuka et al. 1973).

Fomitopsis officinalis

Fomes laricis
F. officinalis
Polyporus officinalis
Boletus officinalis
Laricifomes officinalis
Agaricum officinalis
(QUININE CONK)
(WHITE AGARIC)
(AGARIKON)

> Larche tre . . . giueth also . . . ye famous medicine called Agarick.
> — TURNER

> One dramme of Agaryke and a half dramme of fine Rheubarbe.
> — ELYOT

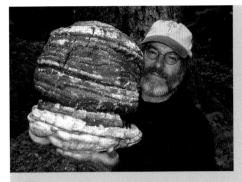
Paul Stamets with *agarikon*

Agaric is thought to derive from Agarus, a town inhabited by Sarmatians along the Agarus River. The Agari were a Scythian people and Agarus was their king around 240 BC.

The Roman Pliny named it *agaricum.*

Quinine conk is found on Englemann spruce, white and black spruce, and occasionally on pine or larch. It has a roasted, tea-like odor that may lend itself to perfumery.

A number of European strains of this polypore are rapidly in decline, and in many areas they are close to extinction. It grows best at temperatures between twenty and twenty-four degrees Celsius (sixty-eight to seventy-five degrees Fahrenheit).

Culture and Folklore

Native tribes of the British Columbia coast carved spirit figures from large, perennial *F. officinalis* polypores. They believed the conks possessed supernatural powers that could be increased through the shaman's arts. These figures often included mouth or stomach orifices, which gave them the capability of catching spirits during a shaman séance. They were often carved into animalistic forms, though Paul Stamets suggests that some of the figures resemble women, similar to the Venus of Willendorf.

After a shaman died, the carved conks were placed at the head of his grave to guard it; the marker let others know the area was sacred and not to be disturbed.

During society rituals, the conks were displayed in the ceiling timbers of special dance houses of the shaman for ritual protective purposes. The Squamish hung them in their homes to protect the inhabitants from evil thoughts. The carved fungi were also believed to redirect evil or malicious thoughts back to the person who sent them.

The fungi were also used to move fire in the form of hot coals, much like the false tinder conk.

Various carved "wooden" objects now found in museums are actually the carved sporophores of *F. officinalis*. G. Emmons collected large numbers of these objects in the late 1800s, sailing up and down the coast of British Columbia and Alaska. He shipped them to the American Museum of Natural History in New York. Notes by Emmons suggest that the grave guardians were made from wood and placed on graves to protect the shaman during his long death sleep. They appear to have been oiled or greased to increase their dark color. Others were painted, and one was ornamented with copper.

The Haida word for bracket fungus is *gyaalgas naan-gha,* which translates as "sea biscuit's grandmother." The Haida personified the mushroom as "fungus man," thought to steer the canoe of Raven (Yaahl) due to his strength.

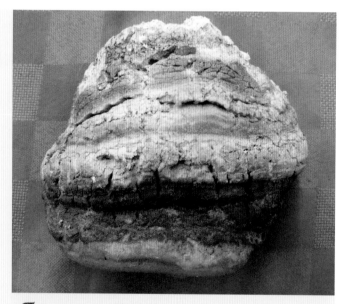

🍃 *Fomitopsis officinalis*

Traditional Uses

Dioscorides used the name *agarikon* to describe what today we call *F. officinalis*. He wrote: "Its properties are styptic and heat-producing, efficacious against colic and sores, fractured limbs, and bruises from falls . . . it is given in liver complaints, asthma, jaundice, dysentery, kidney diseases, and cases of hysteria. In cases of phthisis it is administered in raisin wine, in affections of the spleen with honey and vinegar. By persons troubled with pains in the stomach and by those who suffer from acrid eructations the root is chewed and swallowed without any liquid."

The powdered dry fungus was used for hemostatic application like the powder of puffballs. Thin strips were cut from younger specimens after the hard pellicle and undersurface tubes were removed. These strips were beaten and wetted down until soft, pliable, and thin, and laid on wounds as a dressing, providing protection and antiseptic action.

Dioscorides considered the fungus to have two parts, one male *(Agaricum masculum),* and the other female, but this was simply related to the manner in which it was cut for commerce. The tube layer was called female, and the upper crust male.

Some authors suggest this agaric as the female and *F. igniarius* or *F. fomentarius* as the male agaric.

A pseudoagaricum was identified to be similar but yellow when fresh and mild in taste. This has been identified as sulphur polypore, or chicken of the woods *(Tyromyces sulphureus),* probably a dishonest substitute for true agaric.

Agaric appears in the twelfth-century *Syriac Book of Medicines,* citing remedies on menstruation, excessive urination, repairing nerve damage, and aiding in immortality.

Gerard, in his famous herbal of 1597 recommended "it is good against the shortnesse of breath, called asthma, the inveterate cough of the lungs, the ptysicke, consumption and those that spet blood: it comforteth the weake and feeble stomacke, causeth good digestion, and is good against wormes."

Sauer, an eighteenth-century German American, wrote in his *Compendious Herbal* (quoted in Weaver 2001): "Agaric operates through its divers earthy salts, as well as through a caustic, soft resinous component. It is thus endowed with rather bitter after tasting compounds with the capacity to purge both by stool and urine, and to expectorate phlegm from the chest . . . for persons afflicted by the falling evil (epilepsy), an agaric decoction . . . should be used to scrub the head. Agaric is employed with great favor in laxatives made with wine. But it is also possible to achieve an excellent extraction of agaric's properties by infusing it in brandy and then boiling it to a soft extract that can then be rolled into balls and administered in the amount of twenty to twenty four grains as laxative pills."

In 1965, agaric acid was prohibited as a flavoring agent in food, because animal studies showed large amounts produced skeletal muscle weakness and depression of the central nervous system. And yet artificial monosodium glutamate, under a variety of names, is used widely in prepared foods.

The main indications for use, however, are alternating chills and flushes of heat, with bearing down pain in the back.

The Alberta Cree know it as *wah pah toos.* They powder the dry fungus and apply it with a bandage to treat frostbite.

It was known as *'adagan* or "bread of ghosts," by the Coast Tsimshian, for whom it had important medicinal and spiritual uses. The Tlingit call it *tak'a di,* meaning tree biscuit. They used it as a poultice for swollen and inflamed areas.

Medicinal Use

Chemical Constituents

■ **Agaricic, agaricolic, and agaricinic acid; agaricin (containing 97 percent agaric acid and 3 percent agaricol); ergosterol; cetyl alcohol; ricinolic, eburicolic, dehydro-eburicolic, ricinoleic, and dehydro-buriconic acids; agaricol; phytosterin; dehydromatricaria ester; octadien-(1,7)-diin-(3,5)-diol-(1,2)-carbonic acid-1; ergosta-4,6,8(14),22-tetraenon-(3), 5 lanostane-type triterpenes named fomefficinic acids A-G; fomefficinols A-B; officinalic acid; fomalactone A-C; laricinolic acid; beta-glucans; triterpenoids; dehydrotrametenolic acid; and various gums, resins, and carbohydrates.**

This is the famous agaric of ancient herbals. It has slightly sweet, bitter, and cooling energetics, and was used for strengthening the system, reducing intermittent fevers and night sweats in tuberculosis, and as a mild laxative.

It was part of the famous Warburg's Tincture, also known as *Antiperiodica Tinctura,* of the late 1800s, which was used mainly for relief of sweating at night associated with tuberculosis.

It warms the lungs, removes lumps from the abdomen, soothes the vital energy, allays asthmatic panting, and eases edema and diuresis.

Krzysztof Grzywnowicz (2001) reported on traditional Polish uses to treat coughing illness, asthma, rheumatoid arthritis, and infections.

The Ainu of northern Japan have long used the peeled and dried fruiting body for relieving stomachaches, body pain, and reducing sweats.

Gerard, the famous English herbalist of the seventeenth century, used agaric for cleansing the intestine, jaundice, menstrual problems, asthma, chronic and recurring fevers, and edema.

Quinine fungus from larch has been used traditionally for hemorrhoids, water motions, and vomiting. It helps to cure coughing, asthma, nephritis, urinary calculii, nosebleed, swollen sore throats, and peridonitis.

It possesses a distinct quinine, bitter taste that helps distinguish it from other polypores.

It is not much used today, as it has a slight irritating effect on the bowel. Because it arrests sweating slowly, it was often mixed with ground wild carrot seed.

The fungus dries up breast milk, and in the past was used for certain cases of chorea or epilepsy.

It was an official herb in the Pharmacopoeias of Switzerland, Austria, and Portugal until recent times.

The fungus is used in Unani medicine for coughs and colds, as well as asthma, and as an expectorant. It is known as *ghaariqoon* in this form of medicine that moved from Greece to Arabia and then to India. One compound medicine called *habb-e-iyarij* contains agaric and is used in facial paralysis, epilepsy, as a brain tonic, and for melancholia. The fungus is given with honey to promote the eruption of measles, chicken pox, and other childhood infections. Recent work by Paul Stamets (2005) found anti-pox properties in the polypore, confirming an ancient folkloric use.

More recent work by the National Institute of Health, the National Institute of Allergy and Infectious Disease, and the U.S. Army

Medical Research Institute has screened various mushroom extracts against a variety of viruses.

Agaric shows very strong activity against cowpox, mentioned above, and vaccinia. The mycelium shows promise against smallpox.

Other viruses including influenza B, H1N1 (swine flu), H3N2, and H5N1 (avian flu) strains; yellow fever; West Nile; arenaviruses such as tacaribe and pichinde, and punta toro, a hemorrhagic virus similar to Rift Valley fever virus, all show inhibition by extracts of this polypore.

According to Paul Stamets, a strain of this particular fungus shows high activity against a rare type of drug-resistant tuberculosis.

Practitioners believe it exerts a potent synergistic activity in neurological and inflammatory conditions. Graf and Winckelmann (1960) investigated the transformation of hydroxytriterpene acids in the polypore to 11-keto-corticosteroids.

The fungus may be used medicinally for hemorrhoids, vomiting, excessive sweating, spasmodic coughing, and to slow lactation.

Alcohol extracts of the mushroom appear to have similar effects as atropine, including relaxation of intestinal spasms and smooth muscle and drying up of nasal secretions.

It shows inhibition against sarcoma 180 cancer cell lines of 80 percent (Ohtsuka et al. 1973).

Early work by Robbins et al. (1945) found that this polypore and the related *Fomitopsis pinicola* (below) both inhibit *Staphylococcus aureus* and *E. coli*.

Dehydrotrametenolic acid acts as an insulin sensitizer in glucose tolerance tests and reduces hyperglycemia in non-insulin dependent diabetes (Sato, M. et al. 2002).

Shiuan Chen et al. (2005) looked at the aromatase and 5alpha reductase properties of button mushrooms *(A. bisporus)*. Several strains of *F. officinalis* were found to contain compounds with similar activity, suggesting possible benefit in the prevention of breast and prostate cancers.

Homeopathy

Boletus laricis is made from the triturated dried fungus *Fomes officinalis.*

The main indications are for night sweats and pancreatic and hepatic inflammation. The eyes may be glued shut in morning with dull pain in the eyeballs, painful gums, and a thick yellow coating on the tongue.

There may be a metallic taste in the mouth, with nausea and vomiting or burning pains in area of the gall bladder. Stools may be yellow and thin or bloody, accompanying a high fever, dull pain in the back and legs, shivering up and down the back, hot flushes, and profuse sweats at night.

Burt and Lord identified some peculiar symptoms including the sensation of the teeth being pressed out of their sockets and frightful dreams of water.

Other symptoms include coppery taste in mouth; dry, dark lumpy stools; great weakness and prostration; and restlessness at night.

Dose: 1C to 3C potency, as needed. Burt and Lord did a proving on six males in 1868 (Boericke).

Laricifomes officinalis e mycelio is used for night sweats, asthma, coughs, chronic polyarthritis, and as a laxative. It is produced from the mycelium according to a process developed by Dr. G Enderlein.

Dose: 4C to 5C. Take five to ten drops under the tongue before meals. For polyarthritis, it can be rubbed into the affected area. A commercial product, Larifikehl, is available as drops, ampoules, capsules, or suppositories.

Agaracin is a substance isolated from *Fomes officinalis* and then attenuated for medicine. It is valued for conditions like Sydenham's chorea. This is mainly a childhood condition affecting more girls than boys, and associated with rheumatic fever.

It is recommended by Boericke for night sweats in doses of one quarter to one half gram.

It is used for chorea associated with dilation of the heart and pulmonary emphysema, fatty degeneration, and erythema.

Anxiety and impaired memory and speech are present, as well as contraction of the muscles of the body and extremities. May be helpful in erythema.

Agaracin may also help those prone to epileptic seizure or parasethesia.

In *King's American Dispensatory,* agaritin in doses of one-sixteenth to one-sixth grain show great benefit in colliquative sweating, especially in phthisis, where it allays thirst and controls cough and diarrhea.

Blackwood says that "this remedy is of special service in those patients who have nervous dyspepsia.... In those patients who have been addicted to the excessive use of tea, coffee, or tobacco, or are recovering from some debilitating disease that has greatly weakened the heart; the pulse is weak and irregular, while the heart's action is weak and attended at times by violent palpitations. There is profuse sweating with twitching of muscles and dilatation of the heart."

Dose: 3C to 6C potency, as needed.

Recipes and Dosage

Five to thirty grains of powder per dose.

Decoction, one teaspoon every two hours. Prepare from 0.3 to 0.9 grams in one pint of water.

Tincture: ten to fifteen drops. The official medicine is made from the inner portions of the freshly picked polypore. Prepare at one-to-five ratio and 90 percent alcohol. Agaric acid is best extracted with alcohol.

Fomitopsis pinicola

Fomes pinicola
Polyporus pinicola
P. marginatus
Boletus pinicola
Ungulina marginata
(RED BELTED CONK)

Pinicola means "inhabiting pine," its most common home. I have found it, however, growing on poplar, birch, and spruce.

This beautiful, varnished red-brown shelf fungus is often mistaken for the valuable reishi of Asian fame. It grows on the same dead spruce and pine, throughout the boreal forest, and is a major decomposer of dead spruce. It is one of the most common polypores in the world and has a sweet smell and taste.

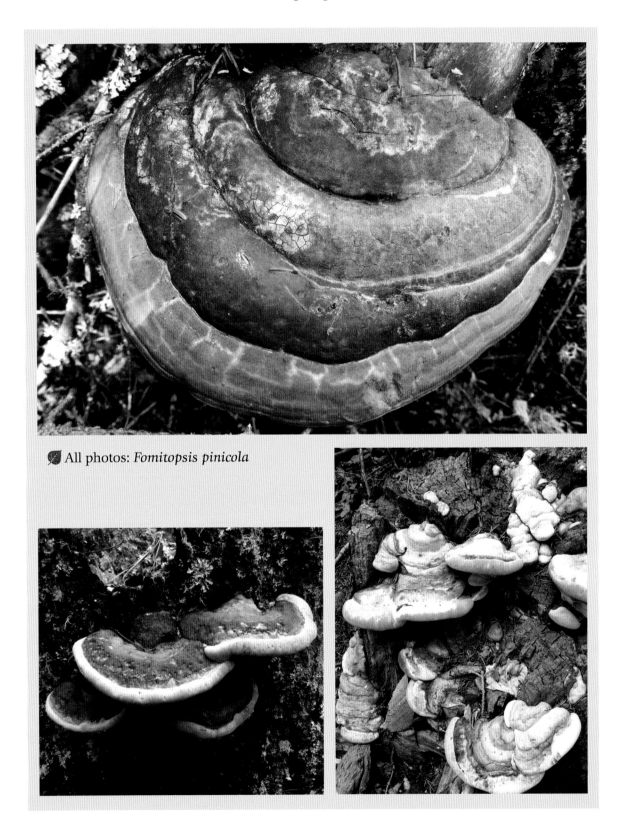

All photos: *Fomitopsis pinicola*

Traditional Uses

The Blackfoot put a dried polypore in a buffalo horn, along with a live coal from the fire, when moving camp. They used a piece of the fungus as a purgative, and thought that too large a dose would turn the hair gray, hence the name *apopikatiss* for "makes your hair gray."

Red belted conk is known as *mech quah too,* or "red touchwood," by the Cree of Eastern Canada. The fruiting body was traditionally dried and powdered and used on wounds to stop bleeding. A half teaspoonful of the powder was put in water and steeped, then swallowed as an emetic for purification.

Traditionally, it has been used as a daily tonic to reduce inflammation of the digestive tract, and to increase general resistance.

The Northern Dene cut the fungi into small chunks and smoke it with tobacco to treat headaches.

The Iroquois differentiated polypores, according to the tree upon which they grow. As a group they were called *unä'sa,* preceded by the tree name. Various polypores including red belted conk, *Grifola frondosa,* and *Laetipo-rus sulphereus* were boiled and used for flavor in soups. There are isolated reports of boiling the conks until edible, but that would be a tough chew, at least with mature specimens. It was probably a case of an alternative to stone soup, with other ingredients providing the nourishment. Or more likely, the polypores act as an antibacterial that preserves the soup from spoilage, and gives everyone an immune boost, especially in winter.

During the 1800s, the polypore was soaked in whiskey as a remedy for ague.

Wagenfuhr et al. (1989) found that fiberboard made from wood chips pre-treated with red touchwood extract showed excellent flexibility, high tensile strength, and little tendency to swell.

Internet sites list the dried tea form of this polypore for $310 per pound. Ridiculously high prices, but it shows the potential for future commercialization. Go pick your own, it is plentiful.

Medicinal Use

Chemical Constituents

- **Ergosterol, 3 compounds related to trametenolic acid, polyporenic acid C, ergosta-7,22-dien-3beta-ol, fungisterol, eburicoic acid, lanosterol, inotodiol, 21-hydroxylanosta-7,9(11)-24-trien-3-on, 21-hydroxylanosta-7,9(11)-24-trien-3b,21-diol, 3a-oxylanosta-8,24-dien-21-oleic acid, 5,6-dihydroergosterol and pinicolic acid. Other constituents include pachymic acid and pinicolol B, polycarpol,**

- **Top crust: lanostane derivatives and triterpenes. Concentration in crust is higher than rest of fungus, and lower in young fungus compared to older.**

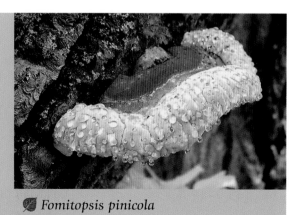
Fomitopsis pinicola

Red belted conk has been found to contain polysaccharides with both moderate tumor-inhibiting and immune-stimulating properties.

A thirty milligram daily dosage showed a prevention rate of 51.2 percent against sarcoma 180 solid cancer cells (Shibata, S. et al. 1968). Given to guinea pigs at the same rate, prevention was 61.2 percent and recovery rate only 33.3 percent.

Cheng et al. (2008) found polysaccharide extracts from mycelium to inhibit tube cell formation in endothelial cells, suggesting anti-tumor potential.

Other studies suggest a beneficial effect on liver enzymes. Mice given crude extracts showed significant retention of bromsulphalein and elevation of serum glutamic pyruvic transaminase induced by the toxic carbon tetrachloride.

It can be used daily as a tonic to reduce inflammation of the digestive tract and increase resistance to diseases, including cancer.

It has been used in herbal medicine for persistent, intermittent fevers, chronic diarrhea, periodic neuralgia, nervous headaches, excessive urination, and jaundice as well as chills and fevers.

In Japan, the mushroom is known as *tsugasaruno-koshikake* and considered a cancer preventative, although not supported as yet by any human clinical trials. The tea is mild and sweet with a slight bitter aftertaste.

Early work by Hervey found activity against both *E. coli* and *Staphylococcus aureus.*

New work by Xue-Ting Liu et al. (2010) found activity from various lanostane triterpenoids and ergostane steroids against *Bacillus cereus.*

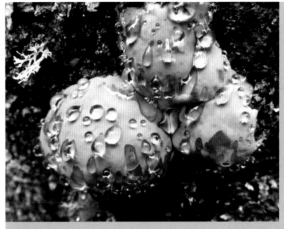

Young, sweating *Fomitopsis pinicola*

Alkaline extracts of the fruiting body show regulation of blood sugar via increased insulin secretion, or prevention of streptozotocin-induced pancreatic damage in mice (Lee, S.-I. et al. 2008).

Fomitopinic acid A inhibits COX-2, suggesting anti-inflammatory activity.

Various lanostane triterpenoids and their glycosides were investigated for their activity against COX-1 and COX-2 (Yoshikawa, K. et al. 2005).

G. Ren et al. (2006) found ether and ethyl acetate extracts of this polypore exhibiting significant cytotoxic effect against human cervical and hepatoma cancer cell lines.

Activity against *Fusarium* species was noted (Guler et al. 2009).

Homeopathy

Pine agaric *(P. pinicola)* is useful in intermittent, remittent, and bilious fevers, with headache, yellow tongue, constant nausea, faintness at epigastrium, and constipation.

There may be a deep, dull, severe pain in the shinbones, preventing sleep.

There may be great lassitude, congestion of the head, vertigo, hot and flushed face, and a prickling sensation all over. There is restlessness at night from pain in the wrists and knee, rheumatic pains, and profuse perspiration. The headaches begin about ten o'clock in the morning, with pain in the back, ankles, and legs, increasing until three o'clock in the afternoon, and then gradually getting better.

Symptoms are similar to *F. officinalis* but appear to affect the joints more, while white agaric is stronger on the gastrointestinal tract.

Fomitopsis pinicola is used for an impaired immune system and prostate adenoma.

Dose: 5C potency. Five to ten drops under the tongue before meals. The product Fomepikehl 5C is injected as one milliliter ampoules intramuscularly or subcutaneously twice weekly. A mycelium preparation, Pinikehl, is also available in 5C capsules and suppositories.

It was first proved by Burt in 1868 with mother tincture and then 1C and 2C, and later by Fuller in 1870, on one to two ounces of the fungus in a pint of whiskey taken three times per day.

Essential Oil

The fungus contains several volatiles including (R)- and (S)-oct-1-en-3-ol (49 percent) octen-3-one and various sesquiterpene hydrocarbons including beta-barbatene, alpha-pinene, camphene, gamma-cadinene, trans-calamenene, and aromatic compounds including furfural, benzaldehyde, phenyl acetaldehyde, and 2-pentylfuran (Fäldt et al. 1999; Rosecke et al. 2000).

Mycoremediation

The related *Fomitopsis carnea* showed 80 percent gold removal compared to that on immobilized calcium-alginate beads (Khoo and Ting 2001).

Cosmetics

The polypore contains a number of antihistamine vegetable sterols with application to skin preparations. The oils exhibit circulatory-stimulating properties and contain C14-C18 fatty acids with moisturizing properties. Various amino acids regulate moisture content and octadecanoate exhibits surface immune stimulation. Various capric/caprilic triglycerides, similar to those found in elm seed oil, are present, and may be used in day and night creams, cleansing milks, and liquid soaps.

The distinct scent is due in part to beta barbatene and (E)-beta-farnescene.

Textile Industry

An oil-soluble red dye can be extracted as well.

Recipes and Dosage

Twenty to thirty grams twice daily in soup or tea. It must be simmered for at least half an hour to extract the active constituents. Larger pieces can be cut into half-inch slices, so that more surface area is exposed.

Tincture: See *Ganoderma applanatum*.

Funalia trogii

Trametes trogii
(TROG TRAMETES)
F. cervina
T. cervina
Polyporus biformis
(DEER TRAMETES)

This polypore looks very similar to *Trametes versicolor,* but has no anise-like odor.

Deer *Trametes* looks similar to trog and even *Antrodia albida.* It is found on hardwood trees including saskatoon, cherry, and poplar.

Medicinal Use

Unyayar et al. (2006) found the fungus to possess compounds with antitumor activity, specifically against HeLa cell lines. The extracts did not affect the proliferation of human lymphocytes.

Unyayar et al. (2005) also wrote about the cytotoxic activity.

Ethanol production residue is an excellent substrate for lectin production by this mushroom (Davitashvili et al. 2008).

Early work by Robbins et al. (1945) found activity against *Staphylococcus aureus.*

It contains polyacetylenic antibiotics such as biformine and biforminic acid that show activity against gram-positive and gram-negative bacteria as well as fungi.

A virulent form of *Mycobacterium tuberculosis* was found somewhat more sensitive to biformine than was *Staphylococcus aureus.*

Yurekli et al. (1999) found this mushroom and *Trametes versicolor* produce indole acetic acid, gibberellic acid, abscisic acid, and cytokinin at a one-to-four dilution of stillage.

Mycoremediation

Trog has been found to be an effective laccase source and pellets are used to decolorize various red and orange textile dyes (Yesilada et al. 2002).

Galerina mutabilis

(see *Pholiota mutabilis*)

> *A chap from the hills of Carolina*
> *Was buried last week in Elvina*
> *After eating some Honeys*
> *He began to feel funny*
> *(He was attacked by a fall Galerina).*
> — OHIO SPORE PRINT,
> NOVEMBER/DECEMBER 1982

Galerina is from the Latin meaning "it resembles a fur cap." They are best left alone as they are considered deadly poisonous, containing phallotoxins and amatoxins.

One species in Germany, *G. steglichii,* was discovered in 1993. It develops a blue stain when pressed and was found to contain psilocybin, psilocin, and baeocystin, the first discovery of psychoactive compounds in the *Galerina* genus.

Hunters of "magic mushrooms" should be able to identify *G. marginata* due to its similarity to the *Psilocybe* species.

Galiella rufa

Bulgaria rufa
(RED CUP FUNGI)

Galiella rufa is a red cup fungus that is hairy and tough on the outside and quite squishy and soft inside.

Medicinal Use

This fungus contains gallielalactone, a compound that may have application in the treatment of prostate cancer. Work in Sweden by Hellsten et al. (2008) have found the compound to be a potent and selective inhibitor of interleukin-6 signaling in HePG2 cells. It has been found to inhibit Stat3 that directly inhibits prostate tumor cells from growing.

Patents are in place and synthetic methods for developing a drug are underway.

Ganoderma applanatum

G. lipsiense
Fomes applanatus
Elfvingia applanata
(ARTIST'S CONK)
G. tsugae
(VARNISHED CONK)
(CEDAR LACQUER FUNGUS)
(GLOSSY GANODERMA)
G. resinaceum
(VARNISH SHELF)
G. oregonense
(WESTERN VARNISH SHELF)

Artist's conk is known to some
As Ganoderma applanatum,
Like its shiny cousin reishi
Helps improve a person's Chi,
A substitute for lucidum.
　　—RDR

Ganoderma is from the Latin *gan* for "shiny," and *derm,* meaning "skin." *Applanatum* is from the Latin for "flattened." *Tsugae* means "of hemlock," derived from the Latin. *Resinaceum* means "resinous." *Oregonense* means "from Oregon."

Artist's conk is commonly found on balsam poplar, spruce, and other trees in the north and on maples and western cedar *(Thuja plicata)* west of the Rockies. Throughout North America it is found on nearly every hardwood tree.

It is, as the name suggests, used for its wide, flat shape with a white spore side that makes a welcoming canvas for painting or sketching. A drawing etched into the surface will almost immediately turn brown and will be preserved for a long time once the surface has dried. Many artists—and would-be artists—have created small masterpieces on the canvas of the artist's conk. One old-timer who drew a likeness of his log cabin claims it was still preserved even after forty years!

The curious thing about the artist's conk is that it is found only on dead, dying, or severely stressed trees. Its presence on a tree is an almost sure sign that the tree will not live. The fungus doesn't kill the tree, but colonizes it once the tree's doom has been sealed.

Artist's conk may be thought of as similar to the related reishi. In fact, the Chinese call it the "ancient *ling zhi,*" meaning "spirit plant," a term usually reserved for its more famous cousin. The ancient *ling zhi* derives from the Chinese name *chih se lao mu chum,* meaning "flesh-colored ancient life source mushroom."

The Japanese medical texts refer to it as *kofukisarunokosshikake,* or the shortened *kofukitake.*

164

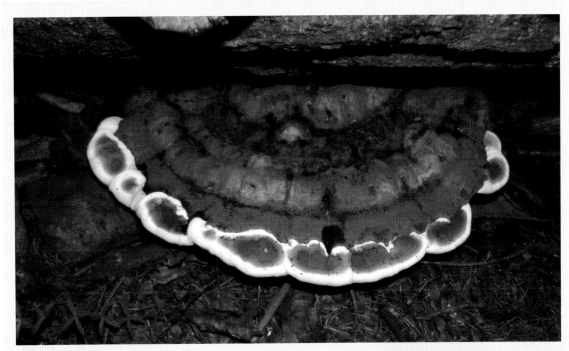

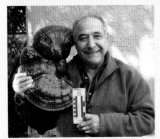

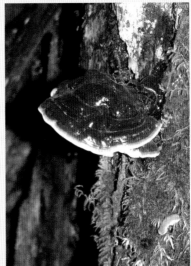

🍃Above and below: *Ganoderma applanatum.* Left: *Ganoderma oregonense.* Right: *Ganoderma tsugae.* Bottom right: Making paper from *Ganoderma.*

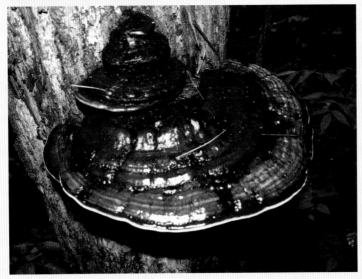

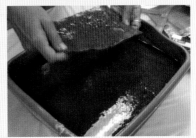

Ganoderma tsugae belongs to the *G. lucidum* complex and looks a lot like it with its shiny red-varnished surface. The Chinese call it *song shan shu zhi,* which means "pine or fir tree fungus," or *sung shan ling chih* with the same meaning.

Cedar lacquer fungus is only found on the trunks of hemlock, western larch, and occasionally douglas fir in the mountains of British Columbia and down the coast. It is commonly found on eastern hemlock on that side of continent, and various trees on the Gulf Coast. Specimens are up to five feet in diameter.

When young, the tender edges are edible, and quite tasty sautéed with butter.

David Spahr mentions their use in English-style ale using the ground fruiting bodies as a replacement for hops.

His first batch was too bitter, but the second was good when used with amber ale malt, adding some red color to the finished product. He suggests two to three heaping tablespoons per five-pound can of malt for a medium to heavy ale like India pale ale or strong ale.

Varnish shelf or resinous reishi is a closely related cousin of *G. lucidum.* In the Quebec publication of polypores, *Les Champignons des Arbres* by Bruno Boulet, it is considered synonymous with *G. lucidum* and *G. sessile.*

It is hoped that one day, DNA will help sort this out, as proper species identification is critical to ongoing medical research.

At the same time, the opportunity for hybridization may one day allow for a reishi hardy enough for more northern climates, and promote wood grown, outdoor cultivation.

A recent article by Jean Marc Moncalvo, at the University of Toronto, asks as many questions as it answers. He writes that DNA studies show that the *G. lucidum* species complex includes *G. tsugae, G. resinaceum,* and others.

He suggests *G. lucidum* is probably restricted to western parts of Europe, but may include Siberia and northwest China. Most collections labeled *G. lucidum* in North America correspond to the taxon labeled *G. resinaceum* in Europe, whereas *G. tsugae* in North America is very closely related, genetically, to the "true" *G. lucidum* from Europe (Moncalvo 2005). I have placed reishi in its own chapter that follows.

Western varnish shelf *(G. oregonense)* is a common polypore of western North America. It is similar to *G. applanatum* but is much larger, up to one hundred centimeters by forty centimeters by five centimeters, with two to three pores per millimeter.

It is closely related to *G. tsugae,* according to rDNA sequencing (S. G. Hong and H. S. Jung 2004). In fact, they are difficult to tell apart and may in fact be one species.

The tender nesting polypore *(Hapalopilus nidulans)* is a cinnamon-brown polypore with gray-brown spores found on birch, fir, spruce, and pine. It is often mistaken for artist's conk.

It is worthy of note that in laboratory germination of spores, glucose alone was successful at 78 percent. Everything else tried, including vitamins and alcohols, were less than 1 percent successful at encouraging growth.

Traditional Uses

Ganoderma applanatum is reported to be in extensive use known as *Phanasomba* or *Phanas alombe* by the Ayurvedic Vedas in the Pine region of India. A paste prepared from the polypore is applied to gums for stopping excessive salivation and is a good styptic.

In traditional Chinese medicine, it is used to reduce mucus production, resolve indigestion, treat hemostasis, stop pain, and remove heat. It is considered a specific for rheumatic tuberculosis and esophageal cancer in China, and used in various antibiotic functions.

In traditional Chinese medicine, the fungus is also used for oxygen deficit tolerance, as in altitude sickness, combining well with safflower seed and chrysanthemum (C. morifolium) flower or Rhodiola rosea.

It is used extensively for radiation protection, and, of course, immune regulation.

The noted herbalist Ryan Drum has reported some success in treating Hashimoto's disease with fungi decoctions. The patient drinks twelve ounces of cooled tea daily for three days and then takes a break.

Martin Osis has found that artist's conk decoctions used as footbaths almost immediately relieve gout conditions.

Medicinal Use

Chemical Constituents

- **G. applanatum: ergosterol and its peroxide, ergosta-7,22-dien-3b-ol, ergosta-7,22-dien-3-one, ergosterol peroxide, beta-D-glucan, fungisterol, alnusenone, friedelin, and various triterpenoids including ganoderenic, furanoganoderic, and ganoderic acids; applanoxidic acids A, B, C, and D; lanostandoid triterpenes E-H, lucidone A, ganoderma aldehyde, 3 linoleic acid steryl esters. Ganoderenic acid and ganoderic acid as a methyl ester are both found in G. lucidum.**

- **The highest amount of triterpenoid acids is found in the tubes (6.4 milligrams per gram of dried weight), followed by the dark context layer of the pileus (2.5 milligrams per gram), and the older white context layer and the upper surface (both with 0.6 milligrams per gram).**

- **Ethanol fractions include D-mannitol, 2-methoxyfatty acids, cerebrosides, daucosterol, 2.5-dihydroxyacetophenone, 2,5-dihydroxybenzoic acid and proto-catechualdehyde.**

- **G. tsugae: 3 alpha-acetoxy-5alpha-lanosta-8,24-dien-21-oic acid; 2beta, 3alpha, 9alpha-trihydroxy-5alpha-ergosta-7,22-diene; 3alpha-acetoxy-16alpha-hydroxy-24É-methyl-5alpha-lanosta-8,25-dien-21-oic acid, tsugaric acid C, tsugarioside B and C, ganoderic acid C2, ganoderic acid B, lucidone A, and various glycans. An immunomodulating protein, FIP-gts, has been recently purified.**

Early work by Ikekawa et al. (1969) found anti-tumor activity in the polypore. This was followed up by Sasaki et al. (1971) who identified the polysaccharides involved. Taichi et al. (1983) isolated the active beta-glucans from the fruiting body.

Bin Gao and Gui-Zhen Yang (1991) found that polysaccharides increase the proliferation of spleen cells in vitro and also possess antitumor activity against sarcoma 180 in mice.

This polypore has shown immune-stimulating properties in many animal studies. It shows interferon-like effect in mice spleens, increasing killer T-cells and inhibiting Epstein-Barr virus-associated activity.

Nucleic acids isolated from this species show

protection against tick-borne encephalitis virus in mice studies (Kandefer-Szerszen et al. 1979).

The conk is readily soluble in water, but no other solvent, producing a yellow-brown extract. It may be, like its more famous cousin reishi, that both the cell wall (chitin) and mycelium are useful. Beta-glucans are water- and heat-soluble, and unchanged by digestion, go right to receptor sites on immune cells in the gut.

The polysaccharides have been found to increase spleen cell proliferation in vitro, and stimulate antitumor activity against sarcoma 180, one laboratory yardstick (Sasaki et al. 1971).

Recent German studies showed water extracts reduced cancer growth by 64.9 percent, with complete regression in 45.5 percent of tested animals.

The compound applanoxidic acid B is the most active of this triterpene grouping to show effect against mouse skin tumor-promoters. Activity against Epstein-Barr virus was shown (Chairul and Hayashi 1994).

Ganoderic acids A and C inhibit farnesyl protein transferase. As this enzyme plays a role in Ras-dependent cell transformation, inhibitors such as these can play a significant role in cancer treatment.

Studies by Kandefer-Szerszen et al. (1979) showed nucleic acid isolated from *G. applanatum* reduced the number of *Vaccinia* virus plaques in chick embryo fibroblast cells and induced small amounts of interferon production. They also found that RNA from this fungus, in vivo, induced a substance showing interferon properties in the spleen of mice.

Bin Gao and Gui-Zhen Yang (1991) reported on the mushroom's polysaccharides and their effect on humoral and cellular immunity in normal and sarcoma 180-transplanted mice.

Rym et al. (1999) found water-soluble extracts exhibited potent activity against vesicular stomatitis virus (VSV) with an EC50 value of 0.104 milligrams per milliliter.

A. Smania et al. (1999) studied the fruiting bodies of *G. applanatum* and found antibacterial properties against *Bacillus cereus, Corynebacterium diphtheriae, E. coli, Pseudomonas aeruginosa,* and *Streptococcus pyogenes.* In general, the gram-positive bacteria were more sensitive than the gram-negative.

Early work by Hervey (1947) found activity against *Staphylococcus aureus.*

Previous work by Robbins et al. (1945) found activity in thiamine-peptone agar plates against *S. aureus* and *E. coli.*

One study found artist's conk cultures, in vitro, inhibited *E. coli* growth completely. It stopped the bacterial growth ahead of the spreading mycelia, suggesting an intracellular antibiotic.

Boh et al. (2004) found triterpenoid levels differ in different layers of the fungi.

Yihuai Gao et al. (2003) suggested that triterpenoids and polysaccharides of *Ganoderma* spp. are the major antivirals, and the polysaccharides are more antibacterial.

Polysaccharides from the mushroom were found to protect gastric mucosa by improving level of PGE2 and other parameters, suggesting the use of the tea in the treatment of ulcers.

Jung et al. (2005) found methanol extracts exhibit potent lens aldose reductase inhibition in vitro, and significant inhibition of serum glucose levels and sorbitol accumulation in eye lens, red blood cells, and sciatic nerves in diabetic-induced rats. Parallel work by Sanghyun Lee et al. (2005) found both methanol and ethanol extracts of the fruiting body exhibit potent aldose reductase inhibition, with IC50 being 1.7 and 0.8 micrograms per milliliter respectively.

Protocatechualdehyde is the most potent inhibitor of fractions found, with possible application to prevention and treatment of diabetic complications.

Byung-Keun Yang et al. (2007) found submerged mycelial extracts lowered blood sugar and cholesterol levels of diabetic rats by over 20 percent in a three-week study. Both alanine transaminase and aspartate transaminase were decreased by 23 percent and 20 percent respectively.

Fatty acids show activity against gram-negative bacteria (Moradali et al. 2008).

Another interesting study, by Davitashvili et al. (2008) found extremely high specific hemagglutinating activity in the biomass of *G. applanatum* after solid-state fermentation of lignocellulose. This suggests an opportunity for lectin production using wheat straw.

Work by Yong-Tae Jeong et al. (2008) found that both protein and carbohydrates significantly inhibited tumor growth and increased natural killer cell activity.

To sum up, artist's conk is antitumor, antiviral antibacterial, immuno-modulating, antidiabetic, anti-inflammatory, and may be useful in eye disease.

Varnish conk has been examined for its medicinal properties. Water extracts have been shown to inhibit the growth of sarcoma 180 and adenoma 755 in white mice. The inhibition rate of sodium hydroxide extract against the growth of sarcoma 180 is 77.8 percent.

Extracts have also been shown to enhance splenic natural killer cell activity and serum interferon production in mice (Won et al. 1992).

Jie Zhang et al. (1994) first reported the antitumor protein containing glycans from the fungi in 1994 .

E. J. Park et al. (1997) suggested that triterpenoids from the mycelium of *G. tsugae* show promise as liver protectives. In the same year, Wen-Huei Lin et al. (1997) identified the immune-modulating protein.

Protein extracts arrest human lung adenocarcinoma cells at the G1 phase.

Ganderic acid B provides protection from carbon tetrachloride-induced liver toxicity.

The following year, K. H. Gan (1998) looked at mediation of the cytotoxicity of lanostanoids and steroids of the fungi through apoptosis and cell cycle.

Recent studies by Huey-Jen Su et al. (2000) showed that various lanostanoids from this mushroom show significant activity against T-24, HT-3, and CaSKi cells.

Shi-Chung Hsu et al. (1998) found antitumor activity against colorectal and adenocarcinoma cancer cells in lab animals with no signs of physiological stress. One possible mechanism is induction of G_2/M cell cycle arrest.

The antioxidant and radical scavenging properties of *G. tsugae* were examined by Yen and Wu (1999). They found methanol extracts more potent than alpha tocopherol, exhibiting substantial inhibition of lipid peroxidation in a variety of tests.

Follow-up work by Jeng-Leun Mau et al. (2002) showed alcohol extracts extremely high in antioxidant activity, reducing power, free radical scavenging, and chelating abilities, slightly weaker, but comparable to its more famous cousin, reishi *(G. lucidum)*. Various phenols are believed responsible.

The fruiting body has been found to increase intracellular glutathione that protects cells from hydrogen peroxide influence (Wei et al. 2009).

X. X. Gao et al. (2000a, 2000b) found polysaccharides (F10-b) from the mycelium both anti-inflammatory and immune-stimulating. This seeming contradiction is dose-dependent and bi-directional suggesting a modulating effect on cytokine production. The production of interleukins is usually associated with an inflammatory response of the immune system, and yet this mushroom and reishi both enhance the immune system and reduce inflammation.

Tsugaric acid B is both anti-inflammatory and antioxidant (Ko, H.-H. et al. 2008).

Mycelia from submerged fermentation of *G. tsugae* and *G. lucidum* inhibit breast cancer cells via apoptosis and mitogenic effect, the latter via estrogen receptor modulation (Chiu et al. 2009).

Chiu et al. (2005) created an artificial fertile hybrid of *G. tsugae* and *G. lucidum*. The idea was based on prolonging the growing season. This hybrid gained anti-proliferative property on colon cancer cells, similar to reishi, in this in vitro study. Oral consumption by mice caused rapid hypoglycemic effect, and enhanced the recovery of ctyokine expression in carcinogen challenged mice. This hybrid vigor may be useful in areas challenged by northern climate. I would be interested to see if *G. applanatum* and *G. lucidum* could be hybridized.

The related sub-species *G. annulare* contains sterols, as well as applanoxidic acids that inhibit the growth of the fungi *Microsporum cannis* and *Trichophyton mentagrophytes* at five hundred to a thousand micrograms per milliliter (Smania, E. F. A. et al. 2003).

The related *G. adspersum* contains polysaccharides that possess immunomodulatory properties (Lakkireddy et al. 2006).

Varnish shelf *(G. resinaceum)* is a close relative of reishi *(G. lucidum)* and hemlock varnish conk *(G. tsugae)*, which it most closely resembles. Paul Stamets suggests that they all "represent a constellation of closely related species, probably stemming from a common ancestry." The polypore shows significant antioxidant activity (Al-Fatimi et al. 2005).

Recent work suggests activity against a trio of viruses, including Punta Toro and Pichinde viruses, and the H1N1 virus associated with swine flu.

The polypore shows 70 percent inhibition of 5-alpha reductase, related to the growth of prostate cancer. Turkey tail *(Trametes versicolor)* is a close second in terms of inhibition, suggestive of a good combination. It also inhibits aromatase associated with breast cancer growth, and is second only to button mushroom *(A. bisporus)* in this activity.

Both of these findings suggest more study for the control of hormone-sensitive cancers and the mechanisms involved.

Ganoderma oregonense, or western varnish conk, shows inhibition of *Staphyloccus aureus* and *Mycobacterium phlei* (Florey et al. 1949).

This is based on unpublished work by Muir from 1947, in which he identified the active substance as oregonensin. Overnight incubation showed inhibition of *S. aureus* at one to eight hundred thousand, *Mycobacterium phlei* at one to one hundred thousand. The active ingredient is quite unstable, as overnight incubation at thirty-seven degrees Celsius found no activity.

Waste from the fruiting bodies of *G. tsugae* was treated with potassium hydroxide and sodium hypochloride to produce a pulp-like white paste that was filtered and lyophilized to produce sacchchitin. Hung et al. (2001) at Taipei Medical University, conducted a six-month study on forty-seven patients with chronic skin ulcers. Approximately 85 percent of patients showed accelerated healing from the sacchachitin treatment. A proliferation and migration of fibroblast cells was noted at 0.01 percent weight per volume of sacchachitin.

Mycoremediation

The polysaccharides of *G. tsugae* in culture appear to be a soluble dietary fiber with some heavy metal detoxification potential, especially effective with copper and mercury, and suggesting mycoremediation potential.

Food Industry

Ganoderma applanatum has been used to cleave beta, beta-carotene into flavor compounds, and yields dihydroactinidiolide. Both *Trametes suaveolens* and *Kuehneromyces mutabilis* produce the same flavor (Zorn et al. 2003).

Artist's conk was inoculated into poplar shavings and incubated at twenty-five degrees Celsius. After four weeks, in vitro rumen digestibility improved to 64 percent, suggesting an alternative source of feedstuff (Reade et al. 1983).

Textile Industry

The fungi can be used for dyeing wool, yielding a dull yellow without mordant, and rust color with ammonia.

David Arora suggests large specimens be used for stools, tables, and shelving.

It was formerly used in Sweden for the manufacture of bottle corks.

More recent work found *G. applanatum* to increase digestibility of wood after decomposition (Zadržil et al. 1982).

Insecticide

Various native tribes use the fungus as mosquito and black fly smudges.

Recipes and Dosage

Weigh chopped fungus and add five times the amount, by volume, of 95 percent ethanol. For example, use one hundred grams to five hundred milliliters of liquid. Let this sit for two weeks. Strain and squeeze reserving the marc. Then make a one-to-twenty decoction of the marc at a slow simmer. Reduce by half. Combine 30 percent alcohol with 70 percent decoction for a 30 percent extract. Easy! This basic recipe may be used with any of the medicinal polypores.

Bits and Pieces

It is estimated that a large specimen releases up to thirty billion spores daily for six months of the year; or more than five trillion spores from a single fruiting body. This works out to twenty-one million spores per minute, and even at fifty tubes or pores per centimeter on the underside, this is a lot of activity. On a still, humid summer day, you can actually photograph the cloud of spores upon release.

Speaking of large specimens, the largest on record has a circumference of 311 centimeters, a height of eighty-one centimeters, and a weight of just over fifty-two kilograms. It was found in the mountains of Kuiu Island, southeastern Alaska, in 1951.

Artist's Conk

The legacy of your life may not be a great achievement or superior success. It may simply be the support you've provided to another whose completed canvas will be your finest eulogy—someone you helped perhaps when you were having tough times in your own life.

— G. Mohammed

Ganoderma lucidum

(REISHI)

(LING ZHI)

They dose themselves with the germ of gold and jade and eat the finest fruit of the purple polypore fungus.... By eating what is germinal, their bodies are lightened and they are capable of spiritual transcendence.

— Wang Chung, 100 AD

Ling zhi (ling chih) means "spirit plant" or "tree of life mushroom" in Chinese. During the Ming dynasty, the fungus was also known as chi zhi, meaning "red mushroom."

Zhi is an ancient name for various polypore mushrooms.

The Chinese character for ling zhi is composed of three calligraphic characters or pictures that together mean "shaman," "praying for," and "rain."

Reishi, meaning "divine or spiritual mushroom," is from the Japanese tradition, where it is also known as the phantom mushroom, or varnished conk. It may be related to the transformation of Buddha into rishi, meaning "forest sage." Another name, mannentake, means "ten-thousand-year mushroom," or "mushroom of immortality." The Japanese also know it as saiwai-take, "good fortune mushroom," or sarunouchitake, meaning "monkey's seat."

Ganoderma is from the Latin gan, meaning "shiny," and derm, meaning "skin." Lucidum also means "shiny" or "brilliant," due to the bright, varnished appearance.

The wild reishi is relatively rare, with almost all commercial products grown in sterilized environments.

It grows well on elm, alder, oak, and some strains are found on conifers. It is found rarely in the Pacific Northwest. The related G. tsugae and G. oregonense grow on conifers, such as hemlock spruce, while this one prefers hardwoods, especially maple.

Reishi (G. curtisii) is a rare yellow form of G. lucidum found growing on maple and other hardwood trees around the Great Lakes and St. Lawrence Seaway of Canada. It is fairly common in eastern North America.

The annual mushroom prefers hardwood hosts, and in Japan, it almost exclusively grows wild on plum trees. In parts of Southeast Asia,

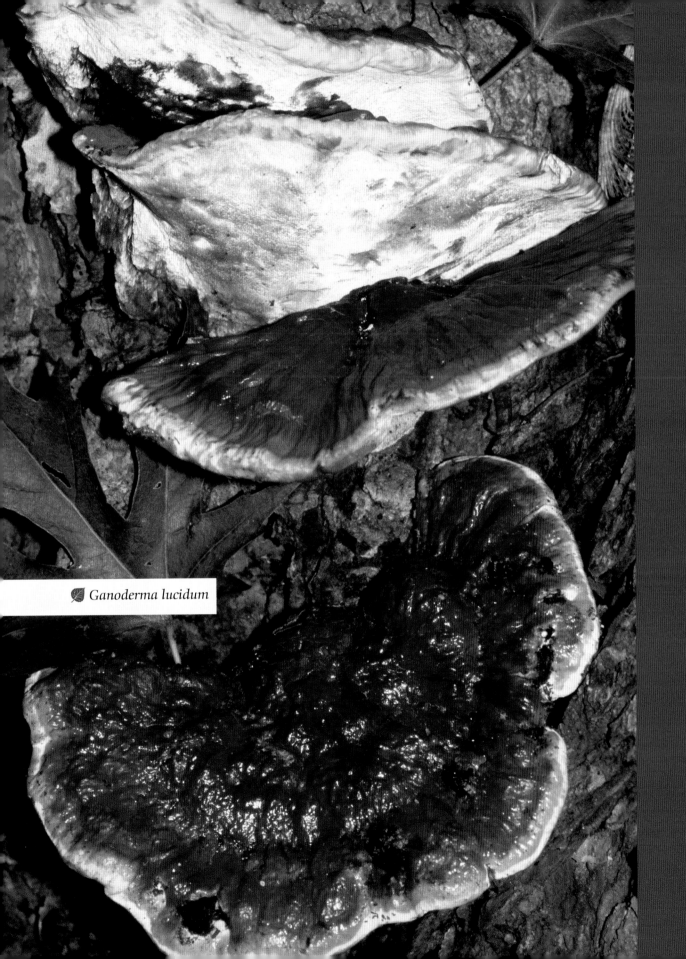

Ganoderma lucidum

the mushroom is commonly found on palm oil trees. The yellow reishi is known as *kishiba,* in Japan.

Cultivation

Reishi is now cultivated in fifteen countries worldwide with annual production of up to fifteen thousand tons. This compares with only two hundred tons just fifteen years ago.

The polypore is not native to my region, but under controlled conditions, reishi can easily be cultivated anywhere.

Solomko et al. (2005) found the husks of sunflower seeds a good alternative substrate for cultivating reishi, as well as shiitake, lion's mane, oyster mushrooms, and others. Potato malt peptones help to stimulate fruiting.

Culture and Folklore

In China, Japan, and other Asian countries, reishi has been used for at least four millennia for medicinal purposes. It is the most widely depicted mushroom in Japan, Korea, and China, and found on temple walls, tapestries, statues, and paintings. The Emporer's official scepter included a carving of a reishi mushroom, and the railings and archways of his residence in the Forbidden City and the Summer Palace depict the fungi.

Kuan Yin, the goddess of mercy and healing, is sometimes depicted carrying a reishi mushroom.

A textile from a first-century AD Mongolian tomb at Noin Ula displays this prized bracket fungus.

The polypore was prized and hung above doorways as a protector from evil. This is very similar to the use of *Fomitopsis officinalis* by shamans in British Columbia. The large fungi were carved and placed on the graves of native shamans to protect their spirits or souls.

Reishi is dried and displayed on mantels or hung on Christmas trees in parts of central Europe.

Traditional Uses

The relative rarity of the mushroom led to its use by those of privilege. Li Shih Chen, the famous sixteenth-century physician, spent twenty-six years writing *The Great Pharmacopoeia,* or the *Ben Cao Gang Mu.* In this text, he relates that the "continued use of *ling zhi* will lighten weight and increase longevity ... it positively affects the life-energy, or *qi,* of the heart, repairing the chest area and benefiting those with a knotted and tight chest. Taken over a long period of time, agility of the body will not cease, and the years are lengthened to those of the Immortal Fairies."

In traditional Chinese medicine, reishi is considered warming, astringent, nourishing, detoxifying, and of course, tonifying.

Reishi has been used traditionally for various liver ailments including chronic hepatitis, lung conditions like asthma and bronchitis, nephritis of the kidneys, nerve pain, hypertension, gastric ulcers, and insomnia.

A formula of various *Ganoderma* species, called Fructificato Ganodermae, has been used as a bronchial tonic for more than two thousand years. Reishi beers and wines are popular in Japan and China.

In 1912, Berthold Laufer wrote: "This fungus is a species of agaric and considered a felicitous plant, because it absorbs the vapors of the earth … as a marvelous plant foreboding good luck, it first appeared under the Han dynasty in 109 BC when it sprouted in the imperial palace. … A hymn in honour of this divine plant was composed in the same year."

In parts of China and Vietnam, the fungus was formerly used as a narcotic by pig thieves to reduce the squealing of poached porcine.

The adaptogenic properties of reishi are like panax ginseng, considered beneficial in stimulating sexual prowess and endurance, as well as balancing endocrine and hormonal levels. The gift of reishi, particularly in the rare antler form, was traditionally given in Asia to men by women, or a neutral courier, as an expression of sexual interest.

Medicinal Use

Chemical Constituents

- **Fruiting body: carbohydrates; amino acids including adenosine, steroids including ergosterols, protease, lysozymes, lipids, triterpenes, alkaloids, vitamins B2 and C, and various minerals including zinc, manganese, iron, copper, and germanium. May contain up to 40.6 percent beta-glucans. High levels of germanium have been found when cultivated using a bed log rich in the mineral.**

- **Mycelium: sterols, alkaloids, lactones, erogone, more than one hundred distinct polysaccharides, and 119 different triterpenoids. These include forty-five lanostane-type triterpenoids such as ganoderic and ganoderenic acids, ganolucidic acid, lucidenic acids, and lucidone. As the mycelium matures into fruiting bodies, the triterpene content increases.**

- **Spores: choline, betaine, palmitic and stearic acid, ergosta-7,22-dien-3b-ol, tetracosanoic acid, behenic acid, nonadecanoic acid, ergosterol, beta sitosterol, pyrophosphatidic acid, hentriacontane, and tetracosane.**

A large number of in vivo, in vitro, and human clinical trials have been conducted on reishi in China, Japan, and elsewhere. Both the mycelium and fruiting bodies contain valuable medicinal constituents and are often combined in products for the marketplace. The red variety, known in Japan, as *akashiba,* is the most prized of all, an observation now confirmed by clinical science. This red-colored variety is considered the most potent and medicinally beneficial.

Reishi has been shown to possess analgesic activity, general immune potentiation, muscle and central nervous system relaxation, cardiotonic activity, and liver and bronchial protection, as well as radiation protection (Chang, H.-M. and P. P.-H. But 1987).

Yun Seon Song et al. (2004) found extracts of the fresh fruiting bodies showed significant anti-angiogenic activity and inhibitory effect on inducible nitric oxide production.

A 1993 study at Shanghai University found reishi enhanced bone marrow nucleated cell proliferation, increased production of interleukin-1 in vitro, and increased white blood cells and hemoglobin in mice studies.

Enhanced natural killer cell activity, improved adrenocortical function, and anti-HIV activity were found both in vivo and in vitro by the researchers. Antiviral, antitumor, and antibacterial activity have all been found, due mainly to increased immune system activation.

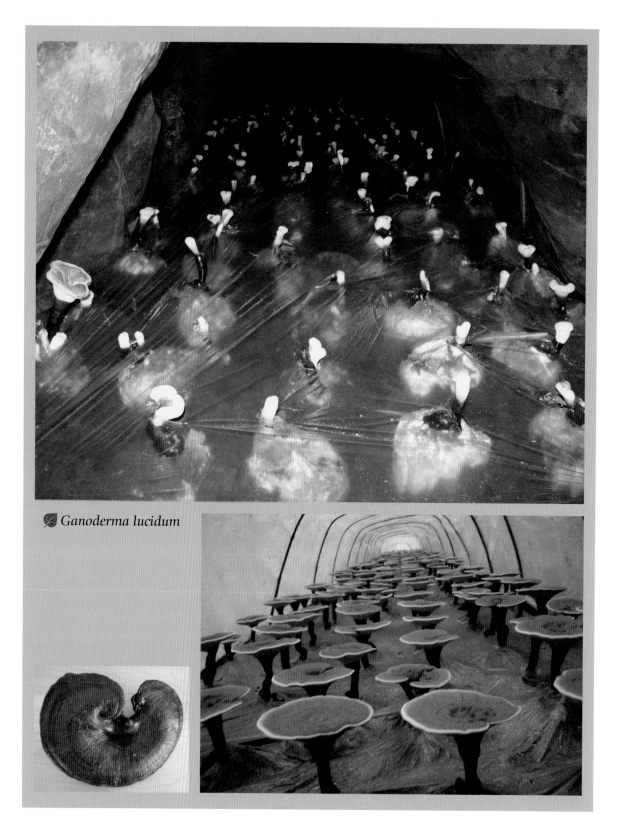

Ganoderma lucidum

Potent inhibition of HIV-1 at low level IC50 of 1.2 micromoles was found from extracts of fresh fruiting bodies at pH two to five at seventy degrees Celsius (158 degrees Fahrenheit) (Wang, H. and T. B. Ng 2006).

Water extracts show activity against *Bacillus, Micrococcus, Streptococcus,* and *Staphylococcus* species. Synergy between the fungi and cefazolin against *B. subtilis* and *Klebsiella oxytoca* was noted (Yoon, S. Y. et al. 1994).

Mice were fed reishi water extract for two days and then injected with *E. coli,* with 60 to 85 percent survival.

Reishi extracts help infertile men with chronic genital inflammation secondary to infection by human papillomavirus overcome this condition. The extract significantly reduces inflammation and improves sperm parameters. Reishi extracts inhibit HPV activity (Lai et al. 2010).

Reishi shows marked antioxidant properties, with super oxide and hydroxyl radical scavenging, as well as lipid peroxidation inhibiting activity, the three main measures of oxidative stress. The super oxide scavenging activity is significantly elevated. Bioactive peptides in the water-soluble fractions have been identified as contributors to the total antioxidative activity of reishi.

Jie Sun et al. (2004) recently identified bioactive peptides responsible for antioxidant activity. These peptides are easily absorbed through the human intestine, at rates 70 to 80 percent higher than free amino acids.

In a study by Wachtel-Galor et al. (2004), reishi supplementation was found to cause an acute increase in plasma antioxidant activity.

Jones and Janardhanan (2000) found extracts exhibit significant antitumor activity against solid tumor induced by Ehrlich's ascites carcinoma cells.

A recent mouse study by Rosalia Rubel et al. (2008) found immune-modulating effect against Sarcoma 180.

Yong-Tae Jeong et al. (2008) found reishi reduced formation of tumors by 40 percent and increased natural killer cell activity of splenocytes by 52 percent.

Cell division, or mitosis, progresses through a number of phases. Reishi helps assist the p53 checkpoint, where genes inspect and then act to destroy abnormal cells. This gene is often damaged in cancer cells, allowing abnormal cells to move on to the next phase and division. Melatonin and IP6 also play a role in helping assist normal functioning of p53.

Some scientists call p53 the guardian of the genome, or master gene. Bert Vogelstein, cancer expert at Johns Hopkins says, "You can call p53 the guardian because it's the common denominator in virtually all human tumors. It's almost impossible to develop cancer in most organs unless p53 is inactivated."

The gene has been the subject of more than three hundred thousand scientific reports since its discovery just twenty-five years ago. Despite this effort, the details of how p53 works are still not fully understood. The gene and protein are the center of a complex network of other genes that detect and prevent cancers. Members cooperate to stop a flawed cell from dividing in order to allow other proteins to try to repair the damage. If not, p53 triggers apoptosis, or cell suicide, eliminating any risk that the cell will turn cancerous.

Stanley et al. (2005) found that reishi inhibits prostate cancer-dependent angiogenesis by modulating MAPK and Akt signaling. This suggests therapeutic possibility for the treatment of prostate cancer.

The balancing effect of androgenic activity exhibited by reishi was noted in a study of nineteen edible and medicinal mushrooms (Fujita et al. 2005). Significant inhibition of 5alpha-reductase inhibitory activity suggests its use in benign prostatic hypertrophy and prevention of reproductive cancers. Similar results with ethanol extracts were observed by Ronghui Lin et al. (2009).

Daniel Sliva (2003) found that reishi demonstrates anticancer activity against breast and prostate cancer cell lines. They found the mushroom inhibits constitutively active transcription factors nuclear factor kappa B and AP-1, which resulted in the inhibition of expression of urokinase-type plasminogen activator and its receptor uPAR.

Urinary tract infections of long standing in eighty-eight males were helped by reishi in a double-blind, placebo-controlled, randomized trial (Noguchi et al. 2008).

A number of human clinical trials have shown efficacy in liver function and hepatitis. In one study of an herbal pill that included the fruiting body of reishi, 92.4 percent of 355 patients with hepatitis B showed positive results (Yan et al. 1987).

Another clinical report from Malaysia, in trials conducted at the MARA Institute of Technology, found mushroom extracts alleviated the symptoms of patients suffering hepatitis B. A significant reduction of serum glutamic oxaloacetic transaminase (SGOT) and serum glutamic pyruvic transaminase (SGPT) levels were found after three months.

In a clinical report by Lui at the same conference, seventy thousand hepatitis patients with "ganoderma detoxification and softening liver soup" showed a 90 percent success rate of improved liver health.

Yihuai Gao et al. (2002) reported on a randomized, placebo-controlled clinical study of hepatitis B patients. The twelve week trial reduced hepatitis B antigen and hepatitis B virus DNA levels in 25 percent of infected patients. After six months, 33 percent had normal aminotransferase value and 13 percent had cleared hepatitis B surface antigen from serum. None of the control patients had normal enzyme values.

Polysaccharides have been found to be effective against indomethacin-induced gastric ulcers, suggesting possible application in both prevention and treatment of peptic ulcers (Gao, Y. et al. 2004c).

The authors suggest that the polysaccharides and triterpenes are the major antiviral constituents and polysaccharides by themselves are important for antibacterial activity.

Triterpenes extracted with alcohol from the mycelium show inhibition of human hepatoma cells suggesting liquid fermentation techniques without the fruiting body have some antitumor use (Yue-Qing et al. 2005).

Ganaderiol-F, ganoderic acid beta, and lucidumol have been identified as antiviral components of reishi. Ganodermadiol is active against influenza virus type A and herpes simplex virus type 1.

Several mechanisms may be at work including some or all of the antioxidant and radical-scavenging activity, modulation of hepatic phase I and II enzymes, inhibition of beta glucuronidase, anti-fibrotic and antiviral activity, modulation of nitric oxide production, or maintenance of hepatocellular calcium homeostasis and immunomodulating effects.

In a study of seventeen medicinal and edible mushrooms, reishi showed the highest level of inhibiting aldose reductase, with significant decrease in galactitol accumulation (Fatmawati et al. 2009).

Muzushina et al. (1998) found two unique DNA polymerase alpha-type inhibitors in the fruiting bodies.

H. W. Kim et al. (2000) found fungus fractions inhibit interleukin-2 secretions, comparable to the effect of cyclosporine A, an immunosuppressive agent. This ability to inhibit proliferation of human blood lymphocytes, and block interleukin-2 secretion suggests immune modulation activity.

For some scientists and medical doctors, there is difficulty with the concept of immune modulation. In the pharmaceutical world, a drug either suppresses or stimulates the immune system. Most anti-inflammatory products suppress immune function.

Recent work suggests enteric mucosal immune response is an important pathway for immune modulation.

Autoimmune illnesses, such as rheumatoid arthritis and lupus, whether in the acute or chronic form, respond to immune modulation, opening a whole new world of treatment possibilities. In Japan and China, the mushroom is approved for the treatment of myasthenia gravis, a serious autoimmune disease. This comes back to the immune modulating effect that regulates and reduces excessive immune response when needed, and stimulates when deficient.

Triterpenoids and steroids exhibit anti-inflammatory activity and protect against UBV radiation.

Ganoderic acids A, B, G and H show stronger anti-inflammatory effect in one study than common aspirin (Koyama, K. et al. 2007).

Patients with diabetes, acute myeloid leukemia, and recurrent nasopharyngeal carcinomas were also found to exhibit positive results. Lovy et al. (1999) found reishi extracts reduced T4 leukemia cells in vitro.

Reishi mushroom helps lower elevated blood sugar levels. Early work by Hikino et al. (1985, 1989) found extracts of the fruiting body induced hypoglycemia in laboratory studies. Compounds such as Ganoderans B and C are involved.

My botanical buddy, Dr. Robin Marles, and his mentor, Dr. Farnsworth (1995), published a paper in *Phytomedicine* suggesting antidiabetic activity.

Yihuai Gao et al. (2004d) looked at patients with type II diabetes mellitus. This condition is reaching epidemic proportions in North America, with an estimated thirty million adults suffering late-onset diabetes. In this study, seventy-one patients with type II diabetes, not yet on insulin, were divided into groups and given either a placebo or reishi extract. Patients underwent four weeks of dosage adjustment and then eight weeks of dose maintenance.

The reishi group significantly decreased glycosylated hemoglobin from 8.4 to 7.6 percent in twelve weeks. Changes in fasting insulin, two hour post-prandial insulin, fasting C-peptide, and post-prandial C-peptide all showed significant improvement for the reishi group over the placebo group.

Shufeng Zhou et al. (2005) reported on several randomized, double-blind, multi-centered, and placebo-controlled reishi studies. In addition to hypoglycemic effect in type II diabetes, improved symptoms of coronary heart disease and neurasthenia were noted, as well as antiviral and liver protection in chronic hepatitis B infection.

Qi et al. (2009) reported that spore extracts are protective in sialoadenitis of non-obese diabetics.

Reishi has a special affinity for the lungs. In a 1986 study reported by Chang and But, more than two thousand patients with chronic bronchitis were given a reishi syrup tablet. From 60 to 90 percent of patients showed great improvement in only two weeks, along with increased appetite. Older patients, especially those with bronchial asthma, responded very well (Chang, H.-M. and P. P.-H. But 1986).

Fructificatio Ganodermae, mentioned above, has been clinically studied and found to alleviate symptoms of bronchial asthma, chronic bronchitis, and other allergy-related respiratory conditions. The active principle or even mode of action has not been identified, but is probably some combination of ganoderic acids, A, B, C_1, and C_2. Animal studies show that mediator release is inhibited, and yet suppressed at high dosage.

It definitely regulates immune response, but has no effect on Immunoglobulin E (IgE) antibody synthesis (Qiu and Wu 1986).

Animal studies show alleviation of allergic reactions and stabilizing immunoglobulin levels, whether low or high. Stabilizing antibody levels probably explains the alleviation of food sensitivities (Kohda et al. 1985).

Japanese researchers, in a 1988 study in *Agents and Actions,* reported that a sulphur compound, cycloctosulphur, inhibited histamine release from mast cells. This particular activity reduces allergenic reactivity associated with chronic bronchitis.

Reishi is cytotoxic to drug-sensitive and drug-resistant human small cell lung cancer and can reverse resistance to chemotherapy (Sadava et al. 2009).

Both clinical and empirical evidence suggests that reishi may be beneficial in patients with viral conditions such as Epstein-Barr Virus or HIV. Work by Hattori, presented at the First International Symposium on *Ganoderma lucidum* in Japan in 1997, found components inhibit HIV and protease activity. Ganoderic acid B inhibits with an IC50 value of 0.17 micromoles.

Acidic protein-bound polysaccharides from reishi have been found to inhibit herpes simplex virus type 1 and 2, responsible for cold sores and genital herpes outbreaks (Kim, Y.S. et al. 2000).

In one study, two patients with postherpetic neuralgia, and two others with severe herpes zoster pain, responded to hot-water extracts, in a dramatic and positive manner. The polypore has been found to help patients with coronary heart disease, and high blood cholesterol, with improvement of dyspnea, edema, and heart palpitations.

A controlled study found reishi extract reduced blood viscosity in patients with high blood pressure and hyperlipidemia. Some of the patients in this study were recovering from cerebral thrombosis, making the results even more striking.

Kanmatsuse et al. (1985) found reishi extracts helped reduce blood cholesterol and lowered hypertension. In this study 240 milligrams were given six times per day, and showed definite hypotensive effect.

A study of 103 patients suffering from coronary heart disease and angina for at least one year were given one gram of *Ganoderma* three times per day for four months at seven hospitals. LDL declined 68 percent, arrhythmia improved 60 percent, insomnia by 78 percent, and angina pectoris by 84 percent.

M. Kubo et al. (1983) reported on reishi's ability to increase fibrin degradation products and to inhibit blood platelet inhibition. This may explain, in part, the anti-inflammatory and anti-allergenic nature of the fungi.

This is due in part to the content of adenosine, also found in *Cordyceps,* wood ear, and shiitake mushrooms. A study of five HIV-positive hemophiliacs taking reishi mushroom extract found no difference in blood aggregation (Gau et al. 1990).

In a double-blind, placebo-controlled trial of fifty-four patients with stage II hypertension, reishi was found to be of benefit. All of the patients had received captopril (twenty-five milligrams three times per day) or nimodipine (twenty milligrams three times per day) for one month, and during this time their blood pressure remained above 140/90. They were then given fifty-five milligrams of reishi or placebo three times per day for one month, with significant lowering of both systolic and diastolic blood pressure over the control group (Jin, H. et al. 1996).

Some research indicates that ganoderic acids are responsible for blood thinning and lowering cholesterol levels. Hye-Seon Choi and Yu-Seon Sa (2000) found ganoderma protease is specific to thrombin and showed anticoagulant activity.

One 1990 Chinese study found that fifteen healthy people and thirty-three heart disease patients taking reishi tea showed reduced blood platelet aggregation, due in part to adenosine and guanosine content.

Arrhythmia relief and other cardiotonic benefit has been reported (Ding, G.-S. 1987).

Ryong et al. (1989) found anti-atherogenic and anti-atherosclerotic activity from reishi, shiitake, and matsutake.

Ganoderic acid B, C_2, D, and F have been found to inhibit angiotensin-converting enzyme (ACE) (Morigiwa et al. 1986); while ganoderic acid S prevents platelet aggregation (Su, C.-Y. et al. 1999). Various other ganoderic acids, as well as ganoderal A and B, are implicated.

Cancer research from Russia has shown positive results, according to Dr. Vladimir Kupin at the Cancer Research Center in Moscow. The extracts have been found to act as host defense potentiators. He has observed normalization of T-cells in Russian cosmonauts.

Shiu-Sheng Lee et al. (2003) found that

hot-water extracts exert an anti-tumor effect through potentiation of the immune system. This means that there is no direct cytotoxic effect, but a mediation of the immune response, enabling the body to defend and repair itself. They also found it works well in combination with cisplatin, adriamycin, fluorouracil, and other chemo-therapeutics.

Polysaccharides can reverse the multi-drug resistance by down-regulating the expression of MDR1 and MRP1 in adriamycin-resistant leukemic cancer cells.

A human clinical trial of 143 cancer patients was conducted by Yinhuai Gao et al. (2004a, 2004b). In this particular randomized, placebo-controlled study, thirty-eight (26.6 percent) of the patients had stable disease for twelve weeks or more when treated with a reishi extract.

A study at the Pritzker School of Medicine, University of Chicago, found both polysaccharide and triterpenoid fractions inhibit proliferation of human colorectal cancer cells.

Work by Jingsong Zhang et al. (2005) suggests reishi exerts antitumor activity by apoptosis as well as the immune pathway.

Calvino et al. (2010) noted activity against human leukemia cell lines.

The water extracts of the fruiting bodies of *G. lucidum* and *G. tsugae* inhibit proliferation of human breast cancer cells and induce apoptosis and mitogenic activity via estrogen receptor modulation (Chiu et al. 2009).

Reishi helps alleviate altitude sickness, combining well with roseroot *(Rhodiola rosea).* In the early 1980s, I hiked the Cordillera Blanca near Huancayo, Peru. Without coca leaf, it was difficult to breath and sleep at night at elevations higher than six thousand meters. I wish I had known about reishi in those days!

Steinert's disease, or myotonia dystrophica, is a relatively rare, inherited disease, characterized by muscular wasting, myotonia, and cataract. The progressive atrophy of muscle spreads from the face and neck to various glands and the entire body. There is no cure at the present time, but reishi has been found to alleviate symptoms.

Fu and Wang (1982) administered water-soluble spore extracts intramuscularly to patients suffering this debilitating disease. Many showed marked muscle strength improvement, reduced insomnia, improved appetite, and weight gain within two weeks. Speech and walking ability improved in many, and some patients who were previously unable to lift their heads were able to after treatment. Three cases of the disease ceased to progress, which is a remarkable and blessed event. The i.m. injection, called *jisheng,* has been used for used for myotonia and polymyositis for many years, helping improve sleep and appetite without the addictive nature of diazepam and other pharmaceutical hypnotics.

Recent work suggests reishi may have a role to play in osteoclasts and bone formation in association with osteoporosis.

Linghong Yu and Huailing Wei (2000) found water extracts of the spores showed hypnotic and sedative activity in mice.

The spores are used to treat liver and stomach cancer in China. The spores, which are really seeds, contain an abundance of *jing* energy, and are considered the elixir of life.

Not all research on reishi has been conducted in Asia. Pharmacology researchers at

Oral Roberts University School of Medicine, in Tulsa, Oklahoma found hypotensive effects were related to the mushroom's sedative effect.

Work by Stavinoha et al. (1995) at Texas Health Center in San Antonio found significant anti-inflammatory activity, similar to hydrocortisone.

Researchers at Indiana University, using a reishi product with cracked spores, found potent inhibition against breast and prostate cell proliferation. Other research at Methodist Research Institute found this same proprietary extract reduced invasion and metastasis of certain breast cells by inhibiting their adhesion, migration, and growth (Zhu et al. 2000).

Min et al. (2000) found spore triterpenes cytotoxic against Meth A and LLC tumor cells. Ethanol extracts of the spores also stimulate T lymphocyte activity. The germinating or cracked spores produce more anticancer cell activity than dormant spores.

The spores contain ganodermasides A and B that extend the replication life cycle of yeast in a manner similar to resveratrol (Weng et al. 2010).

Reishi shows the most significant inhibitory effect on NFkBeta activity in highly invasive breast cancer cells. Other mushrooms demonstrating breast cancer inhibitory activity are *Agaricus bisporus, Trametes versicolor, Grifola frondosa, Inonotus obliquus, Pleurotus ostreatus,* and *Sparassis crispa* (Petrova et al. 2005).

Work by Fujita et al. (2005) at Kyushu University in Japan found that of nineteen fungi, reishi exhibited the highest inhibition of 5-alpha reductase and anti-androgenic activity associated with prostate enlargement.

One study trialed reishi extracts on sixty-eight patients with advanced lung cancer. This randomized, double-blind, placebo-controlled, multi-center trial showed reishi stabled disease in 35 percent of lung cancer patients at twelve weeks, compared to placebo at 22 percent. Related symptoms such as fever, cough, weakness, sweating, and insomnia improved in 43 to 84 percent of reishi patients compared to 10 to 42 percent in controls. Further studies into optimal dosing, efficacy, and safety if used in combination with chemotherapy or radiation are needed.

Previous work on 143 patients with advanced cancers found that reishi extract significantly increased lymphocyte mitogenic reactivity to concanavalin A and phytohemagglutinin by 28 percent and enhanced natural killer cell activity by 25 percent.

Tian-Shung Wu et al. (2001) identified lucidenic acid A, methyl lucidenate, and ganoderic E compounds with cytotoxic effect on HepG2 and P388 tumor cells.

Water extracts of reishi show antimicrobial activity against *Bacillus subtilis, E. coli, Aspergillus niger,* and *Trichoderma viride.*

It is little surprise that reishi is so effective as a calmative, helping alleviate anxiety, insomnia, and nervousness associated with adrenal deficient conditions. It helps relax muscles and reduces the effect of caffeine on the body. It is known as "the mushroom of spiritual potency" by Daoist monks and other people seeking to improve their inner life. It can be helpful for addiction, gradually strengthening the nerves and protecting us on a physical, mental, and spiritual level.

Hence its other name, "the herb of good fortune."

Reishi appears to protect the brain from the harmful effects of beta amyloid associated with Alzheimer's disease.

The polysaccharides in reishi show higher anti-complementary activity than Krestin™ extracted from turkey tail mushrooms *(Trametes versicolor)*.

The related *G. capens* was found beneficial in the treatment of patients with alopecia areata. Nineteen cases of dermal myositis and multiple myositis were treated with this mushroom.

The related European *G. pfeifferi* contains sesquiterpenoid hydroquinones called ganomycins that inhibit MRSA or methicillin resistant *Staphylococcus aureus* (Mothan et al. 200). Whole extracts inhibit various microorganisms related to skin health, such as *S. epidermidis, Pityrosporum ovale,* and *Propionibacterium acnes.*

Spore Oil

The spores of *G. lucidum* are extracted by CO_2 super critical extraction. A 500-milligram capsule of the oil is nine times as expensive as a 300-milligram capsule of the spore powder, but is equivalent to twenty to forty of the powder capsules.

An adsorption column of powdered reishi was used as a polishing treatment unit and removed more than 95 percent of chromium within three hours (Krishna and Phillip 2005).

Cosmetics

Extracts have been found to lighten skin and protect against ultraviolet radiation, suggesting a useful addition to skin creams, lotions, and sunscreens and for the removal of so-called "age spots."

The rich mushroom oil, extracted from the fruiting body's waxes, is applied to warts, swellings, and in formulas to soothe coarse and chapped skin.

Ganodermenonol exhibits anti-histaminic action on the skin, while various sterols stimulate circulation. The unsaturated C14-C18 fatty acids help to moisturize the skin, as do various amino acids and octadecanoate, which stimulates surface cell immunity.

Various caprylic / capric triglycerides present in the oil can be used in moisturizing creams, day and night lotions, cleansing milks, and liquid soaps.

The Xhosa people of Africa call Ganoderma *isibindi,* the word for "liver," related to the dull red color, and use the powder to treat facial imperfections, acne, and as a sunscreen.

Recipes and Dosage

Tincture: five to ten milliliters three times per day. To prepare, see *G. applanatum* above.

Tablets: one one-gram tablet, two to three times per day with meals.

Capsules: three hundred milligram capsules of fifty-to-one extract, take one to three times per day, as needed.

Tea: take three to five grams of fresh conk, break into pieces, and boil for two hours, followed by steeping for another half hour. Drink one to two cups per day. If an instant powder is used, simply infuse in hot water as desired. It is believed that vitamin C helps the body better absorb reishi. Cancer patients taking nine grams per day of reishi and experiencing diarrhea found six to twelve grams of vitamin C per day eased the loose stools. Enzymes found in ginger and pineapple may be used for a similar benefit for patients who cannot tolerate vitamin C supplements.

Do not use before surgery due to its vasodilating effect. Women who suffer heavy menstruation should use with caution, at least during their period. Proceed with caution in patients taking ACE inhibitors.

Geastrum triplex

(COLLARED EARTHSTAR)
(SAUCERED EARTHSTAR)
(TRIPLE EARTHSTAR)
G. fimbriatum
(FRINGED EARTHSTAR)
G. hygrometricum
G. stellatus
Astraeus hygrometricus
(BAROMETER EARTHSTAR)
G. saccatum
(SESSILE EARTHSTAR)

> *Said mycologist Linda verbatim*
> *"When it comes to earthstars, I hate 'em"*
> *So asked by her Master*
> *To key a Geaster*
> *She growled out a curse, "fornicatum."*
> — UNKNOWN

Geastrum is from *geo* for "earth," and *astr* for "star." Triplex means "threefold."

This common ground mushroom is often found in large groupings in forests during the summer and fall. It looks like a puffball ready to launch off its three legged perch. Fringed

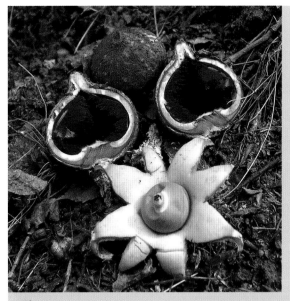

🍃 *Geastrum triplex*

and sessile earthstars are most common in the Pacific Northwest.

Its common name is derived from the way it splits open when mature with the rays bending back under the spore case.

Culture and Folklore

Considering their unique form and name, it is quite surprising that little folklore exists for the fungus. During the seventeenth century, a human-like form was drawn of *G. fornicatum* by Seger, who named it *Fungus Anthropomorphos*. Badham in 1863 alluded that this fungus aspired to occasionally leave this earth, but he may have just been musing about himself.

Traditional Uses

The Cherokee applied the powder spores of *G. triplex* to umbilical cords after childbirth, both to staunch the bleeding and prevent infection.

185

In traditional Chinese medicine, the earthstar is pungent, detoxifying, and tonic to the throat and lungs. It reduces inflammation in the respiratory tract and is mixed with licorice for sore throats, coughs, and laryngitis. The activity is anti-allergenic and anti-inflammatory.

The Mayans of Central America used earthstar spores for staunching wounds.

Fringed earthstar, or *G. fimbriatum,* is prepared like an egg curry in central India and eaten with rice or boiled eggs. It is known as *phutpura,* meaning "erupting out of the ground."

Water measurer *(Astraeus hygrometricus)* was at one time a popular item to foretell weather, as the radiating segments bend back in dry weather and straighten out when wet. *Geastrum hygrometricum* is hygroscopic, meaning it opens its rays to rainy weather, to encourage spore release. The dried sporophore is used to stop bleeding, relieve swelling, and reduce internal heat and fever.

Medicinal Use
Chemical Constituents

- **Barometer earthstar: a number of polysaccharides, including a glucan that combines the (1>6)-beta-D-glucan and the (1>4)-beta-D-glucan known to be so effective as antitumor agents in other fungi. It also contains ergosta steroids, as well as three triterpenes, astrahygrol, 3-epi-astrahygrol, and astrahygrone.**

Research shows purified polysaccharides from barometer earthstar enhance production of nitric oxide and cytokines, with binding on macrophage surface, followed by internalization. Phagocytosis increases two-fold (Mallick et al. 2009).

New work by the same author (2010) found a heteroglucan with potent antitumor activity that reduced tumor growth and apoptosis on Dalton's lymphoma cell lines.

Sessile earthstar *(G. saccatum)* was traditionally used to treat eye inflammation and asthma. Research has found the glucan proteins to possess antioxidant and anti-inflammatory properties by inhibition of nitric oxide synthase and COX.

The related *A. pteridis* contains lanostane triterpenes that show moderate activity against *Mycobacterium tuberculosis* (Stanikunaite et al. 2008).

Barometer earthstar showed immune-stimulating properties with macrophages from treated mice showing higher production of nitric oxide, interleukin-1 NK cell activation, and increased Th1 cytokine levels (Mallick et al. 2010).

Recipe and Dosage

Three grams to a liter of water. Decoct and take twice a day.

Gloeophyllum sepiarium

Lenzites saepiaria
(RUSTY GILLED POLYPORE)
G. trabeum
G. trabea
L. trabea
(POLYPORE de POUTRES)

Gloeophyllum sepiarium
A rhythmic mouthful of words
Every vowel is found if you look carefully;
A, I, O, U, Y and E.
　— RDR

Rusty-gilled polypore is usually found on dead pine, spruce, and fir, but occasionally on birch, where it causes much decay. It can be found on fence posts or other wooden structures in damp areas.

Paul Kroeger of the Vancouver Mycological Society told me he enjoys this mushroom because it contains all the vowels. Now you know!

Medicinal Use

Chemical Constituents

- *G. separium:* **15 alpha hydroxytrametenolic acid.**

- *G. trabeum:* **2,5-dimethoxyhydroquinone.**

Liquid cultures of both polypores have been found to inhibit the growth of sarcoma 180 in white mice.

Jong and Gantt (1987) showed anti-neoplastic activity, while Espenshade and Griffith (1966) found antitumor activity.

Early work by Robbins (1945) found weak activity against *Staphylococcus aureus,* in this species as well as *G. trabeum* and *G. odoratum (G. protractum).*

The *polypore de poutres (G. trabeum)* contains 2,5-dimethoxyhydroquinone, a compound with high antioxidant activity.

This conk plays a role in degradation of lignin as well as 2,4-D and PCP in solid-state culture (Jin, L. et al. 1990).

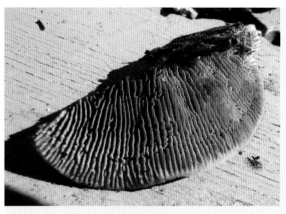

🌿 *Gloeophyllum sepiarium*

Sporophores closely resembling *G. sepiarium,* but found on mangrove wood in Florida, yielded six new sesquiterpenoids, four rearranged illudanes, one rearranged protoilludane, and one sterpurane (Rasser et al. 2000).

Gleophyllols B and C are weakly antifungal, while 1-hydroxy-3-sterpurene exhibits weak antifungal, antimicrobial, and cytotoxic properties.

The related *G. subferrugineum (Lenzites subferruginea)* is used in traditional Chinese medicine for smoothing out vital energy and removing damp conditions.

Rusty-gilled polypore has a slightly spicy odor, due to various unidentified essential oils.

Essential Oil

The related *G. odoratum* has been hydrodistilled and contains 46 percent of the aromatic compound methyl 4-methoxyphenylacetate, as well as linalool, 1-octen-3-ol, and trace of alpha-terpineol, geraniol, daucene, drimenol, and trans-nerolidol.

Fungal Essence

Conifer mazegill (*G. sepiarium*) essence is for sudden, abrupt, and irrevocable changes in life caused by personal trauma. It is when the old has to die and be replaced by something new.
— BAILEY

Mycoremediation

Rusty-gilled polypore mycelium secretes quinone reductases that break down many toxic wood preservatives, suggesting another mycoremediation opportunity. Watch out for accidental fungal infestation of that rosewood dash on your new Lexus or Volvo!

The related *G. trabeum* decays telephone poles, bridge structures, and even automobile woodwork.

Textile Industry

The dried polypore may be simmered with wool to yield a brownish-orange color without mordant.

Gomphidius glutinosus

(SLIMY PEGS)

Despite the name, this is a prized edible mushroom, often found under spruce. The cap is whitish-gray, the upper stalk white, and the lower bright yellow. The stem base should be discarded. *Glutinosus* is from *glutin* or "glue." *Gomphidius* means "a wooden bolt or nail."

David Arora writes, "The hideous *gomphidius* vies with the parrot mushroom, cowboy's handkerchief, and various slippery jacks for the title of 'slipperiest and slimiest fungus among us.' It is interesting to speculate on the function of the slime layer that coats the cap of these mushrooms, for it usually occurs on species with soft flesh. Perhaps it helps them to survive their humid environment. The slime may act like oil, repelling excess water and thereby ensuring that the crucial spore-bearing tissue matures before becoming waterlogged."

It has been found to contain xerocomic acid and gomphidic and pulvinic acid derivatives.

The related *G. viscidus* is used medicinally in China to cure neurodermatitis.

Essential Oils

Breheret et al. identified various monoterpene volatiles in slimy pegs. Alpha thujene, alpha and beta pinene, alpha fenchene, camphene, sabinene, beta-phellandrene, myrcene, 1,8 cineole, limonene, and linalool were all identified (Breheret et al. 1997).

Mycoremediation

Research has found it can myco-accumulate up to ten thousand times concentrations of radioactive cesium, making it a good candidate for tracking the movement of toxins from nuclear plants and other radiation sources. It may be useful to help clean up contaminated sites.

Work by Dr. Solomon Wasser and colleagues found up to 17,117 kBg/kg of cesium in wild specimens in Ukraine.

Gomphus clavatus

Cantharellus clavatus
(PIG'S EARS)
G. floccosus
Turbinellus floccosus
(WOOLLY CHANTERELLE)
(SCALY CHANTERELLE)

Pig's ears are large, firm-fleshed edibles with a mild taste. They are widely distributed under conifers in late summer.

Pig's ears are a suitable edible if pickled or otherwise prepared. Bill Richards, foray coordinator for the Alberta Mycological Society, and his wife Diane make a delicious pickled condiment with this plentiful mushroom.

Woolly chanterelle is not recommended due to severe gastrointestinal upset. I have noted some people eat it without problem, but I haven't been tempted.

Medicinal Use

It contains fatty acids that possess antifungal activity comparable to captan. It shows an inhibition rate of 100 percent against sarcoma 180 and 90 percent against Ehrlich carcinoma.

Other Uses

Pig's ears *(G. clavatus)* were screened for five selected extracellular hydrolytic enzymes and found to exhibit protease, amylase, phytase, carboxy esterase, and lipase activity (Goud et al. 2009). This is significant as these enzymes are widely used in the food, alcohol, paper, leather, and pharmaceutical industries and also have potential for use in biodiesel production and petrochemical degradation.

Grifola frondosa

Polyporus frondosus
Polypilus frondosus
Boletus frondosus
(HEN OF THE WOODS)
(SHEEP'S HEAD)
(MAITAKE)
(DANCING MUSHROOM)
(DANCING NYMPH)
G. umbellata
P. umbellatus
Dendropolyporus umbellatus
(UMBRELLA POLYPORE)
(ZHU LING)
(CHOREI-MAITAKE)
(TSUCHI-MAITAKE)

> *P. frondosus* is the color of smoke. It arises like a phantom from humus at the base of old trees, a ghost banquet, seemingly gauze-petaled, unsubstantial as mist, actually as heavy as a pumpkin.
> — WILLIAMSON

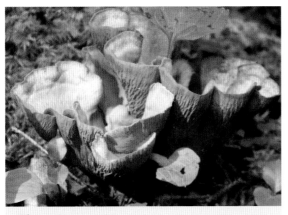
🌿 *Gomphus clavatus*

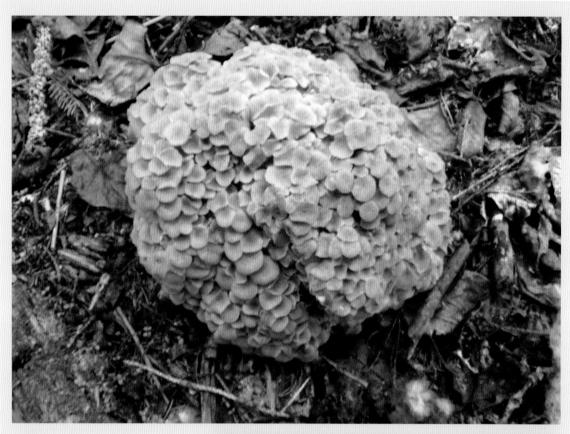

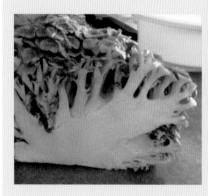

Above and below:
Polyporus umbellatus.
Right: *Grifola frondosa.*

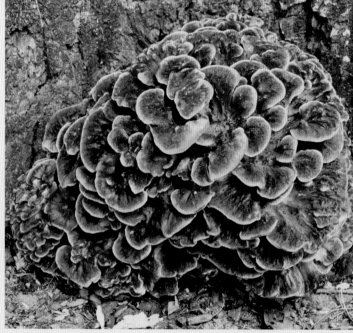

Grifola means "braided fungus," and is the name of another fungus from Italy. Some researchers believe the name is derived from *griffin,* the mythical beast with head and wings of an eagle, and the hind legs and tail of a lion.

Frondosa is Latin meaning "covered with leaves" or "leaf-like," while *umbellata* means "umbrella-like," both in reference to the fruiting bodies.

Maitake, in Japanese, means "dancing mushroom." Some believe the name derives from the shelved fruiting bodies that look like a wild butterfly dance. Others believe it is related to the joy of humans who find the highly prized mushroom, traditionally worth its weight in silver. During the feudal times of Japan, the local lords offered maitake mushrooms to the Shogun, and locals were paid the mushroom's weight in the precious metal.

Hen of the woods is a prized edible mushroom, found mainly in eastern North America. It has a sweet smell that becomes less pleasant with age.

It is one of our tastiest polypores, similar to eggplant in flavor, and usually found on stumps or the base of hardwood trees like oak.

They frequently weigh as much as ten kilograms (twenty-two pounds), resembling small hens covered with leaves. Specimens weighing up to forty-five kilograms (ninety-nine pounds) have been found in Japan. Before commercial cultivation was perfected in the late 1970s, the only source was from the wild.

In Japan, the locations were carefully guarded and known as "treasure islands." The secret location was, in some cases, never revealed by the forager during his entire life and then willed to his eldest son upon death.

In Asia, the mushroom extract is used in teas, tablets, drinks, and powders. Beelman and Royse (2005) have shown enrichment of substrate with sodium selenite can predictably enrich the mushroom with the health benefit of organic selenium.

Work by Qing Shen et al. (2002) suggests that Asian and North American maitake may be different species, based on DNA studies. This is not definitive, but suggests the need to work with the same cultivar when conducting clinical trials.

Umbrella polypore is circumpolar, and more common to eastern North America and Asia. In the summer of 2003, I found a large clump growing from a sclerotium in deep leaf litter of Manitoba maple in the ravine near my home. It may also be found under birch or willow, and there is one report of it growing under spruce in Montana.

It is a lighter color than maitake, and more tender, requiring less cooking time. It is delicious in cream sauce. In eastern France, umbrella polypore sites are protected and kept secret through the generations.

Work by Y. Y. Liu and S. X. Guo (2009) suggests that fructose and peptone ratios play a key role in sclerotial formation under cultivation.

In China, it is known as *Zhu ling* and has been used for thousands of years for its diuretic effect. The name means "hog tuber," due to the black sclerotium resembling pig's dung. A related name for the underground sclerotium is *jia zhu shi,* or simply *shi ling,* meaning "pig's droppings."

In Japan, it is also known as wild boar's dung maitake *(chorei maitake),* and Earth maitake *(tsuchi maitake).* In Korea, it is known as *jeoryeong.*

Cultivation

Work by Job and Schiff-Giovannini (2004) found simple sawdust and wheat straw substrate, complemented with nitrogen, is the best way to cultivate G. *frondosa* commercially. Other research indicates that 10 percent each of wheat bran, millet, and rye gives a short crop cycle, high quality fruiting, with good biological efficiency.

Skim milk added at only 0.2 percent to culture improves exopolysaccharide production by a significant amount (Huang, J. and W. S. W. Ho 2008). A pH of five also appears optimal.

Yukiguni Maitake Manufacturing Corp. has invested $120 million in a plant in New York State that processes thirty tons of fresh maitake mushrooms daily. The company is known as Mushroom Wisdom, Inc.

The spent sawdust substrate used in some production of maitake can be utilized to produce ethanol by saccharification and fermentation (Hideno et al. 2007).

Traditional Uses

The mushroom is found in numerous medicinal combinations, from both traditional Chinese medicine and the Japanese Kampo tradition.

In traditional Chinese medicine, maitake fruiting bodies are used for their diuretic, antipyretic, and anti-gonorrheal therapeutic activity.

It is commonly used for improving stomach and spleen conditions and hemorrhoids, and for calming the mind and nervous system. It also treats neuralgia, palsy, and various forms of arthritis.

Medicinal Use

Chemical Constituents

- **G. *frondosa*: ergosterol, ergostra-4,6,8(14),22-tetraen-3-one; 1-oleoyl-2-linoleoyl-3-palmitoylglycerol, as well as fatty acids such as palmitic, oleic, and linoleic acid; phospholipids, including phosphatidyl choline, phosphatydl serine, both lamarian type and curdlan type Beta-D-glucans and other polysaccharides including grifolin, grifolin-LE, MT-2, LELFD, and grifolan NMF-5N; beta 1,3 glucans with beta 1,6 branches and vice versa. If exposed to six to eight hours of sun after picking, the vitamin D_2 content increases from 460 IU to 31,900 IU per hundred grams.**

- **P. *umbellatus*: ergosterol, alpha-hydroxy-tetraconsanoic acid, biotin, polysaccharides Gu1-4, Ap1-10, 3,4-dihydroxybenz-aldehyde, aceto-syringone, and polyporusterones A-G.**

- **Sclerotium: makisterone derivatives, calcium oxalate, silica, and ergosterols. The highest levels of ergosterol, sugars and polysaccharides are found in two-year-old specimens. Another antitumor polysaccharide contains D-mannose, D-galactose, and D-glucose in the ratio of 20:4:1.**

Recent work by Yanjun Zhang et al. (2002) identifies COX-1 and COX-2 inhibitory activities, as well as antioxidant compounds in the fungus.

COX-2 is a key isozyme in the conversion of arachadonic acid to prostaglandin. The combination of COX-2 inhibitors with radiation or cancer prevention drugs has been reported of benefit to patients.

Studies show the mushroom contains antidiabetic constituents, as well as hepatoprotective properties. One randomized controlled clinical trial of thirty-two chronic hepatitis B patients showed 72 percent recovery rate in the *Grifola* group compared to 57 percent in the control group. More significant was the seroconversion from HBeAg positive to negative in 44 percent of the former, as opposed to only 13 percent of patients in the control group.

A study conducted at the Institute of Health and Environmental Medicine in Tianjin, China, found that D-fraction, in combination with interferon-alpha2b synergistically inhibits hepatitis B virus. Other studies suggest this same combination suppresses the growth of prostate cancer cells.

The dried powder, in lab studies, has been demonstrated to reduce hypertension. Human trials, on eleven volunteers with hypertension, were carried out at the Ayurvedic Medicine Center of New York in 1994. Although uncontrolled and non-randomized, the blood pressure, over six weeks, decreased by 7 percent systolic and 9.4 percent diastolic.

A newly identified compound, SX fraction, has been found to lower blood pressure, cholesterol, and blood sugar levels. These are all associated with Syndrome X, also known as the Metabolic Syndrome or the Insulin Resistance Syndrome.

This fraction is a glycoprotein, or more accurately an oligosaccharide-bound protein. The WS fraction, based on work by Dr. Preuss at Georgetown University, was the starting block for isolation of the SX fraction, which shows remarkable ability to restore normal insulin and blood sugar levels.

Alpha-glucan, isolated from the mushroom, has been found to influence insulin receptors and increase insulin sensitivity (Hong, L. et al. 2007).

A whole powder ether extract shows hypertensive lowering activity due to influence on the renin and angiotensin system (Talpur et al. 2002).

The D-fraction (a three-branched beta-1,6 glucan with 10 percent protein) is garnering the most attention for its interleukin-1-stimulating effect.

Polysaccharide fractions show anticancer and immune-enhancing factors. It appears to enhance the activity of macrophages, N-killer cells, and cytotoxic T-cells, with 86 percent inhibition of tumor growth (Mori et al. 1987).

Interleukin-1 that activates T-cells and superoxide anions that destroy tumor cells are both increased by the D-fraction.

A recent study in *Nutrition* looked at the D-fraction and its ability to enhance the tumor inhibition of Mitomycin-C, while reducing the immune suppression commonly found with this drug.

Noriko Kodama et al. (2002) found the D-fraction suppresses tumor growth via NK cell activity and induced IL-12 release from macrophages.

A sulphated proteo-glucan prevents HIV from killing T-cells in vitro. Research in both Japan and the United States has found maitake compares favorably with AZT for treating HIV, without the negative side effects.

The D-fraction was tested with thirty-five HIV patients over a long period of time, with 85 percent reporting improvement of symptoms and secondary diseases. Twenty of the patients showed increased CD4+ cell counts of 40 to 80 percent and eight patients showed a decrease of 20 to 50 percent (Nanba et al. 2000).

Other work by Ostram (1992) suggests it may stimulate the immune system of those suffering chronic fatigue syndrome.

Lovy et al. (1999) found the mushroom active against human T4 leukemia cells, HeLa cervical cancer cells, and *Plasmodium falciparum*

Various human clinical studies appear to demonstrate anticancer effect in lung, stomach, breast, colorectal, prostate, and liver cancers, as well as leukemia.

The mycelium shows potent activity against the MCF-7 breast cancer cell line (Cui, F. J. et al. 2007).

Human clinical work by Konno et al. (2002) found five patients with type 2 diabetes on oral medications improved glycemic levels with SX fraction caplets. A 30 percent decline in serum glucose levels was found after two to four weeks.

One seventy-five-year-old woman in the study had type 2 diabetes for six years. Average fasting blood glucose was around two hundred milligrams per deciliter, with a glycosylated hemoglobin of 9.1 percent under daily five milligram glyburide therapy. Upon taking three maitake capsules per day with her medication, FBG declined and remained at 110 to 130 for the next ten weeks. Her drug was then cut in half and still it stayed near 130.

A pleasant side effect of the mushroom extract is improvement in abdominal obesity, often associated with Syndrome X and poor insulin sensitivity.

In fact, one study by Dr. Masanori Yokota of thirty patients given two hundred grams of maitake daily (I assume this was fresh in their diets!), for two months, lost an average of eleven to thirteen pounds with no other dietary changes.

Maitake mushroom fractions improve insulin sensitivity (Preuss et al. 2007).

The D-fraction was found highly cytotoxic to prostate cancer PC-3 cells, with over 95 percent cell death in twenty-four hours. This in vitro test found the addition of vitamin C created a significant synergistic potentiation of D-fraction.

One study found maitake reduced the rate of bladder cancer recurrence after surgery from 65 percent down to 33 percent.

Other research has compared maitake, shiitake, and oyster mushrooms for the prevention of bladder cancer. All were very effective, but maitake was the most protective. The same experiment found mushrooms protect macrophages and lymphocytes from being numbed by carcinogenic exposure (Kurashige et al. 1997).

Maitake PET fraction shows antitumor activity against human prostate and bladder cancers. It also suppresses several canine tumor lines including lymph Cl-1, mammary CF33, and connective tissue CF21 (Griessmayr et al. 2007).

PSK, derived from turkey tail *(Trametes versicolor)*, works well in combination with chemotherapy, but maitake shows superiority to both this fraction and reishi extracts in terms of breast tumor growth inhibition.

Grifon-D, a highly purified beta-glucan shows significant activity against hormone-resistant prostate cancer cells. With the addition of vitamin C, the active dose necessary to kill the majority of cells is reduced by 83 percent; and regression of tumors in over 73 percent of patients with breast cancer, 66 percent with lung cancer, and 46 percent with liver cancer.

When interferon-alpha was combined with the D-fraction, growth of prostate cancer cells was slowed by 65 percent. It also reduced interferon to one-fifth of its original dose and was potentiated by D-fraction (Pyo et al. 2008).

In one Japanese study, conducted by Dr. Nanba, of 165 patients with advanced cancer, 90 percent of chemotherapy patients taking the mushroom extract experienced reduced side effects and 85 percent had reduced pain levels.

In a separate non-randomized clinical study of advanced stage breast cancer, tumor regression or significant improvement was found in eleven of fifteen patients (Nanba 1997a).

Other work by the same author found mushroom extracts increased the inhibition of metastasis of transplanted liver carcinoma by mitomycin from 51 percent to 87.5 percent when given together for ten days, compared to the drug alone (Nanba et al. 1997b).

Unhealthy intestinal flora produce D-galactosamine, associated with liver toxicity and inflammation. Testing for certain blood enzymes enables health practitioners to determine how badly the liver is damaged.

Researchers at Shizuoka University found maitake suppressed D-galactosamine in a dose dependant manner, suggesting it may help protect against the effects of bad nutrition (Lee, E. W. et al. 2000).

A study at the same university looked at the amount of blood flow to surface skin in mice, and found maitake may have benefit in cosmetics and skin medicine if applied externally to humans.

Hot-water extracts enhance immune health through induction of IL-8 production by blood monocytes that in turn activate neutrophils (Kodama, N. et al. 2010).

In combination with mitomycin, a chemotherapy drug, it inhibits the growth of breast cancer cells, even after tumors are well formed, and prevents metastasis to the liver. It appears to reduce the pain, nausea, and hair loss associated with chemotherapy.

Work by You et al. (1994) researched the combined effects of this mushroom with mitomycin on liver cancer, with good results.

Mushroom extracts may induce ovulation in women with polycystic ovary syndrome (PCOS). An open trial with eighty PCOS patients found it may be useful alone or as adjunct therapy for patients who failed first-line clomiphene citrate treatment.

The mushroom and drug were compared, with maitake showing tumor inhibition of 80 percent compared to 45 percent for the drug. When both were given together, however, but at half the dosage of each, the rate of inhibition was an astounding 98 percent.

The MD-fraction, combined with D-fraction, has been found of use in treating cancer, HIV, hypertension, hepatitis, and hyperlipidemia (Mayell 2001).

The submerged culture contains polysaccharides such as heteromanans, heterofucans, and heteroxylans. The extract showed marked activity in enhancing phagocytosis of human neutrophils, complement receptor 3 was primed, and NK cell cytotoxicity increased. These relatively low molecular mass polysaccharides, 43-140 and 13-38 kDa, may serve as biological response modifiers.

A case history, reported in *Alternative Therapies,* May/June 2001, by Dr. Eric Scheinbart, is worth noting. "A fifty-six-year-old patient with multiple myeloma and antibiotic resistant pneumonia was presented. Three unsuccessful bone marrow transplants followed three whole-body irradiations. Despite transfusions, red blood cell and platelet counts continued to decline, as did kidney function. Fifteen months later, he was admitted to hospital with vanomycin resistant pneumonia, and told to go home and 'get his affairs in order.' At his family's request, he began taking two droppers full three times daily of maitake D-fraction liquid, along with herbs and nutritional supplements. Within one week he was feeling better and ambulatory. In two months he was pronounced 'miraculously in remission and without pneumonia.' Two years after original diagnosis the patient was playing golf."

Mice studies by Ohtsuru et al. (2000) showed anti-obesity results, but only from the unheated powder. Weight loss was significantly diminished when the powder was heated to 140 degrees Fahrenheit (sixty degrees Celsius) and over, with no results at the boiling point.

Maitake appears to promote absorption of micronutrients by the intestine, making it a potentially useful transport mechanism for herbal combinations.

The mushroom was only available as a wild harvest until cultivation techniques were developed in 1979. In Japan, nearly sixteen million pounds were cultivated in 1990. From 1988 to 1997, the production and consumption rates increased forty-one-fold worldwide.

Paul Stamets notes that vitamin D in mushrooms grown indoors and dried is only 460 international units, but soars to 31,900 international units when the mushrooms are first placed in the sun. This is a significant finding.

Vitamin D_3 receptors are found throughout the body regulating gene expression and healthy function of the nervous and immune systems. It stabilizes the structure of chromosomes and prevents DNA strand breakdown. It induces apoptosis, or programmed cell death in cancer cells, and is anti-proliferative against breast, prostate, bladder, and colon cancers, and inhibits tumor angiogenesis and invasion, helping prevent cancerous growth.

Water extracts of the fruiting body have been found to be anti-angiogenic by blocking vascular endothelial growth factor (Lee, J.-S. et al. 2008).

One study found that maitake may be of benefit in osteoporosis and osteopenia, as well as the later complications associated with diabetes.

Cold-water extracts act as ACE inhibitors, suggesting use in cardiovascular disease.

Maitake appears to be of benefit in sebaceous lipogenesis, suggesting usage in pustular acne or lipomas (Nagao, M. et al. 2009).

It would appear that induction of alpha defensins 1-3 are involved in the protection from infection afforded by the fungi (Kuvibidila et al. 2010).

Zhu Ling or Umbrella Polypore

Zhu ling, or umbrella polypore, is used in traditional Chinese medicine for edema, scanty urine, and various damp heat conditions such as jaundice, diarrhea, and vaginal discharge.

The sclerotium is used for stagnant dampness exhibited by edema and urinary difficulties such as cystitis. It has been found effective, without side effects, for treating pyelonephritis, nephritis, and urologic calculi.

Some studies suggest the fungi may used to prevent kidney stones.

Clinical trials indicate hepato-protection, as well as support for kidney and respiratory weakness.

The underground sclerotium of *zhu ling* contains beta 3 and 6 glucans, with proven antitumor activity.

Its effect is similar to ethacrynic acid, a diuretic drug that causes potassium depletion. *Zhu ling* spares this mineral, making it a safer alternative.

When U.S. researchers visited Beijing in 1983, they were told that the fungal tea was given to lung cancer patients after radiation. Most of these patients recovered in a few years, while a high percentage of control patients died.

One study, conducted in 1957, showed decoctions increased the six-hour urine output by 62 percent, and chloride output by 55 percent in healthy volunteers; probably due to inhibition of electrolyte and water reabsorption by the renal tubules.

One study found that the polypore can promote a better diuretic effect and cause urinary bladder filling faster than a placebo.

Recent work by Guowei Zhang et al. (2010) suggests the diuretic activity is due to down-regulation of aquaporin-2 that, in turn, down-regulates vasopressin 2 receptor.

Both in vivo and in vitro studies have shown antitumor activity against sarcoma 180 and other cancers (Ito, H. et al. 1973).

Various human studies appear to indicate improvement in hepatitis and lung cancer therapies, combining well with chemotherapy, and resulting in better appetite, weight gain, and mental alertness, as well as reduction of leukopenia.

The mushroom extracts appear to increase production of IgM and strengthen phagocytic activity, while improving macrophage activity and proliferation.

Cachexia is common in cancer patients, and associated with loss of weight, muscle atrophy, fatigue, weakness, and loss of appetite. Work by Geng-Shu Wu et al. (1997) found polysaccharides in the mushroom that inhibit cachexia induced by toxohormone-L, which suppresses food and water intake, promotes anorexia in patients, and suppresses a compound secreted by tumors that breaks down fatty acid tissue and uses these compounds to grow new cancer cells.

Various polysaccharides have been shown, in vivo, to be anti-neoplastic, due to a nonspecific immune-stimulating or potentiating activity.

Some studies indicate antitumor activity. One polysaccharide extract remarkably enhanced the effect of other antitumor agents, and suppressed the spontaneous metastasis of Lewis lung sarcoma.

When the sclerotium was combined with mitocycin, the lifespan of mice with tumors was increased (You et al. 1994).

Makisterone derivatives, from ethanol extracts, show inhibition of L-1200 leukemic cells.

The fruiting body contains sterones with cytotoxic activity, showing reduced proliferation of leukemia 1210 cells (Ohsawa et al. 1992).

Mice studies have shown protection against ionizing radiation, with a survival rate of 75 percent for those treated forty-eight hours before exposure, compared to 2.5 percent in the control group.

Sekiya et al. (2005) found triterpenes from the fruiting body that exhibit significant free radical-scavenging effect.

Inaoka et al. (1994) looked at eighty Chinese herbs for hair growth activity. *Zhi ling* placed third, due in part to a unique compound with anti-inflammatory activity.

H. Ishida et al. (1999) found 50 percent alcohol extracts of the mushroom exhibited hair growth activity. Polyporusterones have been isolated and identified (Zheng, S.-Z. et al. 2004).

Maybe the author, who has been follicly-challenged since age twelve, should try it!

Ergone has been found to have an anti-aldosterone diuretic effect, helping balance sodium and potassium levels (Yuan, D. et al. 2004).

Alcohol tinctures exhibit antibiotic effect against both *E. coli* and *Staphylococcus aureus*.

One clinical study found mushroom decoctions showed a 92 percent improvement in patients with liver ascites.

The benefit of *P. umbellatus* in treating chronic viral hepatitis was shown in a clinical study.

In this three-month study, 50 percent of patients showed improvement in ALT enzyme levels. Combining it with red sage *(Salvia spp)* improved this figure to 80 percent. Another study found a combination of the fungus and red sage *(S. miltiorrhizae)* effective against chronic hepatitis. After treatment, 69 percent of patients became HBeAg negative.

The mushroom stimulates bile production, which explains, in part, its benefit in lowering blood cholesterol levels (Sugiyama et al. 1992).

One ingredient, 5alpha,8alpha-epidioxyergosta-6,22-dien-3-ol, is a potentiator of ADP-induced platelet aggregation (Lu, W. et al. 1985).

Lee et al. identified ergosta-4,5,8 (14), 22-tetraen-3-one ergone from the sclerotia. This ergone showed activity against a range of human cancer cell lines including colon, cervix, liver, and stomach, with particular cytotoxic activity against liver and cervix cell lines (Lee, K.-A. et al. 2005).

In further tests, the highest amounts of ergone were found in only two other mycelium, matsutake and maitake, at thirty-eight micrograms per gram. This suggests further study.

Masauda et al. (2006) identified the MZ fraction that possesses antitumor activity. It increases TNF and IL-12 production in clinical trials.

The sclerotium has been found to reduce postoperative recurrence of bladder cancer to 34.9 percent versus the control group's 64.7 percent.

Chlamydia infects an estimated fifty million women each year. It is a bacterial sexually transmitted disease that does not always respond well to pharmaceutical drugs. J. J. Li et al. (2000) found this mushroom to possess inhibitory activity on this nasty STD.

Homeopathy

Grifola frondosa (maitake) is used in neoplastic conditions, diabetes mellitus, hypertonia, and for immune system stimulation.

Dose: ten drops per day of 5C under the tongue before meals. A commercial product, Grifosan or Grifokehl 5X, is available from Germany.

Insecticide

Lovy et al. (1999) found strains of *zhu ling* 100 percent effective against the malarial parasite *Plasmodium falciparum*. Paul Stamets, who was involved in supplying the specific strain, suggests that mycomulch, or wood chips infused with mycelium, could be placed in malaria-infected swamps. This would serve to both consume the parasite and secrete antimicrobials into the environment.

Recipes and Dosage

G. frondosa powder: three to seven grams daily of *G. frondosa* powder.

Capsules: two five-hundred-milligram capsules two to three times per day.

Tincture: fifteen to thirty drops three times per day

D-fraction liquid: up to six milligrams twice a day. Vitamin C increases efficacy of all preparations.

P. umbellatus: decoct six to fifteen grams in one pint of water. Combine with marshmallow root if used for longer than three to four weeks, due to its drying nature. Do not use either mushroom if there is absence of dampness. *Zhu ling* should not be used for extended periods of time as it dries and exhausts bodily fluids and may injure the kidneys.

Maitake extract dose is weight-dependent with half to one milligram per day per kilogram (or per 2.2 pounds) of body weight. That is, an adult weighing 220 pounds (100 kilograms) would take fifty to one hundred milligrams daily. A woman weighing 150 pounds would take thirty-four to sixty-eight drops of tincture daily.

Caution: maitake increases production of interferons, including gamma interferon, that may promote the destruction of nerve damage and aggravate neuromuscular diseases such as multiple sclerosis.

Gymnopilus spectabilis

G. junonius
Pholiota spectabilis
(LAUGHING MUSHROOM)
(LAUGHING JIM)
(GIANT GYMNOPILUS)
(BIG GYM)
(FIERY AGARIC)
Gymnopilus liquiritiae
(BITTER GYMNOPILUS)
(FIR LICORICE GYMNOPILE)
G. sapineus
P. sapinea
(SPRUCE/FIR GYMNOPILUS)
(SCALY RUSTGILL)
G. luteopilus
(GOLDEN GILLED GYMNOPILUS)
G. aeruginosus
G. harmoge

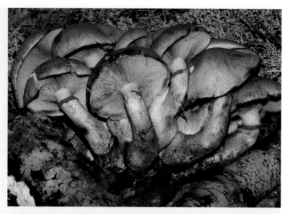

Gymnopilus spectabilis

You should try to give
King Emma several of
The "laughing mushrooms."
— KOBAYASHI ISSA

If you eat *o waraitake*, you cannot stop laughing.
— JAPANESE SAYING

Spectabilis is from the Latin meaning "spectacular."

Gymnopilus is from the Greek meaning "with naked cap." *Sapineus* is Latin for "of spruce," and *luteofolius* for "golden yellow gills."

It is known in Japan as *o waraitakae*. In some texts it is known as *Pholiota spectabilis*.

Laughing Jim lives on the dead wood and bark of deciduous trees, although it is sometimes found on spruce. It could be mistaken for a honey mushroom, as it has a light brown color and grows in clumps around the base of trees. However, it turns green upon cooking, which helps greatly in identification, and is quite bitter and unpalatable.

Arora states that the mushrooms in the West are inactive in terms of hallucinogenic effect.

The very common *G. ventricosus* does not appear to have hallucinogenic properties.

He suggests, however, that the related *G. aeruginosus,* with its blue-green cap when young, is hallucinogenic.

Laughing Jim contains bis-noryangonin (4 hydroxy-styryl-2-hydroxy-4-pyrone) related to the psychoactive ingredients in kava kava. This has been identified in various *Pholiota* and *Polyporus* species.

In Japan, a number of different fungi are responsible for the effects of laughing mushroom including *G. spectabilis, Panaeolus papillionaceus,* and *Psilocybe argentipes.*

Waraitkae (*P. papillionaceus*) is said to be a hallucinogenic mushroom used by Portuguese witches.

An oak growing *G. junonius* is reported in ancient Greek texts to cause clairvoyance, and could be included in the list of possible "laughing mushrooms." In parts of Europe, the young specimen is considered edible, but I wouldn't try it.

Adrian Morgan trialed the mushroom on several occasions, and only once experienced enhanced color vision, with colors floating off objects and hanging in air, with a feeling of euphoria. He states that the effect is like the combined elements of psilocybin and muscimol. Two caps were lightly fried and eaten in this instance, whereas the fresh fungi produced no effect.

Elio Schaechter, cited below, was a consultant for the Boston Poison Center. One day he received a call from an elderly lady who "in the midst of giggles lost no time in coming to the point and wanted to know if she and her dinner guests were about to die" after ingesting *G. spectabilis* mushroom. He suggested they were not in real danger, to which she replied, "You mean, we are not going to die [giggle, giggle]? Goodbye, then!"

Menser, in his *Hallucinogenic and Poisonous Mushroom Field Guide* (1977), mentions research at the University of Washington that identified the presence of bis-noryangoin. This compound is an analogue of yangonin, a weak psychoactive substance found in kava kava. Be careful with this mushroom!

G. liquiritiae is a yellow mushroom that lives in groups on dead conifers; and can be found in the summer and fall.

Culture and Folklore

They encountered in the wilderness a group of four or five Buddhist nuns who were dancing and singing and perceived them to be demons because of their erratic behavior. Upon questioning the women, they were told that these were indeed nuns who had strayed, and, becoming hungry, had roasted and eaten some mushrooms, whereupon they began to laugh and dance about.

The woodcutters were both astonished and hungry. The nuns readily shared their mushrooms, and all became giddy, laughing and dancing about together. The mushrooms were called from that time on maitake or dancing mushrooms.

— ELEVENTH-CENTURY FOLKTALE

Medicinal Use
Chemical Constituents

- *G. spectabilis:* **gymnopilin, cerevisterol (4,6, -decadiyne-1,3,8-triol), bis-noryangonin, ergosterol, ergosterol peroxide, galactitol, gymnopilene (a polyisoprenepolyol), and choline. Psilocybin has been found in some *G. spectabilis* from Michigan.**

In Japan, the mushroom is known as *waraitake,* and has been reported to contain many metabolites. The gymnopilins extracted exhibited a depolarizing activity (neurotoxicity) against rat spinal cords.

It has an inhibition rate against sarcoma 180 of 60 percent and against Ehrlich carcinoma of up to 70 percent.

The related *G. liquiritiae* shows inhibition of 80 percent and 90 percent respectively; and *G. aeruginosus* shows 60 percent inhibition for both.

It possesses anti-carcinogenic activity with inhibition rates of 80 to 90 percent against cell lines.

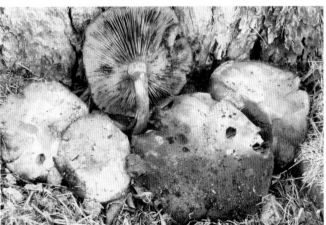

Gymnopilus spectabilis

201

The related *G. aeruginosus* is found mainly on the Pacific side of the Rockies. It has a distinctive blue-green flesh and bitter flavor. It is a definite hallucinogen.

Spruce and golden gilled species contain minute amounts of psilocybin. The former shows activity against *Staphylococcus aureus* (Hervey 1947).

Personality Traits

My first thought when I closed my eyes was actually that I had opened them. I became aware of wide open spaces when I closed my eyes and various curving patterns in pinks. . . . The patterns seemed to be in perpetual motion and to be alive, that is, I sensed they had pulse of their own. . . . My body began to feel numb or as if it were a body but not necessarily my own. This I experienced in a more poignant way when I turned over on my stomach in bed and caught a glimpse of my hand, which had some marks from the pillowcase on it.

It seemed to me the hand of a very aged person and I was startled. I felt some fear and so turned my hand with the palm facing me. It seemed so fleshy and white that I thought of a mushroom and immediately of mortality. I saw that I was made of flesh and that this was corruptible. Yet as I looked at my hand I saw it as a hand, not mine but one lent to me as it were to use in this life. It was meant to help me and I felt great pity on it because it was after all made of flesh and as prone to decay as mushroom flesh.

I craved something raw and colorful so went to the crisper and took out two bright fuschia-colored radishes, and first set them on the table. How much they seemed like sperm or tadpoles, the way their central root shot out like tails. They look comical and I wanted to laugh. . . .

— SCHAECHTER

Gymnopus confluens

Collybia confluens
(TUFTED COLLYBIA)
(CLUSTERED TOUGH SHANK)
C. maculata
Rhodocollybia maculata
(SPOTTED COLLYBIA)
(SPOTTED TOUGH SHANK)
C. dryophila
G. dryophylis
(JUNE MUSHROOM)
(RUSSET TOUGH SHANK)
Collybia radicata
Oudemansiella radicata
(BEECH ROTTER)
C. butyracea
R. butyracea
(BUTTER CAP)
(BUTTERY COLLYBIA)
C. conigera
C. friesii
Baeospora myosura
(CONIFER CONE CAP)
C. tuberosa
(TUBEROUS COLLYBIA)
C. cirrhata
(PIGGYBACK SHANKLET)

Gymnopus is from the Greek *gymos,* meaning "naked," and Latin *pus* for "to rot or stink."

Collybia is from the Greek meaning "a small coin" while *dryophila* means "oak-loving," a misnomer as the mushroom grows under many different trees. *Confluens* means "flowing together." *Maculata,* from the Latin, means "spotted."

Recently, some *Collybia* have been moved to the *Gymnopus* and *Rhodocollybia* genera, just as I was learning the old names!

Because *Collybias* are often misidentified there is a caution regarding edibility. I don't bother personally.

All *Collybias* have caps that are coated with fine, mealy granules. Tufted *Collybia* is often found in spruce forests in clusters, with a red-brown to tan cap that shrivels when dry.

Spotted *Collybia* has a whitish cap and stalk with red stains. It is found solitary or in groupings of two and three in pine forests.

June mushroom *(C. dryophila)* is widespread, growing in forest leaves and debris, under deciduous trees. Some authors say it is edible, but several severe gastrointestinal sufferings have been recorded. Not worth it!

Beech rotter is found in eastern North America under hardwood trees.

Both *C. cirrhata* and *C. tuberosa* have been reported to produce luminescence in germinating sclerotia. They grow on dead fungi and are widespread.

Butter cap, also known as spotted tough shank, is edible, and found under pine. It contains various alkaloids.

Collybia conigera grows on the cones of douglas fir.

Medicinal Use

Chemical Constituents

- ■ *C. confluens*: **collybial.**

- ■ *C. maculata*: **6-methyl purine, 6 methyl-9-beta-D-ribofurno-syl purine, and 6-hydroxy methyl-9-beta-D-ribofurnosly purine.**

C. confluens was studied by Simon et al. in Holland in 1995. They found that collybial, a constituent, is structurally related to koraiol, a sesquiterpenoid from *Pinus koraiensis*. Collybial has been found to inhibit gram-positive bacteria, as well as vesicular stomatitis virus in kidney cells.

Submerged mycelial cultures significantly decreased plasma glucose levels by 26 percent in diabetic rats, as well as total cholesterol and triglyceride levels by over 20 percent in a three-week study (Yang, B. K. et al. 2007).

Inhibition against sarcoma 180 and Ehrlich carcinoma cell lines is 70 percent and 80 percent respectively.

C. maculata contains a number of interesting substances, including 6-methyl purine, 6 methyl-9-beta-D-ribofurno-syl purine, and 6-hydroxy methyl-9-beta-D-ribofurnosly purine. These have been found to be antifungal, antiviral, and cytotoxic, including activity against vesicular stomatitis viruses in BHK cells.

Production of exopolysaccharides from this mushroom in fermentation tanks has been found greatly increased with the addition of toluene (Lim, J. M. and J. W. Yu 2006).

Studies indicate that June mushroom is bacteriostatic against *Bacillus cereus*. Early work by Hervey (1947) found activity against

Staphylococcus aureus. The related *C. marasmioides* exhibits similar activity.

Pacheco-Sanchez et al. (2006) identified a polysaccharide with powerful anti-inflammatory activity. It is similar in structure to shiitake as a 1>3,1>4 beta-D-glucan.

Follow-up work by the same authors found the inhibition of nitric oxide was consistent with decreases in both inducible iNOS protein and mRNA expression (Paheco-Sanchez et al. 2007). This suggests that it exerts its effect by inhibiting iNOS gene expression. At concentrations of four hundred and eight hundred micrograms per milliliter, the polysaccharides show significant increase in prostaglandin E2 production in LPS and IFNgamma-induced macrophages compared to control.

Parish et al. (2004) identified ene-triyne compounds in *Collybia conigera* that show potent activity against gram-positive bacteria. Activity against *Staphylococcus aureus* was only 0.001 micrograms per milliliter MIC, suggesting a powerful substance.

When grown in fermentation tanks, beech rotter produces a liquid that contains oudenone. When injected intra-abdominally in white rats, it lowers blood pressure in a powerful manner.

The mushroom inhibited the growth of sarcoma 180 by 100 percent and Ehrlich carcinoma by 90 percent.

Fungi Essence

Clustered tough shank *(C. confluens)* essence enlarges our radius of perception by stimulating our "mental antennas." We become more sensitive to subtle energies, receiving this information by using our hair as "physical antennas."

— KORTE PHI

Gyromitra esculenta

(FALSE MOREL)
(ELEPHANT EAR)
G. montana
(SNOW MOREL)
G. caroliniana
(BIG RED)
G. infula
(HOODED FALSE MOREL)

Prized in Nordic countries
For the species means to eat
The False Morel is boiled and boiled
To make a mushroom treat.
It looks just like a giant brain
A clue for every fool,
For this mediocre edible
Is packed with rocket fuel.
— RDR

Thus, like rockets, MMH-containing mushrooms have the potential of moving the human body from an early existence to heaven.
— JOHN TRESTRAIL

Gyromitra is Greek meaning "round head covering," due to its twisted, contorted shape. *Esculenta* means "edible."

The genus *Gyromitra*, especially false morel (*G. esculenta*), is found in beds of lichen in the spring, under jack pine. It is considered poisonous, although it is eaten in some parts of the world, such as in Finland, after cooking.

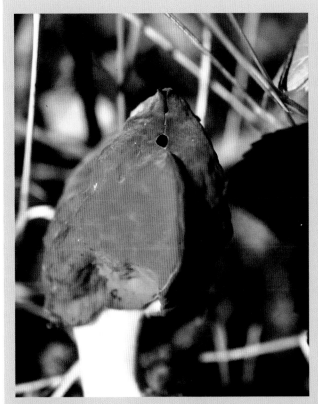

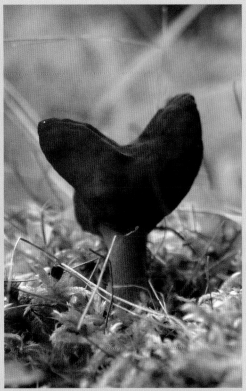

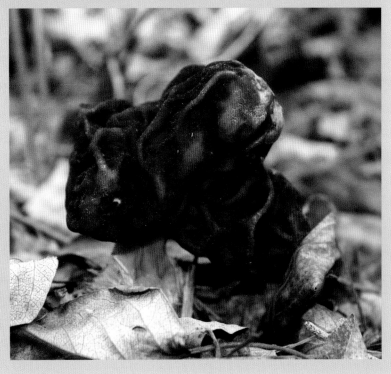

🍃 Above (left and right): *Gyromitra infula*. Right: *Gyromitra esculenta*.

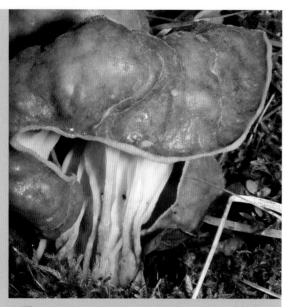

Gyromitra sphaerospora
(Pseudorhizina sphaerospora)

Big red is common throughout Missouri, Iowa, Kansas, and elsewhere. Not recommended.

In 1988, more than 109,000 kilograms (about twenty-four thousand pounds) of false morels were sold in the Finnish marketplace. They are still very popular. Anyone selling false morels has the responsibility to tell customers about the toxic effects of the mushroom and provide instructions on how to cook it. Despite this, the mushroom is still prohibited from sale in both Germany and Switzerland.

In Sweden, it is sold in cooked and canned form in supermarkets. In that country, about two hundred cases of poisoning a year are reported, with few fatalities.

Gyromitra is considered an edible mushroom that sometimes kills. John Trestrail gives this advice: "Persons who decide to continue this gastronomic gamble should have the numbers of their regional poison center permanently engraved on their eating utensils."

The mushroom's toxicity can be variable; most deaths occur after the consumption of raw or insufficiently cooked mushrooms. In spite of its extensive ingestion, serious cases of poisoning are relatively rare. In 2003, seventy-one reports of poisoning from gyromitrin-containing fungi were reported in the United States, with only one fatality.

The volatile constituents are 72 percent oct-1-en-3-ol, a compound that carries the distinct and prized odor. Nine separate volatile N-methyl-N-formyl-hydrazones (MFHs) have been identified from fresh false moral mushrooms, at an average combined level of fifty-seven milligrams per kilogram.

They contain gyromitrin that hydrolyzes to form the toxin, monomethyl-hydrazine (MMH), a substance that affects the central nervous system. Under pH and temperature conditions mimicking the human stomach, monomethyl-hydrazine readily forms, suggesting a carcinogenic and acutely toxic health hazard.

MMH has been employed as a rocket fuel, and gyromitrin-type poisoning was noted in the early days of the aerospace industry. It has a boiling point of 87.5 degrees Celsius (189.5 degrees Fahrenheit) and rapidly dissipates into the atmosphere of a well-ventilated kitchen.

Even drying the mushrooms in an enclosed area can cause nausea and headache. MMH can even be absorbed through unbroken skin.

The toxin is volatile and water-soluble, and the fungi may be made edible by drying or boiling. I don't think they are worth the risk.

Studies in Finland indicate that after prolonged drying, the level of hydrazine residue fell below three milligrams per kilogram, and a boiling time of ten minutes was required to reduce the level below one milligram per kilogram. A change of water and second boiling is even better.

Tests conducted on chickens in a short-term test showed no effect at 0.05 milligrams of MFH. For a seventy-kilogram (154-pound) human, that would translate into 3.5 milligrams; and using a safety factor of one hundred, this would be 0.035 milligrams, the amount contained in only five grams of dried false morel. Caution is advised.

The most active form of B6, pyridoxal 5-phosphate, has been used to antidote *Gyromitra* poisoning and exposure to hydrazine.

MMH interferes with B6, leading to reduced GABA levels, impaired neurotransmission, and neurotoxicity. Pyrodoxine chloride (B6) five times daily at doses of ten milligrams also relieved gyromitrin poisoning.

Work on a cultivated, low poison, or poison-free strain is a possibility, given that the mushroom has been cultivated successfully under glass.

It is known, from studies in Finland, that warmer temperatures reduce the concentration of toxins.

The related snow morel *(G. montana)* is considered edible when cooked. I will pass.

Medicinal Use

A tincture is prepared with vodka at one part dried, powdered mushroom to fifteen parts vodka and used in Latvia as an analgesic rub for osteochondrosis, heel spurs, polyarthritic joints, and the like.

It is said to be useful for pancreatitis, but I cannot verify this.

Homeopathy

Symptoms include wanting to fight; demanding answers; dryness of eyes, nose, and lips; restless sleep; weight gain; and swelling.

Dreams of flood, of rolling stones, accidents, people transforming into owls, vampires, rockets, and traveling to stars.

Symptoms are closest to *Bovista* (wants to fight; epistaxis; dryness; swelling; worse from wine. Some resemblance with *Sticta* (dryness of nose; boring into nose with fingers; knee joints) and *Agaricus* (pains crosswise; penetrating coldness).

Dose: 12C to 30C. This proving was conducted by Bert Breuker and students on nine females. Three of the provers received placebo and had no reactions.

— Vermeulen

Hapalopilus nidulans

H. rutilans
(TENDER NESTING POLYPORE)
(NEST BRACKET FUNGUS)

Mainly found on hardwood trees in Western North America, it is sometimes found on conifers in the west.

Early work by Hervey (1947) found activity against *Staphylococcus aureus*.

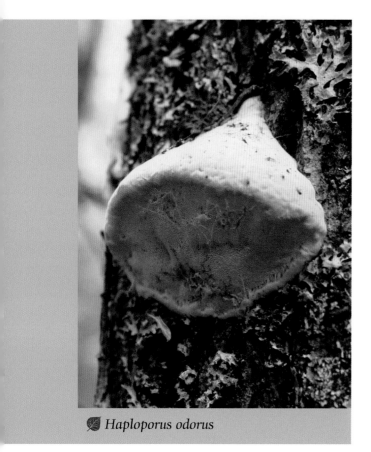

Haploporus odorus

Haploporus odorus

(DIAMOND WILLOW FUNGUS)

Diamond willow fungus has a great deal of special significance to the native people of the northern plains and boreal forest. It grows specifically on diamond willows, and the fungus' size is directly related to the diameter of its host tree.

Traditional Uses

The Cree call it *wiy(h)kimasiygan,* or *wasask-wetiw,* while their northern neighbors, the Chipewyan, know it as *k'ai tlh'elht'are* (willow tinder).

It is smudged as part of special ceremonies, and with its special coumarin/anise-like odor, it is very pleasing to the mind and body. It is a special gift given to healers conducting sweat lodges, as the fungus is believed to guard and protect against unseen forces. The smoke is used in blessings and as part of cleansing and empowerment events.

It was traditionally used to decorate sacred war robes and scalp necklaces as a symbol of spiritual power and protection. It was also used as a part of medicine bundles.

It is considered to have protective powers when taken in infusion that will stop diarrhea and dysentery; or it can be combined in decoction with Indian breadroot (*Psoralea esculenta*) to treat coughs. The smoke is inhaled for treating headaches, or the fresh conk squeezed for juice to treat earaches.

It is a styptic for wounds, making it very valuable in both accidents and battle.

I have often used it as a mosquito smudge when camping in summer. It definitely adds a brightened and vivid element to the dream state. I collect larger specimens, when I find them, as gifts for elders and spiritual leaders.

The smoke is inhaled through the nostrils twice every five to ten minutes for the treatment of migraine headaches.

The Blackfoot wear a white fungus the size of a tennis ball around their neck; while it has often been mistaken for a puffball, it is actually carved diamond willow fungus. It can also be found attached to robes and blankets.

Mors Kochanski supplied diamond willow fungus to Robert Blanchette, at the University of Minnesota. He compared these samples

208

with museum pieces from the Glenbow, to confirm his findings. It is very similar to *Trametes suaveolens* found on aspen poplar and willow, but is a distinct species.

Bruno Boulet, in *Les Champignons des Arbes*, mentions the use of *H. odorus* in parts of Siberia and the Ural Mountains for religious cermonies. *Haploporus suaveolens* may be the same fungus.

Medicinal Use

Morita et al. (1995) identified cryptoporic acid derivatives and similar compounds, such as haploporic acid, from this bracket fungus. See *Cryptoporus volvatus*.

Hebeloma sacchariolens
(SWEET SMELLING POISON PIE)
(SCENTED HEBELOMA)
H. crustuliniforme
(POISON PIE)
H. mesophaeum
(VEILED HEBELOMA)

Hebeloma is from the Greek meaning "with obtuse or rounded margins," or *hebe* meaning "youth" and "loma" meaning "fringe." *Sacchariolens* means "sweet" and *crustuliniforme* is Latin for "the shape of a cookie or pie."

Poison pie is distinguished by its distinct radish odor, and scented *Hebeloma* by a smell variously described as burnt sugar, cheap scented soap, or orange flowers.

They are toxic and should be avoided. Martin Osis has warned me more than once against picking these beautiful looking mushrooms for the dinner table.

Medicinal Use

The related *H. versipelle* contains a lanostane triterpenoid cytotoxic against various cancer cell lines HL60, A549, SGC-7900, and Bel-7402 with low IC_{50} values (Shao et al. 2005).

Mycoremediation

Nussbaum et al. (1997) found the fruiting bodies of *H. sacchariolens* reduce anthranilic acid and some of its analogues to corresponding aromatic aminoaldehydes with a very high efficiency. Anthranilic acid is used in the manufacture of dyes and drugs, and is a common pollutant of waterways in areas where factories manufacture these compounds. Some type of mycofiltration may be possible.

Poison pie *(H. crustuliniforme)* growth was stimulated by up to five hundred micrometers of calcium, while cadmium at twenty-five parts-per-million had no effect on growth (Willenborg et al. 1990).

It reduces the concentrations of cesium in white pine seedlings (Brunner et al. 1996).

Veiled *Hebeloma*, found in northern coniferous forests, has been found to be an excellent inoculant, from either spores or mycelium, of pine forests. It is also useful for mycoremediation.

The related *H. cylindrosporum* and several *Suillus* species degrade chloropropham in culture. This would be exciting news considering the amount of chlorinated herbicides on our planet.

Helvella acetabulum

Paxina acetabulum
(BROWN RIBBED ELFIN CUP)
H. crispa
(FLUTED WHITE HELVELLA)
H. lacunosa
(FLUTED BLACK ELFIN SADDLE)

This mushroom is found under mixed forest. It is sometimes parasitized by *Mycogon cervina*, another fungus. Wilhelm et al. (2004) isolated and identified two petaibols that possess weak bacterial and cytotoxic activity.

Fluted white *Helvella* is common to damp cool patches of the boreal mixed forests of the Pacific Northwest. It is said to be edible, but is indigestible to some people. *Helvella* species may contain small amounts of the toxin MMH found in false morels. Not worth it!

Puttaraju et al. (2006) found it contains significantly high levels of phenolics, 35.5 milligrams per gram in water extracts.

It rated very high among the twenty-three mushrooms tested for free radical scavenging.

Fluted black elfin saddle fruiting bodies contain an alkaline serine protease called helvellisin (Zhang, Guoking et al. 2010).

Hericium

Hericium ramosum
H. coralloides
H. americanum
(COMB TOOTH)
(BRANCHED HERICIUM)
(CORAL HEDGEHOG)
(BEAR'S HEAD TOOTH)
H. erinaceus
H. erinaceum
Hydnum erinaceum
(LION'S MANE)
(POM POM MUSHROOM)
(MONKEY HEAD)
H. abietis
(CONIFER CORAL MUSHROOM)

Hericium means "hedgehog" from the Latin. *Erinaceus* is named after the European hedgehog, *Erinacius eruropeus*. *Ramosum* means "branched." *Coralloides* means "coral-like," in reference to the distinct shape. *Abietis* is in reference to the genus *Abies* that includes both balsam and alpine fir.

Comb tooth must take the prize for most distinctive and beautiful fungi of the boreal forest. It is white, branched, and covered with a multitude of teeth that looks like ocean coral or spongy icicles.

It is edible and delicious sautéed in butter, especially when young, and is one of Laurie's absolute favorites. In fact, I often get to slip away to pick mushrooms on the off chance I will bring some of these home.

Scientists have discovered an interesting compound, erinacine, found to be a kappa opioid receptor-binding inhibitor. These are potent

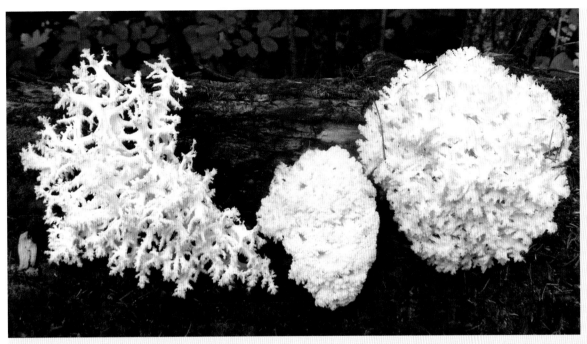

🍃 *Hericium coralloides* (three different structures on the same tree)

anti-convulsants that can be neuro-protective in epilepsy and stroke, as well as brain and spinal cord injuries.

There is considerable taxonomic confusion between *H. americanum, H. coralloides,* and *H. ramosum.* The latter species is believed by some authors to be the fungus formerly named *H. coralloides,* while the first mentioned is considered the new name for *H. coralloides.* Very confusing. On some forays, I have found the brain-like dense version on the same tree as the loose branched ones. I pick them all.

Here is my suggestion. The denser fruiting body may be considered *H. americanum,* the sparser *H. coralloides,* and drop *H. ramosum* altogether. The debate may go on for years. David Arora says that the exact identity doesn't concern him, so I'll leave it at that.

Coral hedgehog and comb tooth are found on hardwood species. According to some authors, *H. coralloides* is found on both coniferous and hardwood trees. I have not seen conifer coral *Hericium* on the plains, but lots on douglas fir trees in British Columbia.

The Gitksan name is *kaedatsots,* meaning "bird hat" or "hat of bird." Paul Stamets calls it a brain food that increases intellect and nourishes the nervous system. It is easy to inoculate conifer logs with plugs, sawdust, or rope spawn.

In Japan, lion's mane is known as *yamabushi-take. Yamabushi* means literally "those who sleep in the mountains," and relates to hermit monks from the Shugendo sect of ascetic Buddhism. The mushroom is said to resemble the *suzukake,* or ornamental garment, worn by these monks, and hence the name. In China, it is known as *shishigashira,* meaning "lion's head," or *houtou,* meaning "baby monkey." Again, there is some controversy with some authors separating *H. erinaceus* and *H. erinaceum* into different species and other authors contending that they are one and the same. Oh please! It is found on oak from California north, but also on beech and maple.

Lion's mane is delicious, with a texture similar to seafood, and is therefore grown commercially on a small scale. When served in French restaurants it is called *pom pom du blanc,* due to the off-white color and shape resembling pom pom balls on the end of stocking caps or toques.

Cultivation

Research suggests that the best medium for growing the fungi commercially is fine beech sawdust with 20 percent wheat bran.

Poyedinok et al. (2005) found that exposing mycelium to helium neon and argon laser irradiation increased growth, shortened the phases of mushroom development, produced more vigorous mycelium, and increased fruit body yields from 36 to 51 percent in work on lion's mane, oyster, and shiitake.

One study found that treating pine with extractive degrading fungi such as *Aureobasidium spp., Ceratocystis spp.,* and *Ophiostoma spp.,* removed 70 to 99.9 percent of extractives. The treated wood chips were then used to cultivate *H. erinaceus,* as well as *Grifola frondosa* and various oyster species.

Those wishing to grow the mushroom medicinally, should note that twenty-six degrees Celsius (seventy-nine degrees Fahrenheit) is the optimal temperature, at 50 to 70 percent humidity, and that carbon dioxide levels can significantly increase growth.

Those interested in liquid culture will find a pH of five, at twenty-five degrees Celsius (seventy-seven degrees Fahrenheit) optimal. The best yields in fermenter cultivation are with twenty grams inoculum per liter of nutrient solution. In two weeks, nearly five hundred grams per liter can be realized. Contamination must be carefully controlled.

Many substrates can be used for *Hericium* species production. For mycelium growth, barley bran was best for *H. alpestre, H. lanciniatum,* and *H. erinaceus,* while *H. americanum, H. coralloides,* and *H. erinaceum* grew better on soybean powder (Ko, H. G. et al. 2005a).

Sunflower seed hulls have been used successfully with a fifty-five-day cycle of growth from inoculation (Figlas et al. 2007).

Hericerin has been found to inhibit pollen growth (Kimura, C. et al. 2005).

The spent compost has been studied for industrial enzyme use, and found to contain alpha amylase (229 nanokatals per gram), cellulase (759 nanokatals per gram) and beta-glucosidase (767 nanokatals per gram) (Ko, H. G. et al. 2005b). This suggests use in mycoremediation.

Traditional Uses

Lion's mane is used in traditional Chinese medicine for digestion and curing gastric ulcers. It has a tonic effect useful for treating neurasthenia and general debility.

Mycelium from various *Hericium* species, extracted with hot water, has been used in a sports drink called Houtou. This was used in the Eleventh Asia Sports Festival in 1990, and believed responsible for several victories.

Various native tribes carried the dried powder in medicine bags as a styptic for cuts and wounds.

Coral hedgehog is used to cure gastric ulcers and has a tonic effect on digestion and the treatment of neurasthenia and general debility.

Medicinal Use

Chemical Constituents

■ *H. erinaceus:* **beta-glucoxylan, glucoxylan, 31 percent protein, galacoxyloglucan protein, hericonene A and B (phenols), 240 international units of calciferol per hundred grams, 381 milligrams ergosterol per hundred grams, polyhydroxysteroids include cerevisterol; six ergostane derivatives including 3 beta, 5 alpha, 9 gamma-trihydoxy-ergosta-7,22-dien-6-one; 3 beta-glucopyranosul-5 alpha, 6 beta-di-hydroxyergosta-7,22-diene, xylan, and glycoxylan. Cyathane derivatives are believed the nerve growth stimulators. Also contains the aromatic compounds erinacerins A and B.**

Lion's mane contains five polysaccharides and polypeptides that enhance the immune system and show significant inhibitory effect on sarcoma 180, as well as cancers of the stomach, esophagus, and skin.

Ingestion of the mushroom in dried pill form has been found to extend the life of cancer patients.

Okamoto et al. (1994) showed antifungal activity against both *Aspergillus niger,* and the yeast *Saccharomyces cervesiae,* and identified antimicrobial chlorinated orcinol derivatives

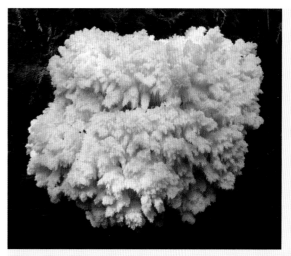

🍃 *Hericium coralloides*

from the mycelium. Kawagishi et al. have a U.S. patent (5,391,544) on cyathane derivatives of this mushroom, after finding it effective against aggressive HeLa cells.

Takashi Mizuno (1999) has identified Y-A-2, a newly discovered fatty acid component with pollen tube growth-inhibiting activity, something shared with *Hercein.* This author has long been looking at this particular fungus, having identified lion's mane antitumor polysaccharides (Mizuno, T. et al. 1992b).

An increase in interleukin-12 and interferon was found using water extracts on mouse splenocytes. This suggests indirect activation of natural killer cells.

Both phenols, Hericenone A and B, appear to be directly active against cancer cells.

The mycelium is used in China to make pills for treating gastric and duodenal ulcers, as well as chronic gastritis.

It produces curative effect on both gastric and esophageal carcinoma. One study found freeze-dried fruiting bodies provide cytoprotection against ethanol induced gastric ulcers in rats.

Lion's mane is immunomodulating, a nerve tonic, and useful in chronic bronchitis (Wasser and Weis 1999).

It is not directly chemotherapeutic, but works by stimulating the immune system, which, in turn, helps control the growth of tumors.

When combined with doxorubicin it treats otherwise drug-resistant human hepatocellular carcinoma (Lee, D. et al. 2010).

Son et al. (2006) found water extracts induce iNOS gene expression followed by NO production in macrophages via enhancing the activation of transcription factor NFkappaB.

One study found it increases human dendritic cells and reinforces host innate immune system function.

Nagai et al. (2006) identified di-linoleoyl-phosphatydl-ethanolamine as a compound that reduces ER stress and protects neuronal cells.

Hericenones C-H, from fruiting bodies, have been found to induce synthesis of nerve growth factor (NGF), which is required by the brain for developing and maintaining important sensory neurons. This may be useful in the amelioration of Alzheimer's and other similar chronic nerve/brain related diseases (Kawagishi et al. 1991). The low molecular weight compounds pass through the blood-brain barrier intact.

Another class of cyathane derivatives from the mycelium, called erinacines A-I, induce NGF production (Kawagishi et al. 1994).

Methanol extracts stimulated an increase in NGF in human brain astrocytoma cells but not the isolated erinacines (Mori et al. 2008).

Kawagishi et al. (2004a) make a strong argument for the use of lion's mane for dementia. He suggests that erinacines are the most powerful inducers of NGF synthesis among all currently identified natural compounds.

A study of one hundred patients in a rehabilitation hospital in Japan looked at the effect of five grams of lion's mane mushroom or placebo in their soup for six months. These patients were elderly and suffered from cerebrovascular disease, degenerative orthopedic disease, Parkinson's disease, spino-cerebellar degeneration, diabetic neuropathy, spinal cord injury, or disuse syndrome.

After six months, six out of seven patients taking the daily dose of mushroom demonstrated improvement in perceptual capacities and all seven had improvements in their Functional Independence Measure. Lion's mane may indeed be a potent inducer of brain tissue regeneration.

A more recent study of twenty-nine men and women aged fifty to eighty with mild cognitive problems was conducted by Mori et al. (2008). This double-blind, placebo-controlled trial showed significant improvement in the mushroom group at eight, twelve, and sixteen weeks, but did not last beyond four weeks after being discontinued. Dosage was one gram of dried fruiting body three times per day. All fourteen showed improvement after three month compared to five of fifteen placebo patients.

One study found in vitro evidence of myelin-generating effect on nerve and cerebellar glia cells.

Work by Moldavan et al. (2007) found extracts

exerted neurotropic action and improved the myelination process in maturing fibers, did not affect nerve cell growth in vitro, and did not exert a toxic effect or nerve cell damage.

The compound 3-hydroxy-hericenone F extracted and identified by Ueda et al. (2008) shows protection against endoplasmic reticulum stress-dependent Neuro2 cell death.

Water extracts of the fresh fruiting body given daily to rats with injured perineal nerves showed improvement.

Submerged mycelial extracts of *H. erinaceus* show antitumor activity on solid lymphoma (Krasnopolskaya et al. 2005).

J. C. Wang et al. (2005) found methanol extracts of the fruiting body to possess hypoglycemic activity in a rat study.

Innovative work by Won-Sik Choi et al. (2005) cultured *H. erinaceus* on *Artemisia* species. When tested, the methanol extract was found to inhibit proliferation of vascular smooth muscle cells. A methanol extract of the fungi showed no such activity, while an extract of *Artemisia iwayomogi* possessed strong inhibitory effects. The change of chemical components took place after addition of the *Artemisia* to the growth medium. The extract also had strong protective effect on carbon tetrachloride hepatic damage in rats, with significant reduction in activity of GOT but not GPT and ALP.

Early work by Hervey (1947) found activity against *Staphylococcus aureus.*

Erinacin E, from *H. coralloides/H. ramosum,* produced in a fermentation broth, is a highly selective agonist of the kappa opioid receptor. It has an IC 50 of 0.8 micromoles,

binding at the m opioid receptor with an IC 50 of >200 millimoles. These compounds may exhibit antinoceptive activity without the side effects associated with agonists like morphine.

Herical, the precursor of erinacin E, was found cytotoxic and hemolytic (Anke, T. et al. 2002).

Total synthesis of this species has been reported (Watanabe, H. and M. Nakada 2008).

Recipes and Dosage

For gastric ulcers, take thirty grams of dried fruiting body and decoct in water. Drink twice a day.

Hericium extracts are standardized to 0.5 percent hericenones and 6 percent amyloban. Two capsules taken three to six times per day.

Tincture: one part fresh fruiting body in three parts 60 percent alcohol; One part dried to five parts 40 percent alcohol.

Heterobasidion

Fomes annosus
Fomitopsis annosa
Polyporus annosus
(BIRCH POLYPORE)
(ROOT ROT)

Despite its common name, birch polypore can be found growing near the foot of a variety of trees including juniper, poplar, pine, spruce, lodge pole pine, and, of course, birch. It is quite prevalent on ponderosa pine. In Britain it accounts for 90 percent of all the decay in conifers.

The fruiting bodies are perennial, woody, and leathery, with white flesh and white to yellow pores. The cap is brown to gray-brown.

Traditional Uses

The dried polypore was used as a kind of moxibustion to burn out and cauterize wounds inflicted by snakes and other venomous animals.

It is a folk medicine for cancer, especially in the Scandinavian countries.

Medicinal Use

Chemical Constituents

- **It contains fomannosin and fomannoxin, two bactericides that are phytotoxic, and hexatriyne, a compound that requires study.**

- **It also contains triacetylene that can detonate violently at room temperature.**

Work in by Hervey (1947) showed activity against both *E. coli* and *Staphylococcus aureus*. Earlier work by Robbins et al. (1945) found activity against only *S. aureus*.

Koch et al. (2002) found the fruiting bodies inhibit in vitro binding of lipopolysaccharide from gram-negative bacteria to CD14 receptor on immune cells. This is what occurs in septic shock when a cascade of inflammatory mediators and reactive oxygen species occurs, causing serious trauma and death.

It may be useful in the development of new drugs for the treatment of pain with activity similar to opioids. See *Daedaleopsis confragosa*.

The fungi produce abnormal pigments on phenol due to oxidases (Rahouti et al. 1999).

It may play a role in lignin degradation, commercially speaking that is.

Bits and Pieces

Because it can be quite destructive, various water plant extracts have been tested to reduce its mycelial growth.

One study tested thirty-one plant extracts for inhibitory activity. The stems and roots of wood anemone *(A. nemorosa)* and lily of the valley gave the strongest inhibition, followed by speedwell *(Veronica officinalis),* hazel leaves (85 percent), mountain ash roots (77 percent), and bilberry leaves (69 percent).

Recent work has found that *Suillus bovinus* suppresses growth of this fungi. *Peniophora giganteum* is a crust lichen that can be painted with water on the stumps of cut pines, outcompeting birch polypore *(H. annosum),* but has trouble establishing itself. The latter is a poor competitor in the fungus race for a tree stump. Pellets of *P. giganteum* or *P. gigantea* are now produced commercially and water suspensions are painted on stumps immediately after felling, a non-toxic approach with novel application.

Heteroporus biennis

Abortiporus biennis
Polyporus biennis

According to David Arora, this mushroom is found under oak and pine in the fall, with misshapen fruiting bodies covered with pores; "The best fieldmark of this otherwise unimposing, profoundly forgettable, pitiful excuse for a polypore."

Heteroporus biennis contains trypsin inhibitors with high heat stability. It exhibits protease, amylase, phytase, carboxylesterase, and lipase enzyme activity (Goud et al. 2009). Phytases are used in chicken feed formulations, for example, to hydrolyze phosphates and decrease their pollution of waterways. The development of phosphatase solubilizers and phytases from basidiomycetes is an emerging and important field.

Hydnellum caeruleum

(BLUISH HYDNELLUM)
(BLUISH TOOTH)
H. suaveolens
Hydnum boreale
Calodon suaveolens
Phaeodon suaveolens
(SWEET SMELLING HYDNELLUM)
H. peckii
C. peckii
(STRAWBERRIES AND CREAM)
(BLEEDING HYDNELLUM)

Hydnellum means "small, spongy plant." *Caeruleum* means "bluish" from the Latin. This is a somewhat rare, but widespread purplish-blue mushroom. It is inedible and has the aromatic odor of drying hay.

Sweet smelling *Hydnellum* is blue-fleshed, inedible, and has a warmer, anise-fenugreek-like odor. It contains thelephoric acid, a terphenyl quinone that has been used as a dye for silks and wools.

Bleeding *Hydnellum* looks, according to Arora, like a Danish pastry topped with strawberry jam. It is found in forests under fir and pine.

Chemical Constituents

- **dihydroaurantiacin dibenzoate, 2-0-methylatromentin, hydnellin A and B, and sarcodonin D.**

- *H. peckii:* **atromentin and leucomelone.**

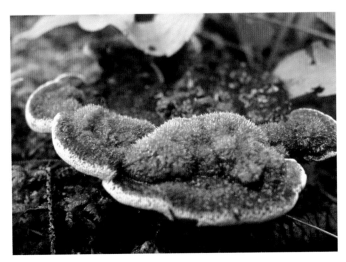

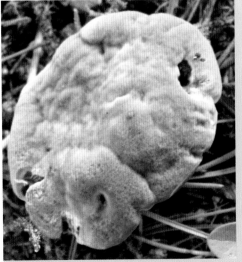

Hydnellum caeruleum

Scientists have isolated aurantiacin, six p-Terphenyl derivatives called thelephantins I-P, as well as dihydroaurantiacin dibenzoate and 2-0-methylatromentin, from this fungus (Quang et al. 2004). Antioxidant activity similar to or greater than vitamin C or BHA was noted.

Hydnellin A and B, as well as sarcodonin D, show moderate antioxidant activity (Hashimoto et al. 2006).

Early work by Khanna et al. (1965) found a 70 percent ethanol extract contained atromentin, an effective anticoagulant similar in activity to heparin. In vitro, one milligram of purified atromentin (or 2.3 milligrams of extract) is equivalent to 5.1 units of heparin.

Atromentin and leucomelone inhibit the enoyl-acyl carrier protein reductase of *Streptococcus pneumoniae* at the very low IC50 rate of 0.24 micrometers (Zheng, C.-J. et al. 2006).

Essential Oil

Sweet smelling *Hydnellum* essential oil contains 30 percent p-anisaldehyde, and coumarins.

Textile Industry

Sweet smelling *Hydnellum* contains thelephoric acid, a terphenyl quinone that has been used as a dye for silks and wools.

Hydnum repandum

Sarcodon repandus
Tyrodon repandus
(YELLOW TOOTHED FUNGUS)

(HEDGEHOG MUSHROOM)
(SWEET TOOTH)
H. imbricatum
Sarcodon imbricatus
(SCALY HEDGEHOG)
(HAWKWING)
(SCALY TOOTH)
(see *Sarcodon imbricatus*)
H. gelatinosus
Pseudohydnum gelatinosus
(FALSE HEDGEHOG)
(TOOTHED JELLY FUNGUS)
H. scabrosus
S. scabrosus
(BITTER HEDGEHOG)

Hydnum means "spongy plant" and *repandum* means "spreading" *Sarcodon* is Greek meaning "fleshy tooth." *Imbricatus* is Latin for "covered with scales." *Repandus* means "bent backwards."

Hedgehog is one of our choice edible mushrooms, and difficult to confuse with any other. This yellow-orange fungus grows in mixed woods in July and August. A pure white form (var. alba) grows later in the season. It may be found into late fall, as it can withstand colder temperatures.

In Italy, the mushroom is called *stecherinos*. Martin Osis considers this his favorite edible. It has a firm, crunchy texture and a slightly fruity odor. The young specimens are best, and those touched by frost tend to be somewhat bitter. It has a very high food value at 434 kilocalories per hundred grams (Colak et al. 2009).

The mature bitter hedgehog is often rated as inedible due to its bitterness, but cooking it

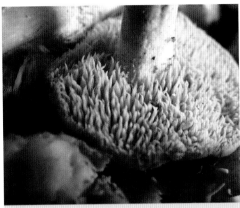
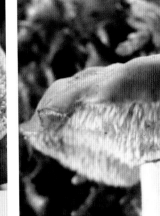

Hydnum repandum

in butter for twenty minutes will do wonders. When young it can be eaten raw in salads, adding a peppery watercress-like flavor.

Members of the Alaskan Mycological Society use the fungus as a pepper substitute. The dried mushroom is ground in a food processor and used, one tablespoon at a time, in soup as a flavor additive. Great idea!

I personally think drying these mushrooms is a waste, as the teeth fall out, and they are fragile and grainy. When reconstituted they are tough and without taste, so enjoy them fresh or pickled.

Swiss mycologists report that the mushroom is psychoactive.

Medicinal Use
Chemical Constituents
- *H. repandum:* **repandiol.**
- *H. scabrosus:* **diterpenoids sarcodonins A-H, scabronines A-F, and scabronines L-M.**

Chloroform extracts of the hedgehog show mild antibiotic activity against *Enterobacter aerogenes, Staphylococcus aureus, S. epidermidis,* and *Bacillus subtilis,* while ethanol extracts show mild activity against only the latter bacteria (Yamac and Bilgili 2006).

Yellow-toothed fungus contains repandiol, a cytotoxic diepoxide potent against tumor cells. The cultured mycelium shows 70 percent inhibition of sarcoma 180 cancer cell lines, while the fruiting body shows 90 percent inhibition of both sarcoma 180 and Ehrlich carcinoma cell lines (Ohtsuka et al. 1973).

The sporophore contains polysaccharide-like substances that lower the blood cholesterol levels in experimental animals.

Scaled hedgehog or hawkwing is a less desired edible, found among conifers in the mountains. See *Sarcodon imbricatus.*

False *Hydnum,* or toothed jelly fungus, is edible, but slimy and chewy.

Pemberton et al. (1994) tested 403 species of mushrooms and only this one showed anti-A serologic specificity.

Inhibition rates against sarcoma 180 and Ehrlich carcinoma are 90 percent.

The related *S. scabrosus (Hydnum scabrosus)* contains cyathane diterpenoids with anti-inflammatory activity (Kamo et al. 2004a).

Bitter hedgehog contains diterpenoids such as sarcodonins A-H, scabronines A-F, and scabronines L-M. These all possess a cyathane skeleton that display activity to stimulate nerve growth factor in vitro.

Sarcodonins are anti-inflammatory, antibacterial, and, as the name suggests, bitter (Shibata, H. et al. 1998).

Scabronines A and G promote secretion of neurotrophic factors, including nerve growth factor from 1321N1 (human astrocytoma) cells, and cause enhancement of neurite outgrowth of PC-12 of rat adrenal medulla cells (Obara et al. 1999).

Later work by same team suggested that scabronine G and its methyl ester might enhance above by activation of protein kinase (Obara et al. 2001).

A series of unusual nitrogenous metabolites with p-terphenyl cores have been isolated from *H. scabrosus* and *Sarcadon leucopus* and found active against tumor cell cultures (Ma, B.-J. et al. 2005; Cali et al. 2004; Geraci et al. 2000).

The related *kootake* mushroom of Japan *(S. aspratus)* has also been found to prevent plaque buildup on arteries and lesions on the blood vessel walls.

One study fed either hedgehog powder or extract to two groups of mice for sixty days. Those fed the mushroom powder exhibited significant physical stamina and delayed fatigue over controls. After exercise, the levels of blood lactic acid were significantly lower than controls, with the rate of elimination much higher.

Other studies by D. H. Kim et al. (1996) show that mushroom extracts inhibit *Helicobacter pylori* urease. This bacterium is associated with formation of gastric and duodenal ulcers.

Textile Industry

Hedgehog mushroom can be used for dyeing, yielding beautiful blue and green colors.

Hygrocybe psittacina

Hygrophorus psittacinus
(PARROT WAXGILL)
H. conica
Hygrophorus conicus
(BLACKENING WAXGILL)
(WITCH'S HAT)

Hygrocybe is Greek meaning "moist head" or "water cap." *Psittacina* means "parrot green," and *conica* means "cone."

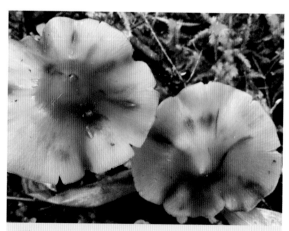
🌿 *Hygrocybe conica*

The parrot waxgill mushroom is edible, but has no distinct taste. The fragrant fungi may contain psilocybin, according to Jonathan Ott. He would know! His early work was a great inspiration to this author.

Blackening waxgill is a yellow, orange, or red color when young, but turns black when touched or becomes older. The latex turns dark on exposure to air. Muscaflavin and L-Dopa have been detected in the blackening fruiting bodies.

It may be edible when cooked, but is not recommended.

Medicinal Use

Blackening waxgill was tested, along with 110 other macrofungi, for inhibition of pancreatic lipase and found to exhibit 97 percent inhibitory activity, the highest of all of the samples tested (Slane et al. 2004). This may well have medicinal application.

The related *H. marchii (H. coccinea var. marchii)* shows inhibition rate of 100 percent against sarcoma 180 and 90 percent against Ehrlich carcinoma cells.

Hygrophoropsis aurantiaca

(FALSE CHANTERELLE)

Hygrophoropsis is Latin meaning "resembles *Hygrophorus*." *Hygros* means "wet or moist" and *phorus* means "bearing" or "combining." It does not resemble *Hygrophorus* and in fact, recent work suggests it is closely related to the *Boletes*.

The Greek *phorus* is from *pherein* meaning "bear." *Aurantiaca* refers to the color orange. It could, by this logic, just as well be called "the orange wet bear."

False chanterelle appears at first glance very similar to the edible chanterelle, with a bright orange color. They are associated with spruce. The gills are regularly forked, thin, and narrow, as opposed to the shallow, thick folds of the edible chanterelle.

They have a mild odor, quite unlike the apricot citrus scent of chanterelle.

It is not a recommended edible, and considered by some authors to cause alarming hallucinations. I cannot find any information on the chemical makeup of the mushroom.

Hygrophorus camarophyllus

(SMOKY WAXGILL)

(DUSKY WAXCAP)

H. eburneus

(IVORY WAXY CAP)

(SLIMY MUSHROOM)

(COWBOY'S HANKERCHIEF)

H. agathosmus

(GRAY ALMOND WAXY CAP)

H. oliveceoalbus

(SHEATHED WAXY CAP)

H. puniceus

(SCARLET WAXY CAP)

H. hypothejus

(OLIVE BROWN WAXY CAP)

H. chrysodon

(GOLDEN FRINGED WAXGILL)

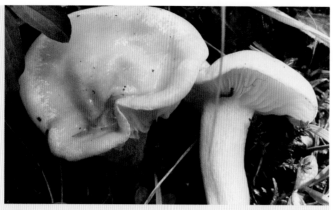

🍂 *Hygrophorus pudorinus*

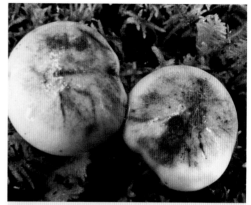

🍂 *Hygrophorus eburneus var. cossus*

Hygophorus means "moisture carrying." *Camarophyllus* is Greek meaning "with arched gills." *Eburnus* is Latin for "ivory."

Smoky waxgill is common to spruce forests of the Pacific Northwest and extremely cold northern Boreal forest.

Slimy mushroom, or kinnickkinnick head, is collected by the Thompson First Nations in British Columbia. It is considered a better edible than *Tricholoma populinum,* despite its slimy head. It has an odor very reminiscent of sage.

Hygrophorus agathosmus has an almond-like scent and is edible, but rather tasteless.

Golden fringed waxgill (*H. chrysodon*) is found near spruce and exhibits a scent like paraffin.

Medicinal Use

Chemical Constituents

- *H. chrysodon:* **chrysotriones A and B.**
- *H. oliveceoalbus:* **hygrophorones, including 4-0-acetyl hygrophorone A.**

Gray almond waxy cap has been found to possess activity against various bacteria and yeast (Yamac and Bilgili 2006).

Significant activity, similar to streptomycin, was found against *Staphylococcus aureus,* and it has been found to be twice as effective as the drug against *S. epidermidis* and *Bacillus subtilis.*

Significant activity was found against *Enterobacter aerogenes, Salmonella typhimurium,* and *Saccharomyces cerevisiae.*

An ethanol extract showed some activity against *E. coli.*

It contains a number of volatiles, including 3 methyl butanol, hexanal, p-cymene, 3-octanone, 1-octene-3-one, 3-octanol, 1-octen-3-ol, and benzoic acid (Ouzoni et al. 2009).

Sheathed waxy cap is common in Northwestern America, under spruce and other conifers.

It contains various cyclopentanone derivatives, known as hygrophorones, that bear some resemblance to the antibiotic pentenomycin.

One hygrophorone, 4-0-acetyl hygrophorone A, has been found most active against *Cladiosporium cucumerinum* (Lubken et al. 2004).

The fruiting body shows 100 percent inhibition against sarcoma 180 and 90 percent inhibition against Ehrlich solid cancer cell lines (Ohtsuka et al. 1973).

Ersel and Cavas (2008) identified high superoxide dimutase activities.

Scarlet waxy cap shows inhibition of 90 percent and 100 percent respectively of above cancer cell lines.

The related *H. hypothejus,* found in pine forests in abundance, shows inhibition rates of 70 percent and 80 percent, respectively (Ohtsuka et al. 1973).

Mycoremediation

Paul Stamets suggests that cold-tolerant mushrooms like this species be investigated for decomposing munitions. The fact that they work at low temperatures lowers the potential for spontaneous combustion, as they continue to secrete enzymes at temperatures below the threshold of danger. He also mentions the potential of *Flammulina velutipes* for breaking down toxic wastes at a lower composting temperature.

Hypholoma

Hypholoma velutina
Lacrymaria velutina
Psathryella velutina
(WEEPING WIDOW)
H. sublateritium
Naematoloma sublateritium
(BRICK TOPS)
(BRICK CAP)

H. fasciculare
N. fasciculare
(SULPHUR TUFT)
H. capnoides
N. capnoides
(CONIFER TUFT)
(SMOKY GILLED HYPHOLOMA)
(CLUSTERED WOODLOVER)
(GRAY GILLED TUFT AGARIC)

Lachrymaria is Latin meaning "tears," and *velutina* means "covered with hair or fleece." *Sublateritium* is Latin for "almost brick color." *Hypholoma* means "mushrooms with threads," or "fringed web," due to the thread-like veil connecting the cap to the stem when young. *Fasciculus* means "a small bundle" and *capnoides* means "smoky."

Brick top (*H. sublateritium*) is common and grows on the stumps of deciduous trees, especially oak. In Japan, it is called *kuritake* or "chestnut mushroom." Another common name is cinnamon cap. The fruiting bodies are nearly 23 percent protein, and are rich in potassium, B5, and niacin.

Weeping widow is a common city mushroom, often found growing in bundles in the grass. It is commonly thought to be edible, despite its name. In Japan, the mushroom is known as *nigakuritake* or "bitter *kuritake.*"

The poisonous, iodine-scented sulphur tuft (*Hypholoma fasciculare*) is more common in Manitoba and the Pacific Northwest.

Conifer tuft has an orange cap with yellow margin, does not have the strong yellow gill color of the sulphur tuft, but instead has smoky brown gills.

It is a choice edible, and rated quite highly for flavor by many fungi aficionados. The mushroom has a fresh, sweet, forest-like fragrance similar to *Stropharia rugoso-annulata*.

It is a true saprophyte, and aggressive conifer stump decomposer. It may be mistaken for sulphur tuft, or even *Galerina autumnalis,* so proper identification is important.

Sulphur tuft is extremely bitter with bright greenish-yellow gills that become dingy yellow-brown with age, and a purple spore print. The edible conifer tuft, on the other hand, has smoky brown gills, a mild flavor, and brown-purple spores.

No resulting deaths have been reported in North America, but Japan and Europe have reported examples of its toxicity. The fungi have a long latent poisoning period of up to ten hours after ingestion. Compounds such as fasciculic acid that inhibit calmodulin are believed responsible. This is a protein that plays a key role in cellular homeostasis and cell signaling.

It causes muscarinic syndrome, and hallucinations, particularly auditory, have been noted. It may contain the toxin yangonin.

In the novel *The Flounder,* by Günter Grass, the sulphur tuft and three *Amanita* species are used for political assassination.

Medicinal Use

Sulfur tuft contains lectins that interact with N-acetyl glucosamine in a binding form. Work at the University of Tokyo, Japan, suggests that the mushroom may be useful in the development of diagnostic tools for rheumatoid arthritis. Earlier work used lectins from this mushroom for acute leukemia tests.

One study found water extractions of the sulphur tuft (fifty milligrams per kilogram) in diabetic rats temporarily created hypoglycemic activity.

Research has found activity against *Bacillus cereus* and *B. subtilis.* Early work by Annette Hervey (1947) showed activity against *E. coli* and *S. aureus.*

Work in China indicates an inhibition rate of 80 percent against sarcoma 180 and 90 percent against Ehrlich carcinoma cancer cell lines (Ohtsuka et al. 1973).

Compounds that inhibit calmodulin have been found in the fungus. This protein plays a key role in cellular homeostasis and cell communication. These compounds have been named fasciculic acids and are worthy of further investigation.

Doljak et al. (2001) found the fungus inhibits thrombin formation by 32 percent, suggesting another medicinal application.

Sulfur tuft was found to produce up to 132 milligrams per kilogram of absorbable organic halogens as dry weight of forest litter substrate in six weeks (Verhagen et al. 1996).

Sulfur tuft has been found to decrease cell proliferation of androgen receptors in dihydrotestosterone-induced cells, as well as inhibition against breast and prostate cancer cell lines, suggesting medicinal application (Zaidman et al. 2007).

Sulfur tuft and conifer tuft are among eight mushroom species that show positive for potential in treating tuberculosis. Work at the University of British Columbia is ongoing into natural therapy for this deadly disease.

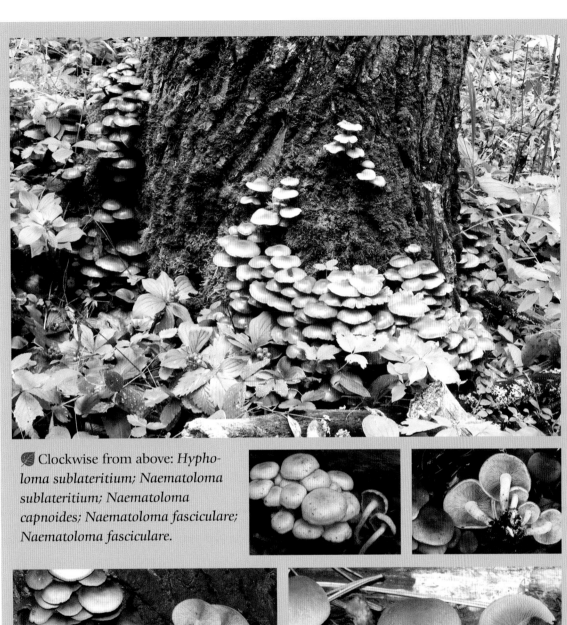

🍃 Clockwise from above: *Hypho-loma sublateritium; Naematoloma sublateritium; Naematoloma capnoides; Naematoloma fasciculare; Naematoloma fasciculare.*

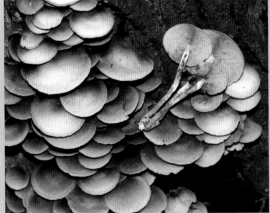

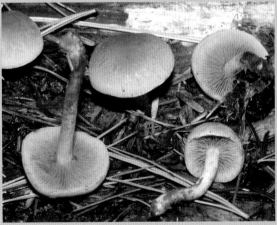

Laboratory studies indicate an inhibition rate of 60 percent against sarcoma 180 and 70 percent against Ehrlich carcinoma (Ohtsuka et al. 1973).

Seeger and Bunsen (1980) identified fascicularelysin that, in vitro, disrupts mast cells and releases marker molecules from both lecithin and sphingomyelin liposomes.

It also contains clavaric acid, an antitumor isoprenoid.

Ethyl acetate extracts show significant inhibition of both COX-1 and COX-2 enzymes (Elgorashi et al. 2008).

Early work by Robbins et al. (1945) found activity against *Staphylococcus aureus*.

Fungi Essence

Sulphur tuft essence will help you when on a spiritual quest. It aids in the integration of knowledge into wisdom. Helps in nervous conditions, skin, nausea, and digestion.

— SILVERCORD

Fungicide

Chapman and Xiao in British Columbia found that inoculation of tree stumps with sulphur tuft controls the growth of honey mushroom *(A. ostoyae)*. The intent is good; it's just too bad it's not a more prized edible or medicinal fungi. Intentional inoculation with the edible *H. capnoides* would be a win-win situation as this prized mushroom outcompetes *Armillaria*.

Cultivation

According to expert Paul Stamets, conifer tuft is one of the few gourmet mushrooms adaptive to cultivation on conifer logs and stumps. He mentions that he has grown it successfully on alder wood chips.

Sawdust spawn can easily be implanted into fresh cuts using wedge or sandwich inoculation. Another approach is to infuse chainsaw oil with the spores, or use rope spawn around old stumps.

Conifer tuft, brown gilled woodlover, and brick top can all be cultivated on forest stumps, and may be some of the most aggressive species for inoculating the millions of coniferous stumps left over from logging. Clusters up to four pounds each have been collected, with annual fruiting occurring over a ten-year time period.

Care must be taken as it is a myco-accumulator of aluminum.

Considerable study has been done on the degradation effect of the related *N. frowardii*. Mineralization of amino-dinitrotoluenes has been demonstrated and a manganese dependent peroxidase isolated from the fungus (Scheibner, K. et al. 1997).

Brick top is a white rot degrader and defender of the forest from blight fungi, like its cousins. Paul Stamets inoculated alder with sawdust spawn, and it fruited for eight years. He has grown the fungi in sawdust mulch added to gardens. Inoculate logs with dowel or sawdust spawn, and lie them down side by side.

Hypomyces

Hypomyces chrysospermus
(GOLDEN HYPOMYCES)
H. lactifluorum
(LOBSTER MUSHROOM)
H. luteo-virens
(YELLOW GREEN HYPOMYCES)

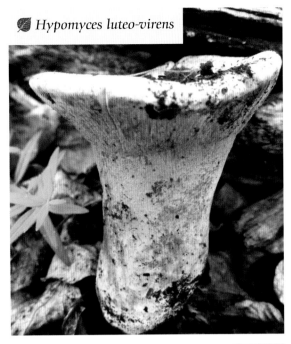

Hypomyces luteo-virens

Hypomyces is Greek meaning "a mushroom underneath." *Chrysospermus* means "with golden seed." *Lactifluorum* is Latin for "flow of milk (sap)" and *luteo-virens* is "yellow, becoming green." The original yellow stage is known as *Sepedonium chrysospermum.*

Golden *Hypomyces* is a creeping hypha that forms a mass of yellow powder on *Boletus, Leccinum, Russula,* and other fungi. It is a fungus on a fungus, and turns from white to yellow to red-brown in stages.

Lobster mushroom is a brightly colored parasite on *Russula brevipes* and *Lactarius piperatus,* and is edible but dependent on the host. The name comes from the perceived seafood flavor. They are delicious and a favorite in our kitchen. They combine well with white wine, but should not be overcooked lest the seafood flavor be lost. They dry well.

They are also a lot of fun to pick.

In the fall of 2008, I went to the Sicamous Mushroom Festival and was treated to a plethora of these giant orange treats. I then went home and filled my freezer.

Yellow green *Hypomyces* is the form found most frequently on *Russula* and *Lactarius* species. Tasty, but with no known medicinal application at present.

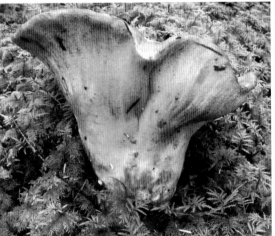

Hypomyces lactifluorum

Medicinal Use

Golden *Hypomyces* is used to cure external bleeding and is especially helpful when sprinkled or applied as a spore powder on cuts or wounds.

Hypoxylon multiforme

(BIRCH HYPOXYLON)

Birch *Hypoxylon* is an irregular-shaped crust or stroma formed on birch bark. It is red-brown when new, becoming black with age. Tiny fruit bodies appear like pimples on the glossy surface.

Medicinal Use

The azaphilone-type compounds multiformins A-D have been isolated from this unusual fungus and tested for antimicrobial activity.

Moderate to strong activity has been found against *Staphylococcus aureus, Klebsiella pneumoniae, Pseudomonas aeruginosa, Salmonella enteritidis, E. coli, Aspergillus niger,* and *Candida albicans* (Quang et al. 2005).

A recent study found *H. fragiforme* contains dihydroisocoumarin derivatives with bacterial and nematocidal activity.

The stem bark of aspen poplars infected with *H. mammatan* contains cinnamrutinoses A and B.

Bits and Pieces

Ethanol extracts of some species have been found to resemble sex hormones of spiders.

Hypsizygus

Hypsizygus marmoreus
H. tessulatus
H. elongatipes
Pleurotus elongatipes
(LONG FOOTED OYSTER)
(LONG STEMMED PLEUROTUS)
(WESTERN HYPSIZYGUS)
(THE BEECH MUSHROOM)
(BUNAPI)
P. ulmarius
H. ulmarius
(WHITE ELM MUSHROOM)
(SHIMEJI)
(ELM OYSTER)

For fragrance matsutake, for flavor shimeji.
—JAPANESE SAYING

Hypsizygus is Greek meaning "carrying high" from *hypsi,* meaning "on high" or "aloft" and *zygus* meaning "yoke." *Marmoreus* is from Latin, meaning "marbled." *Tessulatus* refers to the water spots on the cap. *Tessela* is "a small cube for pavement," according to McIlvaine. *Ulmus* is Latin for "elm." *Elongatipes* refers to the long stems.

These two mushrooms were originally grouped together, then classified separately, but *H. tessulatus* is the older, more valid, and scientifically correct term. Paul Stamets believes they are two different species, so I'll go with that.

Western *Hypsizygus* occurs across North America and up into Yukon and Alaska. It is typically found on poplar, in the crotch of a dead tree or on a tree stump.

It is a good young edible, very slow growing but somewhat woody when older. It has a peculiar aromatic scent like apricots or anise, and has very long stems that help identify it.

The wild mushrooms *(H. tessulatus)* are quite delicious, as I discovered when I found my first group in the river valley in August of 2003. I have revisited the fallen poplar on which it grows many times over the ensuing years.

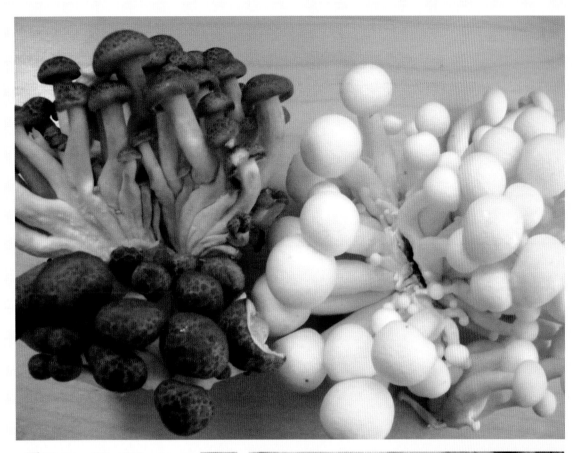

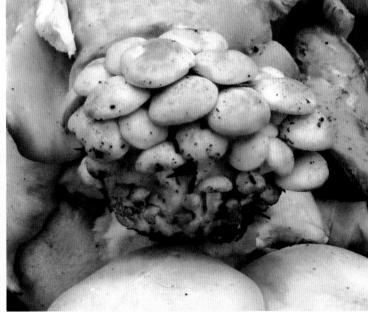

Above: cultivated
Hypsizygus ulmarius.
Right and below:
Hypsizygus tessulatus.

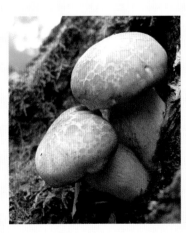

White elm mushroom is very popular in Japan, where it is known as *buna shimeji* meaning "beech mushroom," *tamo-motashi* meaning "elm oyster mushroom," or *yamabiko hon-shimeji* meaning "mountain echo mushroom." A common name is white elm mushroom or *shirotamogitake*.

It is favored as a superior edible mushroom with a firm crunchy texture and a mild nutty flavor.

Elm oyster grows mainly on elm, cottonwoods, maple, and willow. It looks somewhat like an oyster mushroom, but is not related.

Elm oyster is considered by many experts to be superior to the oyster mushroom for both flavor and texture. Both are excellent in stir-fried meals.

Cultivation

Elm oyster has been cultivated in Japan since 1973, using an environment identical to that preferred by shiitake. This produces two-inch tall stems with broad caps. When the light is reduced and carbon dioxide levels are elevated, they grow taller, which the Japanese prefer.

It has taken over some of the oyster mushroom market, due to its firm, crunchy texture and sweet, nutty taste.

It is also cultivated in North America, and goes by the name shimeji mushroom, even though this refers to a number of species in Japan.

When the caps grow the lateral growth continues, increasing the mass of the whole fruiting body. The spore load is much lighter than that of oyster, making it an all-round good choice for cultivation.

Medicinal Use

Chemical Constituents

- *H. tessulatus*: **various polyhydroxysteroids have been isolated from the mushroom, including cerevisterol, 3 alpha, 5 beta, 9 gamma-trihydroxyergosta-7,22-dien-6-one; and two unstable 5 alpha, 9 alpha epidioxides.**

- *H. marmoreus*: **acidic glycosphingolipids, hypsin.**

Recent Japanese research indicates that it retards Lewis lung carcinoma tumor growth when ingested.

Mice were implanted with Lewis Lung carcinoma and given water derived from the fresh mushrooms at the dose equivalent of one gram per kilogram of body weight per day. Tumors were inhibited 100 percent, resulting in total regression. In the absence of the extract, the tumors continued growing.

Motoi (2003) found antitumor activity by the 1,3-beta-glucans of *H. marmoreus* against sarcoma 180.

Matsuzawa (2006) identified antioxidant and potent antitumor activity in dried mushroom extracts.

Cold-water extracts have been shown to inhibit proliferation of human leukemic U937 cell lines. *Flammulina velutipes* also showed inhibition.

Ethyl acetate extracts show activity against human ovarian cancer cell lines (Rouhana-Toubi et al. 2009).

A combination of *H. ulmarius* and seven other mushrooms—including *Panus conchatus*, *Piptoporus betulinu*, and *Trametes zonata*—

was patented by Wasser and others (patent US7258862) in August 2007 for treatment of chronic myelongenous leukemia, acute lymphoblastic leukemia, prostate cancer, and beta-globin disorders such as sickle cell anemia and beta-thalassemia.

An extract of *H. marmoreus* and enoki called EEM, was clinically tested on cancer patients. When compared to MPA on the cachexia in advanced cancer patients, better performance and quality of life was noted. Another trial with EEM and chemotherapy showed better response than with the drug alone.

When investigated for precancerous lesions on the esophagus, a six-month trial showed positive results (Ikekawa 2005).

Hsin Ting Ou et al. (2005) revealed potent antitumor and differentiation-inducing activity of cold-water extracts of *H. marmoreus*. Specifically, proliferation of human leukemic U937 cells was looked at in this study, with tumor necrosis factor (TNF) and interleukin levels stimulated.

It appears that acidic glycosphingolipids contribute to immune homeostasis through minimum induction of invariant NK killer T-cells, at least in vivo (Nozaki et al. 2010).

One study identified compounds in this mushroom with activity against human colon, breast, and hepatoblastoma cell lines.

The mushroom shows activity against liver and colon carcinoma cells with increased glutathione, activation of gluthathione S-transferase, and induction of quinone reductase (Chang, M. S. et al. 2009).

Lam and Ng (2001) identified hypsin, a novel heat-stable ribosome-inactivating protein with antifungal and anti-proliferative activity. Hervey (1947) showed significant activity against *Staphylococcus aureus.*

An as yet unpublished paper from Shizuok State University found arteriosclerosis in mice reduced by 74 percent in a ten-week trial with the addition of 3 percent dried beech mushroom powder. Serum cholesterol levels were significantly better than controls. Maitake reduced arteriosclerosis focus by 52 percent compared to the control.

The mushroom also exhibits anti-allergenic properties. Ethanol extracts have shown activity (Sano et al. 2002).

White elm water-soluble anticancer compounds can be extracted from the waste substrate. It has been found to produce a mycelium-bound toxin against nematodes, explaining the lack of problem with this destructive creature.

Krasnopolskaya et al. (2008) found a two milligram per kilogram dose of artificially grown mycelia fed to mice was a very effective antitumor agent. The yield of mycelia was substantially larger than *H. marmoreus,* and the inhibition rate for lymphoma p388 cells was 80 percent, compared to two strains of its cousin at 38 percent and 59 percent.

Cosmetics

Dr. Andrew Weil, a long time proponent of integrative medicine, introduced mushrooms in a new line of cosmetics by Origins™. One of his favorite mushrooms is *H. ulmarius,* which he includes with reishi and cordyceps in Plantidote™, an internal supplement and external face serum.

Inocybe fastigata

I. rimosa
(DEADLY INOCYBE)
(FIBER HEAD)
(STRAW COLORED FIBER HEAD)

Inocybe means "fiber head" from the Greek. *Fastigata* is Latin for "with a pointed peak or gable."

Deadly *(I. fastigata)* is considered a poisonous mushroom, containing the parasympathetic stimulant muscarine. This is not neutralized by cooking and seriously affects the autonomic nervous system and liver.

Atropine is the antidote for muscarine poisoning, and may be given to individuals who experience discomfort or anxiety.

Despite the common name, this mushroom is valued in China for treating eczema.

The mushroom is said have a mealy, mild, or spermatic odor. According to Michael Kuo (2005), at MushroomExpert.com:

'Disagreeable' was the preferred word in the era of Kaufmann (1918), when Victorian sensibilities still prevailed. The word 'spermatic' began to appear with more and more frequency, however, as the twentieth century progressed, and now it is hegemonic. That's all well and good, I suppose, but now widely accepted use of the term spermatic may underscore the fact that mycology is still an "Old Boys'" network, and still reveals a Victorian hesitation.

The crux of my argument involves *Russula xerampelina*, the so-called shrimp *Russula* which does not smell much like shrimp, to tell the truth, unless you are using 'shrimp' as a synonym, a Victorian coverup, for 'vaginal.'

Why is it okay to call *Inocybe rimosa* spermatic, while heads would turn at a corresponding, genital-secretion-based description of *Russula xerampelina*? The answer is because women mycologists are few and far between, and the Old Boys have not paused to imagine, for example, what must go through *Inocybe* expert Cathy Cripps' mind when she has to type 'spermatic' or what a female graduate student in mycology must feel when she has to discuss the morphology of a species of Phallus with her professor. If these good ole boys had to conjure up with olfactory memory of what is 'vaginal' all the time, things might be different. . . . And anyways, what the hell does sperm smell like? Does anyone know? And are we sure that, for example, one's diet doesn't influence the odor?

Thank you Michael. I could not have put it better.

The related *I. corydalina* has a fruity, jasmine-like fragrance due in part to cinnamic acid methyl esters. Others suggest the smell is more like sweet rotting fruit. This species contains psilocybin.

The related species *I. aeruginescens, I. corydalina, I. haemacta,* and *I. tricolor* all contain psilocybin and baeocystin. They all stain blue-green.

Gartz and Drewitz (1985) say this about *Inocybe aeruginascens:* "The mushrooms taste like ordinary culinary mushrooms. After some thirty minutes, while lying relaxed with no other somatic effects, there gradually appeared an extremely pleasant neutralization of the sense of weight. Abstract hallucinations in the form of sparkling colors and lights slowly developed. When the sense of weight had completely disappeared, there arose a very lively perception of a flight of the soul with corresponding euphoric feelings."

Gartz (1989) elsewhere noted that aeruginascin content is in the same order of magnitude as the amounts of psilocybin or baeocystin, and that it seems to modify the pharmacological action of psilocybin to give an always-euphoric mood during ingestion of the mushrooms.

Jensen et al. (2006) identified aeruginascin, a compound closely related to the frog skin toxin bufotenidine, a potent 5-HT$_3$ receptor agonist.

Inonotus obliquus

Polyporus obliquus
Poria oblique
(CHAGA)
(TSCHAGA)
(CLINKER POLYPORE)
(TSCHAGAPILZ)

Inos means "fiber," *noton* means "back." and *oblique* indicates that the pores are at an angle to the ground.

The mycelium grows best on potato dextrose agar (Tura et al. 2009).

In Norway, the fungus is known as cancer polypore, or *kreftjulce,* and in Finland *tikkatee.* The English call it woodpecker tea.

Nobel Prize-winner Alexander Solzhenitsyn wrote an essay about chaga in 1967 called "White Birch Cancer."

Cree healers call it *posahkan* or *wiskakecak omikih.* Wisakecak is a mythological character that threw a scab, which he had mistaken for dried meat and tried to eat, against a birch tree. To this day, it remains on the tree to benefit mankind.

Chaga or birch mushroom can be collected any time of the year from living trees, usually requiring an ax or saw. These black, porous growths have a sterile orange-brown area. They grow up to two kilograms or more and up to two meters in size. True chaga has a serrated edge on the underside, while false chaga is smooth.

The concept of a sterile conk is of interest as this normally precludes a way to culture the fungus. I know of people who have successfully used a forestry core sampler to extract mycelium from the inner part of infected trees and insert it into a formerly healthy birch.

It has been found occasionally on alder, but in the boreal forest birch is its preferred companion.

The Cree used the fungus as sweet-smelling incense and carried it as tinder for starting fires.

The fungus was also placed in pipe bowls to help keep tobacco and other herbs burning. Mors Kochanski calls this the true tinder conk, as it needs no preparation to help start fires. It is a lot of fun collecting the large polypores with Mors and Randy in early June.

It was used as a counter-irritant in arthritis, like mugwort is used in moxibustion. This entails burning the fungus on specific meridian points to stimulate energy flow. Care must be taken to avoid skin burns.

Robin Marles mentions a divination ritual use of the finely crumbled inner fungus by the Dene of Saskatchewan. Two long piles of tinder that represent two related events are laid

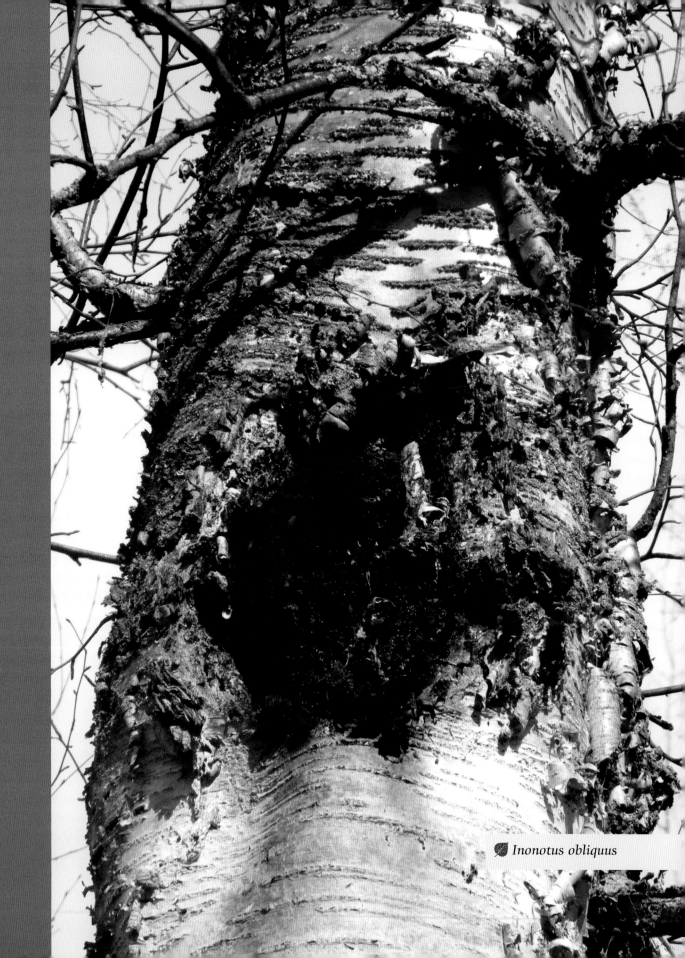

Inonotus obliquus

out end-to-end and ignited at opposite sides. Whichever pile burns through first will signify which activity takes place first. This is known as *etsen dek' on* or "it smells when it's burning."

In Japan, the fungus is known as *kabanoana-take*. It is becoming increasingly popular in the country as more research reveals its full potential.

Traditional Uses

The Gitksan of British Columbia call it *didi-huxw* or *di diyuh* and use the lit fungus to relieve rheumatic pain. The burning polypore was applied as a game between children to test whether they would talk back or not. Probably only once!

Add two heaping tablespoons of chaga powder to a five-gallon wort instead of hops. David Spahr suggests boiling the powder in a separate pot and adding it to the wort at the end. Great idea for all you beer makers.

The Russians have used chaga for various cancers, including Hodgkin's disease, since the sixteenth century. It has been used where operations were problematic or impossible due to the buildup of blood networks (angiogenesis) around tumor sites.

In Western Siberia it is used to treat tuberculosis, liver disease, worms, and stomach problems.

It is a noted blood purifier, tonic, and pain reliever traditionally used to treat ulcers and gastritis. Lower bowel problems were treated with decoctions used as retention enemas.

Medicinal Use

Chemical Constituents

- **More than two hundred constituents including inotodiol; inonoblins A-C; phelligridins D, E, and G; trametenolic acid; 3beta-hydroxylanosta-8,24-dien-21-23-lactone; obliquol; lanosterol; betulin; various triterpenes; vanillic-, syringic-, ferulic (twenty-two micrograms per gram), and p-hydroxybenzoic (263 micrograms per gram) acids; and 21,24-cyclopentalanosta-3beta,21,25-triol-8-ene; and 3 beta,22,25-trihydroxy-lanosta-8-ene.**

- **The wild fungus melanin is known as allomelanins, while the cultured fungus is assigned to eumelanins. The mycelium contains more protein than the fruiting body. The black, charred parts contain up to 30 percent betulin, while the red-brown inside is richer in lanostanes.**

In a study of twenty irritable bowel disease patients versus a healthy control group, reduction of oxidative stress in lymphocytes was noted in both groups (Najafzadeh et al. 2007). Thus chaga inhibits oxidative stress in general.

Chaga may have application in diabetes. Water-soluble polysaccharides inhibit alpha glucosidase, preventing absorption of glucose. No amylase inhibition was noted (Chen, H. et al. 2010).

Chaga has been widely researched for anti-tumor activity, especially in eastern Europe (Kahlos, et al. 1996).

It is beneficial in cases of chronic gastritis and stomach complaints including ulcers. Refined extracts have been manufactured and sold in Russia and its former satellite countries for more than fifty years.

Befungin is an official alcohol extraction, available since 1955 in Russia, containing 50 percent chaga extract for cancer therapy.

It shows definite improvement to the immune system, and has shown to be of benefit in treating psoriasis.

Another chaga extract, available commercially in Finland, is called *pakurikaapa*.

Antitumor activity has been found only in lengthy decoctions, which is the traditional folk medicine preparation. Infusions have been found to be inactive.

Inotodiol was found to be the most active ingredient, able to destroy 100 percent of Walker 256 carcinosarcoma cells and MCF-7 human adenocarcinoma mammary cells (Park, Y. K. et al. 2004).

Some Polish studies indicate chaga has inhibiting effect on tumor growth (Rzymowska 1998).

Water extracts inhibit proliferation and induction of differentiation and apoptosis of B16-F10 melanoma cells both in vitro and in vivo (Youn et al. 2009).

Ethanol extracts show anti-proliferative effect on human colon cancer cell lines (Hu et al. 2009).

Water extracts trigger apoptosis of sarcoma 180 tumor cells while protecting splenic lymphocytes (Chen, C. et al. 2007).

Chaga inhibits oxidative DNA damage in human lymphocytes produced by hydrogen peroxide.

The antioxidant effect of Chaga appears to be the result of polyphenols, with the capacity to scavenge free radicals at concentrations higher than five micrograms per milliliter (Cui, Y. et al. 2005).

Some authors suggest that chaga contains twenty-five to fifty times more SOD antioxidant activity than reishi, *Agaricus,* vitamin C, or blueberries.

In one graph, the oxygen radical absorbent capacity (ORAC), was shown as 36,557 per gram compared to the next closest Wolf Berry (*Lycium* species) at 258.1 and Blueberry at 24.5.

Testing at the USDA compared chaga and other medicinal mushrooms and found the aqueous extract exhibited forty-six times greater superoxide dismutase activity than *Cordyceps,* and 157 times greater than *Agaricus.*

It has, reputedly, four times the antioxidant power of clove bud essential oil, which has an ORAC score of 10,786 per milliliter.

I am not sure of the above claims, as M. Y. Kim (2008) compared antioxidant activity of ten medicinal and edible mushrooms including chaga. *Ganoderma lucidum* scored 70 percent, 74 percent, and 8 percent in the same study; while button mushroom *(B. bisporus)* scored 61 percent, 78 percent, and 47 percent respectively.

I.-K. Lee et al. (2007) identified inonoblins A-C and phelligridins D, E, and G that possess antioxidant activity.

Recent work by Van et al. (2009) found the conk possesses significant anti-inflammatory properties.

Oxidative stress increases the production of phenolics in submerged technology (Zheng, W.-F. et al. 2009).

The fungus contains several immune-stimulating polysaccharides. Submerged mycelial cultures can take advantage of different strains. One study suggests indirect anticancer effect,

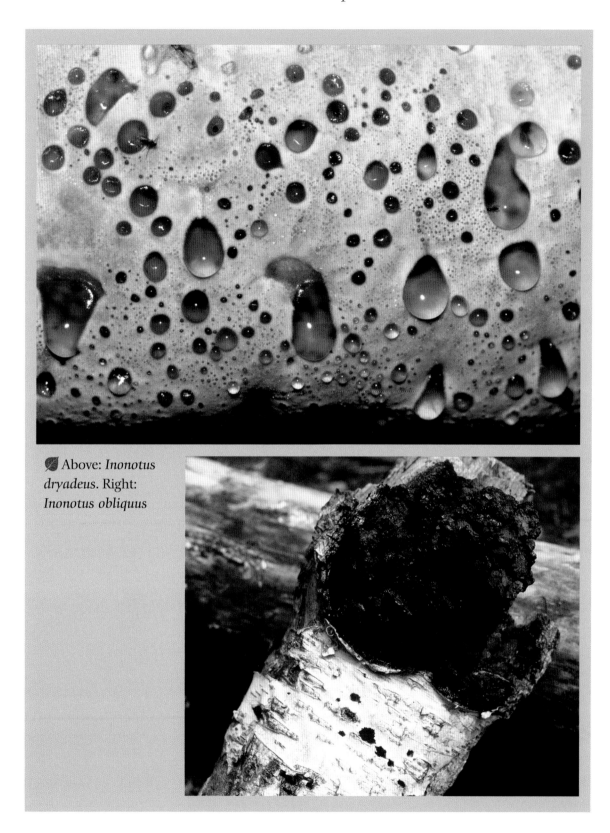

Above: *Inonotus dryadeus*. Right: *Inonotus obliquus*

with endo-polysaccharides as useful immune response modifiers.

A Polish study of forty-eight patients with third and fourth stage malignancies found chaga injections, along with cobalt salts, decreased tumor size in ten patients (Piaskowski 1957).

Water extracts have been found to inhibit human cervix cancer cells at the rate of ten micrograms per milliliter (Burczyk et al. 1996).

A follow-up study by J. Rzymowska (1998) in the same journal two years later confirmed chaga's ability to inhibit human cervical tumor cells HeLa S3, as well as cause a decrease of cell protein amount and mitiotic index value.

Jarosz et al. (1990) found an extract exerts anti-mitotic effect on HeLa cells, mostly in the M, G1, and G2 phases, while at the same time increasing catalase activity.

The water extracts decreased activity of LDH, HBDH, MDH, and GGT and increased activity of catalase.

Water extracts show activity on melanoma B16-F10 cells via cell cycle arrest, apoptosis, and induced cell differentiation. Down-regulation of pRb, p53, and p27 expression levels have been noted (Youn et al. 2009).

Chaga shows activity against non-small cell lung carcinoma and cervical cancer cells (Tepkeeva et al. 2009). A mixture of the fungi with elecampane, greater celandine, and horsetail was particularly cytotoxic.

Methanol extracts (80 percent) of the fruiting body show strong cytotoxic activity against various cancer cell lines including A549, PA-1, U937, and HL60, without affecting normal cells.

A 1997 study showed that betulinic acid is active at a lower pH, similar to the interior pH of tumor tissue. A follow-up study, in the same year, indicated that betulinic acid induces apoptosis in tumors.

Jun-En Sun et al. (2008) found dry matter of culture broth exhibits both hypoglycemic and anti-lipidemic activity.

The wild and cultivated mycelium differ greatly in chemical makeup. Wei-Fa Zheng et al. (2007) found mycelium of wild samples were composed of 45 percent lanosterol and 25 percent inotodiol and ten other sterols. Lab-cultured mycelium was 82 percent ergosterol, but when supplemented with silver nitrate became 56 percent lanosterol.

Studies by Kahlos et al. (1996) indicate the black thin external surface of *I. obliquus* exhibits 100 percent inhibition against the human influenza viruses A and B, and the horse influenza virus A.

The antiviral activity is believed due to the content of betulin, hispolon, hispidin, lupeol, and mycosterols.

Water-soluble lignins from chaga inhibited HIV protease, with an IC 50 value of 2.5 micrograms per milliliter (Ichimura et al. 1998).

Takashi Mizuno (1999) found protein-containing polysaccharides with antitumor and hypoglycemic activity.

Gandodelan A-B lowers blood sugar levels by 60 to 89 percent in only seven hours. Ethyl acetate extracts show significant hyperglycemic and anti-lipidemic activity in diabetic mice (Lu, X. et al. 2010).

These include beta-glucan, heteroglucan, and their protein complexes. Pashinskii et al.

(1998) looked at the anti-ulcer, adaptogenic, and antitumor activities of the mushroom.

Research by Ohtomo et al. (2001) suggests this fungi has strong immune-modulating activity, regulates cytokine and interleukin responses, and stimulates both NK cell and macrophage growth.

They found a dry extract stronger and quicker at protecting gastrointestinal tissue than some well-known drugs. It was more active in blocking the formation of ulcers in response to reserpine, enhanced the physical endurance toward hypoxia, inhibited metastasis, and improved the physical capacity for work.

The mycelium contains novel peptides. Hyun et al. identified a peptide that showed high platelet aggregation inhibition (Hyun, K. W. et al. 2006).

Methanol extracts were used for in vivo and in vitro studies of its anti-inflammatory and anti-nociceptive effect, probably due to inhibition of iNOS and COX-2 expression via the down-regulation of NF-kappaB binding activity (Park, Y.-M. et al. 2005).

Ho Gyoung Kim et al. (2007) suggest that chaga as a 70 percent ethanol extract may have clinical application for the management of inflammatory diseases based on inhibition of NF-kappaB through the phosphatydl inositol 3-kinase, Akt/l_kB pathway and inhibition of JNK activation.

According to Gorbunova et al. (2005) chaga activates the circulation of brain tissue elements and increases bioelectric activity in the cortex of the brain.

Yeunhwa Gu et al. (2005) reported the protective effect of chaga against radiation and in vivo antitumor effects. The authors make the point that the present approaches to tumors are surgery, radiation, and chemotherapy, or what I like to call the slash, burn, and poison approach. They suggest immunotherapy as a fourth therapeutic modality in the future. The first three do take a toll on the body and weaken immune function, and life expectancy could be greatly increased by exploring the potential of this and other medicinal mushrooms.

Bisko et al. found copper ions, pyrocatechol, and tyrosine stimulated the production of melanin in submerged chaga (Bisko et al. 2005). This melanin complex shows high antioxidant and genoprotective effects.

Melanin may play a key role in immune-stimulating function in herbs such as echinacea and ginseng, according to work by Dr. David Pasco at the University of Mississippi. He has found melanin, in mouse spleen studies, to be twenty times more potent than their polysaccharides.

Chaga sulphur soap is marketed in Korea with claims of anti-aging and moisturizing properties.

Essential Oil

Ayoub et al. (2009) found fifty-eight compounds representing 86 percent of the essential oil were found.

Non-terpenoids, mainly oxygenated aliphatic substances with fatty acids, dominate (48 percent).

Sesquiterpenes were dominant, with eighteen of them representing 32.5 percent of hydrodistillate. Beta selinene (16.4 percent) was found, as well as cis- and trans-bergamotene, alpha santalene, beta-sesquifenchene, santalene, photosantalol, and beta- and gamma-eudesmol.

Fungi Essence

Chaga essence is associated with emotional constrictions, where belief systems have sapped an individual's energy and vitality. This may be due to rigid religious doctrine or lasting impressions from early childhood indoctrination. The essence will help promote a more flexible approach to personal and spiritual rewards. It may help ease the suffering that sometimes accompanies perceived betrayals or guilt associated with moving away from old patterns.

When used in conjunction with cancer therapy, it may be useful when emotional rigidity is playing a negative role in immune response.

— Prairie Deva

Agroforestry

Paul Stamets mentions a Quebec arborist that crushed chaga into powder and made a paste that was applied directly to blight caused by *Cryphonectria parasitica* on beech. Over two years, the wounds healed and it became blight resistant. There may be other opportunities to utilize tree fungus species as a means of "inoculating" or protecting other tree species, including commercial fire orchards.

Recipes and Dosage

Decoction: to make chaga medicine, remove the inner orange-brown layers, either cutting them into strips or shredding and crumbling them. Use one tablespoon for each three liters of boiling water and let soak for four hours. Pour off this liquid and save the wet powder. Pour a cup

of water that has been heated and then cooled to fifty degrees Celsius over the fungus and leave at room temperature for two days. Drink up to three cups daily, thirty minutes before meals. This recipe is courtesy of Sherri Anderson, a Cree healer from Flying Dust First Nation.

A Russian recipe is somewhat different. Pour two and a half liters of boiling water over five hundred grams of dry chaga. Cover and let stand at room temperature for four days. Filter and refrigerate. Take the chaga and grind to mush. Add two liters of fifty degree Celsius water and let stand for forty-eight hours. Strain through cheesecloth and combine the two liquids. Drink two hundred milliliters four times per day before meals. This recipe should last four days.

Either recipe is good, but if the final product has 20 to 25 percent alcohol it will last indefinitely. Otherwise it must be prepared every three to four days. Since betulin and betulinic acid are concentrated in "oxidized black coating," my suggestion is to combine one part of a 95 percent alcohol extraction of this part of the fungi with two parts of the decoction made using the first recipe above.

Recent work suggests optimal antioxidant benefit is obtained from a 70 percent ethanol extract.

Steam treatment increases phenolics and antioxidant activity (Ju et al. 2010).

Extract: two hundred fifty to five hundred milligrams of an eight-to-one extract two to three times per day. Many powdered extracts are now standardized to a minimum 0.15 percent inotodiol.

Chaga is apparently non-toxic and without side effects. Some sources, however, suggest stopping intravenous glucose or penicillin-3 during chaga therapy.

Inonotus tomentosus

Polyporus tomentosus
Onnia tomentosa
Coltrichia tomentosa
(TOMENTOSUS ROOT ROT)
(WOOLLY VELVET POLYPORE)
Inonotus cuticularis
P. cuticularis
(CUTICULAR POLYPORE)
I. radiatus
Mensularia radiata
Xanthochrous radiatus
(RADIATED POLYPORE)
(ALDERWOOD POLYPORE)
(ALDER BRACKET)

Woolly velvet polypore is frequently found infesting the root systems of spruce or pine forests. They are polypores and yet this one is found on the ground. Careful eyes will find it attached to roots and wood buried underground.

The related *I. cuticularis* is found on willow, cottonwoods, and other hardwood trees throughout the region. It is woolly and matted with a nearly smooth cap. In folklore, it was considered a panacea for nearly every condition.

Traditional Uses

It has been used medicinally for gastric disturbances, hemorrhage, leprosy, and offensive body and foot odor.

In traditional Chinese medicine, the mushroom is considered sweet. It smoothes vital energy, strengthens the mind and spirit, and removes harmful wind conditions.

Medicinal Use

Research by Ito et al. (1973) in Japan indicated that this fungus contains a substance with B-cell-stimulating activity.

Studies have *I. cuticularis* inhibits Ehrlich carcinoma by 100 percent and sarcoma 180 by 90 percent, suggesting anticancer potential (Ohtsuka et al. 1973).

The related *I. radiatus* also displays antitumor activity (Kahlos, et al. 1989).

Separate studies by Hervey (1947) and Robbins et al. (1945) showed activity against *Staphylococcus aureus.*

It may be found on either birch or alder, and yields pure lupenone, ergosterol peroxide, and other sterols. Water extracts were inactive or only slightly active against Walker 256 and MCF-7, but ethanol extracts killed up to 50 percent of the cells in five days, suggesting moderate activity.

Ergosterol peroxide, when isolated, was 100 percent effective against the cell lines.

Mycoremediation

One study found this mycelium and *Trametes versicolor* both degraded humulones and lupulones from spent hops in only thirty-six hours when exposed to light and in four days in the dark.

Textile Industry

The polypore is dried and used as a source of brownish-orange dye for wool without mordant.

Inonotus hispidus

Polyporus hispidus
(BRISTLY POLYPORE)
(SHAGGY BRACKET)

Hispidus is Latin meaning "rough" or "bristly." This is derived from *hircine* and, in turn, *hircus* meaning "goat." Bristly polypore was once used as a drastic purgative in Germany.

Medicinal Use

Chemical Constituents
- **Hispidin and hispolon.**

The fungi produce styrylpyrones (hispidin) and derivatives of caffeic acid (hispolon) as pigments. Work by Pilgrim (1997) suggested these compounds might be a valuable source of new drugs.

Sure enough, later work by Awadh Ali et al. (2005) found antiviral activity from both hispolon and hispidin. They found ethanol extracts from both fruiting bodies and mycelium to possess considerable activity against influenza virus types A and B.

Hispolon and hispidin were found to inhibit the chemiluminescence response of human mononuclear blood cells and the mitogen-induced proliferation of spleen lymphocytes (Ali et al. 1996).

W. Chen et al. (2006) found hispolon inhibits human epidermoid KB cells with an IC50 of 4.62 micrograms per milliliter. It appears to activate caspase-3 and induce apoptosis via mitochnodria-mediated pathways.

One study found hispolon active against gastric cancer cells causing massive ROS accumulation in them; as well as potentiating cytotoxic effect of chemotherapeutic drugs.

Heng-Yuan Chang et al. (2011) found that hispolon reduces pain and inflammation through suppression of TNF-alpha and nitric oxide.

Hispidin is closely related, chemically speaking, to the kavanins in kava kava and the longistylines in the balche tree from southern Mexico.

Textile Industry

A fine brown dye is obtained from the conk for coloring silk, cotton, and wool, and formerly used by cabinet-makers and joiners for certain woods. It was used traditionally by leather dressers for skins, giving a fawn-chestnut color.

Irpex lacteus

(MILK WHITE TOOTHED POLYPORE)

This white leathery species is widely found on various hardwood trees, including birch and aspen.

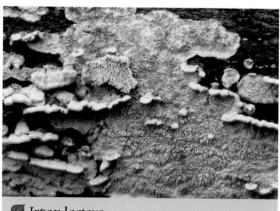

Irpex lacteus

It contains proteinase that makes an acceptable rennet substitute for curdling milk (Kobayashi, H. et al. 1983).

Medicinal Use

It shows activity against a number of bacteria and fungi including *Candida albicans, C. glabrata, C. parapsilosis, Bacillus cereus, E. coli, Staphylococcus aureus,* and *S. typhimurium* (Rosa et al. 2003).

Earlier work by Hayashi et al. (1981) identified the nematicidal compound 5-pentyl-2furaldehyde.

Silberborth et al. (2000) identified a number of irpexans while screening for new inhibitors of AP-1 and NFkappaB pathways that play roles in cancer and inflammation.

One member, 14-acetoxy-15-dihydroxyirpexan, inhibits the phorbol ester-induced expression of dependent reporter gene with IC_{50} values of five to six micrograms per milliliter.

It has been implicated in at least one case of pulmonary abscess in an immune compromised child in Austria (Buzina et al. 2005).

Ischnoderma resinosum

Polyporus resinosum
Lasiochlaena anisea
(LATE FALL POLYPORE)
(RESINOUS POLYPORE)

Late fall polypore is yet another bracket fungus showing medicinal benefit. It is dark brown and velvety, exuding an amber colored fluid when young. The flesh is spongy, with an anise scent.

The polypore is found growing on hardwood and coniferous stumps and logs late in the season. It may, at first glance, appear as a plump artist's conk *(G. applanatum),* and the white pore surface does brown when touched. The young caps are edible and quite tasty when cooked. It has a white spore print.

Traditional Uses

Native tribes of the boreal forest, including the Dene, decoct it for a half hour to treat coughs. About one third of a cup is considered a dose.

Medicinal Use

In studies conducted in China, the mushroom's inhibition rate against sarcoma 180 is 70 percent, and against Ehrlich carcinoma reaches 80 percent.

A beta galactosyl-specific lectin was the first lectin ever isolated from fungi (Kawagishi et al. 1995).

Early work identified moderate activity against *Staphylococcus aureus* (Robbins 1945).

Mycoremediation

The fungus decolorizes both Orange G and Remazol Brilliant Blue R, the former due to laccase, suggesting use in mycofiltration of chemical dye plant waters and industries that utilize these pigments.

Kuehneromyces

(see *Pholiota mutabilis*)

Laccaria laccata

(ORANGE LACCARIA)
(COMMON LACCARIA)
(THE DECEIVER)
L. amethystina
(PURPLE LACCARIA)
(AMETHYST DECEIVER)
L. amethysteo-occidentalis
(WESTERN AMETHYST LACCARIA)
L. bicolor
(TWO COLORED LACCARIA)

Laccaria is from the Persian *laccata* meaning "painted" or "lacquered." *Laccaria* is called "the deceiver" in various languages because of its wide variety of shapes, colors, and sizes.

Bicolor is from the Latin, distinguishing the tan cap and purple stem. *Amethystina* refers to the color of amethyst.

Orange *Laccaria* likes to fruit in cooler weather in bogs, woods, and meadows.

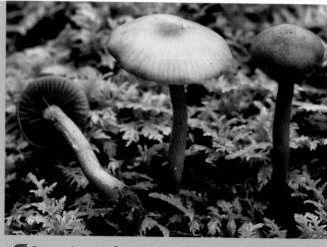

Laccaria amethystina

Raman et al. (1993), from India, have found that furnishing *L. laccata* with tryptophan will produce high amounts of indole 3-acetic acid in an industrial fermentation tank. *Laccaria* respond well to palmitate and oleate lipids for mycelial growth.

Two-colored Laccaria is often found in pine forests. An article in the journal *Nature* (April 5, 2001) found white pine has a mutually beneficial relationship with this mushroom. The mushroom grows among the roots, and preys upon springtails, a small insect, by exuding a toxin that paralyzes them. Like cordyceps, it grows inside them while they are still alive.

Springtails are one of the earth's most plentiful insects, numbering up to a hundred thousand per cubic meter of soil. The nitrogen obtained by the fungus, is then bartered with the pines to get the carbon it needs to synthesize enzymes. This research found that other fungi did not affect springtails in this manner. And when white pine seedlings were grown in controlled environments, without the fungi, they did not grow as well.

In isotope studies, the nitrogen from the insect was traced via the fungi to the trees, and it was discovered that up to one quarter of the nitrogen in the needles originated in the springtails.

Until now, scientists have depicted mushrooms as rather benign, deriving nitrogen from decaying matter and making it available in a passive manner. If predatory relationships such as this turn out to be common, scientists will have to rethink food webs in forest ecosystems. "If this phenomena proves to be widespread, it changes everything," says Klironomos.

The genome, or full DNA mapping of this species is now complete. It shows SSPs or small proteins that connect the fungus and trees in some manner.

Both orange *Laccaria* and amethyst deceiver are excellent, but strongly flavored edibles. They are especially delicious as accompaniments to meat or as an omelet filling.

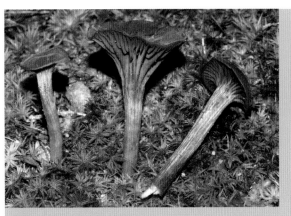

Laccaria amethystina

Purple *Laccaria* is a bio-accumulator of arsenic, up to 146.9 milligrams per kilogram according to Velter, and therefore should not be considered a safe edible. Some people enjoy the subtle, gentle flavor, but there are lots of better tasting and safer mushrooms.

Medicinal Use

The inhibition rate of *L. laccata* against sarcoma 180 and Ehrlich carcinoma is 60 to 70 percent (Ohtsuka et al. 1973).

Laccarin shows phosphodiesterase inhibitory activity (Matsuda et al. 1996).

Purple *Laccaria (L. amethystina)* is relatively rich in lipids, and in particular phosphatydl serine. This compound plays a major role in myelin sheath and brain synapse health.

It is rich in oleic acid at over 32 percent. Inhibition rates are 70 to 80 percent against the two cancer cell lines mentioned above (Ohtsuka et al. 1973).

Fungi Essence

Amethyst deceiver *(L. amethystea)* essence helps us in our inner transformation by bringing hidden inner "poisons" to the surface, then reducing their impact on mind, body, and soul. It opens the third eye chakra, thereby helping us manage the final breakthrough to new, more positive, self-awareness.

— Korte Phi

Mycoremediation

Laccaria species were the most frequently observed ectomycorrhiza associated with pine and poplar in reclaimed oil sands in northern Alberta (Bois et al. 2005). Mycoremediation of this huge industrial site is going to be a major challenge, but a considerable improvement on the present approach of sprinkling brome and native grass seeds and hoping for the best. Suncor, Syncrude, Shell, and other corporations could invest in fungal remediation research and lead the rest of the world by example.

Laccaria bicolor and *L. laccata* show a very high tolerance to creosote (Richter et al. 2003).

Lactarius

Lactarius volemus
(WEEPING MILK CAP)
(ORANGE BROWN MILK CAP)

L. camphoratus

L. fragilis var. rubidus

Lactifluus camphoratus
(SPICY MILK CAP)
(CANDY CAP)
(AROMATIC MILK CAP)

L. uvidus
(PURPLE STAINING MILK CAP)
(MOIST LACTARIUS)

L. deliciosus

L. deliciosus var deterrimus

L. deterrimus
(DELICIOUS MILK CAP)
(SAFFRON MILK CAP)

L. torminosus
(WOOLY MILK CAP)
(PINK FRINGED MILK CAP)
(BEARDED MILK CAP)

L. atroviridus
(BLACK GREEN MILK CAP)

L. glyciosmus
(COCONUT MILK CAP)

L. aquifluus

L. helvus
(WATERDROP MILK CAP)
(BURNT SUGAR MILKY)

L. fumosus
(SMOKY MILK CAP)

L. rufus
(RED HOT MILK CAP)

L. vellereus
(DEADLY MILK CAP)

Lactarius is from the Latin *lac* meaning "milk." *Torminosus* is Latin meaning "full of sharpness," "causing pain," or "suffering from colic." *Uvidus* means "moist," *camphoratus* is "spicy," *glyciosmus* means "sweet scent," and *volemus* is Latin for a type of large pear. Milk cap refers to the lactating nature. *Aquifluus* means "watery."

They are closely related to the *Russula* (see below) and are noted for their waxy gills and cleanly snapping brittle flesh.

They are generally sharp and biting when sampled. The French call them *eau boiront* or "water drinkers," and *poivres* or "peppers" due to the pungency of their milk. The pungent and peppery components are due to sesquiterpenes released when the fungi are damaged.

Many *Lactarius* and *Russula* are considered more unpleasant than seriously poisonous, and most are edible when cooked with several changes of water.

A general rule of thumb is that those with orange or red milk are edible if cooked.

L. camphoratus, also known as curry scented milk cap, has a sweet taste that will later turn bitter. The caps smell like camphor to some authors when fresh, and to others like woodlice. When dry, it is more like curry leaf or ground chicory root.

It exudes white milk but is considered edible. The dried mushroom powder is often used in cakes and cookies, or curry dishes.

Spicy milk cap *(L. camphoratus)* has a distinct fenugreek, maple syrup odor, even when dried. Some individual mushrooms have a coumarin-like odor more similar to sweet clover, celery, or even beef bouillon. It can be used to flavor

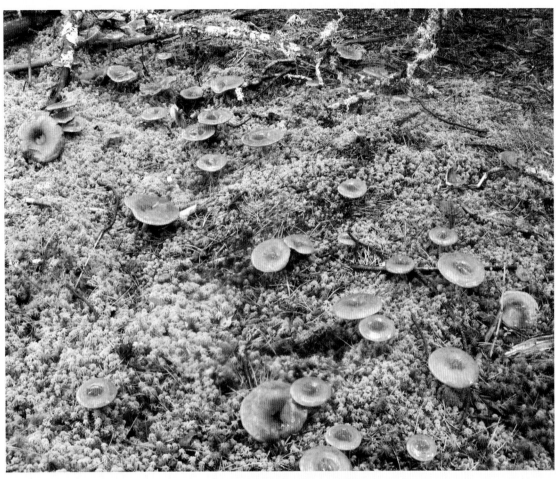

Clockwise from above: *Lactarius rufus; Lactarius peckii; Lactarius corrugis; Lactarius deliciosa.*

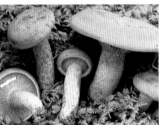

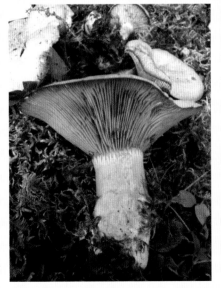

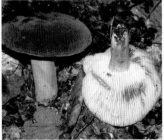

cake icing, giving a burnt sugar, or even walnut flavor to confections.

This same scent is shared by the northern boreal and bog-oriented *L. helvus (L. aquifluus)*, but this species has clear latex. See below.

The related *L. atroviridus,* generally found under oak in eastern Canada, contains powerful mutagenic compounds.

The Northern *L. glyciosmus* is found near birch and alders. It has a distinct scent, somewhere between coconut and bergamot.

Moist *Lactarius (L. uvidus)* is not a recommended edible due to gastrointestinal disturbance.

Delicious milk cap is a safe edible mushroom found in pine or spruce forests. It is bright orange, with the same color latex, and a green discoloration. The popularity of this edible mushroom is told by its appearance on postal stamps from ten different countries. Some authors believe *L. deterrimus* is a variation, while others think it is a separate variety. It has paler gills and the stem is not pitted, but both are edible. It is widely picked and sold commercially in Finland. In my region it is associated with pine, but if you find a species in douglas fir country, it may be the closely related *L. rubrilacteus,* with dark red latex. Both are tasty.

Despite the name, it is not considered that delicious by some mycophiles! Linnaeus may well have confused it with the southern European bleeding milk cap *(L. sanguifluus)*. Personally, I like the sweet, nutty flavor, which is enhanced by cooking it in butter.

In Poland, a piece of bacon is wrapped around the fresh cap and placed in a hot oven until cooked. Yum!

Wooly milk cap is a powerful purgative when eaten raw, but when parboiled may be considered edible. It is widespread and common, especially under birch, and noted for its white, peppery milk. The toxins are unidentified, but are destroyed by heat. I would be cautious!

Muhlmann et al. (2006) found this ectomycorrhizal fungus associates with bearberry *(Arctostaphylos uva-ursi),* as well as spruce.

Waterdrop milk cap *(L. helvus)* is found in wet parts of the boreal forest. It has clear, colorless latex and smells like maple syrup or fenugreek.

It contains two unusual compounds, 13-methylene-L-(+)-norvaline, and 2 methylenecycloheptene-1,3-diglycine.

Smoky milk cap *(L. fumosus)* has a turnip-like odor.

Red hot milk cap is commonly found in sandy areas under pine.

Traditional Uses

Lactarius species have been used for their medicinal benefit in a number of cultures. Saffron milk cap (or the related bleeding milk cap) is depicted on a two-thousand-year-old Roman fresco.

Lactaroviolin is said to be active against Koch's bacillus (TB), and is anti-rheumatic in a manner similar to cartizon, according to a Latvian website. The French physician Dufresnoi, practicing at the beginning of the nineteenth century, reported curing more than thirty cases of tuberculosis using an electuary of *Lactarius deliciosus,* rose petals, spermaceti, washed sulphur, and a syrup of yarrow. A colleague powdered the dried mushroom and mixed it with honey for the same purpose. Dosage was less than a teaspoon at one time.

Some *Lactarius* fungi, prepared into a tincture, have been used for tuberculosis.

L. vellereus is used in Tendon Easing Pills in traditional Chinese medicine.

Medicinal Use

Chemical Constituents

- *L. deliciosus:* **5-methylcytosine; tryptamine; tryptophan; melatonin; indole and indoacetic acid; lectins high in glycogen including lactaroviolin, lactarazulene, lactarovidlin, and lactarofulvene; 37 international units per hundred grams of thiamine; up to 690 micrograms per hundred grams of riboflavin; trehalase; and 300 micrograms per hundred grams of manganese.**

- *L. volemus:* **lactariamide A-B and cerbroside D.**

- *L. uvidus:* **uvidin A and drimenol.**

- *L. camphoratus:* **12-hydroxy-caryophyllene-4,5-oxide.**

- *L. helvus:* **13-methylene-L-(+)-norvaline and 2 methylenecycloheptene-1,3-diglycine.**

- *L. vellereus:* **three novel lactones, lactariolide, and subvellerolactone A and C.**

- *L. piperatus:* **marasmane sesquiterpenoids, as well as lactarorufin and furosardonin, blennin A and D, and isolactarorufin.**

- *L. rufus:* **lactarinic acid.**

Weeping milk cap has been shown to contain substances exhibiting tumor inhibition, as well as the novel compounds lactariamide A and B and cerebroside D. It has a distinct fishy odor. Weeping milk cap has been found to inhibit

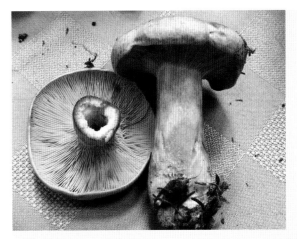

🍃 *Lactarius deterrimus*

sarcoma 180 by 80 percent and Ehrlich carcinoma by 90 percent.

Lactarovidlin is a sesquiterpene aldehyde with moderate cytotoxic activity. It contains a stearic acid ester of sesquiterpene with similar activity, and deterrol, an alcohol with weak antibacterial activity against *Staphylococcus aureus.* All three components have been found to be weakly mutagenic.

Lactaroviolin was found to inhibit tubercle bacilli at concentration of one to 16,000.

Dulger et al. (2002a) found the delicious milk cap active against a number of gram-positive and gram-negative bacteria including *E. coli, Proteus vulgaris,* and *Mycobacterium smegmatis.* Weak inhibition was also noted against *S. aureus, Bacillus cereus,* and *B. megaterium.*

Puttaraju et al. (2006) found this mushroom rated very high among twenty-three tested for antioxidant activity. This was confirmed by Sarikurkcu et al. (2008).

One isolated red-violet pigment, lactaroviolin, has been found mildly antibiotic.

Moist *Lactarius (L. uvidus)* contains fatty acid esters of uvidin A and drimenol that show cytotoxic and insect antifeedant activity. Both of these compounds have been used for the semi-synthesis of biologically active compounds like cinnamodial, cinnamosmolide, and pereniporin A.

Spicy milk cap *(L. camphoratus)* contains anti-carcinogenic substances. Its inhibition against both sarcoma 180 and Ehrlich carcinoma is 70 percent.

The sesquiterpene 12-hydroxy-caryophyllene-4,5-oxide has been isolated from ethanol extracts. This molecule contributes to the spicy taste of black pepper and cloves.

H. Wang and T. B. Ng (2007) found a hot-water extract of *L. camphoratus* inhibited HIV-1 reverse transcriptase activity by 53.5 percent.

New compounds isolated from the related *L. violascens* and *L. rubrocinctus* are two protilludans and four marasmane sesquiterpenes.

Methanol extracts of *L. vellereus* show anti-mutagenic activity, and inhibit in vitro binding of lipopolysaccharides to the C14 receptor on immune cells. This suggests the possibility in development of drugs to address septic shock (Mlinaric et al. 2004) .

This fungus and the related *L. subvellereus* inhibit sarcoma 180 by 70 percent and Ehrlich carcinoma by 60 percent. Jing Zhang and X. Z. Feng (1997) have found that ethyl acetate extracts are cytotoxic and possess antitumor activity.

Three novel lactones, lactariolide and subvellerolactone A and C, have been isolated and identified. Extracts of *L. vellereus* show activity against *Fusarium* species (Guler et al. 2009).

L. vellereus contains velleral and isovelleral, which possess antifungal and antibacterial activity, and an unstable sesquiterpene (velutinal) that reacts enzymatically upon injury. These compounds, including isovelleral and velleral, have strong antibacterial activity against *Escherichia coli* and fungi *(Candida utilis)* that activates within five minutes of mincing the mushroom.

Isovelleral induces calcium uptake or inhibits RTX binding. It appears to influence vanilloid receptors associated with pain control, and the dopamine D1 receptor of the central nervous system. It may prove of some medicinal benefit as an isolated drug.

Inhibition rates of 60 percent against Ehrlich carcinoma and sarcoma 180 cancer cell lines have been found (Ohtsuka et al. 1973).

Mlinaric et al. (2004) found methanol extracts protect against quinoline-induced DNA damage in human-derived cells. The mushroom can be considered a natural source of anti-mutagens with potential application in cancer prevention.

Lactarius sesquiterpenoid alcohols show antiviral activity. One study assessed T and B cell proliferation, interleukin 2, TNF alpha, and interferon gamma in vitro. One compound, isolactarorufin 8-epi, significantly inhibited T lymphocyte proliferation and synthesis of all tested cytokines. Two N-acetyl-phenylisoserinates showed antiviral, cytotoxic, anti-proliferative, and immunotropic properties in vitro. Two compounds inhibit herpes simplex 1 virus growth.

The related *L. badiosanguineus* inhibits thrombin by 31 percent (Doljak et al. 2001). *L. latsudake* contains phospholipase A_2 inhibitors.

Peppery milk cap *(L. piperatus)* contains a number of marasmane sesquiterpenoids, as well as lactarorufin and furosardonin, blennin A and D, and isolactarorufin. It contains natural liquid rubber latex. Hot-water extracts have been found to inhibit Lewis pulmonary adenoma in white mice with an inhibition rate of 80 percent against sarcoma 180 and 70 percent against Ehrlich carcinoma.

Methanol extracts show activity against *E. coli, Proteus vulgaris,* and *Mycobacterium smegmatis.*

Younger fruiting bodies are more potent (Barros et al. 2007b).

The related *L. hygrophoroides* shows inhibition against the two cancer cell lines of 70 Percent (Ohtsuka et al. 1973).

Essential Oil

Waterdrop milk cap *(L. helvus)* has been steam distilled and yields 0.04 percent essential oil composed of 25.6 percent capric acid, 15.8 percent 3-amino-4,5-di-methyl-2(5H)-furanone, and 1.4 percent sotolon. The latter compound is responsible for the fenugreek odor of the mushroom. Sotolon is widely used as a flavoring agent in artificial maple syrup, curry, sherry, old sake, and tobacco. It is found in soy sauce, sugar molasses, and even barley malt for beer.

Insecticide

Acetone and ether extracts of smoky milk cap *(L. fumosus)* have potent insecticidal activity.

Fungicide

Red hot milk cap contains rufuslactone, an antifungal that exhibits great activity against other plant fungi and may be useful in crop protection and greenhouse production. Rufuslactone is particularly aggressive against *Alternaria brassicae.*

Recipes and Dosage

Prepare fresh at a ratio of 1:3 with 90 percent alcohol.

Hobbs suggests preparing the tincture immediately after grinding in a blender to destroy enzymes that might break down active ingredients. Good tip. Use caution.

Take ten to twenty-five drops of tincture twice a day.

Laetiporus sulphureus

L. conifericola
L. gilbertsonii
Polyporus sulphureus
Tyromyces sulphureus
(CHICKEN OF THE WOODS)
(SULPHUR SHELF)

Laetiporus is Latin meaning "a wealth of pores." *Sulphureus* means "a sulphur or bright yellow color," or may allude to the fungi's fragrance.

More than forty compounds are responsible for its odor and taste, including 1-octen-3one, 1-octen-3-ol, 3-methyl butanoic acid, phenyl ethanol and phenylacetic acid (Wu, S. et al. 2005a).

It smells strongly of rotten eggs, but tastes like chicken if eaten when young. Jack Czernacki, a noted chef, writes, "Eating an unfit chicken mushroom is like trying to digest a piece of wood. It never softens and it leaves your mouth feeling dried out and exhausted." I have to agree.

251

This bright lemon to orange-colored fungus is found on the trunks and stems of conifers. When found on birch and other hardwoods they are known as *L. gilbertsonii*.

They can be quite large, with one weighing in at more than a hundred pounds found near New Forest, Hampshire, England.

A recent find, in 1998 at Kew Green, Surrey, has been estimated to weigh 697 pounds and is still growing! As of 2003, it measured more than sixteen feet in circumference. A humongous fungus indeed!

At present, the mushroom is not commercially harvested or marketed and available to health consumers wishing to take advantage of its antifungal, antibacterial, and antitumor properties.

In parts of central Europe, it was reduced to a powder and added to flour to make bread.

Traditional Uses

In eastern Russia, sulphur shelf has a long history of folkloric use as a natural antibiotic and weak disinfectant.

Chicken of the woods is helpful in regulating the health of the human body, improving and defending the body against illness, if taken regularly.

It has been traditionally dried and powdered as a snuff.

Medicinal Use

Chemical Constituents

- **N-phenetyl-hexadecanamide; laetiporic acids A-C; various lanostanoid triterpenes including 3-oxosulfurenic acid, acetyl eburicoic acid, fucomannogalactans,** laminaran (beta-glucan), masutakeside (benzofuran glycoside), and masutakic acid A (a C10 acetylenic acid); egonol; demethoxyegonol; egonol glucoside and egonol gentiobioside; and dehydro-trametenolic acid.

- **Also contains beauvericin, a mycotoxin produced by hypocrealean ascomycetes in grain.**

Water extracts of the fruiting body inhibit Ehrlich carcinoma in white mice, suggesting antitumor activity.

Eburicoic acid produced by the sporophore may be used to synthesize steroids that play an important role in human health.

A useful tool for studying the structures of heterosaccharide chains has been isolated from this mushroom in a highly purified form.

One study suggests inhibition of thrombin formation. In fact, it showed a forty-four-fold inhibition over controls.

Sulphur shelf is unique in that it has the advantage of being almost free of alpha-mannosidase activity.

Lovy et al. (1999) looked at the mushroom and demonstrated activity against human T4 leukemia cells, as well as *Plasmodium falciparum*. Another study found the mycelium strongly antagonistic to *Staphylococcus aureus* and moderately effective against *Bacillus subtilis*.

Further work has noted mushroom cultures destroy *E. coli* upon contact.

The mycelium shows strong activity against *Serratia marcescens,* which is a major source of urinary tract infection in those suffering cystic fibrosis, as well as cuts and burns. This bacterium also causes septicemia and respiratory disease, especially in immune-compromised patients.

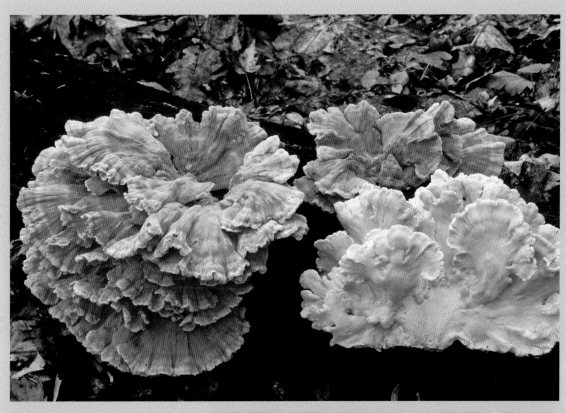

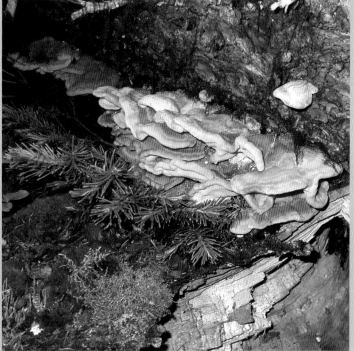

Above: *Laetiporus sulphureus*. Right and below: *Laetiporus conifericola*.

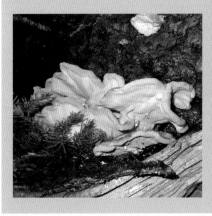

Submerged cultures show a wide range of antibacterial activity against both gram-negative and gram-positive organisms. This includes methicillin-resistant *S. aureus* (MRSA), a growing concern related to previous overuse of antibiotics. Maximal antimicrobial activity was reached after one week of growth (Ershova et al. 2003).

Dehydrotrametenolic acid acts as an insulin sensitizer in glucose tolerance tests and reduces high blood sugar in mice with non-insulin-dependent diabetes (Sato, M. et al. 2002).

Kazuko Yoshikawa et al. (2001) found some compounds in *L. sulphureus var. miniatus* cytotoxic against Kato III cells.

Work in Slovenia by Slane et al. (2004) found chicken of the woods exhibited lipase-inhibitory activity of 83 percent.

Lanostanoid triterpenes have been found to induce apoptosis in HL-60 human myeloid leukemia cells (Leon et al. 2004).

Extracts were found active against HIV-1 reverse transcriptase inhibitors (Mlinaric et al. 2005).

Beauvericin has shown antimicrobial activity.

Chicken of the woods contains alkaloids similar to those found in psychoactive plants like kava kava, as well as sulphurenic acid, trigonelline, and homarine.

The fruiting body contains 15alpha hydroxy-trametenolic acid, as well as sulphurenic acid. Both show dopamine D2 receptor agonist activity.

It has been used to induce strong tryptamine-like hallucination in at least one clinical documented case (Appleton et al. 1988).

Essential Oil

It contains twenty-six volatiles such as 3-methyl cinnamaldehyde, 2 phenylethanol, benzaldehyde, and N-phenylethyl formamide.

Mycoremediation

Wunch et al. (1997) found the extracellular filtrate of this mushroom decolorized 68 percent of polymeric R-478 dye.

Sack et al. (1997) found mineralization of phenanthrene and pyrene compounds. *Trametes versicolor* was shown to be a better degrader but what else is new!

Textile Industry

Sulphur shelf was a source of yellow cloth dyeing in nineteenth-century France.

Insecticide

The older sporophore is burned to drive off mosquitoes and black flies.

Leccinum boreale

(NORTHERN ROUGH STEM)
(REDCAP)
L. insigne
(ASPEN ROUGH STEM)
L. ochraceum
(OCHRE ROUGH STEM)
L. aurantiacum
(ORANGE BOLETE)
L. scabrum
(BIRCH BOLETE)
(BROWN BIRCH BOLETE)

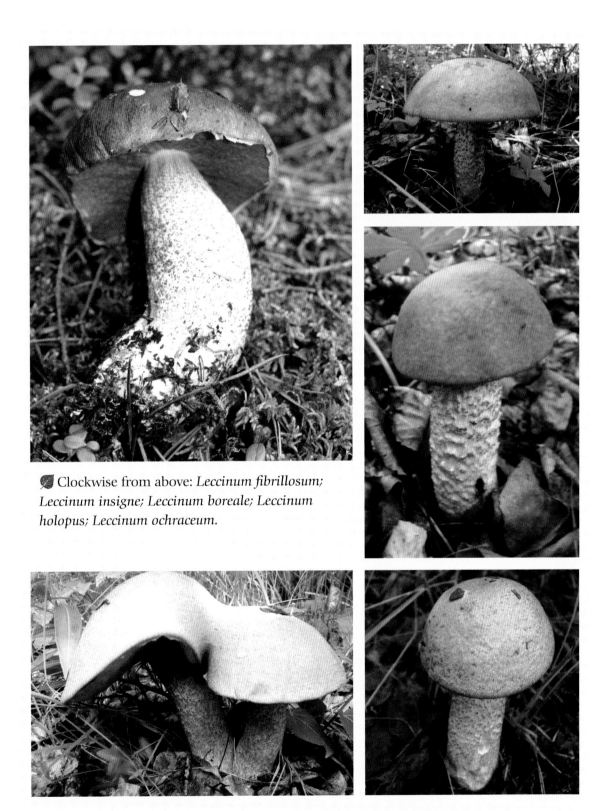

🌿 Clockwise from above: *Leccinum fibrillosum; Leccinum insigne; Leccinum boreale; Leccinum holopus; Leccinum ochraceum.*

The foray was planned to find Leccinum
Through poplar we walked just to find 'em
The mushrooms we brought back
Were cooked up, turned black
But so delicious we again went to find some.
— RDR

Northern rough stem or redcap has been chosen as Alberta's provincial mushroom. Starting in 2003, the Edmonton Mycological Society began a series of consultations and nominations for a fungal emblem. After due process, three mushrooms were selected for the final vote: redcap, oyster *(Pleurotus ostreatus),* and comb's tooth *(Hericium ramosum).* All were worthy nominees, but I am pleased that the regional and distinct redcap was the overall winner. The process for official designation is now underway, and Alberta will soon be the first province in Canada with an official mushroom.

The *Leccinum* genus was a popular substitute for the edible bolete by eastern European immigrants. The *Boletus* contain pulvinic acids that turn the flesh blue upon exposure to oxygen, while the caffeic and gallic acids in *Leccinum* turn a black color. My Polish in-laws, Joe and Olga Szott, grew up near Daysland and in their younger years lived on redcaps summer after summer. When I find a large patch, I send a big box to them by Greyhound, for they really do enjoy the mushroom. They refer to them as *kozoki.*

There can be individual sensitivity to the cooked mushroom, or development of gastrointestinal distress after consumption over extended periods of time. Some find it best to avoid alcohol when consuming them.

Consumption of even well cooked orange cap found under poplar in Colorado has led to some stomach distress, so caution is advised.

As agriculture has become more intense, and the widespread use of fungicides and pesticides more prevalent, their populations have diminished.

Martin Osis notes that *L. boreale* slowly turns light pink to purple-gray after cutting, and has no green tinge. Aspen rough stem *(L. insigne)* has a green tinge around the base of the stalk, and quickly turns mauve or gray upon cutting.

Medicinal Use
Chemical Constituents
- **Orange bolete: 314 milligrams of potassium, thirty milligrams of calcium, and nine milligrams of magnesium per hundred grams.**
- ***L. scabrum:* 740 micrograms manganese per hundred grams.**

Gzogian et al. (2005) found high activity of trypsin inhibitors detected in *L. aurantiacum.*

Lentinula edodes

Lentinus edodes
Tricholomopsis edodes
Cortinellus edodes
C. shiitake
Armillaria edodes
(SHIITAKE)

As they talk, I dream. I am clearing out my clothes and scrubbing my closet as I have never scrubbed it before. I prepare my agar medium of potato dextrose and malt extract, add a dash of alfalfa and pea rinds, and transfer my sterile spores. In days, beautiful, cottony white mycelia appear in my Petri dish. I am scouring the woods for logs, dragging them home and drilling them with holes. Then I plug them with shiitake spawn, and before I can say *Lentinus edodes,* trees filled with shiitake are crowding my backyard. I am queen of the shiitake forest.

— FRIEDMAN

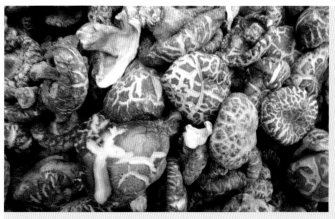

Dried *Lentinula edodes*

Lentinus is from *lent* meaning "pliable" or "supple" and *inus* for "resembling," due to the malleable nature of the fruiting body. *Edodes* means "edible." Shiitake is derived from its relationship with the shiia tree, a Japanese evergreen oak, thus "the oak mushroom."

In China, it is called *shaingugu* or *hsiang ku* meaning fragrant mushroom. It is that as well!

The former genus name, *Lentinus,* led overzealous bureaucrats to ban the mushroom from cultivation in North America until 1972. See *Lentinus lepideus* below.

I love eating shiitakes! Other people obviously enjoy them as well, for it is the second most common mushroom consumed in the world after the button *(Agaricus).* Around 200 AD, the Emperor Chuai was offered, it is believed, shiitake mushrooms by the Kyusuyu, the original aboriginals of Japan.

Shiitake has been cultivated in China since the Song Dynasty in 1100 AD. A woodcutter named Wu San Kwung cut into a log with shiitake and later noticed the mushrooms growing where his ax had struck. This was the beginning of log cultivation, and today his name lives on in festivals and temples throughout the Zhejiang province.

Today, numerous farmers are engaged in shiitake production in China. In 2002, the total production of fresh shiitake topped two million tons. Japan produces more than a billion dollars' worth annually with some 200,000 people employed in the industry.

The United States currently produces about five million pounds annually.

The spicy smell of shiitake is attributed in large part to the content of 1,2,4-trithiolane.

In Japan, there are two general types of shiitake. Donko is a round, thick-fleshed, partially opened cap, while koshin has thinner flesh and an open cap. The former is more highly prized for medicinal value, due in part to the retention of spores.

Be warned that like other mushrooms, shiitakes should be cooked prior to consumption. One case involving daily consumption over a two-week period led to allergic contact dermatitis (Kopp et al. 2009).

Shiitake does not lose its medicinal benefit when cooked at temperatures up to 392 degrees Fahrenheit (200 degrees Celsius).

Shiitake may be eaten sautéed or dried and reconstituted. It may be made into tea by pouring boiled water over the dried, minced caps or by adding dried powder to water and boiling it over low heat until reduced by half.

Fresh shiitake and button *(Agaricus bisporus)* mushrooms in glycerine are used in facial masks for their ability to reduce thread veins.

Cultivation

I have not tried growing them in Alberta, but my colleague and fellow researcher Gordon Steinrath has grown shiitake successfully on alder in British Columbia. They can be grown, with lower yields, on birch logs stacked above ground. Logs must be freshly cut and stacked, with mycelium plugs or sawdust spawn sealed with cheese wax. Newer sawdust plug spawn has a Styrofoam backing and is self-sealing. Both work fine. The logs need moisture and should be watered once a week if nature does not provide timely rains. A number of companies in Scotland utilize birch for shiitake cultivation. Oak is their wood of choice.

Considering the importance of the mushroom, it would be worth running some outdoor trials on various hardwood trees. Shiitake can be easily grown indoors, of course, but I love the idea of picking the fruiting bodies from dead and dying trees during a woodlot walk.

Shiitake, as selected strains, may be cultivated on wheat straw, with best results on sterilized straw at 250 degrees Fahrenheit (121 degrees Celsius) (Mata et al. 2001). It also grows well on vineyard prunings, and fits in well with mycotourism in the Pacific Northwest.

The addition of 0.6 percent calcium carbonate to the substrate produced more consistent yields (Royse et al. 2003).

Shiitake grown on a medium contain L-arabinose as a source of carbon and L-asparagine as a source of nitrogen (9.5-12:1) on days fifteen to eighteen of culturing at pH eight to nine was found optimal for production of lectins.

Paul Stamets has shown that shiitake grown and dried indoors contains only 110 international units of vitamin D per hundred grams, but the same strain grown under diffuse light and sun-dried with gills up increased to 46,000 international units. This is an astounding discovery! Mau and Tseng (1998) noted modest two- to three-fold increases in vitamin D_2 and ergosterol content after exposure to UVB radiation.

Earlier work found a five- to seven-fold increase in shiitake cultivated outdoors, compared to those grown indoors. Higher D_2 levels were found in those harvested on sunny, as compared to cloudy, days.

Traditional Uses

Shiitake has been used in traditional Chinese and Japanese Kampo medicine for centuries to increase stamina and circulation and help to alleviate arthritis, diabetes, high blood cholesterol, and immune deficiency.

The dried powder and purified polysaccharides help stimulate the immune system.

Medicinal Use

Chemical Constituents

- **Twelve different polysaccharides, lentinan, LEM (heteroglucan protein) from mycelia, lignins, KS-2 (alpha mannan peptide) glycoproteins, eritadenine, methyl sulphide, ergosterol, ergocalciferol, 33 percent protein, 47 percent complex carbohydrates, sugars including xylose and arabinose, B12, and thirty-seven enzymes. The molecular structure of lentinan sugars forms a helix that resembles the helix of DNA.**

- **Mycelium: peptide mannans, double stranded RNA, eritadenine, c-AMP modulating endocrines, phyto-hemaglutinine, guanile monophosphate, and ergosterol.**

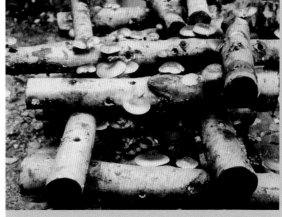

Shiitake cultivated on alder logs

Lentinan is a beta-1, 3-D-glucan that activates the lymphokine activated killer and natural killer cells of the immune system to combat various cancers. It reduces prostaglandins responsible for creating inflammation that would prevent T-cell maturation.

It is medically approved in Japan for the treatment of gastric cancers.

Lentinan is widely used in Japan for breast cancer in women who have had mastectomies without radiation follow-up. When chemotherapy is used, lentinan given prior to treatment prevents further immune system damage.

In one study of sixteen patients with advanced cancer, lentinan was injected directly into tumors. All of the patients died, like the control group, but they lived an average of 129 days, compared to forty-nine days for those given drugs only (Oka 1992).

When shiitake is formed into micelles, it increases lymphocyte proliferation by 40 percent.

An open-label study of sixty-two men with prostate cancer and elevated PSA levels given shiitake extract found no change in their status, suggesting other mushrooms are of greater benefit in this particular disease.

A randomized study of eighty-nine stomach cancer patients showed median survival time of 189 days with chemotherapy and lentinan, compared to only 109 days with chemotherapy alone.

A polysaccharide preparation administered intraperitoneal was found ten times more effective against sarcoma 180 cancer cells than mitocyin C.

Lentinan has been found active against both lung cancer and melanoma.

Work appears to confirm the cytostatic and immune-modulating properties of shiitake, especially around direct inhibition of human breast cancer cells. This work involved water extracts.

One study found lentinan fed to lab mice for seven days before tumor invasion showed a 94.4 percent rate of inhibition.

Lentinan was given to three patients with *Mycobacterium tuberculinum* resistant to drugs. When given by injection, the levels of opsonin toward the bacilli were so greatly elevated that excretion ceased in one patient, followed by great improvement. Resistance to both tuberculosis and *Listeria monocytogenes* was noted in this work.

A study looked at lentinan's effect on twenty-nine bacteria and ten pathogenic fungi. The extracts were 85 percent effective, including 50 percent effective against yeast and mold (Hearst et al. 2009).

A more recent study found intranasal administration of lentinan increased production of alveolar macrophages in the presence of *Mycobacterium tuberulinum*.

Polysaccharides in the mushroom help enhance production of interferon, which reduces blood vessel overgrowth in conditions such as macular degeneration of the eyes.

A polysaccharide, L-II, isolated from the fruiting body showed significant decrease in sarcoma 180, as well as phagocytosis of macrophage, increased TNF-alpha and IFN-gamma, increased NO production and catalase activity.

Eritadenine (lentinacin) helps lower total cholesterol, triglyceride, and phospholipids levels. In one human study, three hundred milligrams per day of eritadenine for seven days decreased bile cholesterol content in choledochostomy patients, while the total bile acid concentration, especially of deoxycholic acid, was increased.

A diet composed of 5 percent eritadenine decreased blood pressure in hypertensive rats, probably due to water-soluble oligosaccharides and content of tyrosinase.

Enman et al. identified shiitake strains with up to ten times the levels of eritadenine, suggesting the use of dried concentrates for therapeutic benefit in removal of blood cholesterol (Enman et al. 2007). This is in contrast to statin drugs that inhibit biosynethesis of cholesterol in the liver.

Follow-up work found eritadenine in submerged mycelial growth, making commercial propagation viable (Enman et al. 2008).

Both eriadenine and ethanolamine showed marked hypocholesterolemic effects (Shimada, Y. et al. 2003).

Shiitake may be of benefit in treating colitis. Shuvy et al. (2008) looked at the mushroom's benefit in liver-mediated immune regulation. This mice study found oral ingestion of fruiting body extracts altered NRT lymphocyte distribution and increased intrahepatic CD8 (+)T lymphocyte trapping, leading to alleviation of immune-mediated colitis.

Fractions from shiitake, enoki, matsutake and hen of the woods have shown in lab studies the ability to inhibit conversion of stem cells into adipocytes, suggesting an anti-fat influence (Ohtsuru et al. 2000).

Eritadenine has been found active against the influenza virus in mice.

Macrophage activation by the high molecular weight glycoproteins from the mycelia was found to suppress liver cancer formation (Sugano et al. 1982).

A freeze-dried extract of mycelia was given

to an AIDS patient with HIV antibodies. After two months, the T4 cell count doubled and symptoms were alleviated.

Water-soluble extracts inhibit the herpes virus both in vitro and in vivo. Lignins known as EP3 and EPS4 inhibit herpes simplex virus types 1 and 2 and western equine encephalitis virus, and partially inhibit the effects of polio, measles, and mumps viruses (Sorimachi et al. 1990).

Cell-free extracts from liquid fermentation of the mycelium inhibited the growth of *Candida albicans, Streptococcus pyogenes, Staphylococcus aureus,* and *Bacillus megaterium* (Hatvani 2001).

Even the mushroom juice inhibits pathogenic and opportunistic microorganisms. A study showed the juice of shiitake had pronounced effect on *C. albicans, S. aureus, E. coli,* and *E. faecalis.* Both lactobacteria and bifidobacteria, the healthy intestinal bacteria, were unaffected.

In fact, water extracts of *L. edodes* demonstrate growth-enhancing effects on both *L. brevis* and *B. breve* due to the disaccharide sugar, trehalose.

Work by Bae et al. (1997) suggests that the extracts can reduce the harmful effects of bacterial enzymes such as beta glucosidase, beta glucuronidase, and trytophanase, as well as reduce colon cancer formation.

Ethanol extracts of the mycelium possess anti-protozoal activity against *Paramecium caudatum.* An alcohol extract of the mycelium known as KS-2 has been found to induce the body's own production of interferon and stimulates macrophages to kill tumor cells.

Another study indicates that lentinan may potentiate resistance to *Klebsiella pneumoniae,*

Listeria monocytogenes, and *Streptococcus pneumoniae* (Chihara 1983).

In vitro studies suggest antifungal activity against *Trichophyton* species (Takazawa et al. 1982).

Sia and Candlish (1999) demonstrated that mushroom extracts enhance production of white blood cells and phagocytosis.

LEM, or *Lentinula edodes* mycelium, is a protein-bound polysaccharide that has been shown to inhibit HIV infection of cultured human T-cells and potentiate the effect of AZT against viral replication. In a phase II study, 107 HIV-positive patients were treated with didanosin for six weeks. After this time, eighty-eight patients were given two milligrams of lentinan per week intravenously, while the control group was given only the drug. The combined treatment significantly increased CD4+ cells after thirty-eight weeks compared to the control.

Lentinan has been found effective in increasing T-cell production when given at low doses, but at increased amounts, patients show lower T-cell counts.

A lignin-rich fraction from LEM called JLS-18 has been found to possess seventy times the antiviral activity of LEM itself.

EP3 is lignin that shows high activity against HIV in the lab. It reduced replication by 90 percent and completely inhibited the toxic effect of HIV to T-cells. Herpes simplex I and II and western equine encephalitis virus were also completely inhibited. Partial inhibition of mumps, measles, and polio viruses was observed.

In one randomized, controlled trial, 275 patients with advanced or recurrent stomach cancer were given chemotherapy with or without lentinan. The best results were found when the mushroom extract was administered before chemotherapy and in those without prior chemotherapy.

A monosaccharide derived from the mycelium of several *Basidiomycete* mushrooms, including shiitake, cultivated in a fermentation tank is known as Active Hexose Correlated Compound, or AHCC. After a series of steps and freeze-drying, a product with an exceptionally low molecular weight of five thousand daltons is produced. The active nutrient is acetylated beta-glucan, which enhances the immune system. More than seven hundred hospitals in Japan use it as part of protocols associated with chemotherapy to reduce hospital infections and support against the formation of abnormal cells. More than eighty research studies have been conducted. It appears to stimulate macrophages as well as increasing their numbers. This leads to increased production of cytokines like IL-12 and TNF, LAK and CTL cells directly, and interferon indirectly.

Animal research suggests it may be more effective at enhancing IL-12 levels in Th-1 dominant individuals.

A prospective cohort study with AHCC from February 1992 to January 2002, was conducted on 269 patients with hepatocellular carcinoma with some on placebo and others on the drug. Survival rate was 79 percent for the AHCC group and 51 percent for the control group.

Another study involved 229 patients with gastrointestinal cancer. All patients received chemotherapy and 127 were additionally given AHCC. After twenty-seven months, survival rate for the AHCC group was 66.7 percent and only 35 percent for the control group. After ten months, AHCC survival rate was 89.9 percent and for the control group was 55.9 percent.

Other work suggests that a combination of the drug UFT and AHCC enhanced NK cell activity, whereas the drug alone suppressed it (Matsushita et al. 1998).

A recent study at Yale on adults over fifty years of age measured two cytokine levels, interferon and TNF, before and after administrating AHCC orally for sixty days. White blood cell counts were elevated after four weeks and continued for the same period after stopping the supplement.

A study of fourteen human subjects given nine grams of AHCC for two weeks, well above normal doses, showed high tolerance by 85 percent with some bloating, diarrhea, and nausea.

A double-blind, placebo-controlled, randomized trial of ten humans taking three grams daily for four weeks found improvement in a number of immune markers. These include circulating dendritic cells and clusters of differentiation and allogeneic mixed leukocyte reaction, with no change in NK cell activity and the proliferative response of T-lymphocytes toward mitogen (Terakawa et al. 2008).

It has been found to have positive influence on influenza, avian flu virus (H5N1), West Nile virus, methicillin-resistant *S. aureus,* and *Klebsiella pneumoniae.*

Ethanol extracts of shiitake significantly decreased cell proliferation of skin carcinoma cells and induced apoptosis but did not affect normal cells. Extracts from the mycelia of maitake, reishi, and hericium showed no such activity (Gu and Belury 2005).

Work by Badalyan and Sisakyan (2007) found mycelium an active anti-protozoal agent against *Paramecium candatum*. Wound healing also improved.

Shiitake glycoprotein from the submerged mycelium reveals hypoglycemic effect in streptozotocin induced diabetic rats. Byung-Keun Yang et al. (2002) found the compound lowered blood glucose by 21 percent and increased insulin by 22 percent compared to a control group. It also lowered cholesterol by 25 percent and triglyceride levels by 44 percent.

Shiitake shows higher anti-complementary activity than krestin from *Trametes versicolor,* and more potent anti-complementary activity than reishi, cordyceps, and *Agaricus campestris.*

Homeopathy

A use for shiitake has not yet been recorded in the Repertories, but several provings have been conducted in India, New Zealand, and Sweden; these have found that it may be used for heavy and sore neck and shoulders, lack of taking responsibility, being pulled in all directions at once, hiding of identity, and the sensation of separation from self.

Physical symptoms include thirst and upward drawing sensation in brain and genitals. The face feels oily or extremely dry and itchy.

Dose: 30C. Provings were conducted by Chetna Shukla in India, Pratibha Dalvi in New Zealand, and Frans Vermeulen in Sweden on a total of fourteen patients, all but one of them female.

Essential Oil

An essential oil may be obtained from the mushroom. It contains lenthionine, a sulphur-based compound that has been found to inhibit platelet aggregation (Shimada, S. et al. 2004).

Fungi Essences

Shiitake essence is for protection against insecurities and will help to ensure a feeling of security and stabilize inconsistent actions. It is an immune regulator, antiviral, and for liver, colds, and flu.

— Silvercord

Shiitake essence is for feeling insecure about changes in life, leading to procrastination and resistance. It is also for discomfort in the feet, ankles, calves, spine, and back. It helps you to become more independent and adaptable.

— Petit Fleur

Mycoremediation

Shiitake secretes enzymes that help break down PCBs, PAHs, and PCPs, all very toxic chemicals. The mycelium has been found to help remove heavy metals and industrial dyes from waterways.

Paul Stamets has used spent sawdust blocks in burlap sacks for mycoremediation. After saturation with toxic effluent and microbial contamination, the burlap sacks often sprout, leading to possibilities for mycofiltration of farm and chemicals waterways.

Spent shiitake compost showed the highest enzyme activity in alpha amylase (229 nanokatals per gram), cellulase (759 nanokatals per gram), and beta glucosidase (767 nanokatals per gram) (Ko, H. G. et al. 2005b).

Oyster mushroom showed the highest laccase activity at 1452 nanokatals per gram, and *Flammulina velutipes* the highest xylanase activity at 119 nanokatals per gram.

One study suggests that manganese peroxidase is mainly responsible for its ability to decolorize synthetic dyes. Hatvani and Mecs (2003) showed the applicability of shiitake in myco-absorption technologies to remove toxic metals from contaminated effluents and in mycoremediation technologies designed to treat complex wastes contaminated with heavy metals and other xenobiotics.

Charles Lee (2005), an ARS scientist at Albany, California, has determined the structure of Xyn11A, a gene instruction for the formation of xylanase, from shiitake. This work has application for biofuel production.

The spent sawdust culture metabolized pentachlorophenol in soil. This activity was markedly enhanced by adding hydrogen peroxide.

PCP is transformed by substrate culture of fungi (Okeke et al. 1997). In soil, Delor 106 was degraded by 24 percent after six weeks.

Shiitake removed 73 percent of color of effluent in five days without an additional carbon source, and when pre-irradiated for ten minutes in the presence of photocatalyst, ZnO and then fungi treatment, effective decolorization resulted in forty-eight hours (Duran et al. 1994).

The laccase of *L. edodes* immobilized on chitosan by absorption and cross-linking with glutarldehyde, eliminated total phenols by 67 percent after twenty-four hours (D'Annibale et al. 1999).

Cosmetics

Shiitake extracts containing about 10 percent ergosterol are used in the cosmetic industry for cell regeneration, wound healing, and skin firming products.

Agriculture

Wasser and Weis (1999) found a protein fraction of the fruiting bodies prevents infection of plants with tobacco mosaic virus.

Recipes and Dosage

Dried powder: six to sixteen grams daily.

Capsule: 400 milligrams three times per day.

Lentinula edodes mycelium (LEM): two to six grams total in three doses.

Lentinan: one to five milligrams injected intravenously or intramuscularly twice weekly. It may decrease metabolism of drugs via the cytochrome P450 system and may act as a vitamin B6 antagonist, in theory. Its safety in pregnancy is unknown as mice studies showed increased spleen weight and weight gain, but normal offspring weight at birth.

Patients on blood thinners should use with caution due to anti-clotting effects of the mushroom. Minor allergies have been noted in advanced cancer patients.

The tougher stems are best decocted and the liquid used in soups, stews, and the like They should not be thrown away as they contain the polysaccharides and other useful compounds. Maximum recovery of polysaccharides is obtained at 10.1 megapascals for seventy minutes at twenty-eight degrees Celsius (82.4 degrees Fahrenheit) (Lo, T. et al. 2007).

Decocting the fresh or dried mushroom for six to eight minutes releases TCA, or thioproline. This is a natural antioxidant found mainly in the liver. Its duty is to neutralize the cancer-making potential of nitrates and nitrites, found in prepared meats like bacon. It also protects against acetominophen, tetracycline, and alcohol toxicity. If the mushrooms are cooked with foods high in cysteine, such as chicken livers, the amount of TCA increases exponentially.

Lentinus lepideus

Neolentinus lepideus
(TRAIN WRECKER)
(SCALY LENTINUS)
L. ponderosus
N. ponderosus
(PONDEROSA LENTINUS)
(LARGE LENTINUS)
L. cochleatus
Lentinellus cochleatus
(COCKLESHELL LENTINUS)
(ANISEED COCKLESHELL)
L. ursinus
(BEAR LENTINUS)
L. vulpinus
(FOX LENTINUS)
L. strigosus (see Panellus serotinus)

Lentinus means "pliable," from the Latin. Lepideus is from the Greek, meaning "scaly." Neo means "new," and strigosus means "hairy." Cochleatus is "cochlea," a snail-like shape. Ursinus means "bear." Ponderosus is Latin for "heavy."

Train wrecker is so named because it grows on dead wood, whether from a windfall, telephone pole, or railway tie. It is commonly found on dead conifers and hardwoods.

They last for a long time, seeming to dry in place rather than decay over time.

It is a chewy, edible mushroom when young, with a distinct anise odor.

Some name confusion comes about from the belief that mushrooms are not able to cause both white and brown rot. For those species that cause brown rot, mycologists created the genus Neolentinus.

Lentinus was the former genus name for the famous shiitake mushroom. The USDA quarantined shiitake for most of the twentieth century based on the mistaken belief that its activity against railroad ties was similar to Lentinus. The ban was lifted in 1972, showing the desperate depths to which bureaucracy, mycophobia, and genus-centricity will sink.

Ponderosa Lentinus is frequently found on ponderosa pine and lodgepole pine in the Rocky Mountains. It has a white spore print, decurrent gills, and a scaly cap.

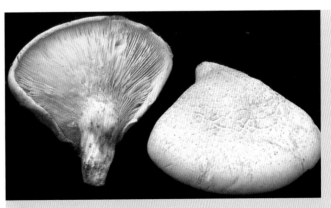

Lentinus lepideus

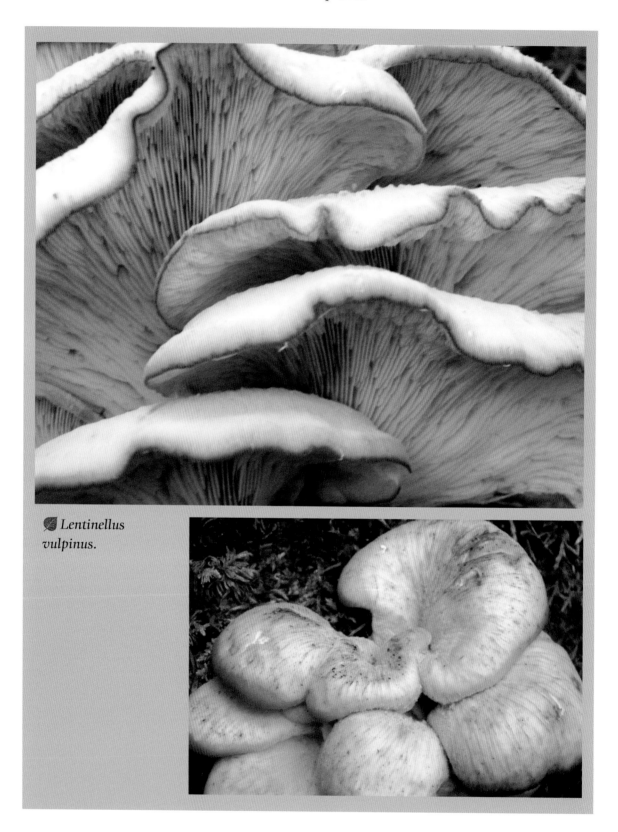

Lentinellus vulpinus.

It has a cinnamon odor similar to matsutake or pine mushroom, but is found on decayed or fallen wood. Lentinus and Lentinellus species are easily identified due to their characteristic saw-toothed gill edges.

Traditional Use

This mushroom is collected and prized by various First Nations healers. It is used for tuberculosis and various cancers.

Medicinal Use

Chemical Constituents

- *L. lepideus:* **eburicoic acid, proteoglycan (PG101), and lepidepyrone.**

- *L. cochleatus:* **deoxylactarorufin A, and blennin A and C.**

- *L. adhaereus:* **2-methoxy-5-methyl-1,4-benzoquinone**

- *L. ursinus:* **isovelleral and lentinellic acid.**

Trainwrecker contains eburicoic acid, which may be used in synthesizing steroid drugs and other compounds.

Such steroids play an important role in the regulation of the human body.

Ehrlich carcinoma was reduced by 70 percent in a study of the mushroom's anticancer activity. Sarcoma 180 was inhibited by only 50 percent, but significant nonetheless (Gregory et al. 1966).

A water-soluble extract of the fungus, PG101, has great potential as an immune enhancer during radiation and chemotherapy. M. Jin et al. (2003) showed that levels of TNF-alpha were elevated in control mice but maintained in the orally treated animals. This suggests it might suppress TNF-alpha related to pathological conditions. The compound increased the levels of IL-1B, IL-6, and granulocyte macrophage colony-stimulating factor over the twenty-four-day period. It significantly reduced level of TNF-alpha, which increases due to tissue injury and anemia caused by radiation. This suggests great potential for immune-compromised or immune-suppressed patients whose bone marrow systems are damaged.

Back in 1996, the same research team identified this proteoglycan as stimulating B-cell proliferation (Jin, M. et al. 1996).

Lepidepyrone, derived from cultivated mycelium, has been found to inhibit hyaluronidase (Hosoe et al. 2007).

Submerged mycelium extracts of ponderosa *Lentinus* show considerable hypoglycemic effect in STZ-induced diabetic rats (Yamac et al. 2008).

The related *L. cochleatus* appears like a yellow-red oyster mushroom with white-pink gills. It is white-spored and edible. It has a licorice-like odor.

It exhibits activity against *Staphylococcus aureus,* as does the related *L. vulpinus.*

Three sesquiterpenoids—deoxylactarorufin A and blennin A and C—are potent inhibitors of leukotriene biosynthesis in leukemia cells and human peripheral blood leukocytes. Lentinellone, a protoilludane derivative, has also been identified.

Methanol extracts show activity against *E. coli* and *Bacillus subtilis,* while dichlormethane extracts are active against these two bacteria, as well as fungicidal against *Candida albicans* and *Cladosporium cucumerinum* (Keller, C. et al. 2002).

The related *L. adhaereus* contains 2-methoxy-5-methyl-1,4-benzoquinone. In vitro studies suggest this compound reduces blood platelet binding. It is a thromboxane A2 receptor.

Work has found antitumor polysaccharides in *L. cyathiformis*.

The related bear *Lentinus, L. ursinus,* contains isovelleral, an anti-feedant compound.

Submerged culture reveals the presence of lentinellic acid, which shows antimicrobial and cytotoxic activity.

Essential Oil

The hydrodistilled oil of *L. cochleatus* has a pleasant anise-like odor. It is composed of 23 percent p-anisaldehyde, 18 percent benzaldehyde, 18.2 percent methyl (E)-p-methoxycinnamate, 13.8 percent methyl p-anisate, 8.8 percent methyl (Z)-p-methoxycinnamate, and minor amounts of nonanal, decanal, 3-octanal, and 2-phenylethanal (Rapior et al. 2002).

In another study of the mushroom grown on a culture medium, the main constituents were trans-nerolidol, fokienol, and 6-formyl-2,2-dimethyl chromene.

Scaly *Lentinus (L. lepideus)* contains forty-three compounds including the two methoxycinnamates above, which explains the anise-cinnamon odor. It also contains nonanol, with a rotten citrus scent, germacrene D (buttery), 2-vinyl malonic acid (walnut), methylpropyl ester, and nonanoic acid (waxy cheese).

Mycoremediation

The related *L. squarrosulus* may be useful for mycoremediation of soil contaminated with engine oil and heavy metals. It is a useful genus indeed, despite the loss of its famous shiitake cousin.

Lenzites betulina

Polyporus betulinus
L. ochraceus
L. variegata
(GILLED POLYPORE)
(BIRCH LENZITES)
L. gibbosa
Trametes gibbosa
P. gibbosus
Daedalea gibbosa
(LUMPY BRACKET)

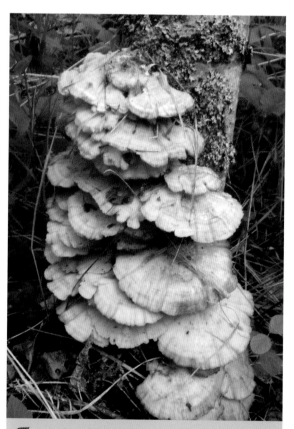

Lenzites betulina

Lenzites is named after the nineteenth-century German botanist, H. O. Lenz. *Betulina* means "of birch." The Japanese call it *kaigaratake.*

Gilled polypore is an oxymoron, like giant shrimp, dry ice, or friendly takeover.

At first glance, it may appear to be *Trametes versicolor* or *T. hirsuta,* and often appears with a green tinge due to algae growth. But again, it has gills, not pores. It is an annual polypore and yet has no tubes. It is very common on birch. The polypore can be easily grown on a medium of malt peptone agar with an admixture of beech or birch sawdust. They must be considered inedible, due to their woodiness.

Lumpy bracket is an introduced bracket polypore with distinct radial, elongated, slotted pores.

Traditional Uses

In traditional Chinese medicine, *Lenzites* is considered warming and supportive of the tendons and veins. It is said to dispel endogenous wind, resolve cold, and stimulate blood circulation.

It is a main ingredient of Tendon Easing Pills.

Medicinal Use

Chemical Constituents

- *L. betulina:* **ergosterol peroxide and 9(11)-dehydroergosterol peroxide; betulinans A and B; ergosta-7,22-dien-3-ol; and fungisterol.**

Water extracts of this fairly common birch polypore showed antitumor activity against sarcoma 180 in mice (Ikekawa et al. 1968).

Early work on polysaccharides derived from mycelium found inhibition against sarcoma 180 and Ehrlich carcinoma of 90 percent (Ohtsuka et al. 1973).

Ether and ethyl acetate extracts have been shown to provide significant cytotoxic effect against cervical and hepatoma cancer cell lines (Ren, G. et al. 2006).

Yamac and Bilgili (2006) found various forms of extracts from the fruiting body active against *Staphylococcus aureus, S. epidermis,* and especially *Bacillus subtilis.*

Mycelium extracted with water showed activity against *S. aureus* and *B. subtilis.* The organic fraction was active only against the latter tested bacterium (Yamac and Bilgili 2006).

The mushroom is considered useful in cardiovascular disorders.

At the present time, the fungus is not marketed commercially for antitumor activity or cardiovascular support. In clinical trials, Fujimoto et al. (1994) showed immune-suppressive effect attributed to ergosterol peroxide and 9(11)-dehydroergosterol peroxide.

In-Kyoung Lee et al. (2002) at the Korean Research Institute isolated two benzoquinone compounds. They showed betulinans A and B to be lipid peroxidation inhibitors, with the former four times more effective as a free radical scavenger than vitamin E.

G. Ren et al. (2006) found extracts to be cytotoxic to cervical and hepatoma cancer cell lines.

The mycelium shows selective anti-proliferating and apoptosis-inducing activity against K562 cells and chronic myelogenous leukemia. An active fraction significantly inhibits the autophosphorylation of native and mutated bcr-abl, which are resistant to imatinib treatment including the T3151 mutation.

Imatinib mesylate is part of standard therapy for CML, but its efficacy decreases with advancement of the disease. This is a great discovery by Yassin et al. (2008).

Methanol extract shows mild inhibition of HIV reverse transcriptase activity (Mlinaric et al. 2005).

Polysaccharides from the fruiting body injected into the arteries of rats showed anti-inflammatory and vasoprotective activity (Czarnecki, R. and J. Grzybek 1995).

Fungi Essence

Birch polypore essence cleans and harmonizes the spirit on the emotional level. It calms down too high emotional activity and is well suited for meditation.

— MARIANA

Recipes and Dosage

Take one or two size "00" capsules twice per day.

A decoction is made at a one-to-two ratio with fruiting bodies, boiled for thirty minutes, and then cooled. Drink six to eight ounces two times a day.

Textile Industry

These mushrooms make some of the best bracket fungi paper. Anna King and Roy Watling (1997) found that they make a soft, silky paper that takes printing ink very well. They are somewhat slow to break down in the blender or Vitamix, but eventually yield copious quantities of a rich, creamy pulp.

Although any polypore will produce paper, the trimitic types produce the best product.

Other conks in this category include *Daedalea quercina, Fomes fomentarius, Ganoderma adsperum, G. applanatum, Trametes hirsuta,* and *T. versicolor.*

Mariam Rice has published a definitive book on preparing mushroom paper.

Lepiota

Lepiota americanum
Leucoagaricus americana
L. bresadolae
L. badhamii
(AMERICAN PARASOL)
L. procera
Macrolepiota procera
(PARASOL MUSHROOM)
L. lutea
Leucocoprinus birnbaumii
L. caepestipes
L. luteus
(YELLOW PARASOL)
Leucoagaricus leucothites
L. naucinus
Lepiota leucothites
L. naucinoides
L. naucina
(SMOOTH LEPIOTA)
L. clypeolaria
(SHAGGY STALKED PARASOL)
L. seminuda
L. sistrata
Cystolepiota seminuda
(LILLIPUTIAN LEPIOTA)

Lepiota means "scaly ear" from the Greek *Lepis* meaning "scaly," as in leprosy. *Procerus* is Latin for "tall." *Caepestipes* is from *cepa* for "onion" and *stipes* for "stem." *Clypeolaria* means "pertaining to a shield."

Many are poisonous and best left alone.

One of interest is the American parasol *(L. americana)* with its dark red to burgundy color. When bruised or cut, the flesh turns yellow or orange. It has a white spore print.

Parasol mushroom is one of our best edibles, with large, woolly, and scaly caps. They appear in large numbers in pastures, and on city lawns. The veil becomes a moveable ring that slides up and down the stem. A mature cap may smell faintly like maple syrup or fenugreek.

They cook up well on a barbecue and are delicious. The immature specimen is known as the drumstick. Coated with egg and breadcrumbs, the fried caps are similar to *weiner schnitzel* in texture and, some say, in taste. They can be sautéed and tempura-fried. The stems are tough, but can be finely chopped for a sauce or soup.

Parasol mushroom is quite high in chromium with some studies showing 0.09 milligrams per kilogram. It accumulates mercury up to 230 times, so caution is advised with regard to your picking site. It also accumulates copper, zinc, rubidium, selenium, and cobalt that play a role in human health.

Yellow parasol appeared one day in my giant Aloe vera that I had recently transplanted. It is bright yellow and appears quite often in greenhouses and flower pots.

Shaggy stalked parasol is commonly found

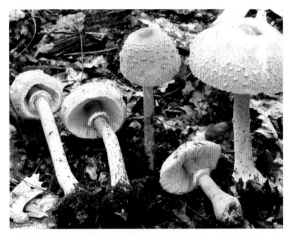

Lepiota procera

under douglas fir in the Pacific Northwest. It should be avoided due to its poisonous nature.

Lilliputian *Lepiota (L. seminuda)* is found very rarely under hardwoods and conifers in fall. It is so tiny and delicate, it may be mistaken for a *Mycena* or *Collybia,* but it has free gills and a veil.

The related *L. humei* contains various lysergamides and N,N-dimethyl-tryptamine. Work by J. Bigwood at Evergreen State College in Olympia, Washington, isolated a new compound in 1983 that had a short life of one to two days, suggesting the fresh mushroom loses potency rather quickly. A psychoactive yellow liquid, derived from the mycelium, and known as "golden goop," can be dried and smoked for hallucinogenic effect. Not that I recommend it.

Also known as Peele's *Lepidota* after a mycology researcher in Pensacola, Florida, the ingestion of five to six fresh carpophores did not produce toxic or hallucinogenic effect.

Only low levels of free tryptophan have been found.

Lepiota genus contains some seriously poisonous species. Michael Beug suggests *Lepiota subincarnata* may be one of the deadliest mushrooms in North America. I wouldn't dispute that.

Traditional Uses

In China, the mushroom is used to promote health and good digestion, if taken regularly. It contains eighteen amino acids, and high amounts of eight that are essential for health.

Medicinal Use

Chemical Constituents

- *L. americanum:* **2-aminophenoxazin-3-one and lepiotaquinone.**

American parasol is edible and contains 2-aminophenoxazin-3-one that inhibits aromatase with an IC50 value of 5.7 micromoles.

Sulfatase was also inhibited by 3-beta-hydroxy-5,8-epidioxyergosta-6,22-dyne at an IC50 value of 0.9 micromoles.

Aromatase is believed to play a key role in the development of estrogen-sensitive cancers. Work by Petrova et al. (2005) shows this mushroom as well as *Agaricus brasiliensis, Trametes versicolor, Grifola frondosa, Inonotus obliquus, Lentinula edodes, Pleurotus ostreatus,* and *Sparassis crispa* exhibit potential in the treatment of breast cancer. This may be as an adjunct therapy to chemotherapy, surgery, or radiation or as part of a natural regime.

Inhibition rates are 70 percent against sarcoma 180 and 80 percent against Ehrlich carci-

noma. Culture broths show antifungal activity against wood-decaying fungi of the genera *Fomes* and *Trametes.*

Smooth *Lepiota* is a choice edible. Basidalin, isolated from the fruiting body, shows activity against lymphatic leukemia cells L1210.

Early work by Hervey (1947) identified activity against both *E. coli* and *Staphylococcus aureus.* Robbins et al. (1945) found the same result.

Shaggy stalked parasol *(L. clypeolaria)* shows 100 percent activity against both sarcoma 180 and Ehrlich carcinoma cancer cell lines.

Polysacchrides from *L. seminuda* mycelial culture were injected into mice intraperitoneally and reduced sarcoma 180 and Ehrlich carcinoma cancer cells by 70 percent and 60 percent respectively.

Fungi Essences

Parasol essence is for psychic protection for those who are too open. It will also help if over the solar plexus. It is an immune tonic, for the central nervous system and bowel complaints.
— SILVERCORD

Parasol essence helps us recognize and develop our full potential. We learn to recognize our true greatness and to accept it for what it really is.
— KORTE PHI

Parasol essence is for self-confidence and to develop courage. It gives backbone and assists in implementing new ideas and freedom from fear of failure.
— MARIANA

Cultivation

In Sweden, Hansson and Hansson developed a technology for garden cultivation of this choice edible. From 1992 to 2000 some three hundred blocks of substrate were planted in lawns and pastures with 95 percent producing mushrooms. The average total yield for a four-kilogram substrate bag was 0.6-1.2 kilograms of mushrooms with 10 percent showing sustained production for up to eight years.

You can slurry old specimens in water for a day or two and then pour over your own lawn for annual harvests.

Lepista nuda

Clitocybe nuda
Tricholoma nudum
Rhodopaxillus nudus
(BLEWIT)
L. saeva
C. saeva
L. personata
T. personatum
(FIELD BLEWIT)
(BLUE LEG)
(PURPLE STEMMED AGARIC)
L. irina
C. irina
(WOOLLY LEPISTA)
(IRIS SCENTED LEPISTA)
L. inversa (see *Clitocybe inversa*)

> The mushroom-scented air of the birch groves is far dearer than the fragrance of the magnolia.
>
> — PAUSTOVSKIY

Lepista is from the Greek *lepis,* which means "scale." *Nuda* is from *nudus* or "naked." The name constitutes a contradiction in terms, literally translating as "the scaly smooth mushroom." An oxymorel if you like. *Irina* means "woolly."

L. nuda should be cooked to destroy traces of thermobile hemolysin that degenerates red blood cells.

Blewit is a corruption of "blue hat." It is a common lilac- to purple-tinged mushroom with a peach-pink spore print helping identification. Blewits are sweet and mild in nature, with a distinct pine rich perfume. This combines well with the flavor of wild game, toasted nuts and cheese. They must be well cooked, as they are slightly toxic when raw. They are best coated in olive oil and grilled, with perhaps a

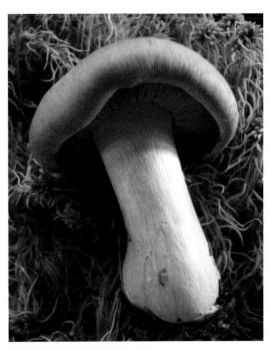

Lepista nuda

273

splash of sherry or tamari. They are good in omelets and soups. They combine well with white wine, particularly Pinot grigio, my wife's summer favorite. It took me until the summer of 2004 to find my first blewit, but I certainly am not going to walk past any future harvests. In the fall of 2008 I found an enormous grouping under red cedar in the Pacific Northwest. They were very tasty.

Care must be taken when picking wild specimens as mercury content up to 3.02 milligrams per kilogram has been found.

Woolly *Lepista* looks very similar to the blewit, but has no purple color. It has a pink spore print, so care must be taken to avoid confusing it with the poisonous *Entoloma*. Also note the similarity of Lepista to the inedible and poisonous Cortinarius on page (124–127). The cortina is often found covered with rusty-brown spores.

Field blewit *(L. saeva)* grows in impressive fairy rings in open fields. The texture is superb, and it is pleasantly aromatic, making it a choice edible.

Medicinal Use

Chemical Constituents
- *L. nuda:* **nudic acids A and B.**

Blewits regulate blood sugar metabolism and support the nervous system; possibly due, in part, to the high thiamine, or Vitamin B1, content. They could be tried as part of a hypoglycemic control diet.

Blewit is resistant to both gram-positive and gram-negative bacteria and inhibit sarcoma 180 by 90 percent, and Ehrlich carcinoma entirely, with 100 percent inhibition.

Suay et al. (2000) found hot-water infusions of blewit retarded the growth of *Candida albicans,* probably due to the content of polysaccharides. Dulger et al. (2002b) identified antimicrobial activities in a 60 percent methanol extract.

Early work by Hervey (1947) found activity against both *E. coli* and *Staphylococcus aureus.* Earlier work by Wilkins and Harris identified substances they called nudic acid A and B. The former was active against *S. aureus* at one part to eight thousand, *E. coli* at one part to two thousand and *Streptococcus pyogenes* and *S. enteritidas* at the same rate. At one part to fifty thousand, it stopped uterus tissue contractions temporarily.

Nudic acid B inhibited *S. aureus* at one part to six hundred forty thousand, and other organisms were also more sensitive.

Badalyan and Gasparyan (2007) found mycelium of *L. personata* exhibiting 26 percent antioxidant activity.

Essential Oils

I-octen-3-ol appears to play an important role in the aromatics of this mushroom, similar to the true morel and common white market mushrooms. It is well known that this compound is formed mainly from the enzymatic breakdown of linoleic acid, which happens when the fruiting body's tissue is damaged.

The aroma of *L. nuda* is also characterized by the presence of linalool and particularly three linalool oxides that give a unique fresh, woody scent. The mushroom also contains a ceramide found in *Amanita pantherina* and *Sarcodon aspratus.*

The monoterpene content of the blewit has

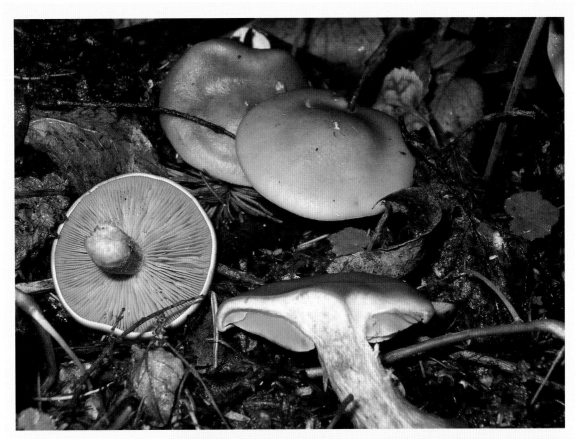

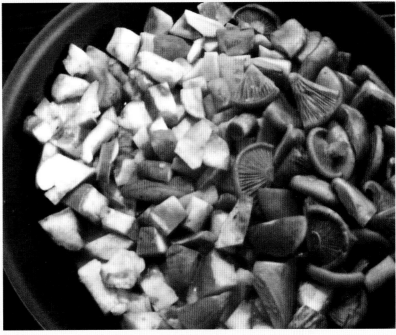

Above: *Lepista nuda*. Right: A bowl of lobsters (*Hypomyces lactiflourium*) and blewits.

been found composed mainly of cis linalool oxide at 45 percent, with minor amounts of linalool, trans linalool oxide, and linalool oxide.

Fungi Essence

Blewit essence is for those who feel depleted of energy. It will help the user focus their energies. It will also you find your true pathway in life. This essence can be used for insomnia, headaches, and to stimulate the metabolism.

— Silvercord

Woolly *Lepista (L. irina)* essence helps us open the third eye (sixth chakra) by cleansing the flow of energy between the physical and subtle bodies via the charkas. It brings us clarity on how to use our intuition and anchors the new balanced energy flow at the cellular level.

— Korte Phi

Mycoremediation

The fungus accumulates mercury by a hundred times or more, suggesting a role for mycoremediation of contaminated mine sites, as the mushroom lends itself well to cultivation.

Cultivation

The blewit is cultivated commercially in France. Its strong and subtle flavor, texture, and violet color present originality that could justify widespread production. Since 1990, *L. nuda* has been commercially produced at the rate of up to eighty tons annually from a specific hybrid cultivar. Yields of 1.25 pounds per square foot in fourteen weeks can be expected.

Isolates of *L. nuda* from Australia appear to have double the growth rate of French isolates.

Leucopaxillus giganteus

Clitocybe gigantea
(GIANT LEUCOPAX)
(GIANT FUNNEL CAP)
(GIANT CLITOCYBE)
L. gentianeus
L. amarus
(BITTER BROWN LEUCOPAXILLUS)
L. albissimus
(LARGE WHITE LEUCOPAXILLUS)

Leuco is Greek meaning "white," *paxillus* is "a small peg or pole." *Albissimus* means "superbly white" from the Latin.

Giant leucopax is widely distributed. It is a choice edible mushroom when young and tender. They last a long time, and often are seen still standing when no other mushrooms are around.

The odor can vary greatly, from turnip-like to slight bitter almond.

You will find them under white spruce and hardwood trees from mid-summer onward. They often will grow in long rows or arcs, creating a fungal frenzy. Hollande noted that the

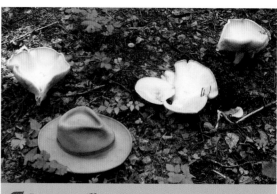

Leucopaxillus giganteus

276

grass inside the rings does not undergo putrefaction after dying.

Bitter brown *Leucopaxillus,* according to Arora, smells like creepy crawlers and tastes like a mildewed army tent.

Large white *Leucopaxillus* is inedible.

Medicinal Use

Chemical Constituents

- *L. giganteus:* **glucans, mannoxyloglucan, heteroglucan, xyloglucan, xylogalacetoglucan, galactoxyloglucan, dehydromatricarianol methyl ether, clitocine, and leucopaxillone A.**

- *L. gentianeus:* **leucopaxillones A and B, cucurbitacin B and its esters, and 16-dihydroxycucur-bitacin B.**

- *L. albissimus:* **2-aminoquioline.**

If the fungi is cut fresh and decocted along with fresh ginger, it helps cure colds—or at least shortens their duration.

The dried fruiting bodies of *L. gianteus* are used medicinally to cure measles, whether the rash is appearing or not, or if the child is feverish due to illness.

It produces clitocybin, which may be useful in cases of tuberculosis.

Clitocybin has been found active against *Mycobacterium tuberculosis, Bacillus.* and *Salmonella typhi,* and bacteria associated with brucellosis or Malta fever as it is sometimes known. The antibacterial activity is greater in an acid solution.

One study identified leucopaxillones with anti-proliferation properties on human tumor cell lines. Clericuzio et al. (2004) found cucurbitacin B to be the active compound against a variety of cancer cell lines, including MCF7, HepG2, A549, and CAK1-1 in vitro. Both epatoblastoma and breast adenocarcinoma cells were particularly susceptible.

In vivo studies on mice found the compound highly toxic to the liver, suggesting a dead end at this point.

Leucopaxillone A, although somewhat less active, exhibited specific activity against the MCF-7 breast cancer cell lines. This compound is present in fruiting bodies and mycelia in fifteen milligrams per gram and thirty milligrams per gram respectively. With an IC50 of only 7.94 micromoles this compound may be worthy of more study.

Some research has found the mycelium of *L. giganteus* to be active against *Staphylococcus aureus* (Barros et al. 2007c).

Bitter brown *Leucopaxillus* contains curcurbitacin B, which exhibits antitumor activity against human cancer cell lines A549, CAKl-1, and is particularly potent against HepG2 and MCF-7 cell lines with an IC50 of 0.7 micromoles (Clericuzio et al. 2004, 2006). The cucubitanes leucopaxillones A and B were much less active. Early work by Coletto (1981) showed inhibition of *Bacillus cereus.*

Large white *Leucopaxillus* contains 2-aminoquioline, a rare compound in nature. Pfister (1988) suggests that the compound possesses antibacterial, anti-parasitic, antitumor, and anti-mutagenic properties, and is a protease inhibitor.

Recipe and Dosage

Ten to fifteen grams of dried *L. giganteus* in water infusion at a ratio of one to ten.

Limacella illinata

(WHITE LIMACELLA)
(SLIME VEILED LIMACELLA)

Illinata is from the Latin meaning "greasy" or "slimy."

This rare member of the *Amanita* family is edible, but the slimy universal veil makes it quite unpleasant. It has a distinctive white spore print. It is often found under douglas fir or pine in the Pacific Northwest.

Fermentation technology has yielded limacellone and illinitone A and B (Gruhn, N. et al. 2007). Limacellone is weakly cytotoxic, and illinitone B is moderately active.

This mushroom also contains 11-desoxyeleganthol, which is relatively rare in fungi and is similar to eleganthol from *Clitocybe elegans* (Arnone et al. 1993).

Lyophyllum decastes

Clitocybe multiceps
Tricholoma aggregatum
L. aggregatum
(FRIED CHICKEN MUSHROOM)
L. connatum
C. connata
T. connata
(WHITE TUFT)
L. semitale
(DOME CAP)
L. carneum (see *Calocybe carnea*)

Decastes means "decade" or "numbers of ten."
Connatum means "born together." *Lyophyllum*
means "with loose gills." *Multiceps* is from *multus* for "many" and *caput* meaning "a head."

Fried chicken mushroom, known in Japan as *hatakeshimeji,* has white spores and the cap color ranges from gray to brown. It occurs in schoolyards and roadsides, usually with some decaying wood underneath. It can be found on dry hummocks in bogs under black spruce. I have seen it frequently on old forestry roads. It is cultivated commercially, and has been shown to grow well on aged, cultured waste of oyster mushroom *(Pleurotus ostreatus)* (Akamatsue 1998). It is pleasantly aromatic, with good flavor.

White tuft is commonly found growing in grassy areas and open forests. It is edible when cooked thoroughly, but may be confused with the white *Clitocybes,* so attention is necessary. The Japanese name is *oshiroishimeji.*

The related dome cap *(L. semitale),* widespread under conifers, stains gray or black with bruising.

Medicinal Use

Chemical Constituents

- *L. connatum:* **(2S,3R,4E,8E,9'Z,12'Z)-N9',12'-octadeca-dienoyl-2-amino-9-methyl-4,8-octadec-adien-1,3-diol, an ergothioneine derivative named beta-hydroxyergothioneine, connatin, N-hydroxy-N',N'-dimethyl urea, and lyophyllin (hydroxy carboxamide).**

Fried chicken mushroom is reported to contain tumor inhibiting properties (Kamasuka et al. 1968).

More recent work by Yeunhwa Gu et al. (2005) suggests that the fungus does not show

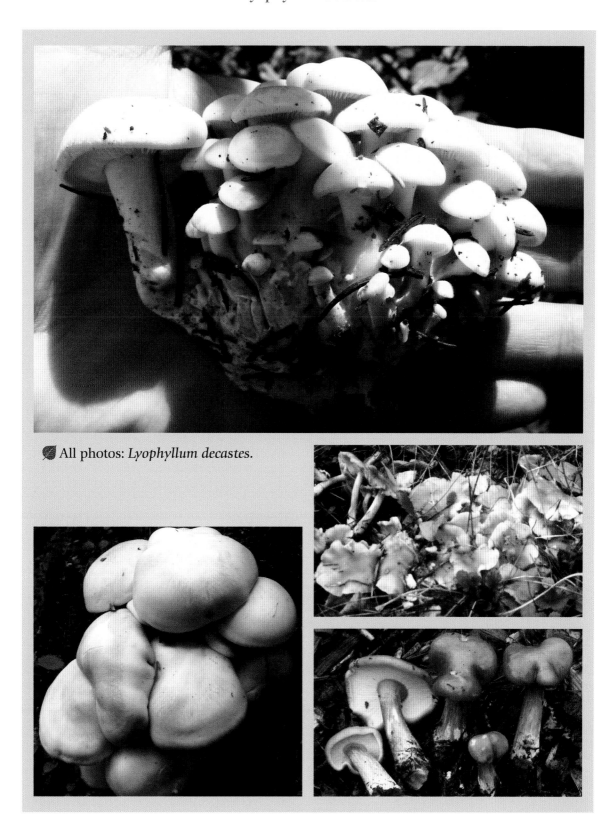

All photos: *Lyophyllum decastes*.

a marked antitumor effect, but combined with radiation therapy it shows an antitumor effect caused by a radioprotective effect on the immune cells, suggesting indirect and yet synergistic activity.

The ability to inhibit ACE and hypertension is not reduced by cooking, even deep frying (Gu, Yeunhwa et al. 2001; Suzuki, I. et al. 2001).

Ukawa et al. (2002) investigated serum lipid levels in rats. As well as lowering total serum cholesterol levels, the mushroom increased the activity of cholesterol 7a-hydroxylase, which converts cellular cholesterol to bile acids.

More recent work identified anti-allergic actions through Th2 and serum IgE responses (Ukawa et al. 2007). Production of IL4 was reduced but the interferon-gamma was not inhibited. The study was based on atopic dermatitis in lab animals, and more study is needed.

The mushroom exhibits antidiabetic activity, in part, due to a decrease in insulin resistance. This is due to an increase of glucose transporter isoform 4 protein content in the plasma membrane of the muscle, as well as a decrease of blood sugar in an insulin tolerance test (Miura et al. 2002).

Significant anti-inflammatory activity is suggested by some tests.

A single incident of hepatitis following oral ingestion of the dried mushroom powder by a sixty-five-year-old diabetic patient was noted in a letter to *Gastroenterology* in 2006.

Submerged cultures grow optimally with 3 percent glucose and 1 percent yeast extract (Pokhrel and Ogra 2007). Barley bran mixed with livestock waste is a good medium for mycelium and fruiting body operations.

White tuft exhibits an ability to scavenge free radicals as well as prevent carbon tetrachloride-induced injury of liver hepatocytes (Kimura, C. et al. 2005).

When aqueous ferric chloride is dropped on white tuft, a characteristic violet color is obtained due to connatin and N-hydroxy-N',N'-dimethylurea.

Dome cap has an inhibition rate against sarcoma 180 of 90 percent and against Ehrlich carcinoma of 100 percent (Ohtsuka et al. 1973).

Macrocystidia cucumis
(CUCUMBER CAP)

This fungi, which smells of cucumber and fish, is found along pathways and in gardens and parks of the Pacific Northwest. Steven Trudell suggests it might at first glance be confused with *Entoloma* species, but its coloration and spore shape are different.

Medicinal Use

Hellwig et al. (1998) identified eight new triquinane-type sesquiterpenoids from fermentation culture; Cucumins A-H, cyclo (phenyl-alanylprolyl), cyclo (leucylprolyl), and arthrosporone. Cucumin A shows strong activity against *Bacillus subtlils*, *Nematospora coryli,* and *Mucor miehei* at low concentrations. Cucumin C inhibits *N. coryli* and the yeast *Saccharomyces cerevisiae.* Cucumins A-C are highly cytotoxic with an IC_{100} of 0.5-1.0 micrograms per milliliter.

Marasmius oreades

(FAIRY RING MUSHROOM)

M. androsaceus

(HORSE HAIR MUSHROOM)

M. scorodinus

(GARLIC MARASMIUS)

*. . . You demi-puppets that by moonshine do the
    green sour ringlets make,
Whereof ewe not bites; and you, whose pastime
    is to make Midnight Mushrooms. . . .*

— SHAKESPEARE

*The forest's erewhile emperor at eve
Had voice when lowered heavens drummed
    for gales.
At midnight a small people danced the dales,
So thin that they might dwindle through
    a sieve
Ringed mushrooms told of them, and in
    their throats,
Old wives that gathered herbs and knew too
    much.
The pensioned forester beside his crutch,
Struck showers from embers at those bodeful
    notes.*

—GEORGE MEREDITH

Marasmius is from the Greek meaning "withered," referring to the ability of the mushroom to revive itself after rain. *Oreades* is Greek meaning "growing in the mountains," which is not always true. *Androsaceus* is from *andro* meaning "male" or "man" and " cheese." Doesn't make sense. Andrus Voitk in *Common Mushrooms of Newfoundland and Labrador* suggests it means "like a certain alga."

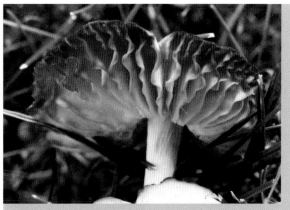

🌿 *Marasmius oreades*

One of the largest fairy rings in the world encircles Stonehenge, and is approximately a millennium in age.

The Blackfoot of Alberta call them *kok-a-tos-i-u*. They are familiar to the grasslands, expanding in larger and larger circles each year. One fairy ring re-discovered in 1969 near Manyberries, Alberta, is a thousand feet in diameter and estimated to be at least seven hundred years old. Considering that they grow twelve to thirteen centimeters a year, it may be even older than that.

Various *Marasmius* species are stimulated to grow faster by small amounts (five parts per million) of taxifolin glycoside, a flavonoid found in pine needles.

The mushrooms contain hydrocyanic acid, which gives the delightful almond odor. It is very volatile and poses no health concern as it dissipates upon cooking. The best storage method is either direct freezing or dehydration at 158 degrees Fahrenheit (70 degrees Celsius).

Fairy rings are, to grassaholics, the bane of pristine urban lawns. Many ingenious attempts have been made over the years to eradicate

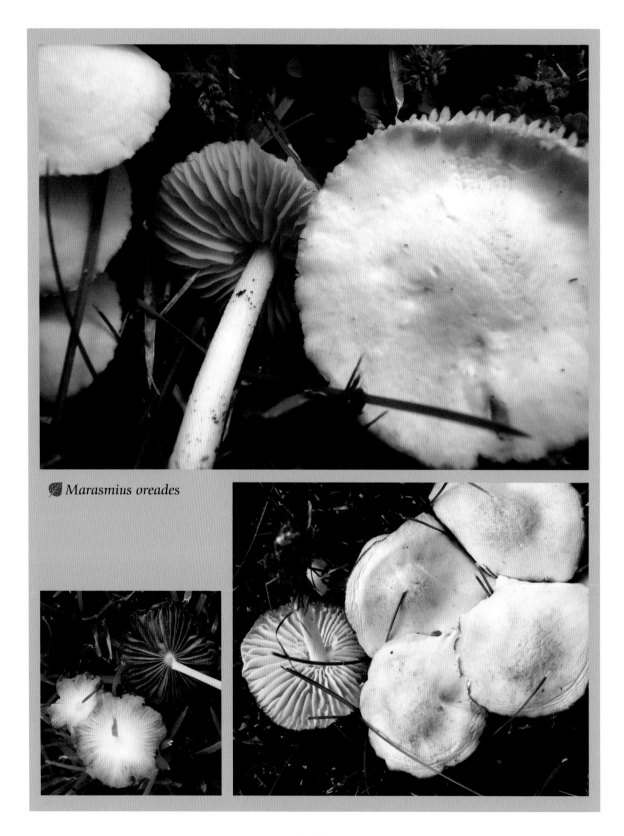

Marasmius oreades

them, but since they are edible, why not just eat and enjoy them? They are good fresh or dried, adding a pleasant oak scent when cooked in butter. Their aroma and taste are out of proportion to their size.

Dried and powdered, the mushrooms can be added to any cookie recipe, or to a soup.

To dry, simply string them on a thread with a button on the bottom and hang them in a warm spot. I use an electric dehydrator with good results.

The closely related horse hair mushroom (*M. androsaceus*) is widespread and common in woods, found on needles, twigs, and leaves.

Culture and Folklore

In Germany, fairy rings are called *hexen* rings, from *hexen* meaning "witches." Folklore there has that on the eve of May Day (Walpurgis Night), the old pagan witches would hold their high revelry; the rings were supposedly formed by the witches' dancing.

The Dutch believed the rings were the resting place of the devil's churns.

In some traditions, it was believed that the rings were formed by lightning strikes, while in others they were thought to be the sites of buried treasure that could only be retrieved with help from fairies or witches.

In France, they are called *ronds de sorcieres* or "sorcerers' rings," said to be sacred circles in which enormous toads with bulging eyes appear. In Tyrol, the rings were believed to be caused by the hot breath of dragons, while the Irish believed they were caused by the devil spilling milk while making butter. Another French name is *faux mousseron,* meaning mushroom scythe.

In parts of Europe, fairy rings were believed formed by spit, urine, or sperm from elves. The Basques of northern Spain speak Euskara, unrelated to any Indo-European languages. Their name for fairy ring fungi is *xapo-perretxiko,* or toad mushroom.

Those individuals interested in the relationship of toads and toadstools will find Adrian Morgan's book by that title a fascinating adventure.

A Native belief is that fairy rings are caused by the dances of the buffalo, the larger by adult animals and the smaller by calves.

Traditional Uses

An old Scottish rhyme tells of its uselessness in agriculture:

> *He wha tills the fairies' green*
> *Nae luck again shall have;*
> *For weirdless days and weary nights,*
> *Are his to his dieing day.*

Young women wishing to improve their complexions were urged to use the dew from within the fairy ring's circle. This dew was also believed to be useful for bewitching a loved one, but would disfigure them if applied to the face during the spell.

In traditional Chinese medicine, fairy ring mushrooms are included in the famous Tendon Easing Powder, which is used to treat lumbago, pain in the legs, numbed limbs, and discomfort in the tendons and veins.

The closely related horse hair mushroom (*M. androsaceus*) is used in traditional Chinese medicine for pains in the joints caused by leprosy, and as a remedy for injuries from falls, including fractures, contusions, and strains, or simply for relieving pain.

Medicinal Use

Chemical Constituents

- *M. oreades:* **4,4-dimethyl-5 alpha-ergosta-8,24 (28)-dien-3 beta-ol, a precursor of ergosterol; agrocybin; drimane sesquiterpenes.**
- *M. scorodinus:* **scorodinin.**
- *M. androsaceus:* **marasmic acid.**

When grown in liquid culture, the sesquiterpenes marasmone, anhydromarasmone, isomarasmone, and dihydromarasmone are produced as well as the norsesquiterpenes 0-formyloreadone, 3.alpha hydroxy oreadone, and dehydrooreadone. Agrocybin has also been isolated, and may be the phytotoxic compound responsible for grass kill (Ayer and Craw 1989).

Both Agrocybin and drimane sesquiterpenes in the fairy ring mushroom possess antimicrobial and phytotoxic properties (Lorenzen and Anke 1998).

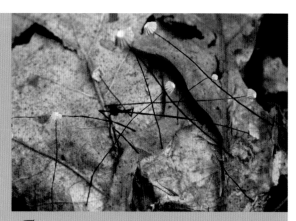

🍃 *Marasmius androsaceus*

A lectin from this species has been found to react with human blood type B (Remple et al. 2002).

Warner et al. (2004) isolated a lectin that caused renal thrombotic microangiopathic lesions.

The molecular structure and carbohydrate binding properties have been investigated (Winter et al. 2002).

Work by Petrova et al. (2007) shows that this mushroom exhibits significant effects on the NFkappa B activation pathway. This has great significance for cancer therapeutics. Further evidence of anti-proliferation and apoptosis was reported by same author (Petrova et al. 2009).

The related horse hair mushroom *(M. androsaceus)* exhibits anti-inflammatory and nerve tonic properties and is used to treat leprous neuralgia, sciatica, trigeminal neuralgia, and migraines, as well as neuralgia in the sockets and rheumatic pain in the joints.

Various *Marasmius* species are cytokine production inhibitors. Marasmic acid is antibacterial.

Two compounds were found to inhibit activity for lipopolysaccharide-induced production of interleukin 1 beta and tumor necrosis factor alpha in human blood (Ichikawa et al. 2001). The IC50 is a low 0.059 to 2.6 micrometers, meaning it has a low toxicity.

Research has found optimal extraction at 78 degrees Celsius (172 degrees Fahrenheit); ninety minutes in a ratio of thirty-six to one yields 11.59 percent polysaccharides.

The mushroom contains the anti-hypertensive compound, 3,3,5,5-tetramethyl 4-piperidone, which works through ganglionic blocking (Zhang, L. et al. 2009).

Garlic *Marasmius* contains scorodonin, a compound with antibiotic properties (Anke, T. et al. 1980).

The fungus contains novel peroxidases MsP1 and MsP2, which are capable of efficient beta-carotene degradation from cultures (Scheibner, M. et al. 2008).

Aliacols A and B, obtained from the related *M. alliaceus,* exhibited weak antibacterial and antifungal activity. The compounds, however, strongly inhibited DNA synthesis in ascites cells of Ehrlich carcinoma.

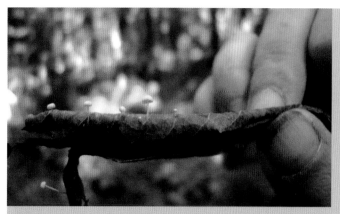

Marasmius epiphyllus

The related *M. ramealis* contains marasin, an antibiotic polyacetylene, as well as mellein, pyrrole-2-carboxylic and p-hydroxybenzoic acid. It shows activity against *Bacillus dentriticus.*

Marasmic acid, isolated from *M. conigens,* is antibacterial, antifungal, and cytotoxic (Abraham 2001). It is closely related structurally to isovelleral found in various *Lactarius* species.

The related *M. candidus,* also known as *M. magnisporus,* is common on the west coast near cedar and oak. It shows activity against *S. aureus.*

The eastern *M. cohaerans* shows an inhibition rate of 60 percent and 70 percent against sarcoma 180 and Ehrlich carcinoma cell lines respectively.

The compound 6,9-dihydroxy-3(15)-carophyllen-4,8-dione has been isolated from tropical *Marasmius* species fermentations. It is strongly cytotoxic on L1210 and HL-60 human lymphocytic leukemia cell lines with $1C_{50}$ values of 1.9 micrometers and 3.8 micrometers respectively.

Aggregation of human thrombocytes stimulated with ADP or collagen was inhibited.

Essential Oil

Marasmius species that have been steam-distilled yield up to 0.2 percent of an oil with a garlic-like odor.

The main volatiles in *M. alliaceus* are 2,4,5,7-tetrahiaoctane and 2,3,5-trihiahexane.

Fungi Essence

Fairy ring essence is for what goes around comes around. It lets us break the circle we feel trapped within. Fairy ring can help you with this, as it is a sedative and calms the nerves.

— SILVERCORD

Mycoremediation

The related *M. troyanus* has been studied for mycoremediation at Tulane University with activity against PAHs, TNT, and other contaminants. A method for encapsulated fungal spore beads has a U.S. patent (6,204,049). This is another interesting approach to cleaning up contaminated sites. A rather rare mushroom, it has the capacity to remove up to 95 percent of benzo(a)pyrene (Wunch et al. 1997).

Meripilus giganteus
(GIANT POLYPORE)

Giant polypore is found at base of hardwood trees in eastern North America.

It has a mild odor and slightly sour taste.

Medicinal Use

Karaman et al. (2009a) looked at several species including this one. Activity against several gram-positive bacteria including *Bacillus* species, *Rhodococcus equi,* and *Staphylococcus aureus* was noted.

The same author noted antioxidant activity, significant activity against estrogen-dependent breast cancer cell line MCF-7, hemolytic potential, and inhibition of acetylcholinesterase, making it of possible benefit in Alzheimer's and related conditions (Karaman et al. 2009b).

Merulius tremellosus

Phlebia tremellosa
(JELLY ROT)
(TREMBLING MERULIUS)
M. incarnatus
P. incarnatum

Meruloid means "folded" as it nearly forms pores. Tremellosus means trembling, quaking, or shaking.

The fruit bodies are flat and narrowly shelved with a hairy to woolly upper surface and pink underneath with shallow pores and net-like folds. The flesh is thin, white, and waxy to gelatinous.

Jelly rot is another bracket fungus found mainly on dead hardwood trees, both widespread and common. In the Kai Yuan County of Lianing, China, people cook it with water and drink the broth or eat the whole preparation as a soup, or eat pancakes made by combining the broth with flour. I would have to be starving to consider this an edible.

Traditional Use

Phlebia species, especially those on the rotten elm, were used in the treatment of dysentery in traditional medicine.

Medicinal Use
Chemical Constituents
- *M. tremellosus:* **merculinic acids A-C.**
- *M. incarnatus:* **5-alkylresorcinols.**

The inhibition rate against sarcoma 180 is 90 percent and against Ehrlich carcinoma is 80 percent. The related *M. aureus* shows 100 percent inhibition against both.

Merculinic acids A-C have been isolated from this mushroom and the related *P. radiata.* They are closely linked derivatives of beta-resorcylic and salicylic acid that exhibit antibiotic effect.

RNA, DNA, and protein synthesis in Bacillus brevis and Ehrlich carcinoma are inhibited shortly after introduction of merulinic acids.

Almost complete hemolysis of human erythrocytes is caused by twenty-five micrograms per milliliter of merulinic acid B (Giannetti et al. 1978).

There is one fatality report in the medical literature of human infection from *M. tremellosus* in a severely immune-deficient patient (Friman et al. 2008).

Merulidial, a compound with antibiotic activity, was isolated (Quack et al. 1978).

The eastern species, *M. incarnatus,* has been investigated for antimicrobial activity (Zjawiony et al. 2005).

W. Jin et al. (2006) isolated 5-alkylresorcinols that inhibit methicillin-resistant *Staphylococcus aureus* (MRSA) and *Leishmania* species.

The related *Meruliopsis corium* is active against *S. aureus.*

Morchella esculenta

M. crassipes
(YELLOW MOREL)
(SPONGE MOREL)
M. elata
(BLACK MOREL)
(FAT HEADED BLACK MOREL)
(TALL MOREL)
M. conica
(NARROW HEADED BLACK MOREL)
(CONICAL MOREL)
M. angusticeps
(BLACK MOREL)
M. deliciosa
(WHITE MOREL)

You may ask for my car, you may even ask for my wife, but don't ask me where I pick morels.
—AN OLD FRENCH PICKER

The morel is truly the food of the gods. It is their exclusive food and it grows in the Elysian fields in plenty; morels are rare among us mortals for the Gods only reluctantly and rarely bestow their blessings on man. We must be content with the crumbs from the tables of the gods.
—ART CONRAD, *FARM QUARTERLY,*
SPRING 1958

Spongy morels in strong ragousts are found,
And in the soup the slimy snail is drowned.
—JOHN GAY

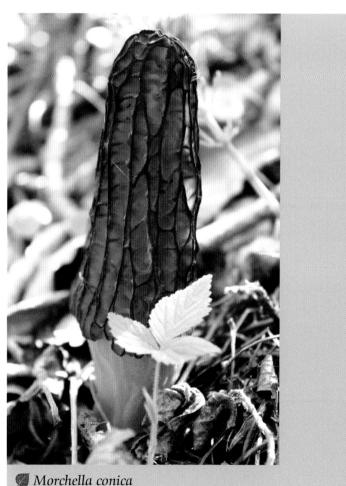

🍃 *Morchella conica*

Morchella is from the French *morille,* in turn derived from the Latin *mauricula.* This is the feminine diminutive of *Maurus* or "little Moor," in reference to the Moors, a dark-skinned group of Arabs and Berbers who settled in Spain and North Africa, and describing the mushroom's yellowish-brown cap.

It may also be derived from the Italian adjective *morello,* meaning "blackish," also referring to the coloring of the cap. Some authors believe *morchella* is simply Greek for "mushroom." Morel may derive from the high German *morhila,* and thus *morchel.*

Esculenta is Latin for "edible." *Elata* means "proud" or "lofty." *Conica* means "conical" and *crassipes* is from *crassus* for "thick" and *pes* for "foot." *Angusticeps* means "narrow head." *Deliciosa* is obvious.

The mushroom was known as *spongiae in humore pratorum nascentes* by Pliny and *spongioli* or *funguli* by Apicius of ancient Rome.

A Mohawk name for morels is land-fish. The neighboring Onondaga call them *uya'gä"da'* meaning "penis." The Cayuga call them *oho'da,* meaning "ear." One native name for the black morel is star sores.

They are found under poplar and pine. It seems that recent burned forests are one of their favorite haunts, but that may be just part of the mythology. Larry Evans (2010), star of Ron Mann's award-winning film *Know Your Mushrooms,* has written a great article on following forest fires for morels for the past twenty years.

They were my late spring favorites when I lived near Lesser Slave Lake, and are, in my estimation, one of the tastiest to be found.

Both are delicious fresh, but the black morel is the only one worth drying.

They have a tobacco-rich scent of sulphur and oak that combines well with eggs, beef, and wild game.

In my part of the world they pop up when stinging nettles are four to six inches tall and ready to eat. City folks may note that they appear when lilacs begin to show color and apple trees start to blossom.

Morel harvest varies with the fire season and rainfall. The year following the eruption of Mount St. Helen's produced huge quantities of morels.

Betty Williamson, in her beautifully illustrated *Reflections on the Fungaloids,* put it like this: "The Morchellian head is pitted with a web of tiny craters, little contiguous caps lined with pre-packaged spores. However primitive biologically, visually the resultant mazes recall the marvels of Celtic calligraphy and outdo the latest in computer-deco."

European morels sold dry are usually the black variety, but have a smoky flavor from being dried over open fires. Both Pakistan and India ship quantities of morels to Europe for packaging and distribution. Morels are also picked in Mexico, shipped to France for packaging, and then shipped back to North America. It is said that the average molecule of food eaten today in North America travels an average of 745 miles (1200 kilometers), so this morel trade is greater than the average.

The yellow morel is the official mushroom emblem of Minnesota, while the black morel is the official mushroom of Michigan. In that state, several morel festivals are held each spring. Merchants with mushroom-related goods set up booths, and a good time is had by all the fun-guys and fun-gals.

It is best to cook both of these mushrooms, in order to destroy a gastro-irritant that they contain. A raw marinade of *M. esculenta* at a Vancouver mushroom dinner several years ago resulted in seventy-seven of the 483 people suffering from vomiting, diarrhea, and, in some cases, rashes and numbness of limbs a week later.

The fumes of cooking morels can be dangerous, due to toxic hydrazines, so cook them in a well ventilated area. Morels, like the *Helvella,* contain small amounts of hemolysins, which destroy red blood cells; however, these are destroyed by cooking.

Morels have an earthy taste that is little enhanced by garlic and herbs. Jack Czarnecki, a chef with considerable fungi experience, says that their flavor reminds him of sweet peppers and caraway. The flavor combines well with roast or barbecued duck and a glass of Madeira wine.

Both *M. conica* and *M. angusticeps* (narrow cap) are believed to be variations of the true black morel, differing only in head shape. The white morel and the so-called red morel are both edible and delicious. They are similar in taste and medicinal value.

Culture and Folklore

In southern Poland, morels were believed to have been created by a devil with a bad temper. He came upon an older woman in the woods and cut her into bits and pieces that fell to the ground and created morels.

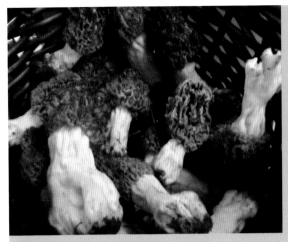

🍃 Basket of assorted morels

In Selisia, morels were also believed to be the work of the devil.

Medicinal Use

Chemical Constituents

- *M. esculenta:* **seventeen amino acids (isoleucine, leucine, lysine, methionine, phenylalanine, phreonine, and valine) and the sterol brassicasterol. Like other mushrooms, morels are deficient in sulphur-containing amino acids.**

- *M. esculenta, M. conica,* **and** *M. crassipes:* **cis-3-amino-L-proline and galatomannan, as well as gold (189 nanograms per gram) (-1), and considerable amounts of magnesium (450 micrograms per hundred grams).**

Black morel *(E. conica)* is used in traditional Chinese medicine for its sweet taste and cold, non-toxic properties. It is considered toning to the stomach and intestines, reducing phlegm and regulating the flow of vital energy in the body. It is decocted for treating indigestion, excessive sputum, and shortness of breath.

Yellow morel *(M. esculenta)* is a tumor inhibitor (Ito et al. 1973).

Recent work by Duncan et al. isolated a galactomannan with immunostimulating activity. At only three micrograms per milliliter, the galactomannan polysaccharide increased NF-kappa B-directed luciferase expression in THP1 human monocytic cells to levels 50 percent of those achieved by maximal activating concentration (ten micrograms per milliliter) of lipopolysaccharide (Duncan et al. 2002). This was also reported by Lull et al. (2005).

This galactomannan comprises about 2 percent of the dry fungal weight, and its glycosyl components include mannose (63 percent) and galactose (20 percent). This suggests indirect immune stimulation via mucosal immune system interaction, as the polysaccharide weight is too large to enter the blood stream.

Work by Nitha et al. (2007) found morel species significantly inhibit acute and chronic inflammation and prevent growth of solid cancer tumors. The fungi were grown on potato dextrose broth for ten days, dried at fifty degrees Celsius (122 degrees Fahrenheit), powdered, and extracted with hot ethanol.

Antitumor activity from a 50 percent ethanol extract of the mycelium resulted in 74 percent inhibition of tumor size and 79 percent of tumor weight in mice studies. Activity against both ascites and solid tumors has been found. The same extract exhibited significant inhibition of acute and chronic inflammation, similar to standard reference drugs (Nitha and Janardhanan 2005; Nitha et al. 2007).

Recent work by Nitha and Janardhanan (2008) suggests the cultured mycelium, prepared as a water alcohol extract, may provide protection against kidney toxicity associated with cisplatin and gentamicin treatments.

Bisakowski et al. (2000) have reported antioxidant activity.

Further work by Mau et al. (2004) confirmed significant antioxidant activity.

One study found *M. conica* to have the highest phenolics levels of all of the *Morchella* species tested, with a radical scavenging activity of 79 percent.

Mature black morels have been found to contain large amounts of beta-alanine. This is a compound found in hydrolyzed human hair, higher in blondes than brunettes. Beta alanine

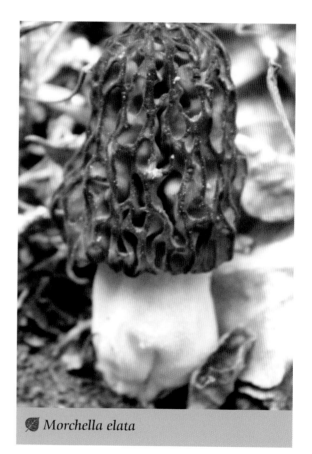

Morchella elata

has been found to be involved in tanning pigments (melanin). The mushrooms have some phospholipids (lecithin) that accentuate this activity. More investigation is needed.

Fungi Essence

Morel essence is to help you to be open-minded, ready to accept new ideas. It is for those looking for change in work and relationships. It will help calm down excessive mental activity.

— SILVERCORD

Mycoremediation

Various *Morchella* species myco-accumulate lead from seventy to one hundred times, suggesting caution with picking sites, including near highways and downwind from industrial plants. A recent article by Elinoar and Efrat Shavit (2010) in *Fungi* found lead arsenate used in apple orchards of the northeastern United States is a significant contributor to morel toxicity.

Cultivation

Black morel *(M. esculenta)* has been successfully cultivated under varying fermentation conditions using peat extracts as the only nutrient source. A patent was granted in 1986 for the artificial cultivation of morels on moistened wheat. From twenty-five to five hundred morels per square meter is claimed by the researchers, headed by Ronald Ower. The rights were sold to a national pizza company, but commercial morel production is still small. An interesting website is www.gorsky.com/~pdilley.

Successful cultivation of *M. esculenta* by Morel Mountain in Minnesota should lead to year-round supplies for restaurants and eventually to your neighborhood grocery store.

Terry Farms in Alabama, using a patented process, runs a production facility for morels year round.

Paul Stamets has found morels growing near a sludge pile of a pulp mill, a composting wheat straw bale, the ashes of an indoor fireplace, a backyard hibachi, and in a basement coal bin! He describes, in *Mycelium Running,* his own method for cultivation involving a fire pit and inoculation with spawn gathered during late summer. The stem butts from these fruiting bodies can be used for respawning as well.

Morels may play an important role in maintaining the health of the new hybrid poplar plantations. Deliberate inoculation trials may be worthwhile.

Recipe and Dosage

Decoct sixty grams of dry fungus in one liter of water and drink one cup twice a day.

Caution: genetically predisposed individuals with deficiency in the enzyme G6PD, which induces favism, making them intolerant of fava beans, are at risk of suffering severe anemia from ingesting morels. This condition is commonly associated with people of Mediterranean ancestry.

Mycena pura

(LILAC MYCENA)
(PINK MYCENA)
M. leaiana
(ORANGE MYCENA)
(LEA'S MYCENA)
M. rorida
Roridomyces roridus
(SLIPPERY MYCENA)
(DRIPPING BONNET)
M. galericulata
(TOQUE MYCENA)
(BONNET MYCENA)
(WRINKLED MYCENA)

Leaiana is named after Thomas Gibson Lea, an Ohio mushroom collector of the early 1800s. *Pura* is Latin for "clean." *Galericulata* is Latin, meaning "with a small hat."

Mycena is named after the ancient Greek city of Mycenae. Perseus severed the Gorgon's head with his sword and named it after the mushroom. In one version of the tale, the tip of his sword scabbard (*mykes* or "mushroom") fell off, and in another the hero's thirst was quenched when he drank from a toadstool issuing a fountain of water. Other tales suggest he was having a picnic with Andromeda and plucked and ate a mushroom from thirst. It was poisonous, and he soon starting hallucinating, seeing visions of a city around him. The city-state Mycenae was one of the great civilizations born because of its connection with a mushroom.

An attic amphora, or two-handled jar, from the third century BC shows Perseus with mushrooms appearing above his head. These appear to represent his emblem, as he slayed Medusa while her sisters slept.

Various *Mycena* species possess bioluminescence similar to the mycelized wood of honey mushroom (*Armillaria mella*). At last count, seventy-one species showed this ability to glow, in both their fruiting bodies and mycelium. Pink *Mycena* exhibits luminosity on the stems and gills, as well.

Sippery *Mycena* (*M. rorida*) appears to have luminescent spores, leading to glow-in-the-dark footprints.

All emit a greenish light with a maximum of 525 to 530 nanometers, based on a luciferin-luciferase type reaction.

Why bother? Insects and plankton have their own bioluminescence agendas involving feeding, mates, and prey, but why fungi?

The glow is steady, like bacteria. One explanation is that bioluminescence may activate DNA repair, or that the oxidation of producing light may help detoxify reactive oxygen. It is a thought!

Lilac *Mycena* is found on withered branches or trunks in dense forest. It appears quite shriveled when dry, and revives when moistened. It has a distinct radish smell that helps in identification.

According to mycologist, Dr. Jaroslav Klan, this species is "slightly hallucinogenic as it contains psychotropic indole substances." Some violent stomach upsets with nerve damage have been reported, while some have eaten it without any problem. It is not an edible, as it contains muscarine.

In 1976, the chemist C.H. Eugster identified the presence of muscarine and epimuscarine.

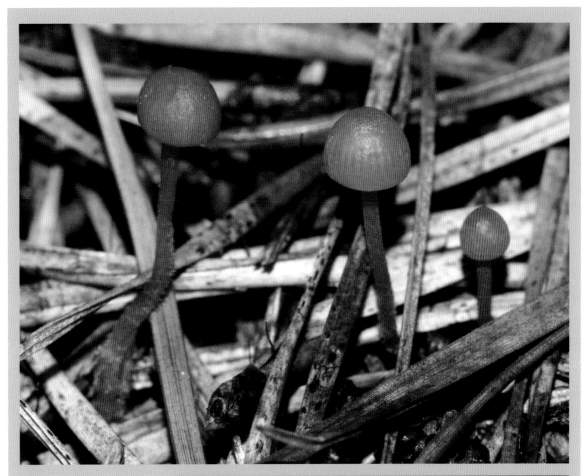

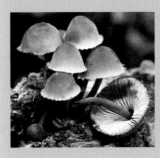

Above: *Mycena stroblioides.* Right: *Mycena leaiana.* Below left: *Mycena haematopus.*

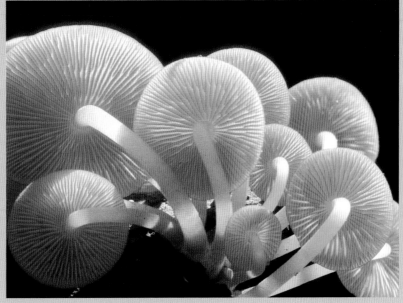

Medicinal Use

Chemical Constituents

- *M. pura:* muscarine and epimuscarine, puraquinonic acid, and strobilurin D.
- *M. leaiana:* leaianafulvene.

The inhibition rates of pink *Mycena* fruiting body extracts against sarcoma 180 and Ehrlich carcinoma are 60 percent and 70 percent respectively, while slippery *Mycena* exhibits 100 percent and 90 percent inhibition respectively. It contains the unusual amino acid L-gamma-propylideneglutamic acid that needs more study.

The novel norilludalane sesquiterpene, puraquinonic acid, has been isolated from mycelial cultures (Becker et al. 1997). This compound induces the differentiation of 30 to 40 percent of human promyelocytic leukemia cells (HL-60) into granulocyte or monocyte/macrophage-like cells at 380 micrometers. At this same concentration U-937 cells, which are blocked at a later stage of development, are also affected, but to a lesser extent.

Strobilurin D, an antifungal metabolite, was also isolated.

Leaianafulvene, a pigment that is cytotoxic and belongs to the cyclohumulanoids, has been recently isolated from the edible orange *Mycena*. The anticancer properties are under investigation.

A 50 percent lysis of Ehrlich ascetic tumor cells was observed. As well, Leaianafulvene significantly increased the number of revertants from *Salmonella typhimurium* TA 100, indicating a mutagenic activity for this compound (Harttig et al. 1990).

The sphaeroane diterpene, tintinnadiol, isolated from *M. tintinnabulum* fruiting bodies, exhibits cytotoxic effect against HL-60 and LI-210 cells at IC values of ten and forty micrograms per milliliter respectively (Engler et al. 1998).

The related *M. viridimarginata* contains 10-hydroxy-undeca-2,4,6,8-tetraynamide, which exhibits strong cytotoxic and antibiotic activity.

The species *M. amicta, M. cyanescens,* and *M. cyanorrhiza* may all contain psilocybin.

The related *M. ramealis* contains marasin, which shows activity against *Bacillus dentriticus.*

The related *M. sanguinolenta* contains sanguinones A and B, which possess a blue coloring. They are closely related to the marine alkaloids, discorhabdins.

Mycena megaspora contains drosophiline, while *M. crocata* contains two metabolites from corismic acid.

Miniscule *Mycena (M. capillaries)* shows activity against *Staphylococcus aureus.*

Mycena laevigata shows inhibition of sarcoma 180 by 100 percent and Ehrlich carcinoma by 90 percent.

Mycena crocata contains strobilurin N, the first strobilurin without antifungal activity (Buchanan et al. 1999).

The recent discovery of several new *Mycena* species with bioluminescence brings the total to seventy-one various species worldwide. Several of these new species, including *M. luxaeterna* and *M. luxperpetua,* exhibit this trait twenty-four hours a day.

Fungi Essence

Mycena polygramma essence assists in giving a better connection with the earth, being here of your own free will. It strengthens the ability to move through difficult situations even when everything seems to be in ruins. It helps in the digestion of hard-to-digest elements and cleans the body. Pluto influence and Gnome energy.

— BLOESEM

Mycoremediation

Work by Paul Stamets identified *M. chlorophos,* a luminescent mushroom, for application in breaking down chemical and biological warfare neurotoxins. This discovery has application for a number of mycoremediation projects.

Mycenastrum corium
(TOUGH PUFFBALL)

Mycena is Greek for "fungus." *Astrum* is from *astro* meaning "star." *Corium* is Latin for "skin" or "hide."

This puffball has a thick, tough inner skin that separates it from the *Bovista* and the thin-skinned *Calvatia,* while the white, felty outer layer distinguishes it from *Scleroderma* and thick-skinned *Calvatia.*

It is found most often in or near livestock pastures, horse corrals, and well-composted soils.

It is edible, like all puffballs, when firm and white inside.

Traditional Uses

In China, the dried sporophore is used to relieve swelling, stop bleeding, and relieve internal heat and fever.

Nectaria cinnabarina
(CORAL SPOT FUNGUS)
N. episphaeria

Nectaria are tiny pink to bright red ascomycetes found on currant, birch, and saskatoon twigs. They are quite common, and often overlooked on forays due to their familiarity and inedible nature.

Nectaria canker is the most common canker disease of hardwood trees.

Homeopathy

Nectrianinum is a clear liquid of a yellowish-brown hue, which has been prepared...and then taken to the autoclave at a temperature of 120 degrees Celsius (248 degrees Fahrenheit).

When this liquid is injected into healthy animals in five milliliter doses several times a week, no result is observed.

In contrast, when injected into cancerous men and animals, the subjects show a rise in body temperature of one to three degrees Celsius within two to four hours. If the dose is increased, the hyperthermia is accompanied by chills, sensation of cold, accelerated pulse, palpitation, headache, and thirst. The crisis terminates after some hours in polyuria and profound sleep. In very advanced cancer, reaction may not occur.

In a summary of the results the researchers say that nectrianinum has caused "arrest or diminution of hemorrhages; suppression of fetid discharges; a tendency at times to epidermisation of the neoplasm with a corresponding well defined arrest in its evolution." The patients were worse when treatment was discontinued and better when it was resumed. A maximum of four milliliters per day was never exceeded.

—VERMEULEN

Omphalina epichysium

O. campanella
Xeromphalina campanella
Clitocybe epichysium
(BROWN GOBLET)

Epichysium is from the Greek meaning "a toasting glass." *Omphalina* is Greek meaning "a small navel or umbilicus." *Campanella* means "bell shaped."

Brown goblet grows in mixed or coniferous forests on rotten, moss-covered logs. They are often associated with lichens. *Gerronema* species are similar but not associated with lichens.

Medicinal Use

Chemical Constituents

- *O. epichysium:* **EL-2 (beta-glucan).**

The related *O. flavida* shows activity against both *Staphylococcus aureus* and *E. coli,* while *O. campanella* shows significant activity against the latter, based on work by Hervey (1947).

Robbins et al. (1945) found *O. campanella* active against *S. aureus.* This small mushroom is found on decaying conifers.

Silberborth et al. (2002) isolated gerronemins that are composed of a C12-C16 alkane or alkene substituted at both ends by 2,3-dihydroxyphenyl groupings.

Gerronemins block the inducible expression of COX-2 and iNOS promotor-driven reporter gene with extremely low IC_{50} values of one to five micrograms per milliliter.

Cytotoxicity associated with inhibition of cell macromolecular synthase was noted.

Omphalotus olearius

O. illudens
Clitocybe illudens
(JACK-O'-LANTERN)
O. olivascens
(WESTERN JACK-O'-LANTERN)

Illudens means "deceiving." Jack-o'-lantern is so called because it glows in the dark, exhibiting phosphorescence or luminescence called foxfire.

The Lakota call it *peta yuhala,* meaning "the one who has the fire that is small."

Some people consider the European *O. olearius,* distinct from *O. illudens,* others as a synonym. The main difference is the larger spore size of the former.

Western jack-o'-lantern is found in California and up the coast.

Jack-o'-lantern is poisonous, with symptoms from ingestion that vary greatly, indicating some constituent variability. In comparing clinical studies, the majority of people who ingested *O. illudens* were feeling well within twelve hours. Perhaps the European species is more concentrated or contains different toxins.

There is one report from Quebec in 2003 when six women cooked the mushroom and within fifteen minutes of ingestion experienced all the unpleasant symptoms of poisoning. All recovered after rehydration.

Nausea, diarrhea, vomiting, and sweating are common symptoms of ingestion, due in part to muscarine derivatives.

David Arora recalls the tale of the shipwrecked sailor who wrote a last message by the light of a jack-o'-lantern mushroom, using the ink of a shaggy mane and an *Agaricus* stalk as a pen. Unfortunately, he starved to death because he was afraid to eat mushrooms!

The silver-green glow is brightest in the autumn at sporulation, thus its association with Halloween.

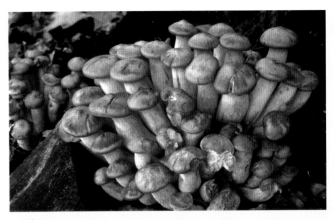

Omphalotus olearius

Pliny noticed this agaric, previously named *Polyporus olearius,* "grows upon the top of the trees and gives out a brilliant light at night; this indeed is the sign by which its presence is known, and by the aid of this light it may be gathered during the night." A fungal signature, as it were.

The eighth-century novel *Beowulf* refers to fire and water, which was probably a reference to luminescence from fungi:

"It is not far from here if measured in miles, that the lake stands shadowed by trees stiff with hoar frost.

A wood, firmly rooted, frowns from the water, there, night after night, a fearful wonder may be seen—fire on the water...that is not a pleasant place."

This source of light from fungal mycelia is also common to *Armillaria mella,* the honey mushroom, as discovered by Hartig in 1874.

Mark Twain mentions "rotten chunks that's called foxfire that just makes a soft kind of glow when you lay them in a dark place."

During World War I, soldiers would fix bits of rotten wood to their helmets, to avoid collisions in the dark.

Young girls in New Caledonia used them as ornaments in their hair when dancing at night.

An American war correspondent reportedly wrote his wife from New Guinea during World War II, "Darling, I am writing to you tonight by the light of five mushrooms." Aren't mycologists just the most romantic?

Medicinal Use

Chemical Constituents

- **Illudens S and M, illudenic acid, illudiolone, isoomphadione, and illudosone hemiacetal.**

Illudens have been investigated as anticancer agents. The number of molecules necessary to kill cancer cells was far fewer than required for cisplatin. Furthermore, illudens exhibited a degree of selectivity in their antitumor activity not seen with cisplatin. Illudens are, however, metabolically activated to unstable intermediates that can cause irreparable DNA damage.

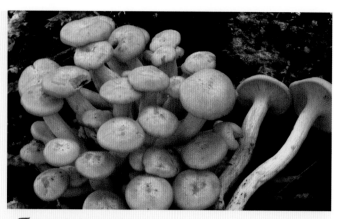

Omphalotus olearius

Some analogs show improved therapeutic index. Deoxyilludin M causes a life span increase of 24 percent when tested for five days against murine leukemia P-388 (Dufresne et al. 1997).

Tumor growth was inhibited by 75 percent when tested on human patients with myeloid leukemia.

Recent work by Dufresne et al. (1997) isolated an illudane sesquiterpene antibiotic with activity against methicillin-resistant *Staphylococcus aureus* (MRSA).

Lehmann et al. (2003) found illudin S to be the sole antiviral component of the fruiting body.

More work is needed to see if this line of inquiry will lead to new drug development. Weis et al. at International Myko Biologics in San Antonio, Texas, are studying the production of illuden S from various strains of *O. olearius*. Depending on the strain, between 0.81 and 3.1 milligrams per milliliter of illuden S is produced in submerged cultivation.

C. illudens contains terpenoids that are effective against protozoa like *Plasmodium gallinaceum* (Coatney et al. 1953; Mayer 1997) and pathogenic nematodes such as *Meloidogyne incognita*.

Under in vitro conditions, omphalotin A outperforms known nematocides, such as ivermectin, in both selectivity and potency. More study is required.

The semi-synthetic illudin analog 6-hydroxymethylcylfulvene (also known as irofluven) shows promise as a tumor growth inhibitor. It has undergone phase-one human clinical trials.

The company MGI Pharma has developed Irofulven, a semi-synthetic compound from illudin S, for the treatment of refractory and relapsed tumors of the ovary, prostate, liver, breast, lung, and colon. Phase II trials were conducted in 2002. Research is ongoing (Paci et al. 2006).

The semi-synthetic antitumor agents called acylfulvenes were derived from illudin s through the mechanism of reverse Prins reaction. In an article by McMorris et al. (1999), they state "acylfulvene is one hundred-fold less toxic in vitro and in vivo than illudin S, but possesses marked antitumor efficacy in vivo, thus displaying opposite properties from illudin S."

Work at Johns Hopkins shows that the drug, when activated by alkenal/one oxidoreductase, has proven chemotherapeutic activity.

Irofluven appears to induce apoptosis in tumor cells.

Studies in France found that irofluven in combination with cisplatin and 5-fluorouracil enhanced cytotoxicity of the drug, while work in San Diego, California, found thiotepa or mitomycin enhanced the activity (Kelner et al. 2002).

Work by Hammond et al. (2000) in San Antonio, Texas, found that combining it with paclitaxel or topotecan enhanced effectiveness.

Side effects are similar to other chemotherapy drugs including bone marrow suppression, nausea, vomiting, anemia, kidney failure, and pulmonary edema.

In a 2005 phase II irofulven trial on women with previously treated ovarian cancer, retinal toxicity began to show. Doses had to be lowered in mid-trial (Shauit 2008).

Combining it with select platinum-derived alkylating agents appears to enhance its effect (Shauit 2008).

The reality is that it helps a number of therapies by potentiating activity of the patient's own immune system. We are sure to hear more about these products in the future.

Panaeolus subbalteatus

P. venenosus
(BELTED CAP PANAEOLUS)
(DARK RIMMED MOTTLEGILL)
P. campanulatus
(BELL CAP PANAEOLUS)
P. sphinctrinus
(PINCHED PANAEOLUS)
(HOOPED PETTICOAT)
P. papilionaceus
(PETTICOAT MOTTLEGILL)

Panaeolus subbalteatus is the classic druid mushroom.

— DANIEL DELANEY

Horse manure also has a chance in the time of giant mushrooms.

— KOBAYASHI ISSA

Panaeolus is Greek meaning "all variegated" or "dazzling," while *subbalteatus* is Latin meaning "darker border on cap." This is from the prefix *sub*, meaning almost or somewhat, and *balteatus*, meaning belt-like, in reference to the darker coloration that forms along margins of the cap as the mushroom dries.

Sphinctrinus is Greek meaning "tied up" or "pulled in." *Venenosus* is based on a previous undeserved reputation of poisonousness. *Papilionaceus* is from *papilo* meaning "butterfly."

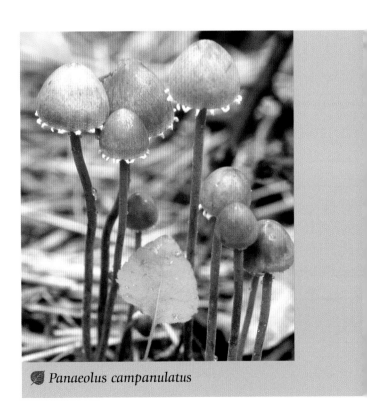

Panaeolus campanulatus

I have found belted cap *Panaeolus* growing on neighbors' lawns in my home city. It is recognized by the dark, marginal band on the cap after which it is named. The spore print is black, the stem pinkish-brown.

The German name, *dunkelrandiger dungerling,* means "dark-banded dung mushroom," while the Japanese call it *magusotake,* or "horse pasture mushroom." The mushroom does like horse ranches and similar environments.

Bell cap *Panaeolus (P. campanulatus)* contains psilocybin, but also ibotenic acid (like *Amanita*) that causes nausea. Not recommended.

Pinched *Panaeolus* has recently been reported to contain psilocybin and serotonin, and is definitely a hallucinogen. It was used by the Mazatec and natives of Mexico, and known as *she-to,* meaning "pasture mushroom," or *to-shka,* meaning "intoxicating mushroom." And while it is not as important as other species of the *Psilocybe* and *Stropharia,* various shamans have used it on occasion.

In China, the mushroom is known as *hsiao chun* or "laughing mushroom."

A number of myths and works of art in ancient Greece depict Nessus, the Centaur, with a mushroom sprouting between his hooves. It may well been the fungal ambrosia associated with Eleusinian and Orphic mystery.

Jonathan Ott wrote than some individuals in Oregon take up to 250 specimens of this species in order to produce a strong hallucinogenic effect.

This common garden mushroom contains psilocybin (1.6 to 6.5 milligrams per gram of dry weight), and baeocystin, but no psilocin (4-hydroxy-di-methyl-tryptamine). Psilocybin, however, becomes psilocin in the body, after phosphorus is stripped away by enzymes. It contains large amounts of serotonin and 5 HTP (5-hydroxytryptophan).

Medicinal Use

Psilocin concentrates in higher amounts in the liver and adrenals, and it has been found to concentrate in the neocortex, hippocampus, and thalamus in rat brains.

This makes it a magic mushroom of the prairies with true psychotropic activity. One thirty-four-year-old Scot ingested more than twenty fruit bodies and experienced mild hallucinogenic reactions without nausea. Within one hour, sensations of detachment were experienced, followed by feelings of unmotivated hilarity.

It is considered more empathogenic and aphrodisiac than mushrooms that contain only psilocybin. Individual visions are observed for longer periods of time and contemplated at a leisurely pace, according to Christian Ratsch. As little as 1.5 grams dry weight produces psychoactivity, while 2.7 grams are considered a visionary dose.

After a forty-year hiatus, psilocybin is again being researched for its benefit in the treatment of addiction, schizophrenia, paranoia, and depression. Dr. David Nichols, at Purdue University, says that psilocybin and psilocin "are some of the most potent compounds we know of that can change consciousness. It's kind of peculiar they have just been kind of sitting on the shelf for forty years. There is no other class of biologically active substances I am aware of that have been ignored like that."

Psilocybin mushrooms might be of further use in improving eyesight, hearing, and circulation, and in activating the self-healing processes within the human body.

Work by J. Gartz, in a publication of the British Mycological Society, suggests that psilocybin, at low doses, is effective against acute migraine and cluster headaches. It likely affects the serotonin receptor (5-HT) in a fashion analogous to Sumatriptan, a drug used for this purpose. Some work in this area could yield a medicine that has low toxicity and fewer side effects for these debilitating conditions.

Spoerke and Rumack, in their excellent book *Handbook of Mushroom Poisoning,* report that migraine headache patients were found to be more sensitive to the hallucinogenic effects of psilocybin in a placebo-controlled study of thirty normal subjects and thirty-six migraine patients. After an oral dose of twenty micrograms per kilogram of body weight, no reaction occurred in 86 percent of the patients in the control compared to 41 percent of the migraine sufferers. Hallucinations occurred in 18 percent of the migraine patients and none in the control group.

Possible mechanisms for this increased sensitivity could be increased blood brain barrier permeability and/or CNS serotonin sensitivity.

Pinched *Panaeolus* produces laccase isoenzymes and manganese peroxide with activity at high pH levels.

Bell cap mushroom is active against *E. coli* (Hervey 1947).

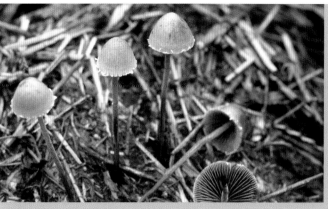

Panaeolus campanulatus

Mukherjee and Sengupta (1985) found *P. papillionaceus* to be a high producer of inulinase and invertase at an optimum pH of 6.5 and sixty degrees Celsius (140 degrees Fahrenheit).

Work by Mukherjee et al. (1986) has found this species resistant to nystatin and amphotercin B.

The related west coast species, *P. retirugis,* contains an antibiotic diterpene. Mycelial culture contains pleuromutilin. Two new illudane sesquiterpenes, paneolic and paneolilludinic acid, show activity against *Staphylococcus aureus.*

Paneolic acid exhibits cytotoxicity against HL-60 cells with an IC50 of 18.9 micrograms per milliliter (Ma, W. et al. 2004).

Both *P. papillionaceus* and *P. subbalteatus* show activity against *S. aureus* (Hervey 1947).

Fungi Essence

P. campanulatus is related to memory loss and gain, reeling about, sudden dimness of vision, slow and feeble pulse, languor and weakness, giddiness, trembling, and great drowsiness.

— VERMEULEN

Panaeolina foenisecii

Panaeolus foenisecii
Psathyrella foenisecii
(HAYMAKER'S MUSHROOM)
(BROWN HAY CAP)
(LAWN MOWER'S MUSHROOM)

Panaeolina means "small *Panaeolus*" and *foenisecii* means "dry hay," both from Latin. *Psathyrella* means "fragile."

This small parasol mushroom is a common lawn mushroom. It has a dark purplish-brown spore print, and fruits in summer on the western prairies.

Small amounts eaten raw are poisonous to young children, according to some authors.

The mushroom contains psilocybin, according to some sources. Studies from Europe indicate no detectable psilocybin or its hallucinogenic derivatives, baeocystin and psilocin. One study found 5-hydroxytryptamine (serotonin) and its precursor 5-hydroxytryptophan. In one test, forty grams of fresh mushroom failed to produce psychotropic effect.

Not all samples have been found to contain psilocybin. Blue staining may or may not mean anything.

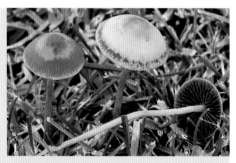

🍃 *Panaeolina foenisecii*

Panellus serotinus

Pleurotus serotinus
Sarcomyxa serotina
(LATE FALL OYSTER)
(GREEN OYSTER)
(OLIVE BROWN PANELLUS)
Panus rudis
(HAIRY PANUS)
P. strigosus
Lentinus strigosus
(GIANT PANUS)
(GIANT OYSTER)
P. stipticus
Panellus stipticus
(STYPTIC PAN)
(LUMINESCENT PANELLUS)
Panus conchatus
P. torulosus
(SMOOTH PANUS)
(CONCH PANUS)

Late fall oyster mushroom is fairly common to hardwood forests. It is edible, although somewhat tough without prolonged cooking over low heat.

The related *Panellus stipticus (Panus stipticus)* is bioluminescent like various honey, oyster, and *Mycena* species.

It grows on old stumps in small, thin, overlapping ear-shaped fruiting bodies that glow a greenish white. Famed mycologist Reggie Buller found that it emitted light when discharging spores, but ceased when it dried. If re-moistened, even after six months, it again becomes luminous. Oxygen is required by all of these mushrooms, as nitrogen, hydrogen, ether, and chloroform all stop the process of bioluminescence.

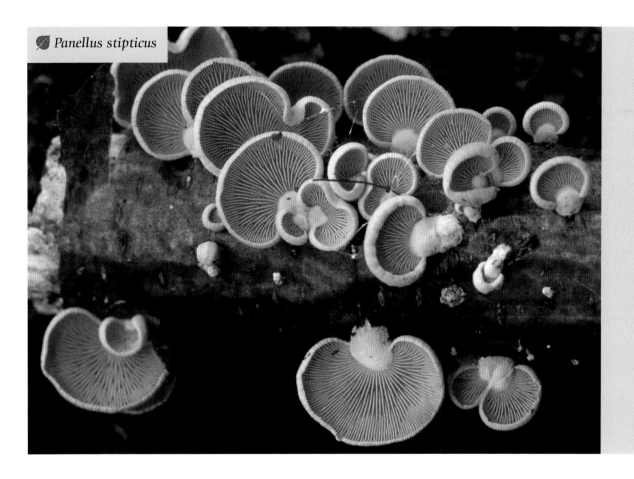

Panellus stipticus

What is interesting is that the North American and European forms are morphologically indistinguishable, and yet the foreign form is always non-luminous. Work by Dr. Buller paired the two forms on agar, and the hyphae fused, producing a hybrid mycelium with luminous and non-luminous sectors.

Dr. Buller was the first professor of botany at the University of Manitoba, and he was considered by many to have been one of the world's finest mycologists. A chapter about his interesting life is found in the excellent book *Mr. Bloomfield's Orchard* by Nicholas Money.

Luminescent *Panellus (P. stipticus)* is found on dead hardwood trees in eastern North America.

Hairy *Panus* grows on hardwood stumps of birch, poplar, and willow, and looks a lot like a hairy oyster mushroom. It is edible, but why bother?

Traditional Uses

Luminescent *Panellus (P. stipticus)*, as the name suggests, glows in the dark and is used to staunch bleeding in parts of Europe, hence the species name.

In parts of China, hairy *Panus* is used to treat various kinds of furuncles. The fungus is decocted and used as a wash on affected areas. The dry sporophore is ground into a powder for staunching external wound bleeding.

Smooth *Panus* is used in China as part of Tendon Easing Powder, used to cure lumbago, pain in legs, numb limbs, and discomfort in tendons and blood vessels.

Medicinal Use

Chemical Constituents

■ *P. serotinus:* **heteroglucan; (1-6)-beta-D-glycosyl-branched (1-3)-beta-D-glucans; two ceramides, (2S,3R,4E,8E)-N-hexadecanoyl-2-amino-9-methyl-4,8-octadecadiene-1,3-diol and (2S,3R,4E,8E,9'Z,12'Z)-N9',12'-octadeca-dienoyl-2-amino-9-methyl-4,8-octadec-adien-1,3-diol. The green color is due to the presence of riboflavin and 3-N-methylriboflavin.**

Late fall oyster contains a human blood type A hemagglutinate (Yagi et al. 2000).

Luminescent *Panellus* shows activity against both *E. coli* and *Staphylococcus aureus* (Hervey 1947).

Inhibition rates against sarcoma 180 and Ehrlich carcinoma are 80 percent and 70 percent respectively.

It contains a human blood type B and O specific hemagglutinate.

Panepoxydone, isolated from *Panus* species, inhibits the phosphorylation of IkB-alpha that, in turn, interferes with NFkB-mediated signal transduction, suggesting use in attacking cancer cells.

The isolated compound has an inhibition rate of 60 percent against sarcoma 180 and 79 percent against Ehrlich carcinoma.

Several compounds, but especially hyponophilin derived from giant *Panus* and *Lentinus connatus,* show significant inhibition of the organism responsible for chagas disease. At only twenty micrograms per milliliter, it completely inhibited *Trypanosoma cruzi* with only minor non-toxic immune modulation on human leukocytes.

Two inhibitors of platelet aggregation have been found in the fermentation of *Panus* species. One inhibitor is identical to naematolon, an antibiotic found in the *Hypholoma* species (Backen, S. et al. 1984). The other constituent, panudial, is a new nordrimane that shows potent inhibition of bovine and human platelet aggregation.

The fermented broth yields panepophenthrin, a compound that inhibits ubiquitin-activating enzyme. This helps regulate cellular events and is linked to serious diseases (Sekizawa et al. 2002).

Ubiquinone, or coenzyme Q10, is a lipid-soluble quinone present in all cells and involved in intracellular respiration.

Smooth *Panus* has an inhibition rate of 100 percent against both sarcoma 180 and Ehrlich carcinoma (Ohtsuka et al. 1973).

Hairy *Panus* fruiting body shows significant blue laccase activity.

Hairy Panus contains panepoxydone, which showed weak activity in a study against the organism associated with Chagas disease.

Panellus nidulans

(see *Phyllotopsis nidulans*)

Paxillus involutus

(POISON PAXILLUS)
(INROLLED PAX)
(BROWN ROLL RIM)
P. atrotomentosus
Tapinella atrotomentosa
(BLACKFOOT PAXILLUS)
(VELVET FOOTED PAX)
P. panuoides
T. panuoides
(FAN PAX)
(STALKLESS PAXILLUS)

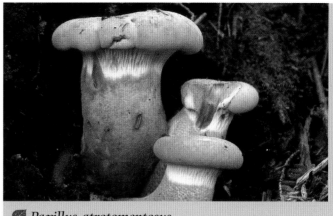

Paxillus atrotomentosus

Paxillus means "a small stake." *Involutus* means "rolled inward."

Poison *Paxillus* is a solo or grouped mushroom found on forest ground or at the edge of forests. It pops up on golf courses, parks, and in cemeteries toward fall.

Blackfoot *Paxillus* is considered inedible and is found in the Rocky Mountains.

Fan Pax *(Paxillus panuoides or Tapinella panuoides)* is found on conifer stumps, with gills that are whitish to ochre, forked, with a buff spore print.

Paxillus is not recommended as an edible. People who have eaten the cooked mushroom, even for years, can suddenly develop a serious allergy that results in kidney failure or even death. It appears to contain a cumulative poison that is not removed or destroyed by cooking.

It is so popular in Poland that this is the third most common type of poisoning reported in that country.

The mushroom is a gastrointestinal irritant when eaten raw or cooked, but appears much safer when salted or pickled, two traditional methods used throughout eastern Europe. I wouldn't chance it.

Recent studies indicate the compound responsible for its poisonous nature is thermostable, and directly produces breaks in the chromosomes of dividing cells, suggestive of mutagenic and carcinogenic activity.

It appears to cause an acute hemolytic anemia, with some fatal poisonings. One forty-nine-year-old male died three and a half days after his last mushroom meal in protracted, unremitting shock. An autopsy showed intravascular coagulation and widespread fat embolism of the lungs.

It can take some time for problems to develop, but for some unknown reason some people produce IgC antibodies to an unidentified compound in the mushroom. During the next meal, antibody-antigen complexes form, agglutination takes place, complement is fixed and the red blood cells undergo intravascular hemolysis. The onset can be rapid, as little as two hours after the meal, with symptoms of vomiting, diarrhea, abdominal pain, and low blood pressure leading to collapse. Kidney failure quickly follows.

The dry powdered mushroom is a different story, used in traditional Chinese medicine.

Traditional Uses

Poison *Paxillus* is part of Tendon Easing Powder, used in traditional Chinese medicine to treat lumbago, painful legs, numb limbs, and discomfort in tendons and veins.

Medicinal Use

Chemical Constituents

- *P. involutus:* **involutone, linoleic acid, crotonic acid, mannitol, ergosterol, as well as methyl-, ethyl-, or butyl-B-D-glucopyranosides and linoleates.**

- *P. atrotomentosus:* **the pigment xerocomic acid, as well as eight ecdysteroids, including paxillosterone, 20,22-p-hydroxybenzyl lidene acetal, atrotosterone, 25-hydroxy-atrotosterone, and atrotosterones A, B, and C.**

- *P. panuoides:* **eight ecdysteroids, 20-hydro-syecdysone, ponasterone A, malacosterone, turkesterone, paxillosterone, panuosterone, 25-hydroxy-panuosterone, and a new phytosphingosine-type ceramide, named paxillamide.**

- *P. curtisii:* **curtisians.**

Extracts have been found to inhibit growth of *Bacillus subtilis.* Robbins et al. (1945) found some activity against *Staphylococcus aureus.*

Recent work by Yamac and Bilgili (2006) found activity in the fruiting body against *B. subtilis,* as well as *Staphylococcus epidermis, Enterobacter aerogenes,* and *Salmonella typhimurium.*

A study found *P. involutus* contains significant anti-spasmodic and papaverine-like activity; it also demonstrated a refrigerant or body temperature cooling effect in mice. The extract exhibited increased dynamic activity and curiosity in the animals, suggesting central nervous system stimulation.

Fan *Pax* contains eight ecdysteroids, 20-hydrosyecdysone, ponasterone A, malacosterone, turkesterone, paxillosterone, panuosterone, and 25-hydroxy-panuosterone. Of these 20-hydroecdysone is the most active.

Ecdysones stimulate the synthesis of proteins in animals and humans and possess adaptogenic, anti-mutagenic, immune stimulating, and nutritive tonic properties.

Two p-terphenyls exhibit strong antioxidant properties. Leucomentin-4 and leucomentin-2 inhibit lipid peroxidation at very low levels (Yun et al. 2000b). These compounds provide neuroprotective activity due to their ability to

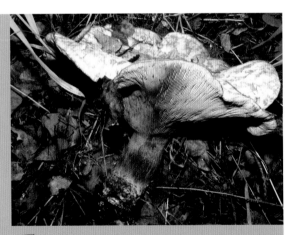
Paxillus involutus

chelate iron, inhibiting oxidative damage to DNA (Lee, I.-K. et al. 2003).

Several of these p-terphenyl ortho-quinones were found active against cancer tumor cell lines (Cali et al. 2004).

A new phytosphingosine-type ceramide, named paxillamide, has been isolated (Gao, J. M. et al. 2004). Ceramides are of considerable interest due to their involvement in signal transduction pathways, cell growth, and apoptosis.

Purified lectins are able to hemagglutinate human red blood cells with an anti-A specificity (Furukawa, K. et al. 1995).

Early work by Hervey (1947) suggests activity against *E. coli* and *S. aureus*.

The related *P. curtisii* contains curtisian R, a strong antioxidant, and curtisians A-D that inhibit lipid peroxidation (Yun et al. 2000a).

Mycoremediation

Poison *Paxillus* degrades PAHs in a manner similar to *Amanita muscaria*. It also transforms TNT after three days of incubation in axenic cultures.

Blackfoot *Paxillus* was found to bioaccumulate radioactive cesium up to twelve hundred times, suggesting its use as a myco-monitor, or mycoremediator of the environment.

Bits and Pieces

One researcher, Fabre, found that poison *Paxilus* emits radiation that passes through a cardboard box and affects photographic film.

Peniophora gigantea
(GIANT PARCHMENT)

Peniophora gigantea is a crust or parchment fungi that covers dead conifers in mats or sheets.

In eastern Europe, the spores or mycelium are painted onto cut tree stumps to prevent annosus root rot and butt rot *(Heterobasidion annosum)* in pine trees. It is an interesting example of a fungi serving to control or neutralize other fungi.

Medicinal Use
Chemical Constituents

- **Xylerythrinin, peniophorin, peniophorinin, peniosanguin, peniosanguin methyl ether, and 5-0-methyl-xylerythrin.**

The related *P. incarnata* showed significant activity against *S. aureus* (Hervey 1947).

Textile Industry

A species of *Peniphora* has been studied in South Africa for application in the pulp and paper industry and found to produce paper with improved strength properties.

Work in Germany cloned pyranose 2-oxidase in *E. coli* to produce an improved method of bioconversion of L-sorbose, D-xylose, and other sugars through enzymatic transformation.

Perenniporia subacida

Polyporus subacidus
Poria subacida
(FEATHER ROT)
P. fraxinea
Fomes fraxineus
Fomitella fraxinea
Vanderbylia fraxinea
(POLYPORE DE FRÊNE)

Perenniporia subacida is, as the name suggests, associated with *Poria,* but is devoid of stem and cap. It is a perennial of the Pacific Northwest, and rarely found on the eastern side of the Continental Divide.

Work by various researchers indicates the fruiting body possesses antitumor, antimicrobial, and anti-leukemia activity.

Medicinal Use

Gregory et al. (1966) found that *Perenniporia subacida* markedly inhibits leukemia L1210 cancer cell lines in mice.

The lectin in polypore de frêne significantly induced nitric oxide secretion in HD11 cells, and suppressed RP9 tumor cell growth (Dalloul 2006).

The related *P. fraxinophilus* showed activity against *Staphylococcus aureus* (Robbins et al. 1945). Feather rot and *P. tenuis* were also found to be active against both *S. aureus* and *E. coli* on thiamine peptide cultures.

Agriculture

One study found that injecting polysaccharides of polypore de frêne into eighteen-day-old poultry helped prevent the development of coccidiosis, a disastrous infection that can decimate commercial chicken and turkey operations. It also suggests effective growth promotion and immune stimulation. A U.S. patent, 7438915, has been issued.

Peziza badia

(RED BROWN CUP)
(BLACK ELF CUP)
(PIG'S EAR)

Badia means "reddish-brown." *Peziza* means "a mushroom without a root or stalk."

Red brown cup is a common mushroom that looks like a small saucer cup and is dark brown inside and red-brown outside. It has no stalk, simply popping directly from the mycelium. It is found along the edges of forest paths, and in the forest under spruce or in sandy soil. They are only edible when cooked.

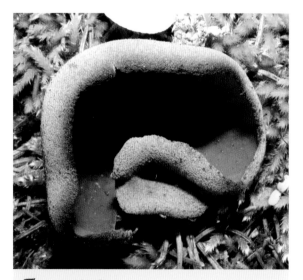
Peziza badia

308

Medicinal Use

This fungus has been found to contain L-fucose, a specific lectin that binds with human thyroglobulin, and mannofuco-galactans that have immunological activity (Antonyuk 1997).

Peziza vesiculosa

(SMALL DUNG CUP)
(BLADDER ELF CUP)
(STRAW CUP FUNGUS)

Vesiculosa is from the Latin meaning "with blisters," referring to the small bulges in the hymenium. *Peziza* was the name given to a mushroom without root or stalk by Pliny. *Vesiculosa* means "full of bladders."

This easily identified mushroom is a soft, fragile, and very small yellowish-brown cup-shaped mushroom. It is often found growing on animal dung. It can be found in the wild,

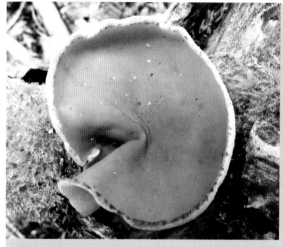

🍃 *Peziza vesiculosa*

or around corrals and old stables. They can be solitary or grow in clusters. They are edible only when cooked.

Traditional Uses

In traditional Chinese medicine, the mushroom is considered sweet, slightly bitter, and cool in nature, and is therefore indicated in cases of low body resistance to illness and tumors.

In Japan, a fungal extract is used to treat tumors and depressed immune systems.

Medicinal Use

Chemical Constituents

- **Vesiculogen, which contains protein (80 percent), carbohydrate (19 percent), and 1,3-glucan polysaccharides, (+)-epipentenomycin I.**

A 1979 study found this fungus to contain a compound that stimulates spleen cell lines but not thymus cells.

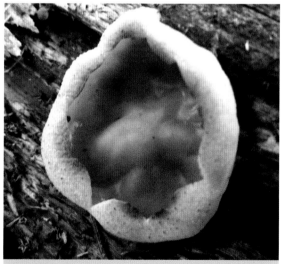

🍃 *Peziza vesiculosa*

A follow-up 1982 study showed that extracts of this fungus act as a B cell mitogen, enhancing the reticuloendothelial system (RES). Specifically, vesiculogen was shown to enhance phagocytosis and inhibit tumor cells in vitro. It has been found to stimulate T-cell production in more recent studies.

The fruiting body inhibits sarcoma 180 in vivo (Mimura et al. 1985). A glucan known as PVG and other polysaccharides from the fruiting body are related to the antitumor activity.

Vesiculogen is a hot-water extracted compound that appears to increase antibody response and thus act as a polyclonal B-cell activator.

The carpophores of various *Peziza* species show activity against gram-positive bacteria. Bernillon et al. isolated (+)-epipentenomycin I as an anti-microbial (Bernillon, J et al. 1989).

Recipe and Dosage

Two to four grams, dried and decocted in water at a 1:5 ratio. Drink one to two ounces twice daily.

Bits and Pieces

Dr. Reginald Buller completed the six-volume *Researches in Fungi* in 1934. This professor of botany at the University of Manitoba was a brilliant mycologist. In one chapter of volume six he investigates and reports on the sounds associated with the release of spores by various fungi. Both *Peziza badia* and *P. vesiculosa*, assigned to a different genus in those days, puffed loudly for one to two seconds. Other genera including *Urnula*, *Rhizina*, and *Aleuria* were found to puff vigorously and discharge

with a distinct sound. *Sphaerobolus* species project spores up to eighteen feet, and are definitely the most powerful and loudest. *Sphaerobolus* means "sphere thrower," which is very descriptive of the shooting spores. To put their power into perspective, shooting their spores eighteen feet would be the equivalent of a six-foot human throwing a baseball one and a half miles high and landing it nearly two miles away.

He suggests that the best fruiting body to use with a microphone is *Coprinus comatus*. It has large spores that discharge at the rate of ten thousand per second and a sensitive microphone could record the faintly audible projections.

This is an example of an obsession colliding with too much free time.

Come to think of it, with the increased sophistication in auditory electronics today, this could well occupy a new generation of fungalphones.

Phaeolus schweinitzii

P. spadicens
Polyporus schweinitzii
(DYER'S POLYPORE)
(VELVET TOP FUNGUS)

The species is named in honor of the mycologist Schweinitz.

Dyer's polypore refers to the fact that the dried fungus can be used as an olive-brown dye for wool.

Velvet top is a good name as it describes the red-brown concentric ring with a spongy leathery texture quite well. It is found on both living

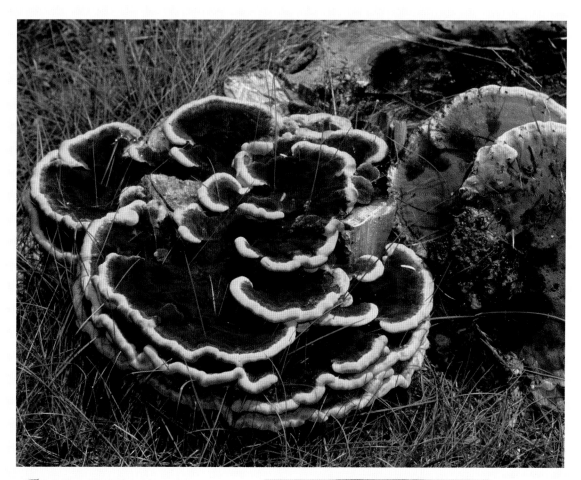

🍃 Above: *Phaeolus schweinitzii*. Right and below: fungal dyes.

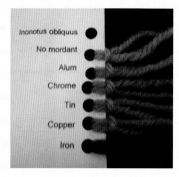

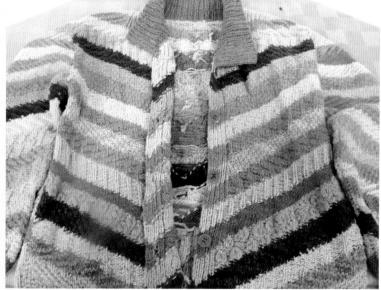

and dead trees, and felled timber on the forest floor of spruce and fir forests.

The annual fruiting bodies form in late summer.

The smell of the polypore resembles beef liver.

According to David Arora, it may be toxic.

Medicinal Use

The culture fluids have been shown to inhibit *Staphylococcus aureus, Salmonella typhi,* and *E. coli,* and are not toxic to guinea pigs. This follows early work that found activity against *S. aureus* and *E. coli* (Hervey 1947).

It does contain a carcinostatic polysaccharide.

The inhibition rate against both sarcoma 180 and Ehrlich carcinoma is 80 percent (Ohtsuka et al. 1973).

Phallus impudicus

(STINKHORN)
(WOOD WITCH)
(STINKING POLECAT)
P. hadriani
(HADRIAN'S STINKHORN)
Mutinus caninus
(DOG'S STINKHORN)
M. elegans
M. bovinus
M. curtisii
(DEVIL'S DIPSTICK)
Clathrus ruber
C. cancellatus
(LATTICED STINKHORN)
Dictyophora duplicata
(NETTED STINKHORN)

As one that smells a foul-fleshed agaric
  in the holt,
And deems it carrion of some woodland
  thing,
Or shrew, or weasel, nipt her slender nose
With petulant thumb and finger,
  shrilling, "Hence."
  — TENNYSON

Oh, 'twas base! To be treated everywhere with politeness and hospitality, and to return invidiously to smell fungus them all over.
  — BARON MUNCHAUSEN

Phallus is Greek for "rod" and *impudicus* comes from the Latin for "shameless," therefore the "unashamed phallus or rod." Mutinus was another Latin name for Priapus, the Roman god of sex, and hence means "small penis or rod." *Caninus* means "dog" and *bovinus* means "of cattle."

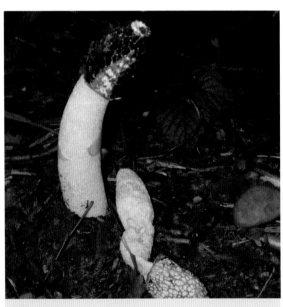

🍃 *Phallus impudicus*

Gerard, in his famous herbal of 1638, called it the "pricke mushroom" or *"fungus virilis penis erecti forma."* Enough already! We get it!

Dog's stinkhorn is commonly found in gardens and parks of western Canada. It is a very foul smelling mushroom found in forests and even on compost heaps. The smell helps attract flies, which it does efficiently. It has been estimated that a single fly "speck" may contain up to twenty million spores.

Stinkhorn begins life as an almost perfect white egg shape, called a devil's egg, that within ninety minutes begins to crack open and expose the complete mushroom inside. The transformation from egg to erection often begins in the night air and is not finished until dawn. When the egg hatches, the central receptacle takes on water and ruptures the skin. This receptacle is surrounded by a green-black cushion of spores called the gleba and encased in a clear jelly, which lubricates the growing shaft.

The top surface is pitted like a honeycomb, all of which quickly turns into a slimy, smelly mass eaten by flies and slugs.

The spores are in slime that contains volatile compounds including hydrogen sulphide, formaldehyde, dimethyl sulphide, methyl sulphide, (E)-ocimene, methyl-mercaptan, and phallic acids.

Methyl mercaptan is found in radish roots, and produced by anaerobic bacteria in the intestine after working on Cabbage family members. Hydrogen sulphide is what produces the smell of natural gas, sulphur springs, and rotten eggs. Formaldehyde is everywhere today, off-gassing from plywood, carpets, cabinets, and numerous disinfectants.

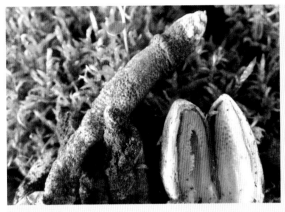

🍃 *Mutinus caninus*

These mushrooms are sometimes sold in the market stalls of Europe, but not widely relished.

Hadrian's stinkhorn is somewhat more pleasant and called purple devil's egg.

Culture and Folklore

The phallic appearance and name of some stinkhorns has given rise to numerous folk beliefs, and was the cause of considerable concern in Victorian England. Such blatant displays of male sexuality were not suitable for the eyes of unmarried women.

"Both *Phallus* and penis swell up due to pressurized fluid and both become flaccid rapidly after performance, having served their purpose," wrote Frans Vermeulen.

They can exert enough pressure that three specimens can lift four hundred kilograms (880 pounds) (Niksic et al. 2008). Pressure exerted was measured at force of two pounds per square foot.

Charles Darwin's eldest daughter would hunt down stinkhorn by scent alone. "At the end of the day's sport the catch was brought back and burnt in the deepest secrecy on the drawing room fire with the door locked—because of the morals of the maids."

In Borneo, the stinkhorn symbolized the penis of a dead hero, returning in spirit form. In graveyards of Germany, it was regarded as the fingers of a corpse pushing up and indicated unrepented sin in the dead. It was known as "corpse finger" or, in German, *leichenfinger.*

In Nigeria, the fungi are used as a charm to make hunters invisible when facing danger.

In 1926, a growth of these fungi led to a surprising incident in France. The local parish priest of Bombon was set upon by twelve fanatical adherents in a sect called Notre Dame des Pleurs. They accused him of sending some birds into the garden of their founder, Madame Mesmin, and that the droppings of these birds produced fungi with an obscene shape and terrible stench.

Traditional Uses

Stinkhorn (*P. impudicus*) has been used worldwide, in powder or ointment form, to treat sore limbs, gout, and rheumatism. In European folk medicine, it has long been used to treat cancer, gout, and epilepsy.

In Germany, where it is known as *stinkmorchel,* village women would collect both mature fungi and the "eggs." The mature specimens were mashed in a mortar and applied to the big toe to relieve gout. The sliced "eggs" were fried and made part of the patient's diet along with cherries, which themselves help remove excessive uric acid from the body.

In central India, where it is known as *jhirri*

pihiri, the fruit bodies are crushed, suspended in water, and given to those suffering typhoid. One teaspoon of the water three times per day for four days is the standard treatment. It is also given to relieve labor pains.

Porcher mentions a tincture to relieve spasms and pain associated with renal colic.

Dr. W. C. Radley, a British physician, recommended a tincture to possess "great remedial power to ally pain in the lumbar region."

According to Helene Schalkwijk-Barendsen, this mushroom was brewed into an aphrodisiac potion. In parts of Europe and in New Guinea, it is given to cattle to encourage reproduction.

Hadrian Junius, in his sixteenth-century *Phalli: A Description with Pictures from Life of the Fungi Growing Occasionally in the Sand of Holland,* wrote "[It] is very effective for intense and unbearable pains in the joints, above all those caused by the passions and limitless debaucheries that exceed the limits of license."

The related netted or veiled stinkhorn (*D. duplicata*) is used in China for treating dysentery.

In traditional Chinese medicine, stinkhorn is used to cure rheumatism.

Dictyophora produces a strong odor to attract insects. *Dictyophora* is included with *Phallus* by some stinkhorn specialists, but has a net-like veil called an indusium hanging from its head. One species, growing on the hot, rocky lava flows of Hawaii, lives for between thirty minutes and four hours. It needs a pungent odor to attract insects in this short time. It is known in Hawaiian as *mamalu o wahine* or "woman's mushroom." This species produces a compound that is identical to or very closely mimics a compound produced in female humans during sexual arousal.

This compound, not yet named, is emitted in increasing amounts during arousal, ultimately triggering orgasm. This fungus species produces a compound millions of times stronger than a woman naturally produces in her body, and when a woman smells this odor, a spontaneous, intense orgasm frequently occurs. More research is presently being carried out, as the market potential is huge.

Ben Sostrin (2002) relates a story of one trial by John Holliday:

> Of twenty males who took part, all found the smell repulsive and declined any further testing. No physiological responses were noted in any of the male test subjects. Women, however, found the smell pleasant. In a controlled clinical trial involving sixteen women, six had orgasms while smelling the fruiting body of the fungus. The other ten [who received smaller doses] experienced physiological changes, most notably increased heart rates.

Medicinal Use
Chemical Constituents
- *P. impudicus*: **sterols (Pl-2 glucomannan) and phenol carbolic acids.**

Early in 1930, it was reported in Germany that the fermentation product of stinkhorn, after being detoxified by ultra-violet irradiation, and the addition of a certain amount of metallic salts, tended to improve the subjective symptoms of cancer in patients.

It has been found to enhance the immune system, and possesses both anti-inflammatory and anti-stress activity. It also shows antitumor activity, especially with regards to cancers of the female reproductive system.

Researchers in Latvia, where the fungus is used for gastric ulcers, asthma, rheumatism, and gout, studied the use of an ointment composed of 25 percent fresh stinkhorn as a treatment for malignant tumors. This ointment showed good application in benign ovarian cysts, uterine fibroids, and cancers of the breast, uterus, and ovaries.

More recent Latvian research at the Medical Academy looked at a fermented succus of stinkhorn. A glucomannan fraction called PI-2, as well as sterols and phenol carbolic acids, were identified.

In animal studies, the succus stimulated T-cells and enhanced NK cell activity. It also showed adaptogenic activity and reduction of stress, as well as antitumor effect against sarcoma 180 and Ehrlich ascites carcinoma of 82 percent and 68 percent respectively.

The juice was found to prolong the lives of mice with cancer. At a juice concentration of 25 percent, life was prolonged by 20 percent; at a concentration of 50 percent, life was extended by 60 percent beyond expectations; and when given at 100 percent concentration, the mice lived twice as long as expected.

In one experiment, the juice was given orally to virgin mice at 0.2 milliliters (ten milliliters per kilogram), and inhibition of adenocarcinoma was 100 percent. In another mouse study, tumors were prevented in 90 percent of animals given the same dose.

The mushroom reduced toxicity of 5-FU, a chemotherapy drug that destroys red blood cells. When given the drug, it took the control mice nine to eleven days for their red blood cells to return to normal levels. The fungal broth reduced this to just three to four days.

Dr. Sergej Kuznecova (2007) of the Latvian Medical Academy presented his results at the Eighteenth International Congress of Chemotherapy in July 1993. Human studies into its usefulness for sarcoma, and carcinoma of the stomach and breast, are ongoing.

Antitumor activity from an extract of the fruiting body in the form of a small particle spray includes prevention of thromboembolic side effects in cancer patients, as well as the reduction of metastases in Lewis lung carcinoma. This was presented as an abstract at the Seventeenth International Congress of Allergology and Clinical Immunology in Sydney in 2000.

Antitumor activity has been connected to strong inhibition of I_kB-alpha by PI-2-glucomannans.

Stinkhorn contains a human blood type O-specific hemagglutinate. A bottled product, Zemesauki, is produced in Latvia.

Dog stinkhorn (*M. caninus*) has been found to be active against gram-positive bacteria.

Devil's dipstick (*M. elegans*) is often mistaken for dog stinkhorn and can be found growing in the same habitats.

One study found it to be active against five bacterium and one fungus tested: *Bacillus cereus, B. subtilis, Staphylococcus aureus, E. coli, Salmonella typhimurium,* and *Candida albicans.*

Dictyoquinazols, isolated from methanol extracts of the related tropical basket stinkhorn or *D. indusiata (Phallus indusiata),* protected mouse cortical neurons from glutamate- and NMDA-induced excitotoxins (Lee, I.-K. et al. 2002). This sub-tropical species has been creeping north and is occasionally found in temperate zones of the United States.

It shows inhibition of sarcoma 180 and Ehrlich carcinoma of 60 percent and 70 percent respectively (Ohtsuka et al. 1973).

Homeopathy

A homeopathic preparation of *Phallus impudicus* is recommended to help prevent blindness and eye disease. It is suggested in vision problems such as colors and shapes in front of the eyes, or when objects appear gray.

Dosage: 6C, both internally and in eye drop form. The original proving was by Kalieniczensko in 1865. He took five or six spoonfuls of an infusion over the course of twenty-four hours.

Fungi Essence

Stinkhorn (*Phallus impudicus*) essence is for those who have strong feminine energy but are unable to access any masculine qualities.

— BRYNAHERB

Recipes and Dosage

In traditional Chinese medicine, the fresh, fruiting stinkhorn is soaked in a ratio of one part mushroom to two parts of a 25 percent alcohol solution for ten days, pressed, and then used. Take twenty to forty drops daily. Alternatively, take nine to fifteen grams of powder three times per day.

Other Uses

The decocted juice of stinkhorn has been used as a short-term preservative.

In parts of France and Germany, stinkhorn is used by veterinarians to treat cattle disease.

Bits and Pieces

Most fungi that produce light, such as the honey mushroom and various *Mycena,* produce light waves that do not penetrate cardboard and other opaque material. The stinkhorn, however, produces radiation that, although non-luminous, will penetrate through a cardboard box and activate a photographic plate inside. This "radiation" may help attract potential sporulators in some unknown manner.

Phanerochaete velutina

(VELVET CRUST)
P. chrysosporium
(YELLOW CRUST)
P. gigantea
Phlebia gigantea
Phlebiopsis gigantea
(GIANT CRUST)
(GIANT YELLOW CRUST)

Velvet crust *(Phanerochaete velutina)* is found in the Pacific Northwest.

Giant yellow crust is widely found throughout North America.

Medicinal Use

A yellow crust strain, CJ-12,954, exhibits potent activity against *Helicobacter pylori* associated with duodenal and stomach ulcers.

Mycoremediation

Velvet crust *(Phanerochaete velutina)* can decolorize azo dyes up to 100 percent by breaking them down into quinone and a phenyl dizine that is then broken down into nitrogen and a phenol compound.

The related yellow crust *(P. chrysosporium)* has been found to be effective in myco-degrading chemicals such as benzopyrenes, pentachlorophenols, and TNT, as well as synthetic dyes such as triphenylmethane, heterocyclics, azo and diazo dyes.

Only white rot fungi have shown the ability to break down TNT and mineralize it to carbon dioxide. Yellow crust, in field studies, is inhibited by high TNT levels, so a two-step process may be necessary to enhance breakdown.

Sublette et al. found that using a rotating biological contactor, water contaminated with TNT at 120 to 175 milligrams per liter, and cyclotrimethylene-trinitroamine at twenty-five milligrams per liter, remediated with more than 99 percent efficiency (Sublette, K. et al. 1992).

2,4-dinitrotoluene, a compound used for explosives and polyurethane production, also degrades in a multi-step process.

Arochlor, a polychlorinated biphenyl, has been found to break down when exposed to *P. chrysosporium* and *Trametes versicolor* (Novotny 1997).

Delor 106, a commercial PCB mixture, was degraded by 25 percent in only three weeks. Turkey tail, in this trial, was twice as effective, with 50 percent degradation in the same time period.

PCP (phencyclidine) is detoxified by *Phanerochaete* species via dechlorination. Field trials suggest that yellow crust and *P. sordida* degrade PCP, in a mixture of creosote, rapidly and extensively, with a mycoconversion rate of 80 percent within six weeks.

DDT (dichlorodiphenyltrichloroethane), aldrin, dieldrin, lindane, and heptachlor have all shown degradation by yellow crust in labs, but in field studies only lindane showed significant breakdown.

These degradations involve fungal peroxidases in several extra and intracellular processes (Hammel and Tardone 1988).

Chlorobenzenes, xylenes, toluenes, and ethylbenzenes are also degraded by *P. chrysosporium* (Yadav and Redy 1993a).

Endosulfan usually shows slow degradation rates, and the primary metabolites are as toxic as the substance itself, but yellow crust breaks it down to less toxic metabolites quite quickly.

Herbicides based on 2,4-dicholorphenoxyacetic acid and 2,4,5-trichlorophenoxyacetic acid; insecticides such as chlordane, heptachlor, lindane, dieldrin, and mirex all are degraded by yellow crust (Kennedy et al. 1990; Ryan and Bumpus 1989; Yadav and Reddy 1993a, 1993b).

DDT (dichlorodiphenyltrichloroethane) has been studied in greater detail and was one of the first compounds demonstrated to be degraded by these fungi (Bumpus and Aust 1987; Bumpus and Tatarko 1994; Bumpus et al. 1985).

It is one of the most persistent insecticides in the environment and because it is lipophilic, it readily accumulates in the food chain. Early work by Bumpus and Aust (1987) found 50 percent degradation in thirty days, but degradation was incomplete and the work was abandoned.

Phellinus igniarius

Fomes igniarius
(FALSE TINDER POLYPORE)
(BRACKET OR SHELF FUNGUS)

Phellinus means "cork." *Igniarius* is from the Latin *ignotus,* meaning "ignition" or "fire."

False tinder polypore is commonly found on willow, birch, and alder throughout the northern woods, and, rarely, on poplar.

The fruiting bodies are hoof-shaped and up to twenty centimeters (about eight inches) wide. Its presence is usually indicative of considerable internal decay of the tree.

Recent work by Robert Blanchette (2001) appears to confirm the true identity of the fungus.

Traditional Uses

Various Arctic tribes boiled the polypore and drank the decoction as a laxative or for stomachache.

Medicinal Use

Chemical Constituents

- **Naringenin, cyclophellitol, sakuranetin, aromadendrin, folerogenin, eriodictyol, coumarin, scopoletin, phelligridins, phelligridimers, igniarius A-D, hispolon, 4-hydroxybenzaldehyde, protocatechualdehyde, syringic acid, protocatechuic acid, caffeic acid, isoergosterone, octadecyl ferulate.**

Studies have shown the polypore to possess good tumor inhibition. It has been used as an emmenagogue for treating uterine bleeding, to

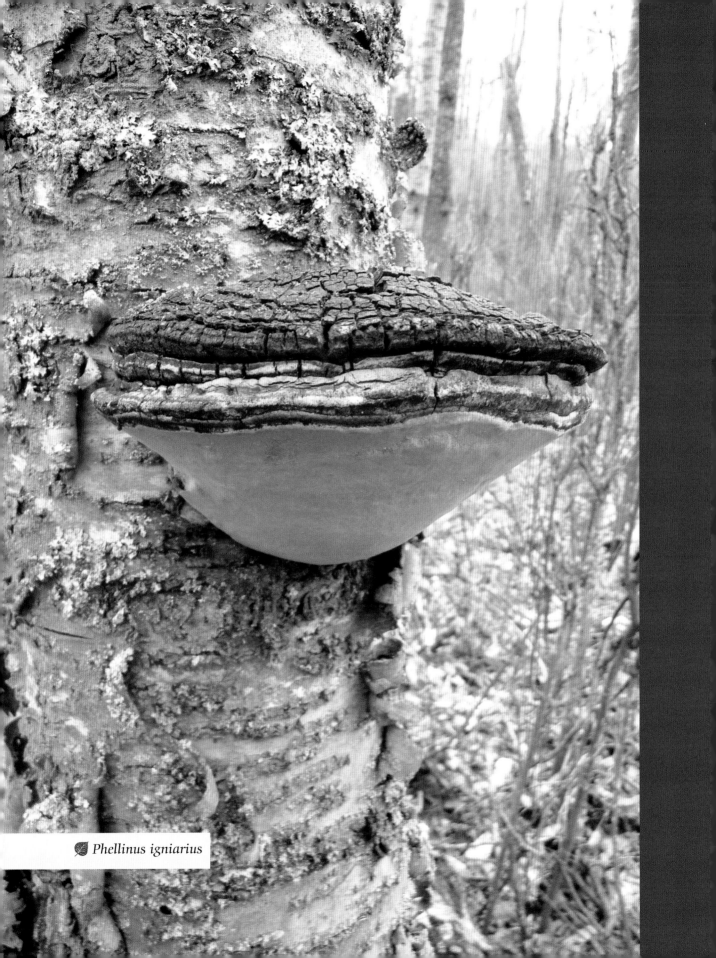

Phellinus igniarius

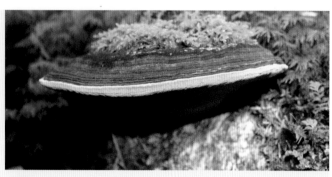

Phellinus igniarius

invigorate blood circulation, to resolve masses of the abdomen, and to stop diarrhea.

It exerts a subtle influence on those addicted to alcohol by normalizing stomach function and strengthening the spleen.

Withers and Umezawa (1991) found that cyclophellitol, a natural product isolated from *Phellinus* species, is a highly specific and effective irreversible inactivator of beta-glucosidases. This unique finding was explored in great depth by Atsumi et al. (1990) who found that as a specific inhibitor of beta-glucosidase, it does not inhibit experimental metastasis. Its structural analogue, 1,6-epi-cyclophellitol, however, inhibited alpha- and beta-glucosidase, as well as metastasis.

Early work by Ohtsuka et al. (1973) found the fungi possessed antitumor activity, but did not identify the specific route of action.

The inhibition rate against sarcoma 180 is 87 percent, and against Ehrlich carcinoma 80 percent.

Jeong et al. shared results of a trial that showed large polysaccharide molecules derived by methanol reduced CCL4-induced toxicity in rats (Jeong, W. et al. 2002).

A study in China has confirmed anti-tumor and immune regulation by this polypore.

Several compounds in *P. igniarius* have been identified that are active against human lung cancer cell lines (A549) and liver cancer cell lines (Bel 7402).

Ying Wang et al. (2005) identified phelligridimer A, a compound that exhibits antioxidant activity.

Polysaccharides from submerged culture show significant antioxidant activity (Lung and Tsai 2009).

Phelligrindin J has been isolated and found to be cytotoxic to various human cancer cell lines (Wang, Ying et al. 2007). The same researchers identified the lanostanes igniarius A-D that possess iNOS-inhibition with an IC_{50} of 37.57.

Shon and Nam (2002) found polysaccharides from *P. igniarius* inhibited the number of TPA-induced skin tumors by 69.7 percent and the number of mice with tumors by 70 percent.

Ethyl acetate extracts show activity against human ovarian cancer cell lines (Rouhana-Toubi et al. 2009).

A site of interest is www.phellinus-research.com. A number of studies involving *P. igniarius* and *P. linteus* are listed, although many of these have never been published in medical journals.

One study found the triterpenoid extracts and ethanol extracts of *P. igniarius* active against prostate adenocarcinoma, stomach ascites SNU638 and antioxidant in nature. Vitamin C improved this potential, and there was no sign of toxicity on normal and fibroblast cell lines.

Yan Yang et al. (2009) found a hetero-polysaccharide that stimulates proliferation of mouse spleen lymphocytes.

R. P. Collins and A. F. Halim (1972) reported an analysis of the odorous constituents produced by the various *Phellinus* species, for those interested. Methyl benzoate was prominent followed by methyl salicylate and benzyl alcohol.

Mycoremediation

Kruger and Pfeil (1976) showed that a peroxidase from *P. igniarius* is an enzyme that can resist extreme conditions (pH, temperature, and salt concentration).

Dombrovska et al. (1998) showed that *Phellinus igniarius* degrades and utilizes cellulose and lignins from oil-bearing crops very efficiently (40 percent cellulose and 24 percent lignins in nineteen weeks).

Recipes and Dosage

Decoct sixteen to thirty grams with water, and take one dose of three to six milliliters two times a day.

To make a tincture, place one ounce of *Phellinus* that has been cut into small pieces in two liters of water and set over high heat. When it comes to a boil, reduce heat, and simmer until liquid is reduced by half. Pour off and reserve liquid. Add another liter of water, return to a boil, reduce heat, and again simmer until liquid is reduced by half. Combine the two liquids and refrigerate.

Place the mushroom pieces into five hundred milliliters of vodka and let sit for one week, shaking daily. Some people reverse the process to avoid spoilage, by using alcohol extraction first and then boiling the marc.

The mycelium is best extracted at seventy degrees Celsius (158 degrees Fahrenheit) for ninety minutes in a ratio of one part mycelium to 6.2 parts water.

Bits and Pieces

Various native tribes from North America use the bracket fungus ash as an addition to smoking or chewing tobacco. It is said to give a powerful kick. Previously, before tobacco was readily available, a chewing mixture was made by combining the fungus ash with the inner bark of cottonwood.

The Yup'ik of western Alaska call the fungus ash *araq,* and they call a mixture of tobacco and ash *iqmik,* meaning "thing to put in the mouth."

It is estimated that more than 52 percent of First Nations adults in the Yukon and Alaska smoke this mixture, even during pregnancy.

Beautiful carved wooden boxes, with ivory and bone ornamentation, were traditionally used to hold the fungal ash.

Edward Nelson wrote in 1899 that "when the tobacco has been cut sufficiently fine it is mixed with ashes obtained from the tree fungus and kneaded and rolled into rounded pellets or quids, often being chewed a little by women to incorporate the ashes more thoroughly. . . . the men do not usually chew the quids, but hold them in the cheek, and rarely expectorate the juice."

Araq is made by placing air-dried fungi in large open coffee cans and placing them over a fire. The ash is then mixed with tobacco and stored for use. The high alkaline mineral content makes nicotine delivery to the brain rapid and powerful.

The Blackfoot used the ash and tobacco in a similar manner, suggesting that tobacco trade moved north, and Phellinus ash was traded south. Today, an eight-ounce bottle of ash sells for about $40.

Phellinus tremulae

Fomes igniarius f. tremulae
F. igniarius var. populinus
(ASPEN CONK)
(FALSE TINDER CONK)
(POPLAR FALSE TINDER FUNGUS)
P. piceinus
P. pini var. abetis
P. chrysoloma
Porodaedalea piceina
Fomes pini
(PINE CONK)
(SPRUCE POLYPORE)
P. conchatus
Porodaedalea conchata
(SCALLOP POLYPORE)
P. robustus
P. hartigii
Fomitiporia hartigii
Fomes robustus
F. hartigii
(ROBUST CONK)
P. ferruginosa
Poria ferruginosa
Fuscoporia ferruginosa
(POLYPORE FERRUGINEUX)
P. gilvus
F. gilva
(OAK CONK)

(CHAMOIS POLYPORE)
Phellinus linteus

Phellinus means "little phallus," which some of these mushrooms resemble, or "cork." Mors Kochanski, a gifted survival expert and personal friend, prefers the former, as it usually elicits a few guffaws on his field trips. Tremulae refers to its relationship with trembling or aspen poplar.

Aspen conk is a common, hoof-shaped perennial parasite on older poplar trees, living and dead. In some texts, P. tremulae and P. igniarius are considered synonyms. In other books, they are treated as separate species. They look similar to me, and the wide variation of shape and size is considerable. They are difficult to tell apart from one another when they are not attached to their host trees. The setae of P. igniarius are smaller, their conks more hoof-shaped, and their pore surface is also at right angles to the trunk.

The conks are inedible.

Phellinus robustus grows into a bright yellow-brown conk on hardwoods of the Rocky Mountains. In the past P. hartigii was named P. robustus, Fomitiporia hartigii, or Fomes robusta. This name is now restricted to hardwoods. Confused yet? I am.

The related P. torulosus, which grows on conifers in Arizona, looks similar to oak conk but has yellow-brown pores.

Traditional Uses

Aborigines in Australia inhale the smoke of burning Phellinus species for sore throat. The scrapings from mildly charred fruiting bodies

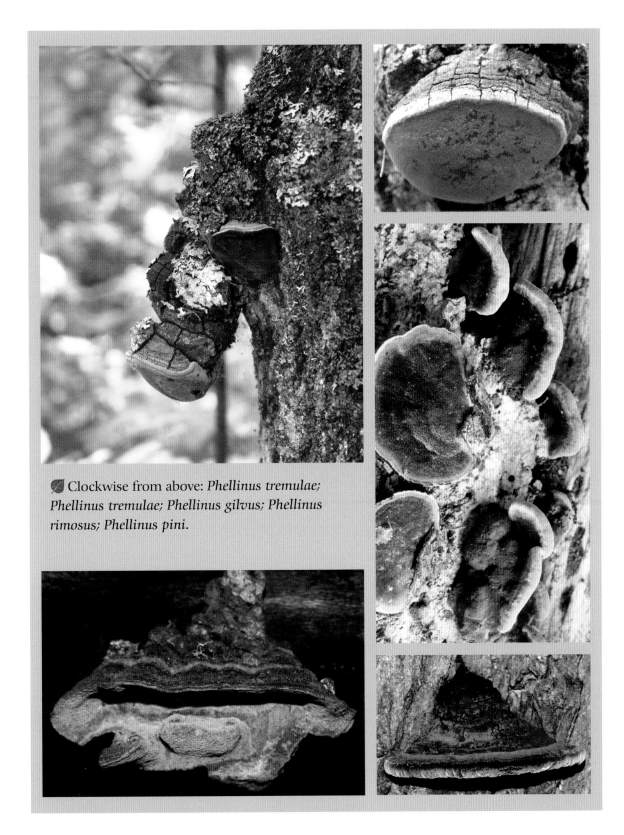

🍃Clockwise from above: *Phellinus tremulae;*
Phellinus tremulae; Phellinus gilvus; Phellinus
rimosus; Phellinus pini.

are taken with water for sore throat, coughs, fevers, diarrhea, and lung problems.

The conk tea is cooling in nature, detoxifying and restoring to the internal organs.

It is a soothing diuretic and a tonic to the digestive system. It will help relieve diarrhea, and it can be sliced into thin pieces, then pounded and softened to create effective external styptic.

The related *P. pomaceus* has been used as a poultice for facial swelling. The hard conk is grated and then heated in the oven before application.

The related *P. gilvus,* or oak conk, is used in traditional Chinese medicine to nourish the spleen, dispel damp, and invigorate stomach function.

P. torulosus is used in traditional Chinese medicine for regulating the flow of vital energy, relieving internal heat, and treating anemia.

The conk is used in China to activate blood circulation, nourish vital organs, resolve indigestion, and relieve hot, inflamed tissue.

Medicinal Use

Serck-Hanssen and Wikstrom (1978) isolated novel fungitoxic products from the Aspen conk. The most common fungitoxin is 7-phenyl heptan-3-one.

Recent clinical trials showed an 87 percent inhibition of tumor growth in test mice, and a recovery rate of 66.7 percent at a dosage of thirty milligrams per day.

E. I. Hwang et al. (2000) isolated phellinsin A, a novel chitin synthase inhibitor from *Phellinus* species broth. The compound shows wide antifungal activity.

In Japan, the mushroom *P. linteus* is called song gen or meshimakobu and in China, mesima or meshima. Mesima is named after the "female island" of the Danjo Islands west of Nagasaki. The fungus has been developed as a medicinal in Korea, where it is known as keumsa sang hwang. Fermentation technology has been developed in Korea, and an analogous poly-saccharide biotechnology from this species has been obtained in Japan (Mizuno, T. 2000). T. Y. Kang et al. (1999) found water extracts protective effects on BNL cl.2 cells, indicating a liver cell sparing mechanism.

C. H. Song et al. (1998) found this mushroom stimulated immune activity by 71 percent, compared to shiitake at 85 percent and *Flammulina velutipes* at 77 percent. This is very impressive company for such a common polypore.

Recent work in South Korea looked at *P. linteus* and adriamycin, a popular chemotherapy agent, and its ability to inhibit tumors. In mice that took only the polypore extract, tumor growth was inhibited and metastases reduced. They had the highest survival rate. In those taking the drug only, tumor growth was significantly inhibited, but metastasis was only slightly inhibited. The combination was effective at inhibiting tumor growth but not metastasis, as the fungus does not directly kill cancer cells. It may, however, prove to be a useful adjunct in chemotherapy and other treatments (Kim, H. W. et al. 1996).

A combination of this mushroom and doxorubicin at low doses resulted in a synergistic effect and brought about the death of prostate cancer cells. It was not only as effective as higher doses of the drug alone, but it also prevented harm to healthy cells (Collins, L. et al. 2006).

Other work indicates increased activity of T-lymphocytes and cytotoxic T-cells, increased activity of natural killer cells and macrophages, and stimulation of B-cells.

In 1995, Korean researchers used hot-water extracts from *P. linteus* to stimulate polyclonal antibody production in vitro. It was shown to be a B-lymphocyte-stimulating polysaccharide. Follow-up research by the same group in 1996 showed large amounts of the amino acids serine and threonine in the extracts.

Shon and Nam (2004) found that polysaccharides fermented from the conk inhibit cytochrome P450 isozymes.

Phellisin A, derived from *Phellinus sp. PL3,* has been shown both to be antioxidant and to inhibit xanthine oxidase with an IC50 value lower than allopurinol, often used for gout (Hwang, E. I. et al. 2006).

Yasuhiro Shibata et al. (2005) found extracts enlarged the prostate, suggesting males with BPH (benign prostatic hypertrophy) use the fungus with caution.

The related *P. rimosus* possesses antioxidant, antitumor, and anti-hepatotoxic activity (Ajith and Janardhanan 2002, 2003). The extract was comparable in effect to cisplatin in ascites and solid tumor models.

Lakshmi et al. (2004) found extracts of *P. rimosus* possess higher antioxidant activity than reishi and various oyster mushrooms. Sheena et al. (2003) found methanol extracts active against *E. coli, Pseudomonas aeuroginosa, Staphylococcus aureus, Salmonella typhimurium,* and *Bacillus subtilis* at levels lower than reishi.

Recent work by Meena et al. (2009) suggests it could be useful for inflammation and conditions such as rheumatoid arthritis.

Mycelium from the related *P. baumii* has been found to possess antidiabetic activity, with blood sugar levels reduced by 52 percent compared to a control group (Hwang, H.-J. et al. 2005). Dai, Y. C. (2003) compared the East Asian *Phellinus linteus* with the holotype and other specimens from Central and South America, and concluded that America, the species are actually *Phellinus baumii.*

Phellinus robustus has been found to have significant manganese peroxidase activity (Songulashvili et al. 2007).

Other work found significant antioxidant activity.

Pereverzev et al. (1993) found the fungi to possess adaptogenic activity, including anti-stress and cytoprotective ability.

The inhibition rate of the water and methanol extracts of the fruiting body against sarcoma 180 is from 68 to 100 percent and against Ehrlich carcinoma up to 90 percent.

The related *P. gilvus,* or oak conk, inhibits sarcoma 180 up to 90 percent and Ehrlich carcinoma to 60 percent. A Korean study found activity against both sarcoma 180 and P388 cancer cell lines.

Found commonly in the Pacific Northwest and elsewhere, this species was found more stimulating than either *P. linteus or P. baumii* (Chang, Z. Q. et al. 2008). Sun drying of the mushroom appears to produce the best product for fighting sarcoma 180 cancer cell lines (Jo et al. 2009). Moderate vasorelaxing effect has been observed (Hosoe 2006).

Phellinus pini contains two interesting ceramides. Inhibition rates of 100 percent have been found against both sarcoma 180 and Ehrlich carcinoma cell lines.

Robbins et al. (1945) found activity against *Staphylococcus aureus* in this species and the related *P. ferruginosa, P. ferreus,* and *P. ribis.*

The related scallop polypore or *P. conchatus,* also known as *Porodaedalea conchata,* shows cytotoxic activity against cervical cancer and hepatoma cell lines (Ren, G. et al. 2006).

The related *P. officinalis,* also known as *Polyporus occidentalis* and *Coriolopsis occidentalis,* has been found to inhibit sarcoma 180 and adenoma 755 in mice studies.

A mini-review of twenty-six *Phellinus* species as medicinal mushrooms has been recently published (Dai 2010).

Food Industry

Various *Phellinus* genus members have been used industrially for helping fermentation of flavor substances, such as methyl salicylate, which is naturally common to birch bark after distillation, but usually found as a synthesized chemical.

Recipe and Dosage

Sixteen to thirty grams as a decoction twice a day.

Phlebia tremellosa

Merulius tremellosus
(TREMBLING PHLEBIA)
(TREMBLING MERULIUS)
(JELLY ROT)

P. radiata
P. merismoides
(ORANGE WAX FUNGUS)

Trembling *Phlebia* is common and widespread on dead wood. The fruiting bodies are light orange buff to pinkish and formed in soft, gelatinous shelves.

The related *Phlebia strigoso-zonata* is similar to *P. radiata* but has concentric furrows and wrinkles instead of radiating ones. The new name is *Punctularia strigoso-zonata.*

Phlebia radiata, also known as *P. merismoides,* is found on fallen conifers and hardwoods. It looks like regurgitated dog food, according to Arora, and ranges from light tan to orange to pink in color.

Traditional Uses

It is used in China to treat dysentery. It is cooked and the soup is then eaten, the mushrooms are eaten separately, or pancakes are prepared from the soup with flour. Nothing is wasted.

Medicinal Use

The inhibition rate against sarcoma 180 is 90 percent and that of Ehrlich carcinoma 80 percent.

Punctularia strigoso-zonata was found by Robbins et al. (1945) to possess moderate activity against *Staphylococcus aureus.*

The related *Punctularia atropurpurascens* contains an antifungal and cytotoxic aldehyde called phlebiakauranol (Anke, T. et al. 1987).

Mycoremediation

Phlebia, Bjerkandera, Trametes, and *Hericium* species produce significant amounts of chlorinated compounds, but are also highly effective in metabolizing or myco-transforming chlorinated pollutants (De Jong and Field 1997).

Trembling *Phlebia* shows great promise in decolorization of textile effluent and well as transformation of alachlor (Ferrey et al. 1994).

Van Aken et al. (1997, 1999) found the annual resupinate to degrade trinitrotoluene and isolated MnP mineralized dinitrotoluene compounds. It degraded DHP in soil with a mineralization rate of 23 percent, while *Trametes hirsuta* mineralized 30 percent in a straw medium without soil (Tuomela et al. 2002).

In pulp bleaching wastewater and pulp mill wastewater, the fungus secretes lignin peroxidase, manganese peroxidase, and laccase. Consumption of glucose and growth of *P. radiata* increases with additional amounts of pulp mill wastewater in the culture medium.

Pholiota

Pholiota aurivella
(GOLDEN SKINNED PHOLIOTA)
P. flammans
(FLAMING PHOLIOTA)
(FLAMBOYANT PHOLIOTA)
P. aurea
Phaeolepiota aurea
Togaria aurea
(ALASKAN GOLD)
P. mutabilis
Kuehneromyces mutabilis
Galerina mutabilis

(CHANGEABLE PHOLIOTA)
(TWO TONED PHOLIOTA)
P. lubrica
(LUBRICOUS PHOLIOTA)
P. alnicola
Flammula alnicola
(ALDER TUFT)
P. spumosa
P. graveolens
F. spumosa
Dryophila spumosa
Gymnopilus spumosus
(SLENDER PHOLIOTA)
(FROTHY PHOLIOTA)
P. adiposa
(FAT PHOLIOTA)
P. squarrosa
(SCALY PHOLIOTA)
(SHAGGY PHOLIOTA)
P. squarrosoides
(SHARP SCALY PHOLIOTA)
P. destruens
P. populina
(POPLAR PHOLIOTA)
P. caperata (see *Rozites caperata*)
P. aegerita (see *Agrocybe aegerita*)

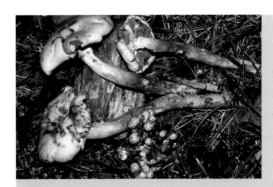
🍃 *Pholiota alnicola*

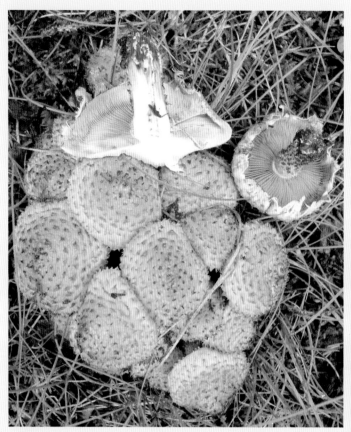

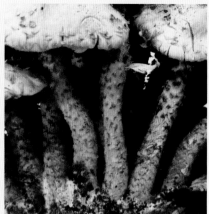

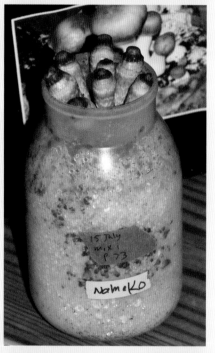

🍂 Clockwise from above: *Pholiota squarrosa;*
Pholiota squarrosa; Pholiota nameko; Pholiota
squarrosa; Pholiota nameko.

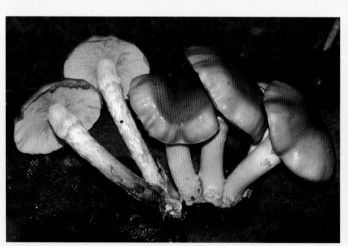

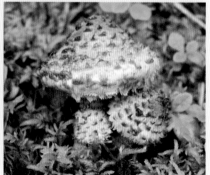

Pholiota is from the Greek meaning "with scaly cap." *Aurivella* is Latin meaning "with golden skin." *Flammans* means "flaming" in Latin. *Aurea* means "golden," *Mutabilis* means "mutable" or "changeable," and *Lucrica* means "lubricated." *Squarrosa* means "scaly" or "scurfy" and *alnicola* means "alder-growing," although it is associated with various hardwoods. *Adiposa* is from *adeps* meaning "fat."

Golden skinned *Pholiota* is found higher in trees, often in the frost cracks of birch. It is said to be edible, but this author has no culinary experience. David Arora does not recommend it, as not only is it slimy, but it sometimes causes digestive upsets. I will pass.

Flaming *Pholiota* is bright yellow with a most unpleasant odor and is considered edible.

Alaskan gold, or golden false pholiota, is a good-sized golden-brown to orange-brown mushroom. It grows in groups or large clumps, usually near alder but not restricted to this tree. It is edible to some but poisonous to others, so avoid serving it at a large dinner party.

Changeable *Pholiota* is common to the mountains of Pacific Northwest and widely distributed elsewhere. The mushroom can be easily cultivated, like the oyster, on pieces of inoculated wood. It is edible, but can be confused with the poisonous *Galerina autumnalis,* a genus to which it was previously classified.

Where found, it will sometimes cover the entire tree stump or log. An alternate name, brown stew mushroom, suggests its suitability in soups and sauces, adding a fruity odor and flavor.

Destructive *Pholiota (P. destruens* or *P. popul-nea)* is common on balsam and cottonwood poplar throughout North America. It has a scaly, white cap and brown spores and is edible, but not really recommended.

The related scaly *Pholiota (P. squarrosa)* has a yellow-brown scaly cap and a ring on the stalk. It is usually found in clusters at the base of live poplar in mid-summer. It has a strong garlic-radish odor and is considered poisonous, or at least appears to cause stomach upset in some diners. Proceed with caution. Pieter Van Der Schoot, a fellow director of the Alberta Mycological Society, says it is a good edible, but I'm not totally convinced. Several books allude to difficult digestion.

The look-alike *P. squarrosoides* is edible and has a mild taste and odor. I avoid both.

Alder tuft, a rusty brown-spored *Pholiota* that is found on decayed alder and sometimes on willow or birch, has shiny, yellow flesh when cut.

Slender *Pholiota* is widely distributed under pine and other conifers. It has a distinct corn or corn silk odor.

Fat *Pholiota (P. adiposa)* is a mediocre edible living on living and dead birch trees. In Japan, it is known as *numerisugitake.*

The Japanese *P. nameko* can be cultivated on sawdust or logs of poplar, oak and other hardwood species. It requires constant moisture, so burying logs works better than stacking. Also known as *P. glutinosa,* nameko is a superior gourmet mushroom. It does have a slimy cap, like other *Pholiota,* that disappears upon cooking. It may grow well in parts of North America.

Medicinal Use

Chemical Constituents

- *P. adiposa:* **15-hydroxy-6alpha, 12-epoxy-7beta, 10alpha H, 11betaH-spiroax-4-ene, 1-linoleic-2-olein, stigmasterol, and 1-(N,N,N-trimethylethylaminophosporyll)-2,3-dilinoleinion.**

- *P. spumosa:* **putrescine-1,4-dicinnamamide, maytenine and pholiotic acid, and fasciculol.**

- *P. squarrosa:* **epicoccamide D.**

Inhibition tests with sarcoma 180 indicate flaming *Pholiota* is 90 percent effective, while Ehrlich carcinoma was inhibited by 100 percent (Ohtsuka et al. 1973).

The inhibition rate of *P. aurea* against sarcoma 180 and Ehrlich carcinoma is up to 100 percent.

Changeable *Pholiota* shows activity against gram-positive bacteria. Mycelium extracts show activity against influenza viruses type A and B (Mentel et al. 1994).

Kuehneromyces species contain the active compound kuehneromycine B, which shows activity reducing blood platelet binding.

Fat *Pholiota (P. adiposa)* contains a number of interesting compounds.

Extracts have been found to decrease retroperitoneal fat in mice fed high-fat diets (Cho, S. M. et al. 2006).

H. E. Yu et al. (2007) found methanol extracts of the fruiting body inhibit HMG-CoA reductase, an enzyme related to cholesterol synthesis, by nearly 56 percent. The purified product is stigmasterol, common to many plants and fungi.

Work in China, where it is cultivated, shows that the sticky substance on the mushroom's surface contains polysacharose A. This has shown an inhibition rate against sarcoma 180 of 80 percent and Ehrlich carcinoma of 90 percent.

Earlier work by Ohtsuka et al. (1973) found extracts of the fruiting body inhibited the above cancer cells by 70 percent and 60 percent respectively.

Two compounds with weak cytotoxicity against murine leukemia cells have been identified: 1-linoleic-2-olein and stigmasterol (Chung et al. 2005).

Yongxun Zhao et al. (2007) identified mycelium polysaccharides with antitumor activity, due to immune function.

It may prevent infection from *Staphylococcus, Pneumonia bacillus,* and *Tuberculinum mycobacterium.* Dulger et al. (2002b) found 60 percent methanol extracts possess significant antimicrobial activity against *Bacillus subtilis, E. coli, S. aureus, Streptococcus pyogenes,* and *Mycobacterium smegmatis.*

The fungi inhibit angiotensin converting enzyme (Izawa et al. 2006). A novel pentapeptide was found, particularly powerful with an IC50 of 0.044 milligrams (Koo et al. 2006).

Guoqing Zhang et al. (2009) reported a lectin with anti-proliferative activity against HepG2 and breast cancer cell lines, and inhibition of HIV reverse transcription, both with very low IC50s.

A novel functional or nutraceutical rice wine containing 0.1 percent fruiting bodies and 1 percent wolfberry shows an ACE-inhibition rate of 82 percent. The idea of fermented drinks, such as wine and beers, with herbal and fungal components opens a whole new arena in the promotion of health and wellness.

Various *Kuehneromyces* species contain kuehneromycine B, which reduces blood platelet binding.

Lubricous *Pholiota* has been shown, in laboratory tests, to lower blood cholesterol levels. It shows 100 percent inhibition of Ehrlich carcinoma and 90 percent inhibition of sarcoma 180.

Studies have shown that slender *Pholiota* is active against the fungus *Botrytis cinerea* (Pujol et al. 1990).

Russo et al. (2007) found the mushroom contains putrescine-1,4-dicinnamamide that inhibits human prostate cancer cell growth and induces apoptosis.

Maytenine and pholiotic acid also show similar inhibitory activity (Clericuzio et al. 2007).

Pholiotic acid is a name given earlier to an illudalane metabolite of *P. destruens* below. This will have to be changed to avoid confusing scientists.

Slender *Pholiota* contains fasciculol, a rare lanostane triterpenoid conjugated to a depsipeptide unit, and two bis-amides derived from cinnamic acid.

Putrescine-1,4-dicinnamamide is common in angiosperm plants, but not in fungi.

The fruiting body of destructive *Pholiota* contains pholiotic acid, an illudalane sesquiterpene, 35-dichoro-4-methoxy-benzaldehyde and its alcohol.

Becker et al. (1994) found the compounds to exhibit weak antifungal and cytostatic activity.

A tetramic acid, epicoccamide D, found in *P. squarrosa,* has been found to exhibit weak to moderate cytotoxicity against HeLa cell lines and human leukemia cell lines (K-562) (Wangun and Hertweck 2007).

Water and sodium hydroxide extracts are 60 percent and 90 percent effective against sarcoma 180 and Ehrlich carcinoma in mice. The fungus protects against *Staphylococcus, E. coli, Baeillus pneumoniae,* and *Mycobacterium tuberculosis* infections.

Alder tuft mycelia exhibits antioxidant activity higher than 44 percent (Badalyan 2003). This suggests further study for the development of natural antioxidant supplements. The same level of activity was found in mycelium from *Schizophyllum commune.* Turkey tail *(Trametes versicolor)* showed antioxidant activity higher than 20 percent in the same study.

The fruiting bodies showed activity against *S. aureus* and *E. coli* (Robbins et al. 1945).

Cosmetics

Kuehneromcyces has a distinctly earthy fragrance that may be of interest in perfume work.

Phyllotopsis nidulans
Claudopus nidulans
Panellus nidulans
(SMELLY OYSTER)

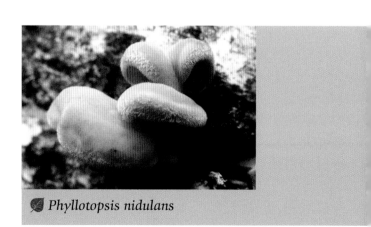
Phyllotopsis nidulans

Phyllotopsis means "looking like a gilled mushroom," and *nidulans* is from the Latin for "nesting."

This beautiful saffron orange mushroom is found on birch, but be warned, it has the smell of rotting cabbage. Eat it only if you have anosmia.

Medicinal Use

The mushroom exhibits activity against *Staphylococcus aureus*.

Piptoporus betulinus

Polyporus betulinus
Placodes betulinus
Ungulina betulina
(RAZOR STROP)
(BIRCH CONK)
(BIRCH POLYPORE)

> *Imagine you're a birch tree, with white, and*
>   *shiny bark*
> *Would you prefer that razor strop or chaga*
>   *leave its mark?*
> *The former's an eraser, gently curved and*
>   *smooth,*
> *The tinderconk a rusty scab you'd rather like*
>   *to soothe.*
> *The betulin cures cancer, and spares Betula's*
>   *life.*
> *While the softer looking razor strop cuts your*
>   *heartwood like a knife.*
>   — RDR

Commonly found growing on northern birch trees, this mushroom was used instead of a leather strip as a razor strop by poor families in Victorian times, hence its common name.

The wood decayed by the fungus, as well as mycelium cultures, have the distinct odor of green apples.

It is edible when very young and fresh and can be sliced and boiled in soups. After only a few days of room temperature storage, however, the taste of the drying polypores becomes quite sour.

Traditional Uses

This mushroom can be roasted until black and then powdered and applied to bleeding wounds as an antiseptic.

In parts of Britain, the inner layer was cut into small strips as a styptic and as corn pads for the feet.

One Australian doctor has reported great success in using this mushroom to treat ingrown toenails (Hilton 1987).

The polypore was used traditionally in Bohemia to treat stomach disease and rectal cancer.

P. betulinus was once used throughout Europe, and is still used today in Italy and Poland, to facilitate the excretion of intestinal parasites.

Oetzi, the Ice Man, who died 5,300 years ago, was discovered relatively intact a few years ago in a mountain pass carrying two walnut sized spheres of the birch conk, mounted on a decorated leather thong; can you explain what this is? (*F. fomentarius*).

"The discovery of the fungus suggests that the Ice Man was aware of his intestinal parasites (*Trichuris trichiura*) and fought them with measured doses of *Piptoporus betulinus*,"

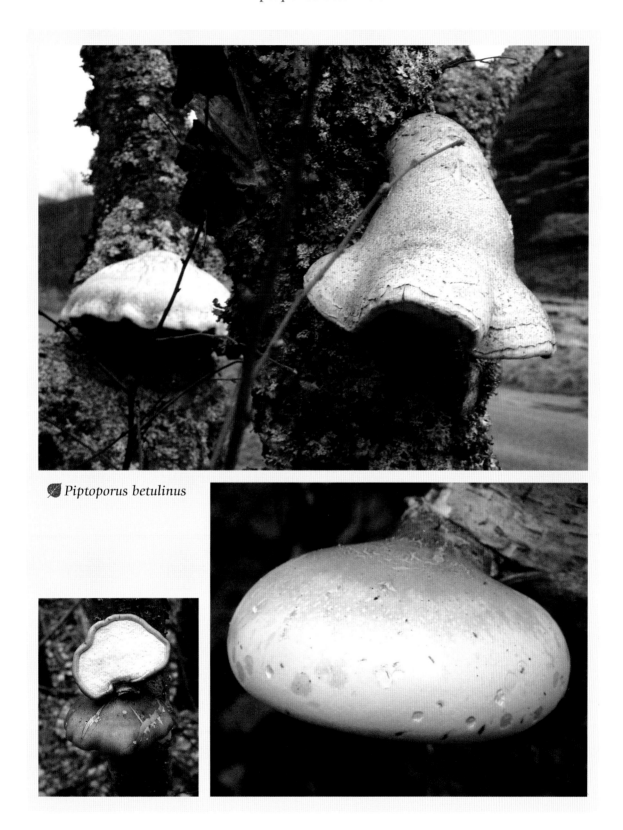

Piptoporus betulinus

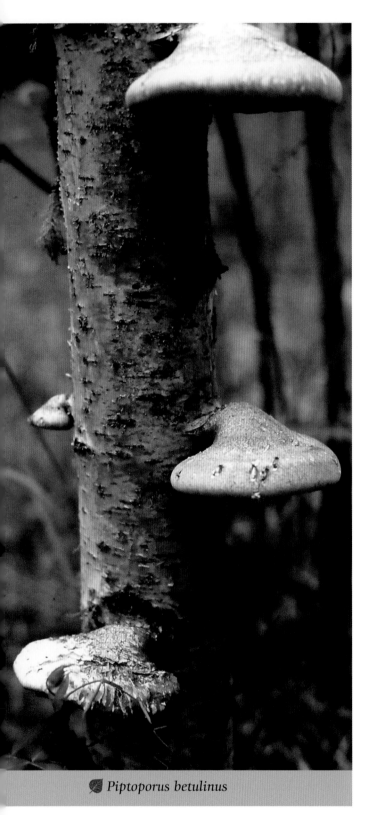

Piptoporus betulinus

wrote Dr. Capasso of Italy's National Archeological Museum, who has studied the use of the polypore *(P. betulinus)* as a powerful but short-acting laxative that contains oils that are toxic to intestinal parasites. "The toxic oils in the fungus were probably the only remedy available in Europe" until thousands of years later.

Medicinal Use

Chemical Constituents

- **Polyporenic acid A and C, 1,3-beta-D-glucopyranan, B ergosta -7,22-dien-3-ol, fungisterol, ergosterol, agaric acid, dehydrotumulosic acid, ungalinic acid, betulinic acid, and tumulosic acid. Also contains 4-methylmorpholine-N-oxide, a methyl sulfoxide soluble glucan, piptamine, and various lanostanoids.**

The birch polypore fruiting body possesses antitumor activity. RNA isolated from this fungi induced interferon production and virus protection when injected in mice (Kawecki 1978).

Polyporenic acid is a bacteriostatic triterpenoid with a wide variety of anti-inflammatory activities. In the early stage of burns on rats, it showed greater activity than cortisone. Pre-treatment of rats with polyporenic acid prevented ammonium chloride-induced inflammation of the lungs, whereas cortisone was inactive under these circumstances.

The pentacyclic triterpenes have shown anti-neoplastic effect. Studies in Poland demonstrated that an extract given orally (three grams per day) to female dogs with Sticker's tumors of the vagina, showed complete remission in five weeks (Utzig and Samborski 1957). Over a half century ago, Wandokanty and Utzig reported the effect of pentacylic triterpenes from the conk on malignant neoplasms. Little follow-up has been done.

Kawagishi et al. (2002) identified a novel hydroquinione with enzyme-inhibiting properties related to the formation of tumors.

Piptamine, a novel antibiotic, has been derived from the polypore (Schlegel et al. 2000). This specific compound shows activity against *Staphylococcus aureus* and *Enterococcus faecalis* at rates of only 0.78 micrograms per milliliter and 1.56 micrograms per milliliter respectively. Early work found activity against *S. aureus* and *E. coli* (Hervey 1947).

The conk contains ungalinic acids that show resistance to *Micrococcus pyogenes* (Ying 1992).

Ten species were recently tested against eighteen bacterial strains, and *Piptoporus betulinus* was the most active (Karaman et al. 2009a).

Work in Germany showed water extracts reduce sarcoma 180 tumors by 49.2 percent. By adding 4 percent sodium hydroxide and ethanol precipitate to a hot-water extract, the rate of inhibition increased to 72 percent.

Betulinic acid and betulin are present in birch bark and concentrated in this polypore, in the same manner as chaga and other fungi on their host tree. Betulinic acid, a pentacyclic triterpene, destroys melanoma cancer cells without affecting healthy cells (Pisha et al. 1995).

Polyporenic acid C has been found able to inhibit the growth of *Bacterium racemosum* (Ying 1992).

Polyporenic acid B is a mixture of tumu-losic acid and dehydrogenated substances, and needs more study.

The compound 1,3-beta-D-glucopyranans is known as schizophyllan in Splitgill *(S. commune)*, and is chemically identical.

When administered to mice intravenously, an extract protected against a lethal infection with tick-borne encephalitis virus strain K5. When tested on mice and monkeys, the polypore was found capable of resisting poliomyelitis (Ying 1992).

In a study by Kandefer-Szerszen et al. (1974) nucleic acids isolated from *P. betulinus* reduced the number of vaccinia virus plaques in chick embryo fibroblast tissue culture. These nucleic acids were found to induce small but detectable amounts of liver and spleen interferon production.

Kawecki et al. (1978) found crude RNA from this polypore can induce human fibroblasts to produce interferon with a specific activity of 400 units per milligram of protein.

Kanamoto et al. (2001) identified a betulinic acid dubbed YI-FH 312 as a novel anti-HIV compound that blocks virus replication. Paul Stamets has filed a patent on an extract of this polypore's mycelium against various viral diseases after studies on vaccinia virus and cowpox.

Further study indicates weaker activity against Pichinde virus, an arenavirus, and the West Nile virus associated and spread via mosquitoes.

In one in vivo study, the fungi showed signs of both excitation and later inhibition of neurons. David Moore, in his excellent book *Slayers, Saviors, Servants, and Sec: An Exposé of*

Kingdom Fungi, says, "*Piptoporus* is known to produce (and accumulate in its fruit bodies) antiseptics and pharmacologically active substances that are claimed to reduce fatigue and soothe the mind."

In reference to the Ice Man, he continues: "I can imagine that with due ceremony and additional magic, these objects may well have been seen as essential to the traveller in the mountains. The conical one could well be a sort of styptic pencil to be applied to scratches and grazes, and perhaps the flattened, spheroidal one was chewed or sucked on when the going got tough."

Suay et al. (2000) found strong inhibition against *Staphylococcus aureus, S. subtilis,* and *Bacillus megaterium.* Paul Stamets suggests it be trialed against anthrax *(B. anthracis).*

Wasser and Weis (1999) confirmed antibacterial activity.

Piptamine is an antibiotic produced by the polypore (Schlegel et al. 2000).

C. Keller et al. (2002) found activity against *E. coli* and *Bacillus subtilis.*

Wangun et al. (2004) found lanostanoids that exhibit anti-inflammatory and anti-hyaluronate lyase activity. Earlier work by Kamo et al. (2003) isolated various laonstane-type triterpene and polyporenic acids and studied anti-inflammatory activity in mice edema. Previous work by Manez et al. (1997) identified triterpenoids that reduce chronic inflammation of the skin.

A fraction of the dried fruiting body was tested, in vitro, against lung (A549), colorectal (HT29), and rat glioma C6 cancer cell lines. A decreased tumor cell proliferation, motility, and induction of morphological changes was noted, with no or low toxicity to normal cells (Lemieszek et al. 2009).

To sum up, Razor strop possesses antifungal, antitumor, anti-inflammatory, antiviral, and antibacterial activity.

Homeopathy

There are several reasons to compare *P. betulinus* with *Carbo vegetabilis* from point of view of the Doctrine of Signatures. The fungus is regarded a "weakness parasite" because it attacks birches with decreased resistance. Since its appearance announces the death of its host, this polypore could be dubbed "deathbed fungus." ... The deathlike condition that the fungus represents brings to mind a remedy with a certain reputation for reviving the near-dead: *Carbo vegetabilis.* [It] is charcoal made of birch. Hahnemann did his provings with birch charcoal. As the residue of birch wood, charcoal has undergone combustion with exclusion of air.

There is still some fire left in charcoal, but not much, it smolders as a slow torch, similar to the *Carbo vegetabilis* condition. *"Op een laag pitje staan,"* the Dutch say, which translates as "simmering on a low flame."

By increasing the oxygen supply the fire will burn higher, which corresponds in the *Carbo vegetabilis* patient with the improvement by fanning. The similarities with *Piptoporus* are interesting. Firstly, the species grow exclusively on birch; secondly, employed as tinder, the fungus will slowly but persistently smolder "if placed in a tin with restricted ventilation."

— Vermeulen

Essential Oil

The hydro-distilled polypore yields an essential oil rich in 1-octen-3-ol (45 percent), and 3-octanol (27 percent), as well as 3-octanone, 1-octanol, (+)-alpha-barbatenc, isobazzanene, (S)-daucene, thujopsene, alpha-chamigrene, and traces of linalool, R-trans-nerolidol, methyl anisate, and benzaldehyde (Rosecke et al. 2000).

Fungi Essence

> Birch polypore essence can help protect you. It is good for those who travel. Hug my friend birch tree. Antiviral, immune tonic, and chi regulator.
>
> — SILVERCORD

Textile Industry

The fungi were cut into long strips and nailed to wood with the pores uppermost. The surface was hardened with siliceous earth and used by barbers, surgeons, and others for stropping sharp knives. The related *Polyporus squamosus* was used in a similar manner.

Lumberjacks in the Pacific Northwest made similar strops but did not powder the surface to finish sharpening of saws and axes.

It may be cut into small strips for tinder in survival packs. The polypore smolders very slowly and can be used as a touchwood for transporting fire from one site to another.

The soft, flexible, and protective nature of the polypore makes it ideal for holding obsidian and other stone for flint knapping spearheads, hatchets, knives, and other cutting surfaces.

Pieces have also been used for sweat pads in hats and by Scottish Highlanders as packing for the back of the circular shield or targets.

Fungal cellulase for denim bleaching and removing surplus hydrogen peroxide during cotton bleaching are two examples. Cellulase decolorizes recycled paper by de-inking.

Other Uses

Beekeepers have used smoldering fruit bodies for calming their hives.

Drawing charcoal has even been produced in the past.

It has been used to polish tarnished silver, and is still used in Switzerland to polish metal watches.

This mushroom possesses one of the highest cellulase activities of any fungi, suggesting industrial use. There are a number of applications for cellulase including detergents, textiles, food preparation, and animal feed.

Phytase and cellulase will become more valuable fungal enzymes as the use of antibiotic growth promoters becomes more restricted.

A wide range of cadmium sensitivity was found in agar and liquid cultures of the fungus (Baldrian and Gabriel 2002). The most resistant strains still showed growth at 250 micromoles of cadmium.

Pisolithus tinctorius

P. arrhizus

P. arenarius

Polysaccum pisocarpium

(DEAD MAN'S FOOT)

(BOHEMIAN TRUFFLE)

(DYEMAKER'S PUFFBALL)

(DOG TURD FUNGUS)

Pisolithus is derived from the Greek *piso* meaning "pea" and *lithos* meaning "stone." *Tinctorius* refers to its use in dyeing.

This is a most unusual fungus. The mature brown, brittle, and dusty mushroom protrudes from the ground like a half-rotted root or ball of dried up dung.

It is found in disturbed soils near trees and shrubs and in old pastures. It has even been known to burst through pavement.

The mushroom has a symbiotic relationship with the rootlets of trees, contributing to their ability to survive in poor soil by helping them to absorb nutrients. This is true of most fungi, but even more so with this species.

The young mushrooms, which resemble puffballs, are known in Europe as Bohemian truffles, and are used when unripe as a flavoring agent.

Traditional Uses

The puffball is used to relieve swelling and stop bleeding in traditional Chinese medicine.

When applied externally, it stops bleeding from wounds, or watery chilblains, and stops running pus. It staunches esophageal and stomach bleeding when taken internally.

The fungus treats heat in the lungs, coughing, swelling, sore throat, and nose bleeds. The mushroom is used medicinally in Japan, too, where it is known as *kotsubutake*.

Medicinal Use

Chemical Constituents

- Pisosterol, leucine, tyrosine, urea, ergosterol peroxide, 9(11)-dehydroergosterol, lipids, calvacin, pisolactone, sodium phosphate, 24-methyl-lanosta-8,24(28)-diene-3beta, 22 idiol; and a mixture of (22S,24R)-24-methyllanosta-8-en-22,28-epoxy-3beta, 28 alpha, and 28 beta diol.

(22S,24R)-24-methyllanosta-8-en-22,28-epoxy-3beta, 28 alpha, and 28 beta diol were isolated and found to possess immunosuppressive activity (Fujimoto et al. 1994).

Pisosterol is a triterpene that strongly inhibited the growth of all seven tumor cell lines tested, especially leukemia and melanoma. Results were comparable to those of doxorubicin and etoposide (Montenegro et al. 2004).

Pisosterol induces a monocytic cell-like differentiation of leukemia cell line HL-60, and shows activity against sarcoma 180 cancer cell lines with a 43 percent inhibition rate at ten milligrams per square meter (Montenegro et al. 2007; 2008).

Textile Industry

It is a good dye mushroom, yielding gold, yellow, brown, dark blue, or black, depending upon the mordant.

An excellent brown dye is obtained from the spores and traditionally used in the Canary Islands, in Italy, and around Nice, France, for the coloring of silks.

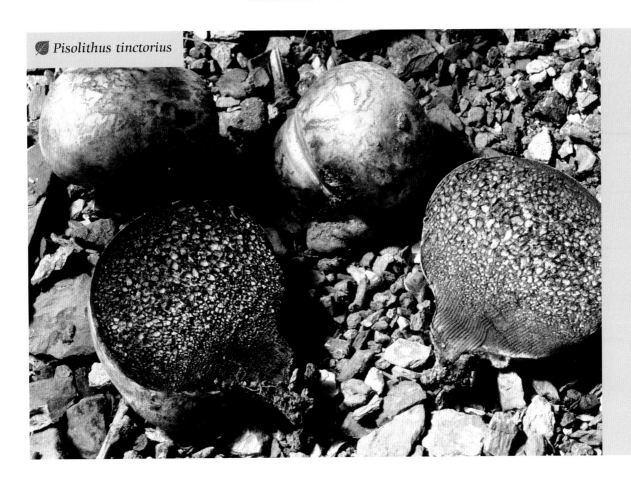

Pisolithus tinctorius

Mycoremediation

It could be useful for growing pine on sterilized soil or to help diversify reclamation projects such as the Athabasca Oil Sands in Northern Alberta. It could help re-establish pine trees on old gas and well sites that are barren due to excess salinity or heavy metals.

Hendrix et al. (1985) found pine seedlings transplanted on a coalmine site naturally infected with this ectomycorrhizal fungus were twice the height and stem diameter of those not infected.

Egerton-Waterton and Griffin found aluminum concentrations up to two thousand parts per million did not affect isolates of the mushroom. The aluminum tolerance was achieved, in part, by increases in calcium and magnesium concentration in the mycelia. Thompson and Medve (1984) found one isolate tolerant of aluminum and manganese.

Other work has noted mercury at a concentration of only 0.1 parts per million inhibited mycelial growth. Macrofungi are very mineral specific.

This mushroom has been found to transform TNT after three days of incubation. It shows promise in biotransformation of 1-naphthalene acetic acid.

Other Uses

It is widely used in experiments and sold commercially as a mycorrhizal inoculum for use in research.

Recipe and Dosage

Six milligrams of powder dissolved in water, with sugar added, taken twice a day.

Plectania nigrella

Pseudoplectania nigrella
(BLACK CUP FUNGUS)

This round-spored mushroom is found under pine in the boreal forest. Its edibility is unknown, but it does have a unique medicinal constituent.

Medicinal Use

Plectasin is a defensin peptide found in spiders, scorpions, dragonflies, mussels, oysters, and now fungi. It is suggested that defensins come from a common ancestral gene more than a billion years old. Mygind et al. (2005) found these cysteine-rich peptides active against bacteria, viruses, and other fungi.

Recombinant plectasin can be produced at a very high, commercially viable yield and purity.

In vitro trials indicate activity against *Streptococcus pneumoniae,* including several strains resistant to conventional antibiotics, and *S. pyogenes.* These organisms are responsible for diseases such as meningitis, pneumonia, strep throat, sepsis, and flesh-destroying skin infections. The exact mechanism of action is yet unknown, but appears to work in a manner quite different from traditional antibiotics.

Dr. Michael Zasloff says that by "utilizing a new genetic approach that allowed the team to discover plectasin, we now know that a whole class of antibiotics has been overlooked."

In humans, defensins are made by specific white blood cells and immune cells that later engulf foreign invaders, and by the skin and mucus membranes to kill microbes before they can invade these protective barriers.

"In mouse studies, plectasin showed extremely low toxicity, and was a effective as vanomycin and penicillin in curing the animals of experimental peritonitis and pneumonia caused by *S. pneumoniae,*" Zasloff continued.

Mice studies showed that ten milligrams per kilogram of weight of intravenous plectasin caused pneumococci levels to fall tenfold in two hours and a thousand-fold after five hours.

It took seventy milligrams per kilogram of weight of subcutaneous vancomycin to produce similar decreases. In mice, the plectasin is excreted without a change in urine.

In another mouse model, strains of *S. pneumoniae* were introduced intranasally and left untreated for twenty-four hours. Treated animals then received a single dose of plectasin or two doses of penicillin totaling thirty milligrams per kilogram of weight. All the mice were killed the next day, and viable pneumococci in lung tissue were counted and found to be at least one thousand-fold to ten thousand-fold lower in the animals treated with either plectasin or penicillin than in untreated control subjects.

Many antimicrobial peptides bind to cellular membranes and directly perturb membrane function, killing target microbes within seconds or minutes of exposure. The slower killing by plectasin suggests alternative mechanisms of action.

Defensins prevent viruses from entering cells, by preventing the virus from merging to cells' outer membrane. These membranes are coated with a layer of molecules called glycoproteins, in a manner similar to bristles sticking out of a hairbrush. Using this analogy, as the viral membrane approaches the cell membrane, the bristles part, leaving bare patches, allowing a fusion to take place. Defensins bind crosswise to glycoproteins, preventing them from spreading apart. It's as if the bristles were bound together by numerous small rubber bands.

Dr. Chernomordik of the National Institutes of Health says that "defensins do not kill the virus, they just prevent it from entering the cell. Viruses that are not allowed to enter the cells can then be destroyed by the cells of the immune system."

Plectasin can be effectively produced at high yields in a fungal expression system of industrial scale (Jing 2010).

Pleurotus ostreatus

P. populinus
P. pulmonarius
(OYSTER MUSHROOM)
P. porrigens
Pleurotellus porrigens
(ANGEL WINGS)
P. cystioliosus

(ABALONE OYSTER)
P. citrinopileatus
(GOLDEN OYSTER)

> The camel is gratefully called the ship of the desert; the oyster mushroom is the shellfish of the forest.
> — McILVAINE

Pleurotus is from the Greek *pleur,* meaning "formed laterally" or in a "sideways position," in reference to the lateral orientation of the stem relative to the cap, and *tus* meaning "ear." *Pulmonarius* is from *pulmo* for "lung," referring to the mushroom's texture.

P. ostreatus spores are whitish-gray to lavender, while *P. populinus* spores are white to slightly gray. *Ostreatus* refers to the oyster shell-like appearance and color, not the flavor of the mushroom.

The wild fungi are widely dispersed on dead aspen poplar throughout the aspen parkland and southern boreal forests of the Pacific Northwest. The *P. ostreatus* complex contains three intersterile strains that differ in morphology, growth characteristics, geography, and host range. Some work suggests that the oyster mushroom found on aspen in the western prairies may be properly called *P. populinus,* while the species found on conifers in Pacific Northwest may be *P. pulmonarius*. Whether they are distinct species or subspecies may require DNA analysis to determine.

In the fall of 1988, a Sicilian farmer collected an oyster mushroom nearly eight feet in circumference, twenty inches thick, and weighing forty-two pounds. What a productive strain this would have been, if the farmer had

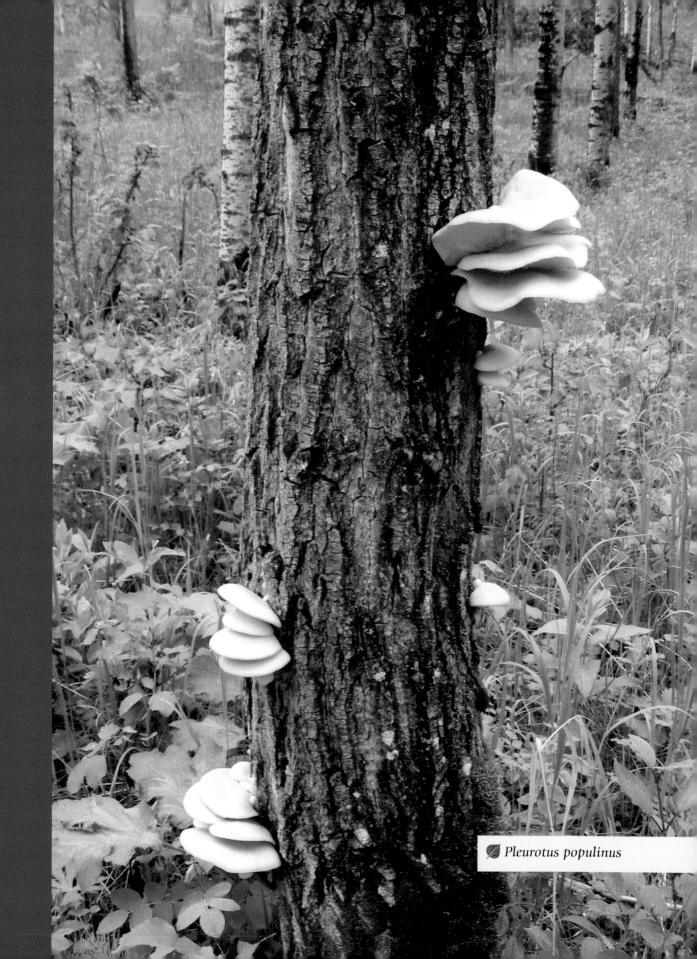

Pleurotus populinus

been a cultivator and not just a mushroom hunter!

On a mushroom forage in June 2001, I found my first wild oyster mushrooms. The multiple clumps were huge and tasty, but a little too wormy for my wife's liking. Oh well. Just more for me! Oyster mushroom is widely available as a fresh product in grocery stores. I recently purchased toasted oyster mushroom snacks, flavored with sugar and seaweed, in an Asian food store. They are a cultivated taste!

Nematodes or eelworms enjoy oyster mushrooms, but the mushroom has found a way to defend itself. The mycelia excrete a substance that numbs the worms, and once knocked out, the fungal hyphae lasso or envelop them to absorb nutrients. This source of nitrogen is essential to allow fruiting to take place. The active toxin is trans-2-decenediotic acid (Kwok et al. 1992).

Tricholomic acid is also present in the mushroom and may also immobilize nematodes, due to insecticidal activity.

Nematodes are the most abundant animals on earth, comprising 80 percent of all living creatures! In his book *The Third Domain,* Tim Friend writes, "If you were to make all of the solid matter on the surface of Earth invisible except for the nematode worms, you still could see its outline in nematode worms. About sixteen thousand species are known to science; the number estimated actually to exist by specialists is over 1.5 million. Almost certainly the world's ecosystems and our own lives depend on these little creatures, but we know absolutely nothing about the vast majority."

Submerged cultures of *P. pulmonarius* were studied and found to contain a number of nematicidal compounds, including S-coriolic acid, linoleic acid, p-anisaldehyde and p-anisyl alcohol (Stadler et al. 1994).

Nutritionally speaking, the oyster mushroom falls between a high-grade vegetable and low-grade meat when considered for biological value, including essential amino acids and nutritional index.

The related angel wings that grows on dead conifers contains eleostearic acid. It is known in Japan as *sugihiratake,* and considered by some to be as tasty as the oyster mushroom.

I would avoid it, as reports from Japan suggest it has caused hemolysis in kidney disease patients.

The related golden oyster mushroom (*P. citrinopileatus*) is Asian, but can be cultivated under controlled conditions. It is very fragile, and quickly loses its bright yellow luster, according to expert Paul Stamets.

The abalone mushroom (*P. cystidiosus*) is sometimes found growing on Cottonwood. Known in Japan as *tamogitake,* it is a dense, upright, ridged mushroom with depressed caps.

Medicinal Use

Chemical Constituents

- **Oyster mushroom contains eight essential amino acids in significant amounts; thiamin; riboflavin; folic acid; sterols, including D_2 and D_4; gamma ergosterol; lovastatin; pigments; carotenoids; bioflavonoid complex; fatty acids; various polyhydroxysteroids; mevinolin; tricholomic acid; trihydroxy-ketones; tetrahydroxy-ketones; tetraol; epidioxide; cerevisterol;**

and triol. Ergosterol content is from 0.124 to 0.469 percent.

Copper and zinc levels are higher than in other cultivated mushrooms. Even when straw substrate, low in zinc, was used, the zinc content of the mushroom was proportionally high. Oyster mushroom is made up of 27 percent protein, 38 percent complex carbohydrates, and only 1 percent fat. It contains twelve milligrams of vitamin C per hundred grams, as well as high levels of potassium (2,700 milligrams), niacin (fifty-four milligrams), and iron (nine milligrams) per hundred grams fresh weight.

Reports of non-starch polysaccharides from mushroom sclerotia are rare, but this mushroom includes beta-d-glycans, heteroglycans, and polysaccharide protein complexes.

Oyster mushroom is used medicinally as a nerve tonic, and to help reduce cholesterol levels.

In traditional Chinese medicine, the sporophore is dried and added to Tendon Easing Powder.

The mushrooms contain the toxin pleurotolysin that have caused hemolysis in various lab animals.

According to Spoerke and Rumack, the composition of pleurotolysin is closer to the bee venom melittin or the *Staphylococcus* delta toxin than other mushroom lytics. The hemolysis induced by this compound is inhibited by liposomes from cholesterol.

Acetone extracts yield water-soluble constituents with high polarity that possess analgesic activity. The pathway is via opioid receptor mediation.

The inhibition rate of water extracts of the sporophore lectin against sarcoma 180 is 88 percent, and hepatoma H-22 is 75.4 percent (Wang, H. et al. 2000).

An antitumor glucan (HA beta-glucan) has been isolated from the neutral polysaccharide fraction (A3) of a hot-water extract (Yoshioka et al. 1985). The glucan shows marked antitumor activity at a dose of 0.1 milligrams per kilogram of body weight. It is a highly branched 1,3 beta-glucan type.

Alcohol extracts of the mycelium possess a high level of antioxidant activity.

Gunde-Cimerman et al. (1995) found *Pleurotus* fruiting bodies contain lovastatin, the inhibitor of 3-hydroxy-3-methylglutaryl-Coenzyme A Reductase.

The extracts stimulated the activity of SOD (superoxide dimutase), catalase, and glutathione peroxidase; and decreased VLDL (very low density lipoprotein) cholesterol levels.

Lovastatin is a well-known pharmacological agent, approved in 1987 for treating high cholesterol. High levels have been found in oyster mushrooms. During the growth of the fruiting body, the constituent is first transferred to the pileus and later the lamellae. Nonetheless, it is fully present in non-sporing mushrooms, and can easily be added to the diet of patients with cardiovascular risk. Lovastatin-like compounds are higher in caps than stems, and more concentrated on mature gills.

Lovastatin has been found effective in reducing and preventing inflammation associated with pancreatitis and stopping progression toward fibrogenesis (Talukar et al. 2007).

Earlier studies on rats by Bobek et al. (1993)

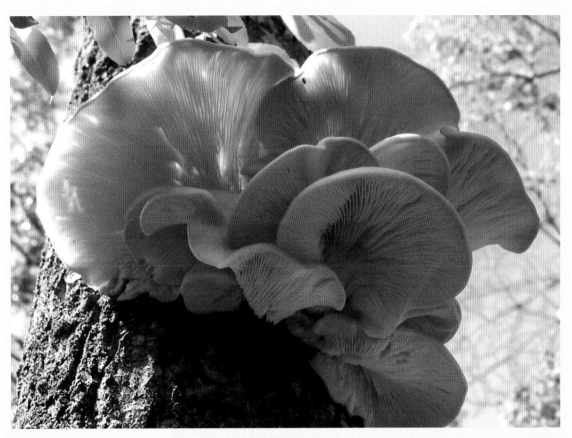

Above and below:
Pleurotus populinus.
Right: Oyster spawn
plugs.

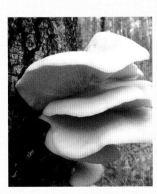

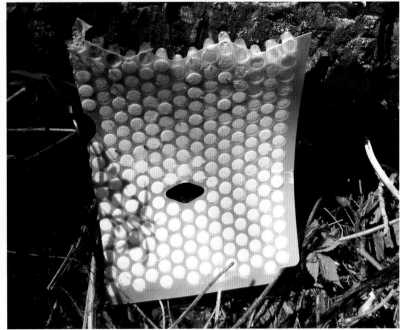

showed that the addition of 2 to 4 percent oyster mushrooms to the hyperlipidemic diet efficiently prevented accumulation of cholesterol. Further work by the same author found a 25 percent decrease in liver compared to control, and a 50 percent plasma cholesterol turnover (Bobek et al. 1995).

Rabbit studies are known to be more accurate indicators of human physiology when it comes to cholesterol issues. Bobek and Galbavy (1999) conducted a rabbit study and found that oyster mushroom lowered serum cholesterol levels and exhibited atherogenic effect.

Mevinolin, a fat-lowering medicinal component, has been detected in the fruiting body, as well.

Plovastin is a standardized extract developed at the University of Haifa in Israel. It contains biologically active statins, which are known inhibitors of cholesterol metabolism in the human body.

The statin drugs, such as Zocor, Lipitor, and Mevacor, are contraindicated in alcoholism, pregnancy, and liver disease, but not so the oyster mushroom.

In the human intestine, the chitin of the hyphal cell wall of mushrooms is changed to chitosan, which helps bind bile salts and influence the absorption of fats.

H. Wang and T. B. Ng (2000) recently isolated a novel ubiquitin-like protein from the mushroom that exhibited anti-HIV or human immunodeficiency virus inhibitory effects. It appears to govern viral cell division.

A clinical trial at San Francisco General Hospital looked at the short-term safety and potential efficacy of oyster mushroom to treat HIV patients with hyperlipidemia who were also taking the protease-inhibitor Kaletra. One issue with these antivirals is that they interfere with lipid metabolism in the liver, which leads to elevated LDL cholesterol levels and increased cardiovascular risk. It may prove that oyster mushrooms are a good adjunct to HIV therapy.

Laccase enzymes from the oyster mushroom inhibit hepatitis C virus from penetrating into peripheral blood and hepatoma cells, at least in the laboratory.

The phospholipids in oyster mushrooms are of interest. Of the seven different components, phosphatidylethanolamines, choline, and phosphatidyl-serine compose the majority. These are all useful in the treatment of myelin sheath and nerve related disease.

Gerasimenya et al. (2001) found submerged mycelium of oyster mushrooms most effective against *Aspergillis niger,* an extremely aggressive mold. It can cause aspergillosis lung disease that severely threatens those with immune deficiency.

Oyster mushrooms were tested against a number of microbes. When exposed to low-intensity laser light the antibiotic activity of *Micrococcus luteus, Staphylococcus aureus,* and *Bacillus mycoides* was increased by 10 to 20 percent (Poyedinok et al. 2005).

Sherbinin et al. (1999) found the dried mushroom powder possesses antacid properties, suggesting another functional food application.

Mei Zhang et al. (2001) showed extracts of the mushroom possess antitumor activity. Based on both in vitro and in vivo experiments, it is suggested that the antitumor activity is host-mediated and cytocidal. Early work by

Ying (1987) found mice tagged with sarcoma 180 and fed a diet made up of 20 percent oyster mushrooms showed a 60 percent inhibition of tumor development after one month compared to the control group.

Zusman et al. conducted research that indicates corn cobs treated with oyster mushrooms may help fight colon cancer. The mushrooms break down the lignins, making the dietary fiber easier to absorb by up to 78 percent (Zusman et al. 1997).

Rats fed an oyster mushroom-treated corn-cob diet had half as many tumors as those in a control group, and only 17 percent of the tumors were malignant. Tumor-associated protein levels were lower than the control group's and levels of the tumor-suppressing gene p53 were significantly increased. The researchers found the diet decreased the tumors' ability to repair its own DNA, and concluded that the fiber produced may be helpful to humans.

A water-soluble extract of the fresh oyster mushroom showed significant cytotoxicity and apoptosis on human androgen-independent prostate cancer PC-3 cell lines (Gu, Y. H. and G. Sivam 2006). Temperatures over eighty degrees Celsius for two hours eliminated the bioactivity, but at forty degrees Celsius it remained stable.

Fruiting bodies inhibit aromatase activity, similar to button mushrooms, with potential for the treatment of hormone-sensitive cancers (Grube et al. 2001).

Lavi et al. (2006) found alpha-glucans extracted by water possess anti-proliferative and apoptosis on colon cancer cells.

Crude mushroom extracts inhibit the proliferation and differentiation of human leukemia cells K562 (Yassin and Mahajna 2003).

Jose et al. (2002) found *P. pulmonarius* to exhibit antioxidant, anti-inflammatory and antitumor activity. Methanol extracts were comparable to the drug diclofenac in their effect, probably due to antioxidant activity.

Glyceride fractions inhibit COX-2 enzymes and lipid peroxidation by 92 percent at only twenty-five micrograms per milliliter (Diyabalanage et al. 2009).

The fruiting body of this mushroom has been found synergistic with glyburide in the treatment of diabetes (Badole et al. 2007).

Oyster mushroom is commercially available as a medicine for reducing cholesterol and as a nerve tonic, but not as yet for antitumor, antiviral, or antibacterial activity.

Water extracts of *P. pulmonarius* show increased glucose tolerance in both normal and diabetic mice, suggesting hypoglycemic activity (Badole et al. 2006).

Approximately 10 percent of North Americans and Europeans show an allergenic response to oyster mushrooms. A study of 701 patients indicates a need for testing before therapeutic application to individual patients (Horner et al. 1993).

Yatsuzuka et al. (2007) found *P. pulmonarius* extracts do not inhibit or increase IgE, and may be helpful in allergic rhinitis through inhibition of histamine release.

The linked beta-glucans show relief of acute and neuropathic pain through inhibition of inotrophic glutamate receptors and interleukin-1beta pathways (Baggio et al. 2010).

Mice fed extracts of golden oyster mushrooms showed a decrease in tumor size and increased longevity. Dr. Minoru Terazawa from Hokkaido University identified mannitol, a sugar alcohol, as the anti-hypertensive agent in this species.

The related *P. passeckerianus* and *P. mutilis* contain anti-carcinogenic and antiviral agents active against influenza.

Oral administration of Remasan, a standardized product made up of nearly two-thirds dried oyster mushroom powder, was found in a Finnish study to cause warts to disappear, and to prevent their reappearance. It is claimed to regulate diabetes and reduce joint pain and growing pains in children.

The related *P. cornucopiae* shows inhibition against sarcoma 180 of 80 percent and Ehrlich carcinoma of 70 percent. It contains tamavidin 1 and 2. These are biotin-binding proteins usually found in birds and bacteria (Takakura et al. 2009).

One intriguing study identified porrinenic acid from angel wings that showed cytotoxicity to human melanoma THP-1 cell lines.

Activity against sarcoma 180 and Ehrlich carcinoma cancer cell lines is 100 percent and 90 percent respectively for oyster mushrooms (Ohtsuka et al. 1973).

Mycoremediation

Oyster mushrooms decompose wood but can also be used to degrade environmental pollutants in both soil and liquid effluent. This includes wastewater from the pulp and paper industry, as well as pesticide-contaminated wastes like chlorinated biphenyls, aromatic hydrocarbons, dieldrin, and the fungicide benomyl. It is not just a matter of degradation but also mineralization of the pollutant, so that it returns to the air and soil as carbon dioxide, ammonia, chloride, and water.

Mycoremediation depends on the number of benzene rings in the structure of polycyclic aromatic hydrocarbons.

Oyster mushroom is effective in mycoremediation of nasty, toxic, cancer-inducing chemicals like PCP, widely used as a wood preservative. Spent mushroom substrates, available after the harvest of crops, absorb, immobilize, and concentrate PCP so that it can be transported from contaminated sites. More important, perhaps, is that it begins to digest the PCP completely.

Ruttimann-Johnson and Lamar (1997) showed it the most efficient (65 percent) in binding to all three fractions of humic materials, followed by *Irpex lacteus, T. versicolor,* and *Bjerkandera adusta.*

Law et al. (2003) found the spent mushroom compost from *P. pulmonarius* degrades naphthalene, phenanthrene, and benzopyrene, suggesting a use in mycoremediation.

It degrades atrazine during solid-state fermentation on wheat straw (Masaphy et al. 1996).

On November 7, 2007, the oil tanker *Cosco Busan* leaked fifty-eight thousand gallons of bunker crude into San Francisco Bay. A group called Matter of Trust laid out isolated squares of saturated soil and inoculated the areas with oyster mushroom mycelium. Several months later the petrochemicals were significantly diminished and the mushrooms that fruited were free of toxins.

Yateem et al. (1998) showed the ability to degrade oil in contaminated soil.

Oyster mushrooms concentrate cadmium and other heavy metals from effluent, due to the fungal wall. The mushroom has evolved over time to accumulate metal ions that it might need for nutrition. It is a chemically reversible binding reaction, so that fungi can take metal from its walls in exchange for a hydrogen ion. Polluting metals can be removed by passing the effluent through a column of fungal material.

Mercury, for example can be concentrated up to 140 times in mushroom substrates (Bressa et al. 1988).

Precious metals, such as silver from photographic processes and gold from electronic chips, can also be recovered. The simple treatment of the fungi with sodium bicarbonate removes the metals, and the process starts all over again. No large-scale industrial applications are yet operating.

Jauregui et al. (2003) found *P. ostreatus* transforms a variety of organophosphorus pesticides. Their study suggests that some intracellular origin of the transformation activity takes place, rather than simply being an enzymatic effect. Sesek et al. tested oyster mushrooms on two industrial sites contaminated with polycyclic aromatic hydrocarbons. The fungus degraded fluorine 41 to 67 percent, phenanthrene 24 to 42 percent, anthracene 29 to 49 percent, fluoranthene 29 to 57 percent, pyrene 24 to 42 percent, chrysene 0 to 42 percent, and benzoanthracene 0 to 13 percent at the two sites respectively (Sasek et al. 2000).

P. ostreatus, P. pulmonarius, and *P. citrinopileatus* have been found to be able to decolorize a commercial blue dye, suggesting mycofiltration of effluents containing this dye.

The related *P. eryngii* sometimes attacks the endophyte *Gliocladium roseum* (Chen, J. T. and J. W. Huang 2004).

Work by Gary Strobel and others found a strain of this fungus in Patagonia that breaks down cellulose and synthesizes liquid fuel. The volatiles are dubbed myco-diesel, due to their resemblance to components of crude oil. Patents are pending.

Paul Stamets, whose work I greatly admire, has this to say:

> If one mushroom can steer the world on the path to greater sustainability, fighting hunger, increasing nutrient return pathways in ecosystems, destroying toxic wastes, forestalling disease, and helping communities integrate a complexity of waste streams, oysters stand out. . . . Oyster mushrooms are well positioned to lead the way for rebalancing vast waste streams that currently overload our ecosystems.

Cosmetics

High concentrations of sphingo-glycolipids (vegetal ceramides), according to Dr. Yasuyuki Igarashi, lend themselves to skin moisturizing and protection, suggesting a cosmetic application.

Building Materials

The mycelium is used to create organic insulation, suitable for housing. Panels are filled with buckwheat or rice husks, natural silica, hydrogen peroxide, water, and inoculants. After ten to fourteen days, the mycelium, at rate of eight miles of strands per cubic inch, fills the entire panel, which is then oven-dried for completion. Greensulate, developed by Eben Bayer and Gavin McIntyre of Ecovative Design, is comparable to polystyrene but uses ten times less energy and eight times less carbon dioxide to produce. Very exciting!

Other Uses

The conversion of alpha pinene by basidiomycetes for flavor and fragrance compounds has huge potential due to the wood waste associated with pulp and paper, and the lumber industry in general.

Fungi Essence

Oyster essence is a transporter that changes and brings into action spiritual ideas, grounding them into matter. It provides trust, safety, and joy. Good for circulation of blood, tumors of the throat, and muscle tension.

— SILVERCORD

Cultivation

Work by Tudor (1998) found that substrates based on waste from hemp and flax plants, amended with 6 percent calcium carbonate and incubated at fifteen to twenty-five degrees Celsius (fifty-nine to seventy-seven degrees Fahrenheit), worked as well as a combination made up of 80 percent corn husks and 20 percent straw.

The waste from dill processing produced high quality oyster mushroom fruiting bodies, another value added possibility for farm producers.

In various studies, wheat straw has been found to be a suitable substrate for oyster mushroom production. It is often produced in vertical containers, like a tree, with a number of holes optimally distributed.

The spent mushroom compost is high in laccase at 1,452 nanokatals per gram (Ko, H. G. et al. 2005b).

Mycelial growth was best in a mixture of 0.5 percent yeast and 0.5 percent glucose in distilled water. Cheese whey also worked well.

They may be harvested in the wild, and encouraged by spreading mycelium; or you can take an inoculated log section and set it in your backyard or basement for a more long term harvest. It is one of the easiest mushrooms to grow, using substrates from paper, straw, wood, and other spent materials. Inoculated poplar stumps produce, on average, more than one pound annually for more than three years. Work by Pagony published in 1973 found that of two hundred poplar stumps averaging six to twelve inches in diameter, inoculated in spring, all were fruiting by the fall of following year. Each and every one!

Recent work has shown that the cultivation of oyster mushrooms on spent barley grain husks left over from beer production is quite feasible. The spent grains that were larger than one millimeter were found to be the best. And after cultivation, the substrate can be used for mycofiltration or mycoremediation, really adding value to the grain.

Using nitrogen as a medium maximizes the lovastatin production in the oyster mushroom. Mannitol is the best carbon source for both this mushroom and *Phlebia radiata*.

Mycelium grown on wheat straw- and wheat germ-based substrates work well.

Mikiashvili and Isikhuemhen (2009) found 10 percent solid waste from poultry on wheat straw, 10 percent millet, and 80 percent wheat straw produced the optimal yield of fruiting bodies.

Oyster mushroom can be grown on poplar wood waste and, when supplemented with a low concentration of dextrose, will form fruiting bodies within three to eight weeks. The contribution of 3-0-octyl and 3-0-decyl-D-glucose was found to stimulate oyster mushroom fruiting.

Oysters can be grown on "old" growth systems previously used for commercial button mushrooms *(Agaricus bisporus)* (Danai et al. 2008).

Ostreolysin, a cytolytic protein, strongly induces the formation of primordia and its development into a fruiting body (Berne et al. 2007).

Muller et al. (1986) found oyster mushroom *(P. florida)* helped delignification of straw and helped it ferment anaerobically to biogas with a fruit yield nearly double.

Grape pomace and vineyard prunings also make an excellent substrate for mushroom propagation. Vineyards may wish to look at the related economic spinoff from essentially a waste product with low nutritional value. Many vineyards have tasting rooms and restaurants that could take advantage of another agri-tourism/ fine dining opportunity by growing and serving oyster mushrooms. Slightly charred, they go well with balsamic vinegar in salads, or with cardamom and leeks in soup. Wine-pickled oyster mushrooms—say a cup of dry white wine, two cups white wine vinegar, and a pound of oyster mushrooms, along with some spices—would make a good condiment for a high-end restaurant. Bill Jones, author of *The Savoury Mushroom* and a food consultant on Vancouver Island, has expertise on wild mushrooms and edibles for the hospitality industry.

The straw of both astragalus *(A. membranaceus)* and Job's tears *(Coix lacryma-jobi)* work as efficient substrates for oyster mushroom production.

Recipe and Dosage

The dried powder can be added to just about anything, from smoothies to breads. Take three to nine grams per day. The benefit is not reduced by heat, so baking and cooking are fine.

Pluteus atricapillus

P. cervinus
(DEER MUSHROOM)
(FAWN PLUTEUS)

Pluteus is from the Latin meaning "bracket," "shed," or "shield." *Atricapillus* means "dark hair," while *cervinus* means "deer."

There are a number of species of pink-spored deer mushrooms in the northern boreal forest, usually found on decaying birch and poplar logs.

The blue-staining willow *Pluteus,* or *P. salicinus,* and *P. nigroviridis* (black-green) contain up to 1.57 percent psilocybin, and psilocin as well as small amounts of the biogenetic precursor bacocystin and tryptophan. These mushrooms can be considered hallucinogenic, due to their psilocybin content.

The deer mushroom *(P. atricapillus)* has a radish odor that disappears with cooking. It also contains psilocybin, as does the related *P. glaucus.*

Podaxis pistillaris

(FALSE SHAGGY MANE)
(DESERT SHAGGY MANE)
(ABORIGINAL PAINTBRUSH)

Podaxis is Greek meaning "strong foot." *Pistillaris* means "like a pestle."

This mushroom is found in dry, desert regions of the world. They are found as far north as Kamloops and in the hot, dry valleys of the Canadian Rockies.

Like the common name suggests, it looks a lot like shaggy mane *(Coprinus* species), but with a tough stalk. It does not digest itself at maturity like the shaggy mane. It is highly prized in India for edibility. It contains 21 percent protein.

Traditional Uses

In China, the mushroom is used to staunch wounds and aid in detoxification.

In both Afghanistan and South Africa, the mushroom was used traditionally to heal cancerous sores, and to relieve sunburn. It is used for diaper rash of babies in Yemen.

Medicinal Use

The antimicrobial activity is due to epicorazines, belonging to an important group of active fungal metabolites known as epiolythiopiperazine-2,5-diones. More research would be welcomed.

The fungus appears to exhibit antibacterial activity against *Staphylococcus aureus, Micrococcus flavus, Bacillus subtilis, Proteus mirabilis, Serratia marcescens,* and *Escherichia coli.* Epicorazine A-C have been identified and assumed responsible for the antibacterial activity (Al-Fatimi, et al. 2006).

Cultivation

Work by Dr. Jiskani at the Sindh Agriculture University, Tandojam, found that the spores of mature mushrooms could be directly sown in soil, and watered twice daily. A crop appears within thirty days, suggesting a desert crop possibility.

Cosmetics

In Australia, the purple spores have been used for body paint and to darken the white hair of old men's whiskers.

Insecticide

It may have been burned as a fly repellant.

Podostroma alutaceum

(SOFT LEATHER PILLOW)

Podostroma is from the Greek meaning "pillow on a base." *Alutaceum* is Latin for "like fine leather."

This is a relatively rare member of the order Sphaeriales. It looks like a puffball or *Spathularia* species but is not.

The related *P. yunnanensis* is dried and ground into a powder for external wounds and bleeding.

Polyozellus multiplex

(BLUE CHANTERELLE)
(BLACK CHANTERELLE)
(MAGPIE MUSHROOM)

This beautiful mushroom looks at first glance like a deep violet *Craterellus,* but the caps are spoon or fan shaped, rather than trumpet-like. It is found under spruce and fir in the Montane region of the Rocky Mountains and throughout North America.

Edible and delicious, it has a decidedly earthy smell and taste when dried.

Medicinal Use

Chemical Constituents

■ **Polyozellin and kynapcin-12.**

Polyozellin enhanced quionone reductase, glutathione S-transferase activity and glutathione content in a dose dependent manner. These compounds quench free radical damage.

Polyozellin also promotes differentiation of HL-60 human leukemia cells and should be studied further for potential in preventing cancer (Kim, Jeong Hyun et al. 2004).

The water extract is chemoprotective of gastric cancer cells by increasing glutathione and SOD as well as p53 tumor suppressor gene (Lee, I. S. and Nishikawa 2003).

Both compounds inhibit PEP (prolyl endo-peptidase), which is implicated in memory loss and senile dementia (Lee, H. J. et al. 2000).

Polyporus elegans

Melanopus elegans
(BLACK FOOT)
(ELEGANT POLYPORE)
P. squamosus
Melanopus squamosus
(DRYAD'S SADDLE)
(PHEASANT'S BACK POLYPORE)
(THE SCALY POLYPORE)
P. badius
Royoporus badius
P. picipes
P. durus
Melanopus picipes
(BAY BROWN POLYPORE)
(PITCH COLORED POLYPORE)
P. alveolaris
P. mori
Favolus alveolaris
Favolus canadensis
(FRINGED POLYPORE)
(SPRING POLYPORE)

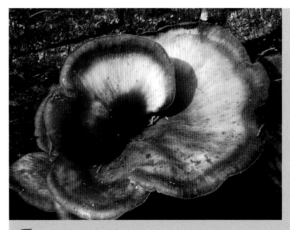

🍃 *Polyporus badius*

Polyporus means "many pores" and was the genus to which all bracket fungi were once assigned. *Elegans* means "elegant" and *squamosus* means "scaly." *Squamosus* is from *squama*, meaning "a scale." *Badius* means "bay-brown; and *picipes* means "pitch foot."

Black foot is widespread and common on poplar, alder, and willow. It is recognized by its tan-white cap and distinctive black foot.

Bay brown polypore *(P. badius)* is a kidney-shaped bracket fungus common to poplar and other hardwood trees in the Pacific Northwest.

Polyporus croceus has a narcissus fragrance while *P. obtusus* is more jasmine-like in scent.

Fringed or spring polypore is commonly found on decayed aspen poplar throughout the region. The honey color and large angular spore openings make identification easy.

The related dryad's saddle *(P. squamosus)* is said to be edible when young, and with good honey-like flavor.

Nicholas P. Money, in his delightful *Mr. Bloomfield's Orchard,* recalls his attempt to make a saffron-flavored dryad's saddle stew for some colleagues:

> The fresh fruiting bodies emitted a strong perfume, akin to the smell of a very cheap cologne. This didn't bode well, but I reasoned that the threads of saffron would dominate the final flavor.
>
> But as the broth simmered, the scent from the brackets intensified until it matched the pungency of a disinfectant used in a slaughterhouse. Removing the lid of the casserole when my guests arrived, I forced a mouthful down and attempted a feeble smile. Everyone was horrified. I remain revolted by dryad's saddles and never touch them in the woods. Even the scent they leave on my hands is sufficient to provoke stomach contractions.

To me, it has a cucumber-like odor, and may be better in a cold salad, after steaming.

David Spahr, in his wonderful book on mushrooms of New England, suggests the odor is like watermelon rind.

Use young specimens only and cook them immediately for best results. Spahr suggests sautéing thin slices hard and fast, as overcooking will make them tough. Spahr also suggests drying them into white, crunchy chips.

In Asia, where bitter flavors and chewy textures are more popular in wild mushrooms, dryad's saddle is prized.

Traditional Uses

The polypore is valued in traditional Chinese medicine for dispelling endogenous wind and cold, stimulating blood circulation, and easing pain in tendons. It is one of the many ingredients in Tendon Easing Powder.

Medicinal Use

Chemical Constituents

- *P. mori:* **Isodrimenediol, drimenediol, and related sesquiterpenes isocryptoporic acids H-I.**

One study found dryad's saddle to possess cholagogue and choleretic activity in laboratory animals. Cholagogues stimulate gallbladder contraction, and choleretics help aid excretion of bile by the liver, both activities helping promote bile flow that aids breakdown of fatty acids and ensures antiseptic and healthy bowel function.

Lectins from this species may be a useful tool for histochemical detection of 12,6-linked NeuAc5 in asparagines linked oligosaccharides.

Extracts from the fruiting body of bay brown polypore inhibit binding of lipopolysaccharide (LPS) from gram-negative bacteria to the CD14 receptor on immune cells. The binding of LPS is part of the septic shock syndrome that releases a cascade of inflammatory mediators and reactive oxygen species leading, in some cases, to death (Koch et al. 2002). *Trametes versicolor, Piptoporus betulinus,* and *Heterobasidion annosum* also exhibit this property.

Many polyporus species contain ergosta-4-6-8 (14), 22-tetraen-3-one, a compound found to possessing anti-aldosteronic diuretic properties, suggesting a role in urinary and prostatic complication in elderly males, as well as PCOS (polycystic ovary syndrome, also known as Stein-Leventhal syndrome) in women.

Fleck et al. (1996) identified isodrimenediol, drimenediol, and related sesquiterpenes, called isocryptoporic acids H-I in fringed polypore. The latter are isomers of cryptoporic acids with drimenol instead of albicanol as the terpenoid fragment (Cabrera et al. 2002).

Both water and organic fractions from extracts of the mycelium show activity against *E. coli, Salmonella typhimurium Staphylococcus aureus,* and *Bacillus subtilis.*

Cultured mycelium extracts inhibit sarcoma 180 in mice by 80 percent, and fruiting body extracts inhibit sarcoma 180 by 72 percent and Ehrlich carcinoma cells by 60 percent (Shibata, S. et al. 1968).

The spring polypore *(P. mori)* is high in amylase and lipase activity.

Polyporus tuberaster

Boletus tuberaster
(STONE FUNGUS)

You must grow like a tree not like a mushroom.
—JANET STUART

Tuckahoes are black, tuber-like structures that are white and translucent inside when dried. The term *tuckahoe* or *tockawhoughe* is a native North American name used for several edible bulbs and tubers, such as wake robin or other *Trillium* species. *Tuberaster* means "like a truffle," referring to its underground sclerotium.

Theophrastus, a pupil of Aristotle, was the first ancient Greek to mention the stone fungus.

"In the sea around the Pillars of Hercules, fungi are produced close to the sea, which

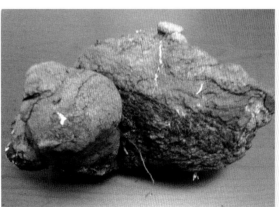

🌿 *Polyporus tuberaster*

people say have been turned into stone by the sun." Many scholars believe he was referring instead to coral's calcareous plates, which resemble fungi.

In early Roman times, the fungus stones were prized and traded under the name *lapideus*. This continued into the sixteenth and seventeenth centuries.

Early mycologists, such as Mattioli, referred to the sclerotium as *lapis lyncuris,* meaning "the fossilized feces of lynx."

Another name, fossil pemmican, from the Cree *pimikkan,* may be derived from the thought that it was a petrified food.

Stone fungus is common to the mixed aspen woods of western North America. They are of a hard, rubbery texture when fresh, but dry out to the hardness of stone. They are referred to as Indian bread, and, at one time, were mistaken for fossilized pemmican.

Tuckahoe is a large, black sclerotium, or a resting stage for a fruiting body. It is usually found at the base of conifers or birch in our region.

The external surface is usually marked with lines or ridges. When cut in half the internal mass has grains of sand and even, encased small stones.

Below the black crust the interior of fresh tuckahoe is olive green. When older and dried, the interior looks marbled gray and white.

The mushrooms that grow above ground, either planted or wild, vary from two to six inches in diameter and height.

They can be found up to several feet below the surface and are usually the size of a clenched fist, but some specimens as large as four and a half kilograms (about ten pounds) have been found and described.

The scent has been described as floral, fruity, and cinnamon-like.

When an old dried specimen is soaked in water, it absorbs up to 50 percent of its weight, but is still too tough to chew. If boiled, it becomes slightly softer, but hardly edible.

When fresh, the sclerotium is moist and easily cut. It contains pectin, and has been used as an arrowroot substitute after boiling.

Traditional Uses

Eastern Canadian tribes used the root for food, while the Cree used it for poultices and rheumatism. Various native groups used the underground tuber as a poultice for treating rheumatism. It is called *medicin de terre,* or "ground medicine" by the Cree or Métis of my area.

In Italy, the underground tuber, or sclerotium, is placed in a flowerpot of earth and watered to produce the edible fruit. There it is known as *pietra fungaia,* meaning "mushroom or fungus stone."

The fruiting tops are used medicinally in both Italy and China for treating fevers and a variety of eruptive diseases.

Christopher Hobbs notes the fungus is considered in traditional Chinese medicine to be sweet and bland, with mild energy that affects the heart, spleen, and lung meridians.

Medicinal Use

Work by Ayer et al. (1992) at the University of Alberta investigated metabolites in the sclerotium. They found a ten-membered unsaturated lactone and tuckolide, as well as erogsterols, ergosterol peroxide, an unidentified disaccharide, and triacetyl tuckolide.

A compound of similar constitution to tuckolide, isolated from a fermentation culture of *Penicillium,* has been reported in the patent literature.

Tuckolide potently inhibits cholesterol biosynthesis. One group of researchers have identified and synthesized the compound. They found the configuration comparable to the lactone portion of the HMG-CoA reductase inhibitor compactin.

Essential Oil

Polyporus tuberaster contains various volatiles, with benzaldehyde accounting for 61 percent. Another aromatic compound is 3-methyl-1-butanol.

When l-phenylalanine is added to the medium of cultivation, both benzaldehyde and benzyl alcohol increased in yield.

Kawabe and Morita (1994) showed that *P. tuberaster* can produce benzaldehyde and benzyl alcohol in high yield from L-phenylalanine, under cultivation. This has commercial potential.

Cosmetics

In a sensory evaluation of 117 mushrooms by ten sniffing panelists, *P. tuberaster* was the most highly rated. The strain has a fruity and floral odor suitable for beverage or perfume work.

The related *P. mylittae* from Australia has a number of chemicals that apply to cosmetic and haircare formulation. It was used traditionally for dandruff and hair preparations, and contains salicylic acid and organic sulphur compounds, which give keralytic and antifungal effect respectively. Volatile oils stimulate the scalp and organic acids that are astringent provide additional support.

Recipe and Dosage

Nine to sixteen grams in decoction three times per day.

Polyporus umbellatus

(see *Grifola umbellatus*)

Poria monticola

Both of these polypores are identified by their resupinate appearance, with a layer of tubes on sitka spruce, douglas fir, and redwoods further south. Resupinate means they lack caps and stems and lie on dead logs. They are brown rot decayers.

Medicinal Use

Mlinaric et al. (2005) found *P. monticola* showed 86.1 percent inhibition of HIV-1 reverse transcriptase.

The related *P. vaillantii,* found on the same species of trees, showed a moderate activity of 53 to 68 percent.

Psathyrella candolleana

(SUBURBAN PSATHYRELLA)
(CRUMBLE TUFT)
P. velutina
P. lacrymabunda
Lacrymaria velutina
L. lacrymabunda
Hypholoma velutina
(VELVET PSATHYRELLA)
(WEEPING WIDOW)
P. spadicea
P. sarcocephala
(DATE-COLORED PSATHYRELLA)

Psathyrella is from the Greek meaning either "fragile" or "straw-like." *Candolleana* is named after A. P. de Candolle, a French mycologist of the early 1800s. *Spadicea/spadiceo* is from the Latin meaning "the color of fresh dates."

Suburban *Psathyrella* has worldwide distribution, occurring in yards among dead grass and on old tree stumps. It is said to be edible, and does possess a delicate mushroom odor.

Velvet *Psathyrella,* or weeping widow, is found on lawns and is edible. It may not look tasty, but its firm flesh is prized by many mycophiles. It should be picked before the spores mature.

Koike determined that *P. candolleana* contains psilocybin. Ohenoja later identified psilocin.

Medicinal Use

Research found crumble tuft to possess activity against gram-positive bacteria, including *Staphylococcus aureus, Bacillus cereus, B. subtilis,* and *Salmonella typhi,* as well as the fungus *Candida albicans.*

Coletto et al. (1981) found *P. spadiceo-grisea* exhibits activity against *Bacillus subtilis, Staphylococcus aureus,* and *E. coli.*

Crumble tuft shows hypoglycemic activity.

Inhibition rates against sarcoma 180 and Ehrlich carcinoma are 70 percent and 80 percent respectively (Ohtsuka et al. 1973).

The related *P. gracilis* shows inhibition against sarcoma 180 and Ehrlich carcinoma of 60 percent (Ohtsuka et al. 1973).

Bits and Pieces

A recent discovery of the first gilled underwater mushroom was made in Oregon, by Robert Coffan. It has been named *Psathyrella aquatic.* One unusual feature is the formation of gas bubbles on the cap.

Psilocybe

Psilocybe coprophila
Stropharia coprophila
(ROUND DUNG MUSHROOM)
S. merdaria
P. merdaria
(DUNG MUSHROOM)
P. coronilla
S. coronilla
(GARLAND STROPHARIA)
S. semiglobata
S. semiglobata var. stercoraria
P. semiglobata
(HEMISPHERICAL STROPHARIA)
(ROUND DUNG HEAD)
P. semilanceata
Panaeolus similanceata
(LIBERTY CAP)
(PIXIE CAP)

S. aeruginosa
Psilocybe aeruginosa
Pratella aeruginosa
(BLUE GREEN STROPHARIA)
(VERDIGRIS TOADSTOOL)
P. cubensis
S. cubensis
(MAGIC MUSHROOM)
S. cyanescens
(POTENT PSILOCYBE)
P. caerulescens
(LANDSLIDE MUSHROOM)

The little mushroom comes of itself, no one knows whence, like the wind that comes we know not whence nor why.

— MAZATEC SAYING

In my experience, psychedelic mushrooms, such as *Psilocybe semilanceata* . . . have the potential, if used carefully with knowledge and awareness, to be useful for developing sensitivity to the cycles of nature, to learn how we can be in harmony with its processes.

— CHRISTOPHER HOBBS

Let us cheer for dung fungi!
Dung fungi—unsung fungi!
Never-touch-the-tongue-fungi!
High-strung, ever-young fungi!
Freely flung across the dung
Freshly sprung with ho so gung!
Stench a song so plainly sung!
— R.C. SUMMERBELL, *MYCELIUM*,
APRIL 1983

Psilocybe is from the Greek meaning "bare head." *Coprophila* means "dung loving." *Merdaria* is from the Latin, also pertaining to dung.

Stercoraria is derived from the minor Roman god Stercutus, the son of Faunus and the patron of manure. Liberty cap is derived from the emblem worn by the figure of Liberté during and after the French Revolution. It was originally associated with the Phrygian bonnet.

The mushrooms are widespread and common, often found growing on manure.

Round dung is one of the few *Psilocybes* on the Great Plains east of the Rockies. It contains low amounts of psilocybin, but no psilocin when fresh.

Liberty cap is the most common West Coast "magic mushroom," and fruits during the rains of autumn.

Dung mushroom is believed to contained small amounts of hallucinogenic compounds by some authors. Paul Stamets suggests both are non-psilocybin species.

Round dung head grows on horse or cow dung in pastures and is identified by a bright yellow gel covering them when young. It does not stain blue. According to Arora, it is edible but slimy and mediocre.

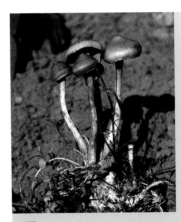

Psilocybe azurescens

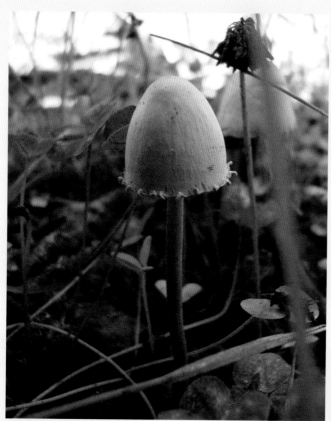

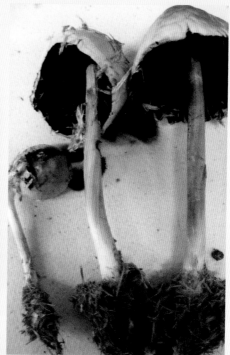

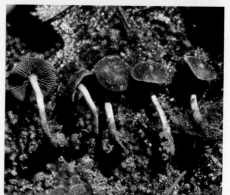

🍂 Clockwise from above: *Panaeolus sphinctrinus;*
Psilocybe drying; *Psilocybe cyanofibrillosa;*
Psilocybe pelliculosa; Panaeolus campanulatus.

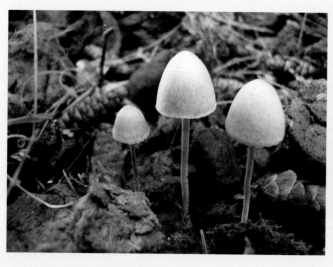

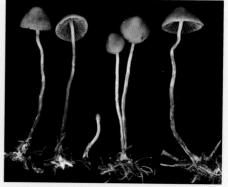

In one experimenter, the mushroom caused dizziness, loss of coordination, unprovoked hilarity, depression, and space and time distortion.

A small species, *P. angustispora,* grows on marmot and elk dung in the Cascade Mountains. It is psychoactive.

The related *S. coronilla* may contain psilocybin, but is of dubious edibility and may be considered poisonous. Two teenagers seeking a hallucinogenic experience only received intense "bone pain" upon ingestion.

Some sources cite malaise, headache, ataxia, dizziness, vomiting, hallucinations, and confusion.

Blue green *Stropharia* or *Psilocybin* is common in the Pacific Northwest. It has a heavy layer of green slime that washes away to expose the ochre yellow cap. It has the distinct odor of fresh tomatoes.

It has not caused any poisonings in North America, or at least none reported. I wouldn't bother.

The related *P. pelliculosa* and *P. stuntzii* are both weak to moderate psychoactive species common to the Pacific Northwest.

There are some 180 species of mushroom that contain psilocybin and/or psilocin, not all in the *Psilocybe* genus.

Culture and Folklore

The fourth chapter of the *Eiriks Saga Rautha* gives a fairly detailed description of the woman named Lill-volvan, a "seeress" who travels from farm to farm predicting the future for the landowners. She was one of ten sisters who did this work. Unlike earlier Scandinavian shamanistic myths, this account is filled with intriguing mushroom motifs that are highly suggestive of *Psilocybe* mushroom metaphors.

The seeress is dressed in a very special way. She wears a blue cloak, jewels, and a headpiece of black lamb decorated with white cat skins, and she carries a staff. I would suggest not only that her outfit is clearly a shamanic ritual costume, but also that it serves as an entheogenic metaphor. To begin with, Lill-volvan wears a black and white fur cap. It may be merely coincidental, but the cap of … the most common and most potent of the *Psilocybes* found in Scandinavia is frequently black and white, as well as furry looking. The seeress also wears a blue mantle (or cloak), which immediately brings to mind the tendency of *Psilocybe* stems to turn blue when they are handled. Furthermore, she sits on a cushion of chicken feathers. When a mushroom is picked, one often sees white, downy material at its base, which is part of the mycelium. …

It is stated that the seeress wears a belt with mushrooms hanging from it. Moreover, on her belt hangs a pouch in which she keeps a "magical substance" that she reportedly uses in order to go into trance. It is not difficult to imagine what this substance might be.

— STEVEN LETO, *SHAMAN'S DRUM* (#54)

Traditional Uses

In traditional Chinese medicine, *Psilocybe* is used to treat Kashin-Beck disease, a form of polyarthritis believed caused by eating grain contaminated with another fungus, *Fusarium sporotrichiella.*

Also in traditional Chinese medicine, it is one of the main components of Pine Mushroom Elixir.

Medicinal Use

Round dung mushroom shows activity against *Bacillus subtilis*, *S. aureus*, and *E. coli*.

Liberty cap has been found to inhibit *Staphylococcus aureus* bacteria (Svay 2000).

The body apparently hydrolyzes psilocybin, the indole alkaloids, into psilocin, the bioactive compound. The psychic activity is based on interference with the neurotransmitter, serotonin, which is structurally similar to psilocin. They are also closely related to dimethyltryptamine (DMT).

Psilocin binds to the serotonergic receptor, 5HT2a, and acts as a partial agonist. That is, it stimulates some neurons and not others. The exact pathway to psychedelic experience is unknown, but one hypothesis is that an increased activity of the sensor motor gating system of the brain is involved. This system normally suppresses the majority of sensory stimuli from conscious awareness, so we can operate at a normal level.

The conscious mind is overwhelmed by sensory stimuli and cognitive processes normally hidden in the conscious part of the mind.

All species vary in their effects and due to a variety of constituents may well react differently in individuals. The species *P. cubensis* and *P. caerulescens* are found on the Gulf Coast region. The former is widely cultivated.

Paul Kroeger, one of British Columbia's finest mycologist, notes there are ten *Psilocybe* species with hallucinogenic properties in that province.

Richard Haard, in *Poisonous and Hallucinogenic Mushrooms,* relates his experience with six different species of *Psilocybe*.

P. cyanescens generally lets me look into the order which my inner mind forces on the rest of me; *P. semilanceata* is a model builder allowing me to look into the past, present and future of my life and activities, even into the very nature of life and eternity; *P. strictipes* and *P. baeocystis* both give a visual adventure, with baeocystis the most visual mushroom thus far.

This makes sense, as *P. cyanescens* was found to be the most potent (thirteen milligrams per gram psilocybin plus psilocin) in a study of Pacific Northwest species. *Psilocybe semilanceata* (ten milligrams per gram) was second and *P. stunzii* (two milligrams per gram) the weakest. Variation within species varied as well, by factors from two to six.

There appears to be great bias toward mushroom species containing psilocybin. It may surprise readers to find that research by Dr. Adrian North found 12.3 percent of opera lovers have used magic mushrooms at one time or another. His research involved twenty-five hundred people.

Charles Schuster, former director of the National Institute of Drug Abuse, notes a return to the study of certain hallucinatory compounds that showed potential into the nature of human consciousness and sensory perception.

Human consciousness . . . is a function of the ebb and flow of neural impulses in various regions of the brain—the very substrate that drugs such as psilocybin act upon. Understanding what mediates these effects is clearly within the realm of neuroscience and deserves investigation.

A news release from Reuters, dated July 3, 2008, noted "the 'spiritual' effects of psilocybin from so-called sacred mushrooms last for more than a year."

An article on the potential religious experience of states of consciousness induced by psilocybin, written by William Richards, is worth a read.

In 2006, Roland Griffiths of Johns Hopkins University in Baltimore, Maryland, and colleagues gave psilocybin to thirty-six volunteers and asked them how it felt. Most reported having a "mystical" or "spiritual" experience and rated it positively. "More than a year later, most still said the experience increased their sense of well-being or life satisfaction."

In the same year, another study found the mushroom aborted cluster migraine headaches in twenty-two of twenty-six patients and eighteen of nineteen had extended remissions from the debilitating head pain.

Studies of psilocybin for treating schizophrenia and obsessive-compulsive disorder have been conducted.

Dr. Charles Grob of the Los Angeles Biomedical Research Institute is conducting a study to measure the effectiveness of psilocybin on the reduction of anxiety, depression, and physical pain in stage IV cancer patients.

In 2009, Johns Hopkins began recruitment for a psilocybin study involving cancer patients.

Inhibition rate against Sarcoma 180 is 80 percent and Ehrlich carcinoma cancer cells 70 percent.

The tetraprenylphenol Suillin has been identified as the principle responsible for the mushrooms cytotoxic activity. Suillin is also found in *Suillus* species.

Alarcon et al. found that this mushroom biotransformed 5-hydroxytryptophan to 5-hydroxy-tryptamine.

Stropharia stercoraria is a variant of *S. semiglobata*.

Blue green *Stropharia* or *Psilocybin* contains some interesting fats and lipids.

Early work suggests antitumor activity with inhibition of sarcoma 180 and Ehrlich carcinoma cells at 70 percent and 60 percent respectively.

Both water and ethanol extracts cause inhibition and excitation of impulse activity of neurons in the hippocampus stratum pyramidale region of the brain (Moldavan et al. 2001).

The related *P. argentipes* has been studied and may have application for the treatment of obsessive-compulsive disorder (Matsushima et al. 2009).

Homeopathy

Absentminded when conversing, delusions of ants, changing suddenly, creative powers, alternately God and the devil, or in communication with God. Other delusions include possessing infinite knowledge, hearing beautiful music from a primitive source, vertigo with blurred vision, head pain, drowsiness, metallic taste in the mouth.

Dose: a proving of *P. caerulescens* was carried out in 1968 by David Flores Toledo, using mother tinctures of 5C, 6C, 12C, and 30C.

— Vermeulen

Psilocybe (*P. semilanceata*) is for symptoms of the mind including fear of death, euphoria, feelings of unreality, withdrawn and uncommunicative, obsessive compulsive behavior, distortion of time and space, numbness and tingling of limbs, dizziness, hyper-reflexia in deep tendon reflexes, dilated pupils, blurred vision, lively colors, increased auditory acuity, flushing of neck and face, yawning, incontinence, and temporary erythema-like chest eruptions.

Dose: low potency.

— VERMEULEN

Spiritual Properties

Henry Munn wrote a fascinating paper called "The Mushrooms of Language". It can be found in *Hallucinogens and Shamanism,* edited by Michael Harner (Oxford University Press, 1973). In it, he writes:

Language is an ecstatic activity of signification. Intoxicated by the mushrooms, the fluency, the ease, the aptness of expression one becomes capable of are such that one is astounded by the words that issue forth from the contact of the intention of articulation with the matter of experience.... The spontaneity the mushrooms liberate is not only perceptual, but linguistic, the spontaneity of speech, of fervent, lucid discourse, of the logos in activity. For the shaman, it is as if existence were uttering itself through him."

— HENRY MUNN

The principle gift of the psilocybin mushroom is that it allows one to commune directly with the vastly powerful intelligence that is located within all of Nature.... With psilocybin-enhanced perception, I saw the trees without the usual mechanistic associations. They were no longer trees in the mundane sense, but something quite different. It was as if I were seeing for the very first time. And, once again, I was graced with the overall impression, the principal insight, that trees and plants are slowly moving organismic expressions of intelligence. Oaks manifest one kind of intelligence, pine trees another, but both are manifestations of natural intelligence....

I am convinced that the paradigm of natural intelligence, forged in me as a result of my numerous encounters with Nature's wilder side, could play a useful role in restoring our planet's health and healing our dysfunctional relationship with the rest of Nature.... By encouraging extreme ecological sensitivity, psilocybin mushrooms may serve as a kind of medicinal antidote to the poisonous impact of rampant materialism. At the least, the mushrooms can show us how we have severed ourselves from the natural system of intelligence that birthed us and that still sustains our existence.

— SIMON G. POWELL

Much to my surprise and occasional dismay, I was pulled into the heaviest psychic experience I have ever encountered. I was possessed by the mushroom spirit almost as if it sought to teach me a lesson. It now seems that I was drawn into a psychoanalysis, which allowed me to act out my personal conflicts by alternately becoming the conflicting selves and always observing myself at the same time.

Something had suddenly appeared out of the creative depths of my mind, something of which I was previously unaware. I underwent an awesome, fear-filled, but enlightening experience. Without respect you may be pulled into a vortex which you have no desire to enter. If you insist on stepping through the door of ecstasy, then prepare yourself with the writing of such people as John Lilly and Carlos Castaneda.

— RICHARD HAARD

Mycoremediation

Manganese ions at two hundred micromoles increased the effect by four and twelve times respectively. A study of sixteen different polycyclic aromatic hydrocarbons found the higher molecular mass ones more easily converted (Steffen et al. 2003).

Recipes and Dosage

From 0.25 grams of dry mushrooms to 0.75 grams depending upon sensitivity of ingester. Up to two grams or more can be used by more experienced people.

Toxicity is very low. Therapeutic index is 641, compared to aspirin at 199 and nicotine at twenty-one. This index is a ratio of the ED50, or effective dose in 50 percent of subjects versus the LD50 that kills 50 percent of subjects.

The greatest danger is mixing them up with other LBMs, or little brown mushrooms that are lookalikes. Do not combine with MAO-inhibitors or alcohol.

Recent work suggests that the level of psilocin can vary by up to a hundred-fold when grown in dark versus light conditions. This is significant (Rafati et al. 2009).

Bits and Pieces

Psilocybin mushrooms have been declared illegal by a number of countries in the last while. These include Denmark in 2001, Japan in 2002, Britain in 2005, Ireland in 2006, and Holland in 2007. Yet one more example of petty politics getting in the way of good science.

Pulveroboletus ravenelli
(VEILED SULFUR BOLETE)

Widely distributed, the unusual looking veiled sulfur bolete has a bright yellow cottony veil that covers both cap and stalk. It looks like a bolete, but the bright yellow, tall, and slender stalk help in identification.

Traditional Uses

In traditional Chinese medicine, it is used as one of the ingredients of Tendon Easing Powder, which is used to treat lumbago, painful legs, numbed limbs, and even tetany. The yellow powder on its surface is used to stop bleeding from any external wound.

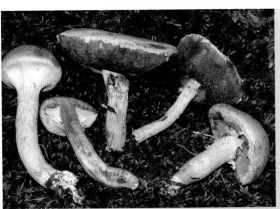

Pulveroboletus ravenelli

Medicinal Use

Chemical Constituents

- **Vulpinic acid; two novel butenolides, isoravenelone and ravenelone; and as pulveraven A and B.**

Duncan et al. (2003) evaluated pulveraven A and B for antimicrobial and COX anti-inflammatory activity, and on mouse mammary cultures at the University of Mississippi.

Pycnoporellus alboluteus
(ORANGE SPONGE POLYPORE)

Pycnoporellus is Greek meaning "countless spores." *Alboluteus* is from the Latin for "yellow and white."

Orange sponge is a soft, spongy polypore growing on the bark grooves of conifers in the Rocky Mountains.

It looks tooth-like, with its large pore openings. They can be surprisingly large considering they grow as annuals. This is a significant decomposer of conifers, starting to grow under snow in the spring.

The polypore starts out orange, then turns yellow, then white, and finally black at end of its life.

Medicinal Use

Early work by Robbins et al. (1945) found activity against *Staphylococcus aureus* on thiamine peptone agar.

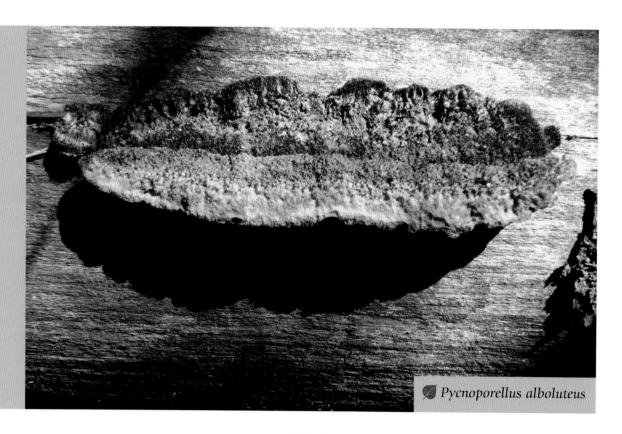

Pycnoporellus alboluteus

Pycnoporus

(see *Trametes*)

Pyrofomes demidoffii

Truncospora demidoffii
Fomes juniperinus
P. juniperinus
Fulvifomes juniperinus
(JUNIPER POLYPORE)

This polypore looks a lot like a *Phellinus* conk, but only grows on juniper, and thus the species name.

Medicinal Use

Early work by Robbins et al. (1945) found activity against *Staphylcoccus aureus* and *E. coli*.

Other work found one compound, pleuromutilin, to possess antitumor activity in clinical studies. To my knowledge, no follow-up work has been conducted.

Radulum orbiculare

Basidioradulum orbiculare

According to David Arora, this fungi "has an irregularly lumpy or warty spore-producing surface that is distinctly reminiscent of regurgitated dog food."

Medicinal Use

Early work by Robbins et al. (1945) found significant activity against both *Staphylococcus aureus* and *E. coli*.

Ramaria botrytis

Clavaria botrytis
(CLUSTERED CORAL)
(PURPLE TIPPED CORAL)
R. aurea
Clavaria aurea
(GOLDEN CORAL)
R. abietina
R. ochraceovirens
(GREEN STAINING CORAL)
R. formosa
(PINK CORAL)
R. flava
(YELLOW RAMARIA)

Clustered coral, like the name suggests, is a brittle, pink-white or purplish fungi with brown tips, found in mixed forest. It is edible and widespread.

Golden coral is greatly prized in many parts of the world. It must be eaten young, as the older specimens are just too leathery and chewy, even for me. After first boil throw away

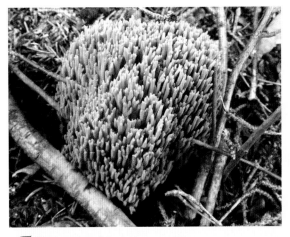

🍃 *Ramaria abietina*

367

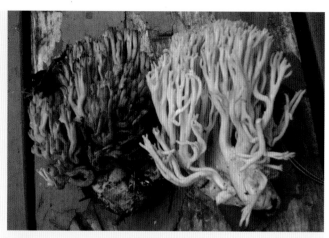

Ramaria stricta (left) and Ramaria flava (right)

the water, and then boil a second time, which helps digestibility. I enjoy the chew.

Green staining coral mushroom is found under coniferous trees. It is common, sometimes difficult to identify, but has a coconut odor and bitter taste.

R. formosa is poisonous and known to cause severe stomach upset and laxative effect.

Yellow *Ramaria* has a high food value at four hundred fifty calories per hundred grams (Colak et al. 2009).

Medicinal Use

Chemical Constituents

- *R. botrytis:* **ergosterol peroxide, cerevisterol, 9alpha-hydroxycerevisterol, (2S,2' R,3R,4E, 8E)-N-2'-hydrooxyoctadecanol-2-amino-9-methyl-4,8-heptadecadiene-1,3-diol, and 5a,6a-epoxy-3beta-hydroxy-(22E)-ergosta8(14),22-dien-7-one.**

Other *Ramaria* species, including *R. flava, R. apiculata,* and *R. formosa* show similar cancer-inhibition rates. The inhibition rate against sar-

coma 180 and Ehrlich carcinoma is from 60 to 70 percent (Ohtsuka et al. 1973).

The fruiting body contains nicotianamine, an amino acid that inhibits angiotensin 1-converting enzyme, and may be useful in cardiovascular disease (Izawa et al. 2006).

Methanol extracts have been found to be hepato-protective via cytochrome P-450 and antioxidant activity (Kim, H.-J. and K.-R. Lee 2003).

Yellow Ramaria *(R. flava)* was a name traditionally given to any yellow species, but is now considered inadequate. One study found *R. flava* to possess antioxidant properties similar to synthetic BHA, and antimicrobial against several *Micrococcus* species and *Yersinia enterocolitica.*

Resupinatus applicatus

Pleurotus applicatus
(BLACK JELLY OYSTER)

Resupinatus is Latin meaning "bent backwards," while *applicatus* means "fixed against something."

Black jelly oyster is a small, black, rubbery bracket fungus that looks like an upside down cup on the underside of logs.

Medicinal Use

Chemical Constituents

- **The mushroom genus contains a number of bioactive sesquiterpenes including 1 (10), 4-germacradiene-2,6,12-triol, and 1,6-farnesadiene-3,10,11-triol, a nerolidol derivative.**

These are the first natural compounds discovered that inhibit cAMP induced appressorium formation in *Magnaporthe grisea* and show cytotoxic activity.

Rhizopogon
(FALSE TRUFFLE)

These small, potato-like fungi are found in sandy soil under douglas fir and pine in late summer and fall.

Traditional Use

In China, spores of the related *R. piceus* are used to stop bleeding by sprinkling the powder directly onto wounds.

Medicinal Use

Recent research has derived the semi-synthetic drug 9 beta-hydroxy anhydro dihydro-artemisinin from this mushroom. This compound is used for anti-malarial activity.

Rhizopogon roseolus, which turns pink with age, has been found as ethanol extract to exhibit activity against *Saccharomyces cerevisiae.* Methanol extracts showed activity against *E. coli, Bacillus subtilis,* and *Enterobacter aerogenes.*

Yamac and Bilgili (2006) found no activity against *S. cerevisiae,* but results showed activity against *Pseudomonas aeruginosa, Staphylococcus aureus,* and *E. coli* from fruiting body extracts.

The mycelium water extracts showed activity against *E. coli* and *S. aureus.*

Mycoremediation

Rhizopogon vinicolor has been found to degrade 2,4-D when supplemented with one mM nitrogen concentration (Donnelly, P. K. et al. 1993).

Experiments with the fungi show some interesting capabilities with regards to the degradation and breakdown of herbicides like atrazine and 2,4D. Is this another possible mycoremediator for northern climates?

Rickenella fibula

Omphalina fibula
Mycena fibula
Gerronema fibula
Hemimycena fibula
Marasmiellus fibula
(ORANGE PIN MUSHROOM)
(PIN MYCENA)

Rickenella is named for the French mycologist A. Ricken. *Fibula* means "hairpin."

This small orange fungus grows in mossy areas across northern Canada. It contains minute amounts of psilocybin.

Ripartites tricholoma
(BEARDED SEAMINE)

This small white fungi appears throughout North America in the fall. Edibility is unknown.

Medicinal Use
Chemical Constituents

- Mycelial culture: illudane riparols A and B and proto-illudane riparol C; psathyrellon A; 5-desoxyilludosin; and 5-demethyllovalicin.

5-demethyllovalicin is a sesquiterpene that inhibits the human methionine amino peptidase-2 and growth of human endothelial cells (Son 2002).

Psathyrellon A (illudane C) is found, as well, in *Psathyrella pseudogracilis* and *Clitocybe illudens* (*Omphalotus olearius*).

Riparol C possesses weak antifungal and antibacterial properties. Riparol A inhibits the growth of MCF and MDA-MB-231 human breast cancer carcinoma at only one microgram per milliliter (Schüffler 2009).

Rozites caperata

R. caperatus
Cortinarius caperatus
(THE GYPSY)

Rozites is named after the nineteenth-century French mycologist Ernest Roze. *Caperata* means "wrinkled." The mushroom has been re-classified to the *Cort* genus, but placed here as most people still know it as *Rozites*.

The gypsy is widespread and common throughout the forests of North America, found singly or in groups on the ground. It is one of my favorite edibles, with a pleasant odor and minty flavor.

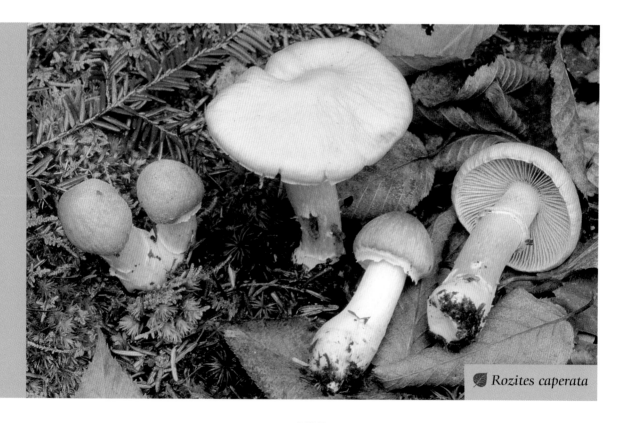

Rozites caperata

Medicinal Use

Chemical Constituents

- **S-2-amino ethyl-4-cysteine.**

A new antiviral, RC-183, has been found to show in vitro activity against herpes simplex I and II, as well as varicella-zoster virus, influenza A virus, and respiratory syncytial virus (Piraino and Brandt 1999).

RC28, an antiviral drug based on a protein molecular weight of twenty-eight kD has been shown to be active against a number of enveloped viruses. Activity against cytomegalovirus has been noted.

It is not active against non-enveloped viruses such as coxsackie and strains of ECHO viruses (Piraino 2005). Work is ongoing.

The fungi contain anti-carcinogenic substances, with inhibition rates against both sarcoma 180 and Ehrlich carcinoma of 70 percent (Ohtsuka et al. 1973).

Bits and Pieces

The related *R. gonglylophora* is cultivated in Brazil by leaf-cutting ants that eat the mycelial hyphae.

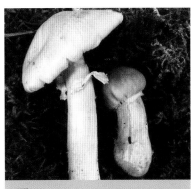

🍂 *Rozites caperata*

Russula

Russula alutacea
(LEATHERY LOOKING RUSSULA)
R. decolorans
(GRAYING RUSSULA)
R. densifolia
(REDDENING RUSSULA)
R. emetica
(THE SICKENER)
R. laurocerasi
(ALMOND RUSSULA)
R. brevipes
(SHORT STALKED RUSSULA)
R. nigricans
R. elephantina
(BLACKENING RUSSULA)
R. xerampelina
(FISHY SMELLING RUSSULA)
(SHRIMP RUSSULA)
R. virescens
(QUILTED GREEN RUSSULA)
(GREEN CRACKING RUSSULA)
R. claroflava
(CHROME YELLOW RUSSULA)
(YELLOW SWAMP RUSSULA)
R. cyanoxantha
(VARIEGATED RUSSULA)
(THE CHARCOAL BURNER)
R. paludosa
(BOG RUSSULA)
(RED TINTED RUSSULA)
R. subnigricans
(RANK RUSSULA)
R. aeruginea
(QUILTED GREEN RUSSULA)

Russula is from the Russian meaning "red," as many members of this genus have red caps.

Alutacea is Latin for "resembling thin leather." *Xerampelina* is Latin "resembling dried grapevine leaves." *Emetica* means "to cause vomiting." *Laurocerasi* is Latin for "the odor of bitter almonds." *Flava* means "yellow" and *virescens* is "greenish." *Paludosa* means "of the bog or swamp."

Rank *Russula (R. subnigricans),* at least the Japanese version, has led to seven deaths in that country. The toxic compound cycloprop-2-ene carboxylic acid has recently been found for the first time in nature (Matsuura et al. 2009).

Graying *Russula* is edible and so named for the change of color after exposure to air. This mushroom contains various proteinase compounds that have pronounced milk-clotting activity.

Reddening *Russula* is found in groups under jack pine. It has a sharp taste and is not recommended as an edible.

The sickener *(R. emetica)* smells fruity, and is usually associated with pine forests. In parts of Slovakia and Hungary, the skin is separated and used to flavor goulash. The rest of the mushroom is discarded. Good idea!

Short stalked *Russula* is closely related to *R. delica,* originally described in Europe and rare in North America. It is pickled or marinated in Russia, but never eaten raw.

Blackening *Russula,* found regularly in the boreal and mixed forests of the west, is inedible.

Quilted green *Russula* has been found in Montana, and in Alberta at the 2006 NAMA foray in Hinton. It is choice and edible, despite its unusual green color. Many experts con-

sider it the best-flavored *Russula,* despite small amounts of hydrazine derivatives that dissipate with cooking.

Variegated *Russula,* known as the charcoal burner due to its large dark green, gray and violet patches that resemble flames, has a faintly nutty flavor and odor. It is edible and best eaten when young.

Bog *Russula (R. paludosa)* is a rosehip-colored species that fruits early and has an unpleasant fresh odor. It grows in moss and is a choice edible when cooked.

In northern Europe, several of the *Russulas* are eaten after parboiling and careful preparation. The toxic chemicals are heat sensitive, but not all species are recommended or choice edibles.

In 1986, Jeff Donaghue wrote in *Toadstool Review:*

> Some books have said that any *Russula* which does not taste acrid is edible. Others will say that even acrid species are OK after being parboiled. While these last two statements may sound a bit careless, there is no *Russula* known that can even come close to killing you. The worst that can happen is that you may be sick to your stomach or have a bit of looseness in the lower digestive tract. But hey, good chili does that!

Culture and Folklore

When the sea had dried so that men appeared, the first two beings, after planting trees and creating food plants, made two mushrooms. The first man threw one of the mushrooms high into the sky, creating the moon, while

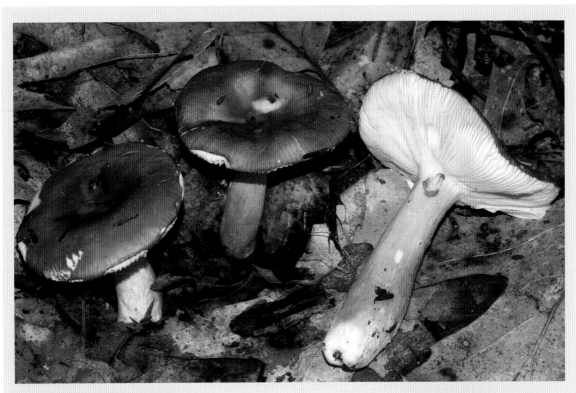

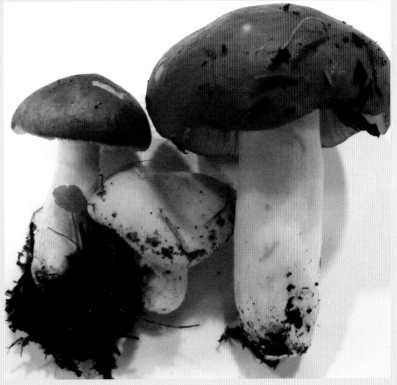

🍃 Clockwise from above: *Russula peckii;* various Russula species; *Russula aeruginea.*

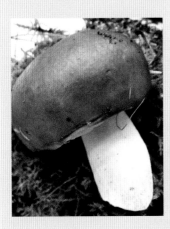

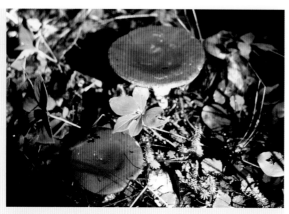

🍃 *Russula borealis*

the first woman tossed the other mushroom upward and formed the sun.

In the Waghi highlands of Papua, New Guinea lives the Kuma tribe, isolated from the rest of the world until the 1930s.

The Kuma have a "mushroom madness" cult that involves the consumption of various species of *Russula* and *Boletus*. The mushrooms are boiled in pots and consumed by the whole community, but only a few individuals appear affected by a "shivering madness" called *komugl tai*. *Komugl* roughly translates as "deafness (to reason)" and *tai* to "the shivering bird of paradise."

A pageant called *kai tamb* is performed prior to ingestion, with the men dressing up in headdresses decorated with yellow bird of paradise feathers. On the second day of the mushroom brew, the women dance the *ndadl*, during which they feel free to vent frustrations with their husbands and boast of their sexual exploits. In a sense, it is a ceremonial opportunity to discuss pent up feelings and issues in a socially acceptable manner. An article by Marie Reay (1977), "Ritual Madness Observed: A Discarded Pattern of Fate in Papua New Guinea," reveals more.

Traditional Uses

Leathery looking *Russula* and reddening *Russula* are used in traditional Chinese medicine as a component of Tendon Easing Powder, for curing lumbago, painful and numb limbs, and discomfort in bones. The related *R. integra,* also known as *R. polychroma*, is also used in Tendon Easing Powder.

The fungus is used effectively for the treatment of dysentery in China.

In China, where it is classified sweet and slightly sour, the dried fungus is used to cure ophthalmocopia, or eyestrain, remove fire from the liver meridian, dissipate heat, and ease constriction of vital energy. It is often given to women suffering poor energy circulation, and is recommended to be taken with ginger in decoction.

The fruiting body of *R. vinosa,* also known as *R. obscura* and *R. decolorans var. obscura,* is cooked in Asia to cure postpartum anemia.

Medicinal Use

Short stalked *Russula* possesses strong antioxidant activity and antimicrobial activity against a variety of gram-positive bacteria including *Salmonella* and *Yersinia* species, *Klebsiella pneumoniae,* and *Staphylococcus aureus*.

The four fungi mentioned above all possess inhibition rates against sarcoma 180 ranging from 60 to 100 percent, and Ehrlich carcinoma from 60 to 90 percent (Ohtsuka et al. 1973).

Almond *Russula* inhibits the cancer cell lines 90 percent and 80 percent respectively (Ohtsuka et al. 1973).

Various *Russula* contain russuphelins that have shown activity against leukemia P388 cells lines (Takahashi 1993).

Blackening *Russula* contains more than eighty percent ergosterols.

Research found *R. nigricans* to possess strong anti-mutagenic activity.

Inhibition of sarcoma 180 and Ehrlich carcinoma is 60 percent (Ohtsuka et al. 1973).

Work by Mao Xiaolan (1998) suggests the fruiting bodies possess antitumor activity.

Nigricanin is the first ellagic acid from higher fungi, and was isolated from the fruiting body by Tan et al. (2004). Ellagic acid is found in strawberries, raspberries, and various nuts, and possesses both antioxidant and antitumor properties.

A dichloromethane extract has been found active against *Biomphalaria glabrata* (Keller, C. et al. 2002).

One rat study of quilted green *Russula* suggests it may be helpful in blood cholesterol reduction. The same study showed reduced liver enzyme markers related to liver and oxidative stress, as well as increased levels of SOD.

Galactomannan content is believed responsible for free radical scavenging (Sun, Y. et al. 2010a).

Studies in laboratories show an inhibition rate of 70 percent for both sarcoma 180 and Ehrlich carcinoma (Ohtsuka et al. 1973).

Chrome yellow *Russula* is a bright yellow, edible species with a pleasant vanilla or coumarin-like odor. Studies have found gold levels of 136 nanograms per gram in the fruiting body. Organic gold has a number of medicinal properties, including the treatment of various forms of depression and rheumatoid arthritis.

The similar looking *R. ochroleuca* contains termitomycesphin E. As the name suggests, these compounds are commonly found in *Termitomyces* species associated with termite nests. A Chinese edible, *T. albuminosus,* contains various termitomycesphins that induce neuronal differentiation in rat PC12 cells.

Variegated *Russula* contains a ceramide with an unusual sphingoid base and could hold the basis of a new medicine, as sphingolipids help anchor lipid-bound carbohydrates to cell surfaces and create an epidermal water permeability barrier; participating in both antigen-antibody reactions and biological information transmission (Kolter and Sandhoff 1999; Gao, J. M. et al. 2001). Early work found this mushroom inhibited growth of sarcoma 180 and Ehrlich carcinoma cell lines by 70 percent and 60 percent respectively.

Lepidamine, isolated from the related *R. lepida,* is the first aristolane-type sesquiterpene alkaloid isolated from nature. Lepidolide has also been identified (Tan et al. 2002, 2003).

A novel lectin in this species exhibits activity against Hep G2 and MCF-7 breast cancer cell lines.

Inhibition rate of cultured mycelia against sarcoma 180 is 100 percent.

The related *R. adusta* shows 80 percent inhibition of both sarcoma 180 and Ehrlich carcinoma cell lines, and the related *R. crustosa* 70 percent inhibition. *Russula lilacea* inhibits the cell lines 60 to 70 percent, comb *Russula (R. soraria)* by 60 percent, and *R. sanguinea (R. rosacea)* and *R. vesca* up to 90 percent.

Blushing red *Russula (R. rubescens)* shows inhibition of 70 percent and 60 percent respectively, while *R. sanguinea,* another red *Russula,* shows 90 percent inhibition against both cancer cell lines.

The related European species *R. foetens* has been found to inhibit sarcoma 180 and Ehrlich carcinoma cancer cell lines by 70 percent. Likewise for *R. aurea.*

Work by H. Wang and T. B. Ng (2007) found extracts from *R. paludosa* inhibit HIV-1 reverse transcriptase by 97.6 percent. One fraction, SU2, showed an IC50 of eleven micromoles, suggesting further investigation in regards to a natural product for AIDS.

Shrimp *Russula (R. xerampelina)* demonstrated activity against malaria-inducing *Plasmodium falciparum* (Lovy et al. 1999).

Homeopathy

Russula emetica (Agaric emetic) is used for severe vertigo, indicated in part by a longing for cold water, which relieves symptoms. There may be gastritis, with an ice-cold sweat, vertigo, weakness, sneezing, vomiting, and a sensation as if the stomach was suspended on a string. Sensations of deadly nausea and dislike of wine and meat are noted.

Dose: low potency as needed (Boericke).

Sarcodon imbricatus
(SCALY HEDGEHOG)
S. aspratus
(KOOTAKE)

Sarcodon is Greek meaning "fleshy tooth" and *imbricatus* is Latin meaning "covered with scales."

Scaly hedgehog is found throughout the Pacific Northwest and north to the Yukon and Alaska amongst coniferous forests. It is a very popular edible with mycophiles from eastern Europe.

The young specimens can be eaten after cooking, and the older, slightly bitter caps are better when boiled first and then fried. I find them an excellent edible.

This mushroom contains nearly 26 percent protein, with seven essential amino acids making up nearly 43 percent of the total. It is high in potassium, calcium, and magnesium.

Medicinal Use

The sphorophore of scaly hedgehog lowers blood cholesterol levels in lab animals.

The fruiting body shows antibacterial activity against *E. coli, Enterobacter aerogenes, Salmonella typhimurium, Staphylococcus aureus, S. epidermis,* and *Bacillus subtilis* (Yamac and Bilgili 2006).

Four different solvent extracts have been found to be active against *B. subtilis.*

The related *S. aspratus* has been studied and found active in reducing inflammation, lesions, and plaque associated with cardiovascular risk (Ryong et al. 1989).

Takei et al. (2005) found acetone extracts markedly inhibited the growth of HL-60

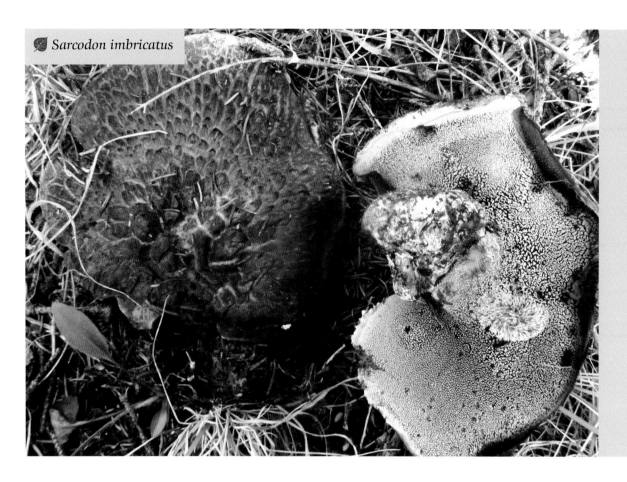

Sarcodon imbricatus

human leukemia cells and induced apoptosis after twenty-four hours of incubation. The main active component was identified as ergosterol peroxide, with complete inhibition at twenty-five micrometers.

A fucogalactan, isolated from the fungus, elicited the release of TNF-alpha and NO in macrophages. The TNF-alpha production with one-tenth the amount of lentinan was approximately 4.3-fold. The author suggests that the immune modulating effect may contribute to antitumor activity in tumor-bearing hosts as well as various immunomodulating effects.

One study identified a sterol, 9(11)-DHEP, that is a very effective inhibitor of HL-60 cell growth and strong apoptosis. It also inhibits HT29 colon and adenocarcinoma cells but not normal cells by inducing CDKN1A expression.

A water-soluble polysaccharide stimulates cultured mice spleen lymphocytes, suggesting immune enhancement.

The related *S. cyrneus* contains cyrneines A and B, both of which significantly promote neurite outgrowth. Neither showed cytotoxity at one hundred micromoles. The same author identified cyrneine C and D, as well as claucopine C.

Activity on neuritis suggests nerve growth factors at play.

Sarcoscypha coccinea

Plectania coccinea

(SCARLET CUP FUNGUS)

This cup fungus, more common in cold weather, has a bright red surface on fertile interior, with a whitish exterior. It is associated with willow, alder, and poplar forests.

The coloration is due to carotenoids such as beta-carotene and plectaniaxanthin. The mushroom does contain lectin-binding lactose, N-acetylatosamine, N-nitrophenyl-beta-D-gluco, and galacto-pyranosides.

Schizophyllum commune

(SPLITGILL)

Split gill (*Schizophyllum commune*) is a fan-shaped, grayish-white, and unusual fungi found on living and decaying poplar, sometimes on birch, and occasionally on spruce and pine.

It has unique, lengthwise, split gills that fold back in dry weather, with no stalk to speak of. The fungus is very common, and found worldwide, as the species name infers.

It is used in Mexican cooking, with sesame seed and beans.

In Zaire, it is first boiled for several hours with vegetable salt to tenderize, and then served with peanuts, salt, and oil for seasoning. It is also consumed throughout India and Southeast Asia.

It is probably prudent to avoid eating raw. People who have done so have been found to have abnormal growths in the mouth and throat that, upon isolation, were shown to be schizophyllum.

Traditional Uses

In traditional Chinese medicine, the fungus is considered to have a sweet taste and be very mild in nature. It is recommended for general weakness and debility.

In China, it is sometimes cooked with eggs to make a preparation for leucorrhea.

In Mexico, it is considered by natural healers to have a cold energetic quality, reducing fevers and inflammation.

Medicinal Use

Chemical Constituents

- **Cysteine and glutamine, 17 percent protein, schizophyllan or sizofiran (SPG) (1-3-alpha-D-glucarin- polysaccharide), cholesterol oxidase, schizostatin, a novel phenylalanine specific amino peptidase, a branded D-glucotetraose, multiple proteases, invertase and ferulic acid esterase activity, acid phosphatase isozymes, schizoflavins, various cerebrosides, glucoceramide, and two amino-isobutyric acids.**

- **The dried fungus contains, per one hundred grams, 280 milligrams iron, 646 milligrams phosphorus, and ninety milligrams calcium.**

Schizophyllum shows antitumor activity against both the solid and ascites forms of sarcoma 180, Ehrlich carcinoma, as well as Yoshida and sarcoma 37 and lung carcinoma (Komatsu et al. 1969; Yamamoto, T. et al. 1981).

In Lithuania, the mushroom is noted for its antitumor activity. One German study found it decreased sarcoma 180 tumors by 99 percent at the rate of only one milligram per kilogram (2.2 pounds) of body weight.

It has been shown to increase immunity by restoring suppressed killer-cell activity to normal levels in mice with tumors.

The fungus is anti-infective against *Pseudomonas aeruginosa, Staphylococcus aureus, E. coli,* and *Klebsiella pneumoniae.*

Schizophyllum is structurally similar to lentinan, an active component of shiitake, but differs in that it does not directly activate T-cell production.

In 1992, Dr. Uchida at Kyoto University announced he had tested the beta-glucans in eleven chronic fatigue syndrome patients, with ten showing improvement. Of these, three were able to return to work, and the other seven, some so ill they could not walk a flight of stairs, resumed "a regular life." For all ten patients, their NK-cell activity levels were restored to normal.

By the summer of 1993, thirty more patients, including some Americans and Canadians, were treated with twenty milligrams per day of SPG. After one to two months, more than 90 percent found their debilitating fatigue reduced or gone entirely, without any side effects.

Serum levels of interleukin 2, which previously were elevated, returned to normal. Elevated levels would tend to indicate immune activity, since these receptors are found on the membrane of T-cells in an activated state. However, the responsiveness of T-cells to activations by interleukin-2 only returned to CFS patients after SPG therapy. It is worth noting that patients with major depression also show higher than normal levels of interleukin-2.

In a normal, healthy person, interleukin-2 causes NK-cells to become active. But Dr. Uchida (1995) found that interleukin-2 receptors on the NK-cells of CFS patients were normal, and yet the NK-cells would not respond to the interleukin 2 signals to become active. After administering SPG, they did. This is exciting news for long time sufferers of chronic fatigue syndrome and related autoimmune conditions of unknown origin. A patent

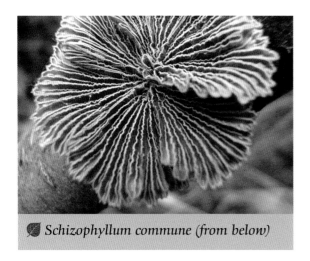

Schizophyllum commune (from below)

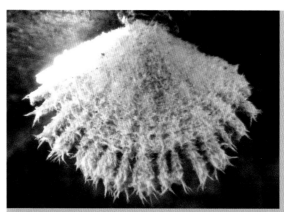

Schizophyllum commune (from above)

was issued in the same year for proprietary preparation.

Beta-D-glucans bind to membrane complement receptor type 3 on immune effector cells. The ligand receptor complex can be internalized, and the intracellular events that occur have been poorly understood to this point. Schizophyllan has been shown able to bind the mRNA poly(A) tail. The molecular weight, branching pattern, and presence of single and triple helices all significantly alter the activity of beta-glucans. In general, and with some exceptions such as the MD fraction of *Grifola frondosa,* higher antitumor activity is associated with higher molecular weight, lower levels of branching, and greater water solubility.

The greatest improvements with SPG were reduction of swollen lymph nodes, sore muscles, neuropsychological problems and pharyngitis.

It is distributed in the body in macrophages, tissues next to tumors, and in the bone marrow, lymph nodes, liver, and spleen.

In the bone marrow cells of mice, it has been shown to inhibit chromosomal damage caused by chemotherapy drugs and radiation.

The best results were obtained when administered shortly after radiation, and restored mitosis of bone marrow cells previously suppressed by drugs.

Human studies with recurrent and inoperable gastric cancer on 367 patients showed significantly longer life span when schizophyllan was combined with chemotherapy.

In combination with radiation, it significantly prolonged the five-year survival rate of stage II cervical cancer patients, but not stage III patients. However, those given the fungi extract showed more "significantly rapid" restoration of T-lymphocyte levels following radiation than controls.

Schizophyllan when injected intra-tumor to cervical cancer showed significant infiltration of Langerhans' cells, as well as T-cells (Nakano et al. 1996).

Schizophyllan increases interferon-g production, making it beneficial to hepatitis B patients. This is due to enhanced response to the virus through production of interferon-g.

Yo Kimura et al. (1994) showed schizophyllan an assistant to immuno-therapy in the treatment of neck and head cancers, increasing survival rates of patients receiving the compound.

Enhancement of Th1 immune response from mycelium has been shown.

C. H. Han et al. (2005) identified a novel homodimeric lactose binding lectin with potent mitogenic activity, anti-proliferation to tumor cell lines, and inhibition of HIV-1 reverse transcriptase. This was from the fresh fruiting body of split gill, with stability up to forty degrees Celsius (104 degrees Fahrenheit).

Schizostatin, another derivative, is a potent squalene synthase inhibitor.

D-glucotetraose is an interesting component as it is part of the repeating unit of extracellular polysaccharides found in maitake, a very well researched fungi with antitumor activity.

In Japan, cultured broth products are produced, called Sizofiran, Sonifilan, SPG, or Schizophyllan. Produced by Kaken Pharmaceutical of Tokyo, SPG is now mainly used in the treatment of cervical cancer.

One study identified a lectin that exhibits potent mitogenic activity toward splenocytes and anti-proliferation against tumor lines, and inhibits HIV reverse transcriptase (Han, C. H. et al. 2005).

Schizophyllan (1-3-alpha-D-gluco-pyranan) is found in razor strop *(Piptoporus betulinus),* a much larger and more common bracket fungus in northern boreal forests.

Cosmetics

A U.S. patent (5320849) involves liquid cultivation for isolated branched glucans with applications for skin aging, whitening, and repairing skin damage.

Mycoremediation

This mushroom has been well researched by the pulp and paper industry for de-colorization of mill effluent.

It removed nearly 80 percent of the color in five days in one study. Other work, by Belsare and Prasad (1988), also found efficacy in decolorization of effluent from pulp.

It has application in L-malic acid fermentation production.

Cultivation

Growing the mushroom under controlled conditions is best achieved at twenty-five degrees Celsius (seventy-seven degrees Fahrenheit) and 5.5 pH, with a mannitol or sorbitol substrate and sufficient B2 and B6.

Recipe and Dosage

Nine to sixteen grams as a decoction up to three times per day. Prepare at a 1:5 ratio.

Bits and Pieces

It is a very hardy fungus. Dr. Buller, a famous Canadian mycologist, showed that specimens enclosed in glass tubes for thirty-five years were still able to sporulate!

Like most fungi, *S. commune* fungal filaments pair with another. These must be of differing "mating types," and in this particular mushroom some twenty-eight thousand kinds of pairings are possible, since unlike humans, there are more than two genders.

Cerebroside A on rice leaves induced the accumulation of antimicrobial compounds (phytoalexin), cell death, and increased resistance to subsequent infection by compatible pathogens.

Scleroderma geaster

S. polyrhizon
(DEAD MAN'S HAND)
(EARTHSTAR SCLERODERMA)
S. verrucosum
(EARTHBALL)
(WARTED DEVIL'S SNUFFBOX)
(ROOTING TOUGHSKIN)
(SMOOTH EARTHBALL)
S. citrinum
S. aurantium
Lycoperdon aurantium
(PIGSKIN POISON PUFFBALL)
(COMMON EARTHBALL)

Scleroderma is Greek meaning "tough skin." *Citrinum* means "lemon yellow" and *verrucosum* means "full of small warts."

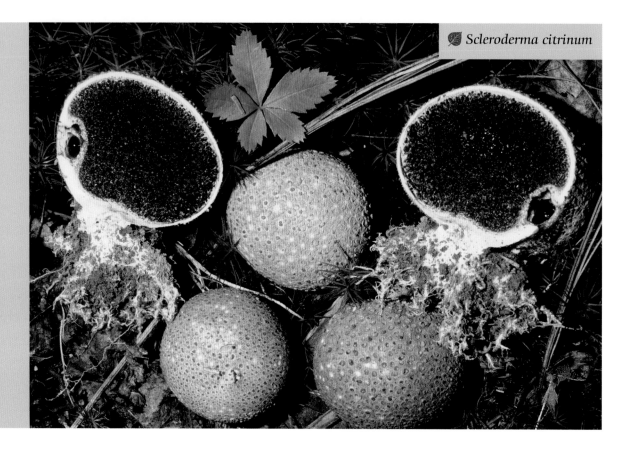

Scleroderma citrinum

Dead man's hand resembles a hard puffball. It matures and splits open like a *Geastrum* and takes on the look of the outstretched palm of a buried corpse.

They can be mistaken, initially, for puffballs but have a hard, thick skin with a purplish to black interior. This species is poisonous, not edible. Another difference is that puffballs are saprophytic, while this one is mycorrhizal.

Some *Scleroderma* species, such as *S. citrinum* or pigskin poison puffball, are considered poisonous, and yet they have been used in several cultures to cause narcosis and visual disturbance.

It is sometimes canned in central Europe and sold as a substitute for truffle. It is way too pun-gent to be used as a condiment. Although not recommended, the dose is one half of an unripe fruiting body. It has a distinct rubbery smell.

In Germany, it is known as *kartoffel bovist,* or "potato bovist."

According to Adrian Morgan, his personal experience ingesting one half a small specimen resulted in a deep sleep of two hours, followed by a period of restlessness and pupil dilation. The chemical structure has not been identified.

The related *S. verrucosum* is believed to contain psychoactive compounds, as well.

Traditional Uses

In China, the mushroom is used to counteract swelling, stop bleeding, and cure hemorrhage from external cuts or wounds. It is used for watery chilblains, with an appropriate amount of powdered spores applied to the wound.

Medicinal Use

Chemical Constituents

- *Scleroderma citrinum:* **contains norbadine A, sclerocitrin, badione A, xerocomic, methyl 4,4'-dimethoxyvulpinate, 4,4'dimethoxyvulpinic acid, and a lanostane-type triterpenoid. Sclerocitrin, which provides the distinct yellow color, is found up to four hundred milligrams per kilogram. It is also present in** *Chalciporus piperatus.*

The lanostane-type triterpenoid exhibits significant antiviral activity against herpes simplex, while vulpinic acid derivatives exhibit activity against *Mycobacterium tuberculosis,* as well as cytotoxicity against the NCI-h187 cell line.

Fungi Essences

Earthball *(S. citrinum)* essence is for those who think they are not good enough, lack self-worth, or boundaries. It helps to sustain grounding when life becomes difficult when working through transformation.

— BYRNAHERB

Earthball essence is for difficult life situations, for crises and helping one maintain and review so that one does not fear it and has possible solutions.

— MARIANA

Frans Vermeulen speculates that "on the basis of analogy / signature *Scleroderma* might be considered for scleroderma (thickening of the skin caused by swelling and thickening

of fibrous tissue) and cellulite. The Dutch name for the latter condition, *sinaasappelhuid* ('orange peel skin'), wonderfully matches the specific name *aurantia,* orange peel."

Sclerospora graminicola

Millet hosts a pathogenic fungus that infects both the leaf blades and flowers. The chlorophyll of infected blades disappears and the blades break up into spreading, thin-stranded filaments called "white hair disease."

The flowers also change into long-leafed floral buds that are hairy.

The diseased spikes are collected in the fall and dried in the sun.

Traditional Uses

In traditional Chinese medicine, the diseased spikes are prized for their diuretic and antipyretic properties.

For debility and edema, agitation, thirst and lack of urine flow, it will increase diuresis.

Agriculture

Chloroform extracts of *Ganoderma applanatum* have been found to inhibit growth of this pathogen in greenhouses.

Recipe and Dosage

For urethritis and prickly pain during urination, decoct six to fifteen grams chaff of infected grain with water and drink at body temperature two times per day.

Sclerotinia species

These small cup-shaped fungi are often found in vegetable gardens, where they injure members of the legume, cabbage, or nightshade families.

They produce spores from a hard black fungus or sclerotium in a manner similar to tuckahoe.

Medicinal Use

In Japan, researchers have been fermenting and culturing *S. sclerotiorum* for many years and have isolated a dextran or polysaccharide that inhibits the growth of sarcoma 180.

They contain sclerin and sclerolide, which are co-metabolites of sclerotinin A and B, related to citrinin, and other isocoumarins. These are plant growth promoters. Sclerothionine is a sulphur containing imidazole isolated from *S. libertiana* cultured on bran.

Studies indicate *Sclerotinia* species may possess tumor inhibition.

Serpula lacrymans

Gyrophana lacrymans
Merulius lacrymans
(DRY ROT FUNGUS)

This is a serious, destructive fungus in older wooden houses, often developing in poorly ventilated areas under floorboards. Dry rot is so named because it extracts moisture from the wood and cracks it into small cubes that eventually crumble into a fine, dark dust.

Medicinal Use

Studies have shown the fungus to inhibit the growth of sarcoma 180 by 70 percent and that of Ehrlich carcinoma by 60 percent.

Early work by Hervey (1947) found significant activity against *Staphylococcus aureus.*

A culture of the related *S. himantiodes,* often found on dead conifers, produced antibiotic metabolites as well as himanimide C, which exhibits antifungal activity against *Alternaria porri, Aspergillus ochraceus,* and *Pythium irregulare.* It is cytotoxic to HL-60 and L1210 human cancer cell lines.

The vaguely related wet rot *(Coniophora puteana)* shows moderate activity against *S. aureus.* Robbins et al. (1945) found the related *C. cerebella* and *C. suffocata* active against both *S. aureus* and *E. coli.*

Essential Oil

Gas chromatography of *S. lacrymans* essential oil reveals nineteen constituents, including 1-octen-3-ol and 2-methylbutanal.

Mycoremediation

Research has found activity against various chemical toxins, including chromated copper arsenate and polycyclic aromatic hydrocarbons.

It shows tolerance to copper citrate.

Bits and Pieces

Culture growth is greatly increased by exposure to infrared rays.

Sparassis crispa

S. radicata

S. ramosa

S. spathulata

Manina crispa

Masseola crispa

(SPONGE FUNGUS)

(CAULIFLOWER FUNGUS)

Sparassis is from the Greek meaning "torn apart," while *crispa* means "curly." The French call it fall morel.

This unusual fungus grows at the foot of coniferous trees, looking just like a wild cauliflower, hence the common name. They can be quite large, up to nearly a meter across and weighing more than thirty kilograms (sixty-six pounds). You will most frequently find them on the east side of pine or spruce facing east and protected from the prevailing winds.

It is a prized edible, with a very fragrant tea-like scent; but it must be cooked for a long time unless you enjoy chewy food. The initial scent of latex and ammonia changes with cooking, resulting in a good textured addition to dishes.

For best results cook for at least one hour in chicken broth and then remove and slice thinly. Individual leaflets can be battered with tempura and deep-fried. I prefer the chewy texture in stir-fry.

The western species is considered to be *S. radicata* and the eastern species, *S. spathulata*. *S. crispa* is found in Europe and parts of eastern North America. All are delicious.

Medicinal Use

Chemical Constituents

- **Sarassol, 348 micrograms benzoic acid per gram, eighteen micrograms caffeic acid per gram, thirty-six micrograms narigenin per gram, twenty-four micrograms quercitin per gram, and thirty-eight grams p-coumaric acid per gram, as well as xanthoangelol and 4-hydroxyderricin.**

Antifungal metabolites have been identified.

One constituent, sparassol, possesses antifungal and antibiotic activity. Unknown, and unnamed constituents inhibit various *Bacillus* species.

Sparassol was isolated and named by Falck in 1923 and is one of the earliest crystalline antibiotics to be examined.

Work by St. Pfau, Spath, and Jeschki in 1924 found the substance identical to the methyl ester of everninic acid, obtained from the lichen *Evernia prunastri,* isolated in 1848 by Stenhouse.

C. Keller et al. (2002) found dichloromethane extracts active against *B. subtilis* and *E. coli,* and molluscicidal on *Biomphalaria glabrata.* Early work by Hervey (1947) and Robbins et al. (1945) showed activity against *E. coli* and *S. aureus.*

A novel bioactive compound and another also present in *Antrodia camphorata* inhibits melanin synthesis by melanoma cancer cells and inhibit the growth of MRSA, or methicillin-resistant *Staphylococcus aureus* (Kawagishi et al. 2007)

Research by Ohno et al. (2002) looked at this edible and medicinal mushroom that is cultivated in Japan, and known as *hanabiratake.*

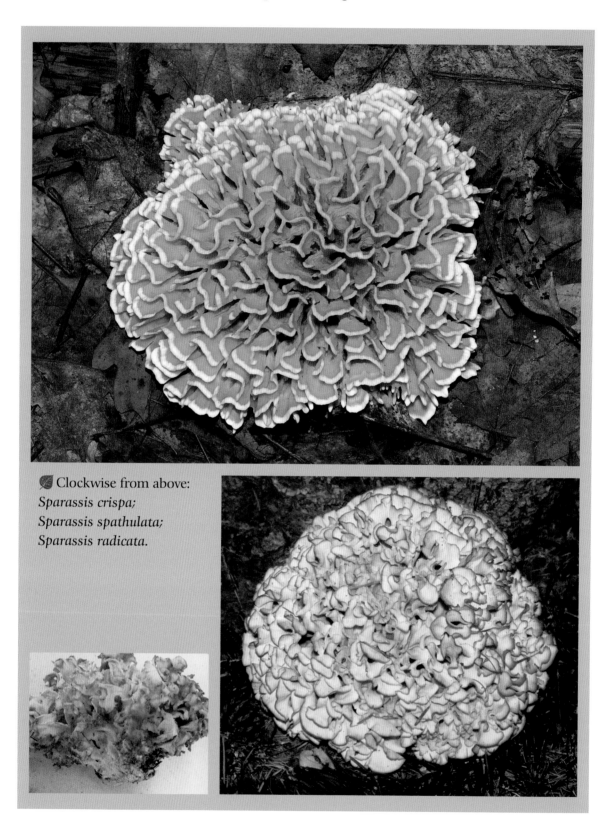

Clockwise from above:
Sparassis crispa;
Sparassis spathulata;
Sparassis radicata.

It contains over 40 percent of six-branched 1,3-beta-glucans, which show antitumor activity. The beta-glucan fraction can be extracted with cold dilute sodium hydroxide.

One research team identified a polysaccharide with antitumor activity. Both sarcoma 180 and Ehrlich carcinoma were 100 percent suppressed during in vitro studies, and the hematopoietic response was enhanced.

Petrova et al. (2007) found a diethyl ether extract inhibits the degradation of IkBalpha, associated with anticancer potential.

K. Yamamoto et al. (2009) found *Sparassis* helps suppress angiogenesis and metastasis in lung cancer cell lines.

Mouse studies found the extract modulated recovery rates in cyclophosphamide-induced leukopenia. In Peyer's patches, recovery of the T-cell/B-cell ratio was faster than controls, and in vitro, both interleukin-6 and interferon gamma production are enhanced. This strongly suggests improved hematopoietic response due to enhanced cytokine production (Ohno et al. 2002).

Ohno et al. (2003) looked at the enhanced cytokine capacity of the beta-glucan extract in healthy volunteers. Three hundred milligram capsules were given orally to several cancer patients, with improvement after several months in nine of the fourteen patients, suggesting possible application to human cancer immunotherapy.

Human NK cell cytotoxicity was enhanced without increasing the number of NK-cells, suggesting that oral intake activates Th1 cell, and inhibits Th2 cell activation, promoting a shift toward Th1 dominant immunity.

One study showed activity on human leukocytes, including enhancement of IL-8 synthesis, release of complement fragment C5a, and induction of anti-beta-glucan natural antibody in human plasma.

Harada et al. found six branched 1,3 beta D-glucans induced cytokines by granulocyte macrophage colony stimulating factor (Harada et al. 2004). Earlier work in by the same research team found the glucans enhanced the hematopoietic response in mice treated with cyclophosphamide (Harada et al. 2002a).

Harada et al. (2006b) also found polysaccharide fractions show strong antitumor activity against sarcoma 180 and in cyclophosphamide induced leukopenic mice. Sodium hydroxide treatment of the hot-water extracts decreased the hematopietic response of cytokine induction. Immune-modulating effects of the mushroom are significantly modified by the method of preparation.

The same author found SCG from this mushroom completely abolished cytokine activity in dendritic cells from dectin 1-knockout mice (Harada et al. 2008).

The mushroom appears to relieve rhinitis through induction of IFNgamma but at the same time inhibits IL-4 and IL-5 secretion. Serum IgE levels were also reduced.

Harada et al. (2002b) found polysaccharides induce interferon gamma and interleukin-12 p70 production. They earlier identified tumor necrosis factor alpha and granulocyte-macrophage colony stimulating factor by the beta-glucans.

Further work found the glucans synergistic with soy isoflavones, suggesting a model for

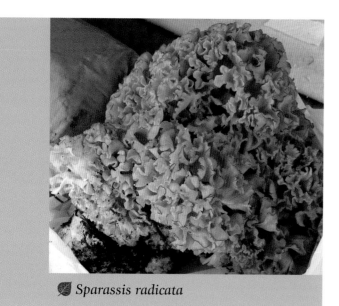

Sparassis radicata

hormone sensitive cancer cell lines (Harada et al. 2005).

More recent work by Harada et al. (2006a, 2006c) suggests that cell-to-cell contact and soluble factors are important for cytokine induction by the beta-glucans, and specifically that increased levels of GM-CSF and dectin-1 (a beta-glucan receptor) expression are crucial to this induction.

It appears that the mushroom supports innate immunity through activation of macrophages, induction of dectin-1 receptor and inflammatory cytokines, and secretion of inflammatory cytokine influence by TLR4 stimulation (Kim, S. I. et al. 2009).

Petrova et al. (2005) suggest that the mushroom inhibits breast cancer activity.

Compounds other than beta-glucans from hot-water extracts were found to suppress tumor growth, increase IFN-gamma production, and reduce the growth of new blood vessels that accompany tumor growth (angiogenesis). These low molecular weight compounds enhance the Th-1 response, at least in mice studies (Yamamoto, K. et al. 2007).

Three antifungal compounds have been found in submerged culture, including sparassol, ScI, and ScII; the latter two show the greatest activity against *Cladosporium cucumerinum.*

A hot-water extract of the mushroom inhibits HIV by over 50 percent at a concentration of only one milligram per milliliter (Wang, H. and T. B. Ng 2007).

Kodani et al. (2008) were screening for MRSA (methicillin-resistant *S. aureus*) activity and found two chalcones previously isolated from *Angelica keiskei*. This is the first report of chalcones from the fungal kingdom, and may have potential for production of these two compounds, xanthoangelol and 4-hydroxyderricin.

Xanthoangelol has been found to lower blood pressure and reduce lipid metabolism and LDL levels in stroke-prone hypertensive rats.

The mushroom may ameliorate cerebrovascular and othelial dysfunction and may be useful for preventing stroke and hypertension (Yoshotomi 2011).

It induces apoptosis of stomach cancer cells. The compound inhibits gastric H(+)-ATPase.

Xanthoangelol D improves vascular health via NFkappaB activation.

One study found the compound effective for neuroblastoma and leukemia apoptosis via activating capase 3, but not involving Bx/Bcl-2 signal transduction.

It has the same antibiotic effect as gentamicin on *Micrococcus luteus* (Inamori et al. 2008).

Xanthoangelol is anti-metastatic and antitumor in activity (Kimura, Yoshiyuki and Kimiye Baba 2003).

Oral consumption of the mushroom helped promote healing of impaired diabetic wounds. It appears to directly increase synthesis of type 1 collagen.

The fungus has been found "effective in suppressing blood sugar levels," according to a recent Japan Scan Food Industry bulletin. No commercial products are presently marketed and available in North America.

Hyuk-Gu Park et al. (2009) found nanoparticle extraction of beta 1>3-D-glucans very efficient with 90 percent water soluble after only ten minutes of incubation.

Cultivation

Their growth can be promoted by inoculating tree stumps with spored dowels or simply burying the stem butts in the ground near a tree base with a fresh root wound. According to Paul Stamets, the long taproot can be replanted and will regrow. He believes it a valuable ally in preventing the spread of honey mushrooms (*Armillaria* species) by outcompeting for the tree without killing the host.

Stamets plans to inoculate the perimeter of a clear-cut forest populated with *Armillaria* to research whether fungal barriers can be effective reforestation tools.

Mycoremediation

The fungus uptakes arsenic in affected zones, suggesting mycoremediation potential.

Stereum hirsutum

(HAIRY STEREUM)
(HAIRY PARCHMENT)
S. subtomentosum
S. ostrea
(FALSE TURKEY TAIL)

Hairy parchment (*Stereum hirsutum*) is a cinnamon-colored bracket fungus found on birch and other deciduous trees. It shelves and overlaps in two-centimeter by two-centimeter strips leathery strips that become gray with age. It often shares logs with witch's butter (*Tremella mesenterica*). It has an affinity for felled logs, often found growing on the cut face.

False turkey tail is often mistaken for *Trametes versicolor*. Some authors consider *S. ostrea* and *S. subtomentosum* to be the same mushroom while others disagree. I can't tell.

Stereum complicatum is found on branches and twigs of hardwood trees in eastern and central North America. They are plentiful and beautiful to the eye.

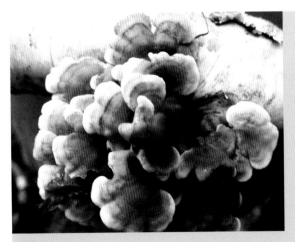

Stereum hirsutum

Medicinal Use

Chemical Constituents

- *S. hirsutum:* **hursutic acids, sterin A and B, ergosta-7,22-dien-3b-ol, mycosporine, sterelactones, stereumin A-E, and epidoxysterols 1-4.**

- *S. vibrans:* **vibralactone.**

- *S. complicatum:* **vibralactone.**

Stereumin A-E are canadine sesquiterpenoids grown in culture broth. The D fraction showed particularly aggressive nematicidal activity against *Panagrellus redivivus* (Li, P. et al. 2007).

The fungi produce hirsutic acids, among which the A version inhibits the growth of suppurated *Micrococcus pyogenes,* and the N version inhibits the growth of *Diptheria bacilli* and *Neisseria meningitidis.*

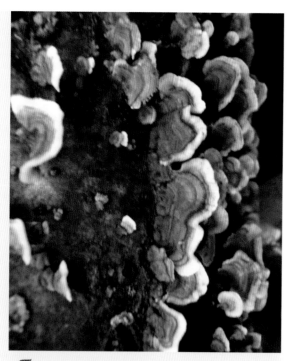

Stereum hirsutum

The whole mushroom possesses antibiotic activity. One study showed activity against *Bacillus cereus.* Another study showed activities against *B. subtilis, E. coli, Staphylococcus aureus,* and *Salmonella typhimurium.*

Hirsutic acid A has been found to inhibit *S. aureus* at a ratio of one in eight thousand.

Sterelactones, new isolactaronetype sesquiterpenoids, show antifungal activity (Opatz et al. 2008).

The mushroom contains ergosta-7,22-dien-3b-ol and hirsutic acid C, an inactive precursor of antibacterial activity with an unknown structure.

The compounds sterin A and B inhibit lipid peroxidation, suggesting antioxidant properties (Yun et al. 2002b).

The same author identified hirutenol F with an EC_{50} of 0.39 micromoles.

It contains mycosporine, with yet unknown properties. Cultured broths contain tricyclic sesquiterpenes, hirsutenols A-C (Yun et al. 2002a).

Work by Hervey in 1947 suggested moderate activity against *S. aureus* and *E. coli.*

Epidoxysterols 1-4 show significant activity against *Mycobacterium tuberculosis.*

A dry extract inhibits thrombin by 34 percent in a docking manner similar to phosphonate thrombin inhibitors.

The mycelium of the related *S. subpileatum,* or *Lloydella subpileata,* has shown antagonism to the growth of sarcoma 180.

The oak-loving *S. gausapatum* shows inhibition of sarcoma 180 by 90 percent and Ehrlich carcinoma by 100 percent.

The related *S. fasciatum (S. ostrea/S. lobatum)* contains laricinolic and methoxylaricinolic acid.

Related species, such as *S. rugosum, S. sulcatum, S. gausapatum, S. fuscum,* and *S. fasciatum* show moderate to significant activity against *S. aureus* (Robbins et al. 1945).

The related *S. vibrans (Boreosterum vibrans)* contains vibralactone, a potent inhibitor of pancreatic lipase.

The bright orange spore-bearing *S. complicatum* contains a closely related compound, percyquinnin that is also a potent lipase inhibitor. This compound has turned out to be identical to vibralactone.

The inhibitory mechanism of vibralactone may be similar to orlistat, a derivative of the streptomycete compound lipstatin, which is a prescription drug for obesity.

Another relative, *S. murrayi,* has a vanilla-like fragrance, while *S. rugosum* is fruity and banana-like. The former shows activity against both *E. coli* and *S. aureus.*

The closely related *Aleurodiscus amorphous* shows inhibition against sarcoma 180 and Ehrlich carcinoma of 100 percent.

Mycoremediation

Two strains of *S. hirsutum* were investigated in South Africa for use in the pulp and paper industry, and found to produce paper of improved strength.

Stereum hirsutum is a lignin degrading fungi that was used in one experiment to degrade bisphenol A in culture. It showed high resistance to the chemical and in seven to fourteen days completely degraded the toxin. Estrogen activity was tested upon completion and found very effective at clean up (Lee, S.-M. et al. 2005).

The related *S. subtomentosum* has been found to contain protease, amylase, phytase, carboxyl esterase, and lipase enzyme activity, suggesting a wide application of use in various industries (Goud et al. 2009).

Strobilomyces floccopus

S. strobilaceus
(OLD MAN OF THE WOODS)

If dignity can be attributed to a mushroom, then the old man of the woods would get the "Most Dignified" award.
— WALT STURGEON, NORTH AMERICAN MYCOLOGICAL ASSOCIATION MEMBER

Darkly knobbed with warts he stands
Close to the ground. His cap, a coffee cup
Drained of its brew; his mouth hangs
  open loosely…
No armor against foul weather
His suit, threadbare and shaggy
Wears thin. Black knight of fast
Declining years, he has been vulnerable
  All his life.
— JESSIE KEIKO SAIKI, WISCONSIN MYCOLOGICAL SOCIETY NEWSLETTER, FALL 1983

Strobilomyces is from the Greek meaning "a cone-like fungus."

Although mainly an eastern species, found under oak, it is occasionally related to conifers. It is a rather distinctive bolete, with a shaggy black or gray fruiting body. The flesh is white, but becomes red and then black after exposure to air. It is edible, but not highly rated.

Medicinal Use

Ethanol extractions inhibit both Ehrlich ascites tumor and Yoshida sarcoma growth.

Strobilurus occidentalis
(WESTERN CONE MUSHROOM)

S. trullisatus
(DOUGLAS FIR CONE MUSHROOM)

Both cone mushrooms grow on old, and often buried, cones of pine, spruce, and douglas fir.

The former may sometimes be found on the leaf stems of poplar species.

Medicinal Use

The compounds show antitumor activity in vitro when tested on Ehrlich carcinoma cell lines. They can also shut down respiration.

Fungicide

The related *S. tenacellus* contains strobilurins. One active metabolite, strobilurin A, identical to mucidin, has been used as a blueprint for synthetic strobilurins, a broad-spectrum fungicide widely used in agriculture.

They accounted for nearly half the UK market for cereal crop protection in 1999. Evidence of a resistant strain of mildew is already appearing however.

Strobilurins A and B are active against yeasts and filamentous fungi.

The natural product degrades quickly in sunlight, and is very volatile, with a short life when sprayed on leaves.

Stabilizing this compound would be useful for organic producers.

Mycoremediation

Strobilurus species are one and a half to three times more powerful a lignin degrader than *Trametes versicolor*.

Stropharia rugoso-annulata

S. ferrii

S. imaiana

Naematoloma ferrii
(THE WINECAP)
(KING STROPHARIA)

Stropharia means a "ring," sword," or "belt." *Rugosa-annulata* is Latin, meaning "with wrinkled ring." Both names refer to the membranous ring on the stem.

The fungus enjoys being around people, and is found in areas of cultivation, old compost, and greenhouse environments.

It has a prominent ring on the stem that splits into re-curved triangular segments and looks like an oversized diamond clasp with up to a dozen prongs. The brown caps of the cultivated forms do not seem to suit the common name winecap. The winecap can become quite large, a single cap growing up to five pounds!

Winecap is believed to have come west from Russia, with Napoleon's army. Some say it came from Peru, with the potato. In fact, they have a taste similar to potato or turnip. It is a choice edible with mild taste. The mushrooms should not be eaten for more than two to three days in a row, as some individuals experience nausea or indigestion. They should be well cooked.

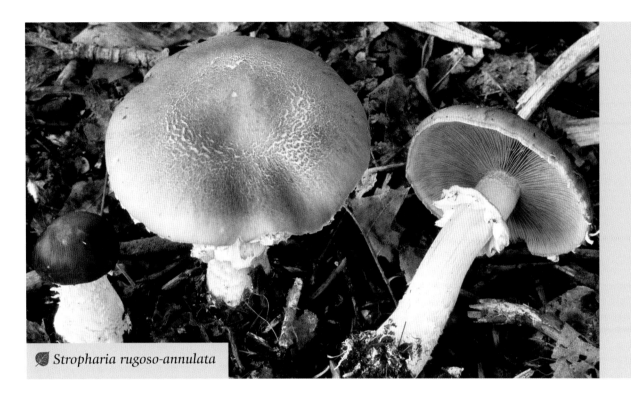

Stropharia rugoso-annulata

Cultivation

It is an ideal mushroom for outdoor cultivation, breaking down alder wood chips that are used for garden mulch. When grown with vegetables, the arrangement is complete. The vegctables give needed shade, and the mushrooms provide rich humus for next year's crop.

The mycelium produces buttons after eight to ten weeks, with the full-grown mushrooms following in another week. Yields of two to three pounds per square foot over eight weeks can be expected. Fruit bodies are produced between fifteen and twenty-one degrees Celsius (fifty-nine to seventy degrees Fahrenheit)—a considerable range and a low temperature for commercial mushrooms, making it ideal for northern temperate climates.

In Hungary, the king stropharia is grown in rows of baled wheat straw simply wetted down and inoculated.

Domestication of the winecap was first proposed for Germany by Puschel in 1969. Since that time, many refinements have been suggested for the cellulose substrate necessary for optimal growth. Because of the high levels of soluble nutrients, the substrate must be presoaked in hot water. The yields, up to 220 grams per kilogram, are higher and more regular than when conventional substrates are used. By contrast, corn stalk yields were poor, with higher contamination rates.

Fruiting and yields were greatly increased when wheat straw was enhanced with 30 percent *Lolium perenne* grass chaff. This is believed due to beta-adenosine identified in methanol extracts. When twelve milligrams of beta-adenosine was added to one kilogram of wet wheat straw, the fungi fruited eighteen days earlier than the pure wheat straw control, with a 220 percent increase in yield. When twenty-five milligrams was used, the yield increased by 258 percent (Domondon et al. 2004).

Paul Stamets found these mushrooms were a good companion for corn in Washington State.

Mycoremediation

Preparations of extracellular manganese peroxidase from *Stropharia rugoso-annulata* have been found to rapidly convert and breakdown the explosive amino nitro-toluenes.

A study by Steffen et al. (2002) found the mushroom to be an efficient degrader of benzopyrene, polycyclic aromatic hydrocarbons, and other toxins, especially in the presence of manganese, which may stimulate the production of manganese peroxidase. The breakdown of these chemicals within six weeks suggests a role in mycoremediation.

Work by Grodzinskaya et al. in Kiev, Ukraine, showed that both water and ethanol extracts of the fruiting bodies are non-toxic (Grodzinskaya et al. 1999). This is good news, as a commercial strain (*Gelb,* with yellow caps) has long been cultivated in the Ukraine as an edible mushroom. It helps enrich the soil and appears attractive to earthworms and other friends of good ecology. About four million pounds are produced annually in France.

Fungi Essence

King *Stropharia* essence brings new insight into what you do. Instead of focusing only on problems and difficulties you now learn to notice the pleasure and nice things in life. This especially when you have seen things the old way for a long time. No more hesitating when you have considered doing things so long, this essence helps you to just do it. Act from your heart, because you like it, not because you need to. Perhaps old traumas made this kind of pleasure disappear from your life, and the outside world still reflects your old soul trauma. The essence grounds and helps you to let go of energies and tension right behind your eyes.

— BLOESEM

Bits and Pieces

The mushroom shows some activity against coliforms, but no serious studies have been yet conducted.

The mushroom contains a human blood type A hemagglutinate.

Suillus

Suillus grevillei
(TAMARACK JACK)
(LARCH BOLETE)
S. cavipes
Boletinus cavipes
(HOLLOW STEMMED LARCH BOLETE)
S. luteus
(SLIPPERY JACK)
S. granulatus
(MILK BOLETE)
(DOTTED STALKED SUILLUS)
S. tomentosus
(WOOLLY PINE BOLETE)
S. reticulatus

Boletus reticulatus
(SUMMER CEP)
S. tomentosus
(POOR MAN'S SLIPPERY JACK)
(BLUE STAINING SLIPPERY JACK)
S. serotinus
S. aeruginascens
S. laricinus
S. viscidus
Fuscoboletinus ssp.
(VISCOUS BOLETE)
S. salmonicolor
S. subluteus
(SLIPPERY JILL)

> *Slippery jack's a type of Suillus*
> *You can't mistake for other fungus.*
> *First remove the slimy cap*
> *Then add to soup, or stews and zap!*
> *A tasty meal with little fuss.*
>   — RDR

Suillus is Latin for "little pig" while granulatus means "dotted."

Grevillei is named after the English mycologist R. K. Greville. *Cavipes* means "hollow foot." *Luteus* is Latin for "golden yellow," a misnomer in that it is considerably less yellow than many other species. *Tomentosus* means "covered with hair."

If you look carefully, you will see that instead of gills there is a lacy network that some mycologists consider an intermediate stage between gilled mushrooms and the pored boletes.

Tamarack jack is often, as the name suggests, found in tamarack forests. Hollow stemmed tamarack jack is found in the same tamarack or larch woods, but is not slimy and

the hollow stalk is noticeable. It is edible but not especially tasty.

Slippery jack is found in the cool of fall and common in northern pine forests. It has even been found in Cotopaxi National Park in the highlands of Ecuador, after hitchhiking in on some imported monterey pine.

It has bright yellow flesh with some red or purple spots.

Slippery jack is a popular dried wild mushroom that is exported in significant amounts from Chile to worldwide markets. It is sold extensively in Europe under the name pine bolete.

Milk bolete is common to mixed or pine forests in summer and fall.

Dotted slippery jack *(S. granulatus)* is an edible found under jack pine and black spruce.

Poor man's *Suillus* contains toxins that largely cook off, but why bother.

Woolly pine bolete is common in the mountains.

Viscous bolete is edible but mediocre. It stains blue.

Suillus are edible when the caps are peeled, but can cause some diarrhea symptoms in many people. All *Suillus* should have their slimy caps removed to avoid this purgative effect. Many species contain thiaminase, which can create B1 deficiency over time, but more importantly, can trigger swift movement of the bowels.

Traditional Uses

The Roman Pliny said that "*Suilli* are dried and transfixed with a rush and are good as a remedy in fluxes from the bowels which are called rheumatisms . . . and they remove freckles and blemishes on women's faces. A healing lotion is also made of them for sore eyes. Soaked in water, they are applied as a salve to foul ulcers and eruptions of the head, and to bites inflicted by dogs."

Tamarack jack and hollow stemmed tamarack jack are added to the traditional Chinese medicine formula called Tendon Easing Powder, which is used to treat lumbago, painful legs, numbed limbs, and discomfort in the tendons and veins.

Slippery jack is used in traditional Chinese medicine to treat Kaschin-Beck disease and is one of the main ingredients in Pine Mushroom Elixir.

Medicinal Use

Chemical Constituents

- *S. grevillei:* **dibenzofuran, thelephoric acid, and the flavanone, 3',4,4'-trihydroxy-pulvinone.**

- *S. granulatus:* **suillusin, suillin, and flazin.**

- *S. cavipes:* **boleletins A-J, 16-hydroxy geranyl geraniol, and cavipetin.**

- *S. luteus:* **suillumide.**

Tamarack jack has an inhibition rate of 60 percent against both sarcoma 180 and Ehrlich carcinoma cell lines.

Work by Kamo et al. (2004b) on hollow stemmed tamarack jack identified boleletins A-J, 16-hydroxy geranyl geraniol, and cavipetin, the latter a strong antioxidant with low cytotoxicity.

The related *S. lakei* is host specific to douglas fir. Keep in mind that douglas fir may be able to form ectomycorrhizae with as many as two thousand different species of fungi.

When found under black spruce, dotted slippery jack markedly reduces the effect of the pathogen *Mycelium radicis atrovirens,* probably due, in part, to competition for nutrients. It contains suillusin, a unique benzofuran that is probably a derivative of polyporic acid (Yun et al. 2001).

Tringali et al. (1989) identified suillin as the antitumor principle from this mushroom. Both in vitro and in vivo activity against P388 leukemia cell lines was found.

Flazin, a highly fluorescent compound, has been identified recently. It is found naturally occurring in fermented soy sauce.

Slippery jack is used for the same purposes as other *Suillus.* Inhibition rates are 90 percent and 80 percent respectively for sarcoma 180 and Ehrlich carcinoma.

Suillumide has been isolated from the fruiting body and inhibits the growth of SK-MEL-1 human melanoma cells with an IC_{50} of ten micrometers (Leon et al. 2008).

Both *S. luteus* and *S. granulatus* possess cytotoxic activity against L1210 and 3LL cancer cell lines.

Work by Badalyan (2003) in Armenia found significant antioxidant activity in this mushroom and *Pholiota alnicola.*

In studies by Geraci et al. (1992) suillin was found to possess significant in vivo antitumor activity against P388 leukemia cell lines.

Suillin, from *Suillus placidus* of eastern North America, has been found cytotoxic against human liver cancer cells.

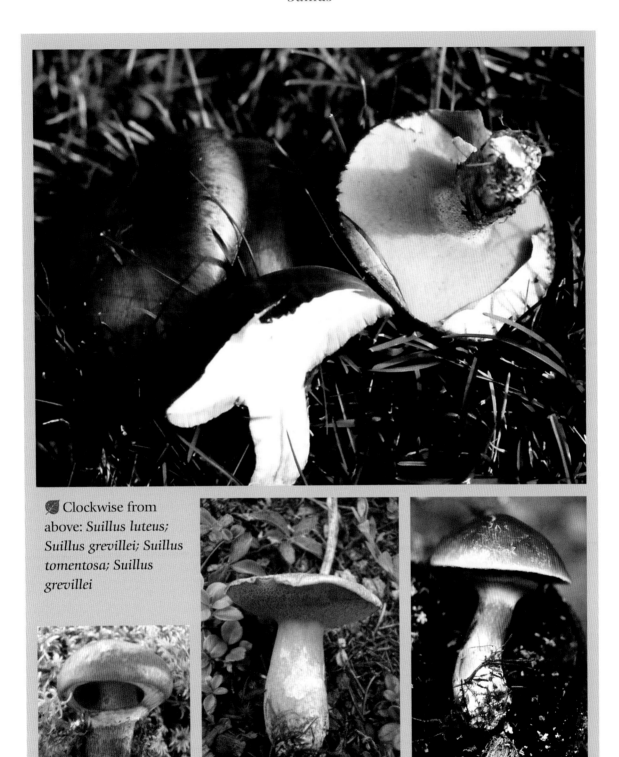

🍃 Clockwise from above: *Suillus luteus; Suillus grevillei; Suillus tomentosa; Suillus grevillei*

Related compounds in milk bolete include dimethoxysuillin that shows cytotoxic activity against KB cells (human naso-pharyngeal cancer), P388 cells (murine leukemia), and NSCLC-N6 (human bronchopulmonary carcinoma) (Tringali 1989).

Inhibition rate against sarcoma 180 and Ehrlich carcinoma is 80 percent and 70 percent (Ohtsuka et al. 1973).

Four distinct tetraprenyphenols have been identified by Tringali et al. (1989) with two of the compounds possessing antimicrobial activity.

Methanol extracts were found to exhibit significant cytotoxicity against two murine cancer cell lines with an IC50 lower than twenty micrograms per milliliter, for both this species and the related *S. luteus*.

The related *Suillus collinitus* shows activity against *E. coli, Enterobacter aerogenes, Salmonella typhimurium, Staphylococcus aureus, S. epidermidis, Bacillus subtilis, Candida albicans,* and *Saccharomyces cerevisiae.* The dichloromethane extracts showed higher activity than standard antibiotics (Yamac and Bilgili 2006).

Viscous bolete shows an inhibition rate of 100 percent against sarcoma 180 and 90 percent against Ehrlich carcinoma.

Fungi Essence

Summer cep *(S. reticulatus)* essence grounds and anchors us within the strength and power of Mother Earth. It provides energy protection for the entire organism.

— Korte Phi

Slippery jack *(S. luteus)* essence brings any unexpressed feelings of shame and guilt up to conscious awareness. It helps release blockages that are caused by deep-seated negative feelings that deny self-worth.

— Korte Phi

Mycoremediation

Various *Suillus* species, including *S. grevillei, S. luteus and S. variegatus* remove benzo pyrene at a rate of 50 percent in four weeks (Braun-Lullemann et al. 1999).

The latter species degrade TNT under nitrogen-deficient conditions.

Suillus granulatus completely metabolizes catechol, 3,4-dihydrobenzoic acid, and vanillic acid, due to tyrosinase activity. Mycelium transformed para-cresol in just five hours.

Woolly pine bolete is a significant mycoaccumulator of lead by sixty-seven times, and a minor accumulator of mercury by up to six times. It may have a role in mycoremediation of contaminated oil and gas sites, and cleaning up industrial accidents.

Numerous authors have noted the concentration of oxalic acid in *Suillus* and other ectomycorrhizal fungi when exposed to heavy metals. This appears to be somehow related to disease suppression.

Suillus granulatus shows darkened hyphae when grown on copper-amended media (Gruhn, C. M. and O. K. Miller Jr. 1991). *Suillus tomentosus* growth was reduced at 370 micrometer levels of soil.

The related *S. bovinus* can be adapted to zinc-rich soils.

Thelephora terrestris

(EARTH FAN)
(COMMON FIBER VASE)
T. vialis
(GROUNDWART)

Thelphora is Greek for "bearing nipples," due to the warty nature of this leathery genus. It looks at first glance like a *Ramaria* or *Clavaria*, but grows on the debris of pine needles.

Earth fan is inedible.

Traditional Uses

The related groundwart *(T. vialis)* is used in traditional Chinese medicine as part of Tendon Easing Powder, which is used to treat lumbago, pain in legs, numb hands and feet, and uneasy tendons and veins.

Medicinal Use

Chemical Constituents

- *T. terrestris:* **terrestrins A-G and pregnane-type steroids terresterones A-B.**

- *T. vialis:* **vialinin A and B, thelephorin A, and ganbajunins.**

Earth fan contains terrestrins A-G and pregnane type steroids, terresterones A-B. These compounds exhibit antioxidant activity equivalent or stronger than vitamin C or BHA (Radulovic 2005).

The related *T. ganbajun* and *T. aurantiotincta* have been shown to contain various p-terphenyl compounds that show very strong antioxidant properties (Liu, J. et al. 2004).

Thelephantins A-H have been found in *T. aurantiotincta.*

Thelophoric acid possesses antitumor and anti-allergenic activity.

Vialinin B in *T. vialis* potently inhibits TNF-alpha production and may be a promising anti-allergenic (Xie, C. 2006).

The IC50 value of 0.02 nanomoles is comparable to the immunosuppressant tacrolimus.

Vialinin A is a powerful antioxidant but also strongly inhibits cytokine production such as TNF-alpha and may have application for treatment of inflammatory conditions such as rheumatoid arthritis. The IC50 is also stronger than tacrolimus, used for organ transplantation.

Vialinin B is a potent inhibitor of TNF-alpha with an IC_{50} of 0.02 nanomole (Xie, C. 2006).

This eastern North American species also contains various ganbajunins and thelephorin A that possess ten times the antioxidant activity of ascorbic acid (Tsukamoto 2002).

Mycoremediation

Thompson and Medve (1984) found the fungus tolerant of aluminum and manganese,

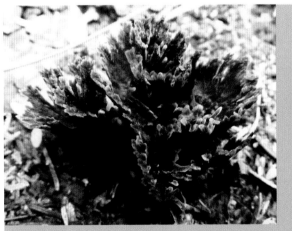

Thelephora terrestris

suggestive of a use in myco-monitoring associated industries. Cadmium inhibited growth at 350 parts per million.

It degrades 4-fluorobiphenyl by more than 65 percent.

Trametes

Trametes suaveolens
Boletus suaveolens
Coriolellus suaveolens
(ANISE POLYPORE)
(SWEET TRAMETES)
T. hirsuta
Polyporus hirsutus
Polystictus hirsutus
Coriolus hirsutus
(HAIRY TURKEY TAIL)
T. versicolor
C. versicolor
P. versicolor
(TURKEY TAIL)
(VELVET STALK)
T. cinnabarina
Pycnoporus cinnabarinus
(CINNABAR RED POLYPORE)
T. cinnabarina var. sanguinea
P. sanguineus
(RED POLYPORE)
(VERMILION POLYPORE)
T. pubescens
Tyromyces pubescens
(SOFT TRAMETES)
T. conchifer
Poronidulus conchifer
(LITTLE NEST POLYPORE)

Trametes means "one who is thin" and *versicolor* means "various colorings."

Pycnoporus is from the Greek meaning "the pores are close together." *Cinnabarinus* means "red," as in cinnabar red. *Suaveolens* means "sweet smelling."

Anise polypore *(T. suaveolens)* found growing on willow and aspen poplar contains a substance with a pleasant odor reminiscent of anise. The smell is especially evident when the fungus has been cut and is drying. The smell is very similar to that of *Haploporus odoratus,* a species found only on diamond willow.

It is used by the Laplanders of Finland as an aphrodisiac, due to the spicy fragrance, which is attributed to methyl anisate.

Hairy turkey tail *(Trametes hirsuta)* is widespread and common. It is a similar, but thinner polypore with variations of gray and a yellow to light brown color.

A related fungus, *Trametes versicolor,* grows throughout North America. Known as turkey tail, this is one of the most important medicinal mushrooms in the world. It is also known as *Coriolus versicolor* (a name still preferred by Chinese and Japanese scientists), *Polyporus versicolor,* and previously *Polystictus versicolor.* In Japan it is called *kawaratake,* meaning "mushroom by the riverbank," while in China, it is called *yun zhi* or "rain cloud mushroom."

In Holland, turkey tail is known as *elfenbankje,* or "fairy bench," and in Germany, *schmetterlingstramete* meaning "butterfly tramete."

The fruiting body is fan shaped, resembling a turkey tail, and is blue, brown, gray, and white.

Although not reported in the literature, the mushroom has been found with frequency

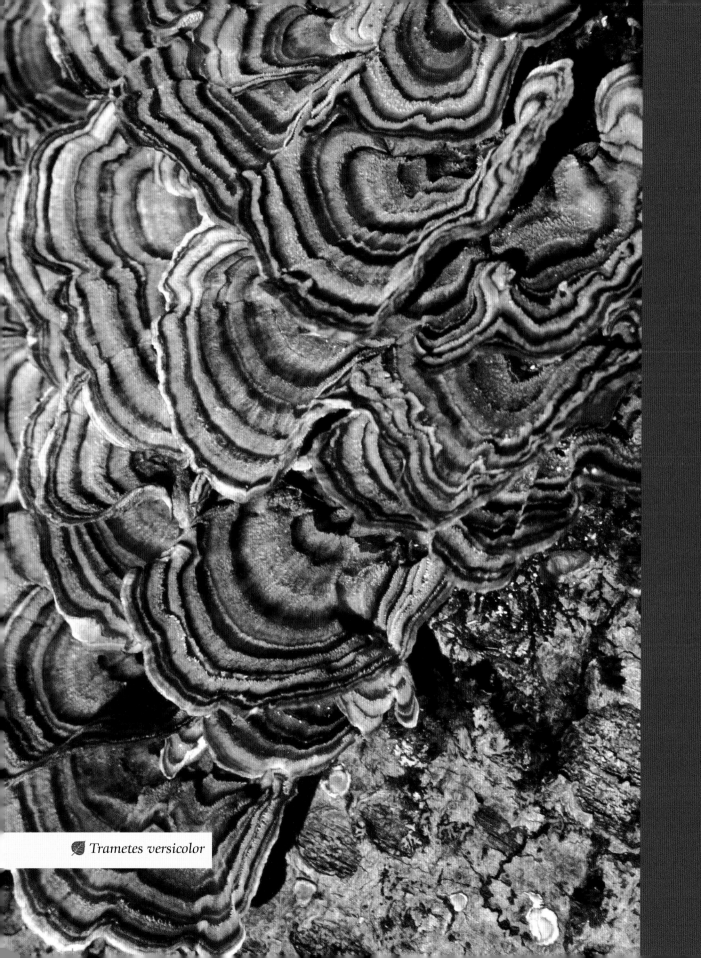

Trametes versicolor

in Alberta, including several patches by this author.

The Dakota were reported to eat the somewhat fibrous fungi. They may have been added to soups and stews and used as a preservative to prevent spoilage.

Cinnabar polypore is named for its intensely bright red color. Cinnabar is derived from the Persian *sangarf* meaning "red lead" or "mercuric sulphide." It is known as *shutake* in Japan.

Trametes, or *Tyromyces pubescens,* is another shelf bracket that is common on birch and other hardwood trees. It is both smaller and lighter than turkey tail.

Culture and Folklore

Linnaeus, in his 1737 *Flora Lapponica,* had this to say:

> The Lapland youth, having found this Agaric (*T. odora),* carefully preserves it in a little pocket hanging in front of his pubes, that its grateful perfume may render him more acceptable to his favorite one. O whimsical Venus! In other regions you must be treated with coffee and chocolate, preserves and sweetmeats, wines and dainties, jewels and pearles, gold and silver, silks and cosmetics, balls and assemblies, music and theatrical exhibitions; here you are satisfied with a little withered fungus!

Traditional Uses

Badham, in *A Treatise on the Esculent Funguses of England* written in 1847, tells of

> a young man of twenty-one, [who] was seized at the beginning of autumn with inflammatory cough and haemoptysis. . . . But the

cough, coming on again with renewed severity during the winter, was accompanied by the expulsion of glairy mucus, which was sometimes specked with blood.

> Toward the spring the young man had become much thinner, and was continuing to waste away; the expectoration also had changed in color, and had become fetid and green; his nights were feverish and disturbed; he had no desire for food, and ate but little; his ankles had begun to swell; he had copious night sweats and diarrhea. A teaspoonful of an electuary of the *Polyporus suaveolens* in honey was given three times a day, and nothing else; and extraordinary as it may appear, under this treatment his sweat speedily began to diminish with the cough, and after three months' continuance of the medicine the patient entirely recovered.

Anise polypore has been used for night sweats associated with tuberculosis and various other lung ailments.

Porcher reported on several medical cases given up as incurable that recovered. Two drams of the powder were given morning and evening to effect a cure.

Ancient Taoists prized the fungi, partly because they can grow on evergreen pine trees, and therefore must have the staying power of the trees. They believed the fungus collected yang energy from the roots of the tree and prescribed it for patients with yang-deficient energetics.

The polypore is applied topically in Mexico as a treatment for impetigo and ringworm.

In China, the polypore is used medicinally

for increasing circulation and clearing heat and damp. It is often prescribed by herbalists in rheumatism and to cure fevers.

Cinnabar polypore is dried and powdered as a styptic.

The fungi are used in Malaysia for skin complaints including acne, probably due to the plant signature of red for inflamed skin and blood problems.

In Johore, it is powdered and added to *eau de cologne* to heal leprous tubercles, according to Hobbs. His book, *Medicinal Mushrooms,* has been a great inspiration to me in my own exploration of local species.

It is decocted and used as a wash for eczema, and extracted in warm oil for knotty swellings.

According to Ying et al. (1987), cinnabar polypore was used traditionally for its hemostatic and anti-inflammatory properties.

Hairy turkey tail is used in traditional Chinese medicine to dispel wind and damp, cure lung disease, stop coughs, resolve suppurations, and promote the growth of muscle.

In traditional Chinese medicine turkey tail is considered sweet and slightly warming, entering the spleen and heart meridians. It is used for infection and inflammation of the upper respiratory, urinary, and digestive tracts. The mushroom is used to increase energy and stamina, and benefits patients with hepatitis B and chronic active hepatitis. It can be used for general immune weakness and tumors.

In Mexico, *Trametes* or *Tyromyces pubescens* is used to cure ringworm and impetigo of the skin.

The red or cinnamon polypore is recommended in traditional Chinese medicine for reducing fever, swelling, and dampness, and as an antidote for toxins.

Decoctions are used for arthritis, rheumatism, and gout, as well as fungal disease.

In Malaysia, where it is known as Chendawan Merah, the fungus is used to treat dysentery.

A powder is made for external application to wounds to stop bleeding and prevent infection.

The fungus is said to invigorate vital energy, improve blood circulation, and stop skin itching. It is said to promote muscle growth.

Aborigines of Australia sucked on the polypore to treat sore mouths; they also rubbed it inside babies' mouths to treat oral thrush and to alleviate pain from teething.

Medicinal Use

Chemical Constituents

- *T. versicolor:* **PSK (polysaccharide krestin), PSP (polysaccharide peptide), lipids (1.7 percent) containing ergosta-7,22,dien-3(ol), a major sterol of many polypores, as well as ergost-7-en-3(ol) and ergopsterol (provitamin D2), polyhydroxysteroids, cerevisterol, tetraol, sitosterols, coriolan; 3 beta, 5 alpha, 9 gamma-trihydroxyergosta-7,22-dien-6-one, 11 percent protein, 76 percent complex carbohydrates, and various B vitamins and minerals.**

- *P. cinnabarinus:* **cinnabarin, cinnabaric acid, and tramesanquin.**

- *T. versicolor* **and** *P. sanguineus:* **4-hydroxymethyl-quinoline.**

- *T. versatilis:* **1 percent eburicoic acid.**

- *T. menziesii:* **trametenamides A and B.**

Turkey tail has been widely studied in China and Japan for its immune-stimulating poly-

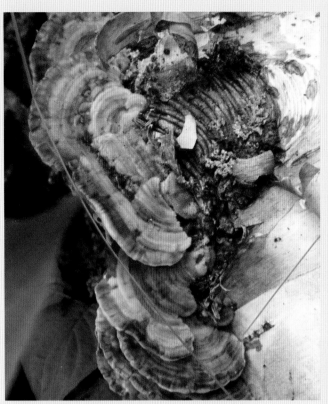

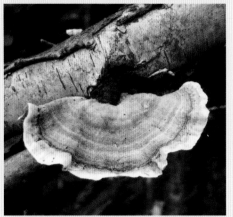

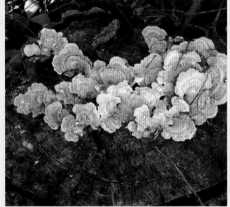

🍃 Clockwise from above: young *Trametes hirsuta,* older *Trametes hirsuta, Trametes pubescens, Pycnoporus cinnabarinus, Trametes pubescens.*

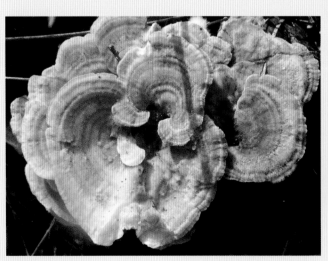

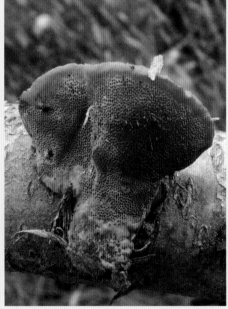

saccharides and its use in the treatment of cancer. More than four hundred clinical studies have been published in Japan in the past thirty-some years, showing benefits to the immune system, with or without chemotherapy and radiation.

In 1987, more than 25 percent of the money spent on natural anticancer agents in Japan, were for PSK, a polysaccharide fraction of turkey tail. The P is for polysaccharide and K is the first letter of Kureha, the company that developed both PSK and Krestin.

Another active component is a protein bound polysaccharide (PSP) consisting of six kinds of monosaccharides, glucose, mannose, galactose, xylose, arabinose, and rhamnose connected with a small molecular protein polypeptide.

Krestin was the first mushroom-derived anticancer drug approved by the Japanese government, and all healthcare plans in that country cover its cost.

In 1965, a chemical engineer working for Kureha Chemical Industry Company observed a neighbor taking the remedy to cure himself of gastric cancer. He was in the late stages and had been rejected for treatment at all clinics and hospitals. He took the treatment for several months and then went back to work. The engineer convinced his workers to investigate the mushroom. The success of Krestin inspired Chinese researchers to look into other extracts, and they developed PSP, or polysaccharide peptide, from a different culture strain.

PSK is a water-soluble protein-bound polysaccharide with 1,4 glucan as a main component, 1,3 glucan linkages, and 38 percent protein. PSP is 10 percent peptide and 90 per-

cent polysaccharides. It lacks fucose, but contains arabinose and rhamnose, which PSK does not have. They are quite different.

To manufacture PSP, the PSK is precipitated with alcohol to reduce the protein links to peptide links. The glucan structures are left unchanged.

Coriolan is an antitumor polysaccharide that does not contain any nitrogen. This reminds me of the sundew, venus fly trap, and other carnivorous plants that trap insects for survival in nitrogen-depleted bogs and swamps. These nitrogen-deficient herbs are also used for treating cancer.

PSK improves the function of blood vessels, normalization of spleen index, immune enhancement, and possible prevention of liver cancer. It prolongs the activity of antibiotics and increases sensitivity in antibiotic-resistant bacteria, working in a synergistic manner in cases of MRSA and other resistant strains.

PSK, derived from mycelium, is immune enhancing, and has broad neoplastic activity. It has been shown to restore antibody (IgG) production in mice with sarcoma 180, but not in normal mice.

It acts directly on tumor cells, prevents metastasis, and enhances the effects of radiation or chemotherapy. It stops the spread of tumors by disabling enzymes that allow tumor cells to break out of the matrix that holds healthy cells in place. This is very useful in radiation therapy for endometrial cancer.

PSK is antiviral, inhibiting HIV by either modifying the viral receptor or stopping HIV from binding with lymphocytes. It also stimulates interferon production.

One study found thirty-six patients with chronic fatigue syndrome who took the mushroom supplement for two months showed a 35 percent increase in natural killer cells.

Dr. Andrew French reported a case study of a pregnant patient whose chronic genital herpes were alleviated with turkey tail mushroom extracts.

PSP is immune stimulating, and although similar to PSK, it has no fucose, while PSK has no rhamnose or arabinose. At least sixteen papers have examined the ability of PSK or PSP to stimulate immune cells or inhibit cancer cell proliferation. More than forty studies have looked at their ability to inhibit metastasis, angiogenesis, and/or tumor growth in animal studies.

PSP has been found to alleviate symptoms and prevent decline in immune status.

Thirteen studies looked at interactions with radiation or chemotherapy, or the ability to decrease immunosuppression caused by these therapies. Fifty-four studies focused on their ability to inhibit cancer progression in humans.

Twenty-four randomized controlled, multi-centered trials found adding PSK to treatment regimes improved patient survival rates.

PSP induces gamma interferon, interleukin-2, and T-cell proliferation.

In tumor-bearing mice, PSP has been shown to stop thymus atrophy and increase IgG values. It has shown tumor-inhibiting activity in animals with sarcoma 180, P388 leukemia, human lung carcinoma, and various cancers of the liver, stomach, nose, and throat.

In one study of 185 patients with stage III lung cancer, the five-year survival rate for those who received radiation and PSK exceeded the radiation-only survival rate by 400 percent (Hayakawa 1993).

In colorectal cancer, it checked advancement and increased survival rate in a trial involving 221 patients treated with mitomycin. PSK reduced the depth to which the cancer invaded the intestinal wall and curtailed its spread to lymphatic nodes and blood vessels.

In one randomized study, 111 patients with curatively resected colorectal cancer received either chemotherapy or chemotherapy plus PSK. The latter group increased the eight-year survival rate from 7.8 percent to 28 percent and the ten-year survival from 19 to 36 percent.

Work with 124 gastric cancer patients showed similar benefit (Nakazato et al. 1994).

Patients without cancer but suffering from leaky gut syndrome may also benefit.

In a pilot study of thirteen patients, nine improved and one patient with hypothyroid made a full repair of tissue in only three months.

One study found PSK increased the survival rate of seventy-four patients receiving a chemotherapy combination of 5-fluorouracil, cyclophosphamide, mitomycin C, and prednisolone following breast cancer surgery.

A recent discovery is that PSP exhibits S-phase cell cycle arrest-specific activity, in addition to immune modulation (Hui 2005).

Reduction of toxicity from radiation and chemotherapy accounts for much of the extract's popularity.

One glycoprotein from turkey tail shows activity against hypertension, diabetes, thrombosis, and rheumatism. The protein inhib-

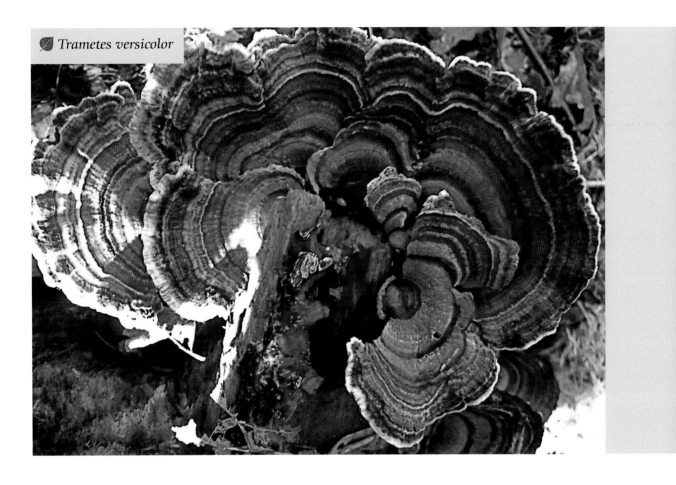

Trametes versicolor

its blood platelet aggregation and exhibits analgesic, antipyretic, anti-hyperlipemic, anti-arrhythmic, anti-inflammatory, and vaso-dilating activity.

Studies by Ikuzawa (1985) showed that it reverses conditions associated with nephron (kidney) disorders, including proteinuria and proteinemia, and regulates prostaglandin formation and degradation.

The whole mushroom has been shown to lower serum cholesterol and in combination with *Astragalus root (A. membranaceus)* enhances neutrophil function and speeds recovery from burns.

Numerous human clinical trials have been conducted on PSK and have shown it to be effective against many human cancers.

PSK reduces cancer metastasis by inhibition of tumor invasion, adhesion, and the production of cell-degrading enzymes. It suppresses tumor cell attachment to endothelial cells by inhibiting platelet aggregation and tumor cell migration by limiting motility. It suppresses tumor growth by inhibition of angiogenesis.

Ethanol extracts of the fungus show promise as an adjunct therapy for prostate cancer, by slowing tumorigenesis (Hsieh, T. C. and J. M. Wu 2001).

A 1982 study on the survival rate of cervical cancer patients in Tokyo showed that PSK, when given orally with radiation, showed no tumor cells in 36 percent of patients as opposed to 11 percent in the control group.

The two-year survival rate was 94 percent with PSK, and 74 percent without. The rate of cancer deaths within five years was 21 percent with PSK, and 52 percent without.

A year-long double-blind study of human papilloma virus and cervical dysplasia involving forty-three patients showed a 72 percent decrease in low-grade squamous intra-epithelial lesions compared to a control group at 47.5 percent. Dosage was three grams daily.

One ten-year study of 185 lung cancer patients who underwent radiation showed that stage I or II patients taking Krestin had a 39 percent survival rate compared to placebo at only 16 percent. Those with stage III showed 22 percent survival rate in the Krestin group and only 5 percent in the control group.

A randomized, controlled clinical trial of 227 patients with breast cancer involved one group taking PSK and chemotherapy, the other chemotherapy only. The ten-year study found an 81.1 percent survival rate in those taking PSK, compared to 64.5 percent in the control group receiving only chemotherapy.

Improved symptoms have been observed in patients suffering systemic lupus, chronic rheumatoid arthritis, sclerosis, Bechet's disease, and other autoimmune disorders, suggestive of immune modulation.

The polysaccharides enhance alkaline phosphatase in osteoblast cells, suggesting use in osteoporosis and degenerative bone disease.

In melanoma, it reduces the rate at which cancer cells spread to the lungs and increases the effectiveness of cyclophosphamide and interleukin-2.

In ovarian cancer, it helps maintain the body's own production of IL-2.

It appears that PSK in higher concentrations (five to eleven micromoles) inhibits cancer cells, due to hydrogen peroxide produced when SOD activity is increased (Kobayashi, Y. et al. 1994a, 1994b, 1994c).

This increased production of SOD and hydrogen peroxide may explain PSK induced enhancement of cisplatin activity against cancer cells in vitro (Kobayashi, Y. 1994d).

PSK stops the invasion of normal cells by leukemia cells, and reduces the likelihood of relapse in childhood acute lymphocytic leukemia after chemotherapy is discontinued.

One study found that PSK cured both primary and metastatic tumor in a double-grafted tumor system.

When given as a maintenance therapy with 6-mercaptopurine, fourteen patients with various leukemias increased survival times or had complete remission (Nagao, T. et al. 1981).

A controlled clinical trial on PSP was conducted on 485 patients with cancer of the esophagus, stomach, and lungs. The PSP group suffered fewer side effects of conventional therapies such as pain, poor appetite, tiredness, weakness, and dryness of the mouth and throat. Body weight remained higher, as did T-cell ratio, natural killer cell activity, and IL-2 levels (Yang, Q. Y. 1999). The rate of remission in esophageal patients receiving PSP was 72 percent, compared to a control group receiving chemotherapy only, which showed a remission rate of just 42 percent.

A ten-year clinical trial involving fifty-six post-surgery colon or gastric cancer patients receiving PSP evaluated the patients every three months. Their survival rate was considerably higher than the fifty-five patients in the control group who received a placebo.

In a study by Shiu W. C. T. et al. (1992) breast cancer patients treated with 4'epidoxorubicin and cyclophophamide, the addition of PSP stabilized and practically prevented white blood cell decreases due to chemotherapy. The polysaccharide peptide (PSP) taken three times daily prevented a significant drop in white blood cell count following three courses of chemotherapy when used as pre-treatment in eleven patients and taken with vincristine, cyclophophamide, and 4'epidoxo-rubicin in human clinical trials.

Animal trials suggest significant restoration of immune-suppressing effects of cyclophosphamide.

The polysaccharopeptide PSP also suppresses the expression of vascular endothelial cell growth factor associated with anti-angiogenesis and antitumor growth.

The oral LD50 of PSP is ten milligrams per kilogram, with no toxicity or side effects reported.

Turkey tail is effective when kidney or liver function is impaired, as about 70 percent of the break-down products is excreted through the lungs.

Jeng-Leun Mau et al. (2002) found turkey tail possesses some antioxidant properties, but it is only one-third as powerful as *Ganoderma tsugae*.

Mikiashvili et al. (2004) found *T. versicolor* shows high carboxymethyl cellulase (4.29 units per milliliter) and xylanase activity (5.54 units per milliliter).

Polysaccharide extracts were found to increase macrophages 7.2-fold over controls (Jeong, S.-C. et al. 2006).

Methanol extracts of turkey tail also exhibit activity against B16 melanoma cells. Extracts have been found to be directly cytotoxic and anti-proliferative to tumor cells and indirectly via macrophage activation.

Hairy turkey tail *(T. hirsutus)* possesses anti-tumor and anti-neoplastic activity (Jong and Gantt 1987).

It inhibits sarcoma 180 in white mice by 65 percent (Ikekawa et al. 1968).

Studies indicate that red polypore is active against sarcoma 180. This could be due in part to the significant content of organic germanium (eight hundred to two thousand parts per million) in this shelf fungus.

It is considered an antidote for toxins and is used for arthritis, including gout, as well as for antibacterial and antifungal activity.

Trametes sanguinea is used in the alkaloid transformation of thebaine to 14-hydroxy-codeinone with a 40 percent yield. Theabaine poppies are being developed in Canada to replace dependency on sources from Afghanistan. It is easy to transform thebaine into morphine and codeine but extremely difficult to produce heroin.

The cinnamic acid ester of this product is 177 times more potent than morphine as an analgesic and five hundred times as potent as morphine in a test involving pentobarbitol potentiation of grip on a forty-five degree plane.

The cultured red or cinnamon polypore mycelium, which contains polyporin, as well as water extracts of the fruiting body, have been found active against *Staphylococcus aureus, S. albus, Streptococcus salivarius, Pseudomonas aeruginosa, Salmonella paratyphi, E. coli, Klebsiella pneumoniae, Vibrio cholerae,* and *Shigella paradysenteriae.*

Callow and Chain, in unpublished work, identified polystictin as active against *S. aureus.*

Water extracts show antitumor activity in vitro. Inhibition rates against sarcoma 180 are up to 90 percent.

Both *T. versicolor* and *T. sanguineus* contain an unoxidized quinoline compound, which is active against malaria (Abrasham and Spassov 1991).

Silva et al. (2009) found activity against chloroquine-resistant *Plasmodium falciparium,* as well as inhibition of nitric oxide and immune-modulating activity.

Cinnabarin acid shows activity against gram-positive bacteria including *Streptococcus* species. Cinnabarin is antibacterial, antifungal, and antiviral. It has a basic ring-like structure similar to acitomycin D, an antibiotic used in cancer treatment. Cinnabarin at only 0.31 milligrams per milliliter reduced the rabies virus levels by four-fold (Smania, A. et al. 2003). It does not cause any toxic effects in mice at concentrations of one thousand milligrams per kilogram.

Meyer described an antibiotic substance from *T. cinnabarinus* that inhibited bacteria at a concentration of one part in five thousand. It was active against *Staphylococcus* and *Streptococcus* species.

The fruiting bodies of *P. cinnabarinus* have antibacterial activity. The mycelium showed activity against *Bacillus subtilis.*

Cultured fluids also show activity against *Streptococcus* species, due in part to the content of cinnabarinic acid, mentioned above.

Culture filtrate of the fungi is active against *E. coli* and *Pseudomonas aeruginosa,* as well as *Staphylococcus aureus* and various plant pathogenic fungi.

Early work found polysaccharides from the mycelium culture inhibit sarcoma 180 and Ehrlich carcinoma cell lines by 90 percent (Ohtsuka et al. 1973).

T. conchifer has been shown to possess antitumor polysaccharides in the polypore.

The related *T. gibbosa* has an inhibition rate of 49 percent against sarcoma 180 with both hot-water and ethanol extracts. It is a very strong inhibitor of both 1 kappa B-alpha degradation and phosphorylation.

Trametes versatilis, in the form of cultured mycelia, produces 1 percent eburicoic acid (Ma, B.-J. et al. 2007).

Trametes menziesii contains two ceramides, trametenamides A and B. The former is cytotoxic to SK-MEL-1 cells at low concentrations due to apoptosis. Ceramides induce self-programmed death in cells by permeabilization of the mitochondrial membrane, which allows the exit of pro-apoptotic factors such as cytochrome (Leon et al. 006).

The inhibition rate of a hot-water and ethanol extract of *Trametes* or *Tyromyces pubescens* on the growth of sarcoma 180 is 59.5 percent (Shibata, S. et al. 1968).

Lau et al. (2004) found water and alcohol

extracts of the fungus inhibit the proliferation of lymphoma and leukemic cells by apoptosis, or programmed cell death.

The fruiting body and mycelium exhibits activity against various bacteria, including *Staphylococcus aureus, Enterobacter aerogenes, Pseudomonas aeruginosa,* and the yeast *Saccharomyces cerevisiae* (Yamac and Bilgili 2006).

Homeopathy

Picnoporus sanguineus is related to irritability and feelings of frustration, accompanied by an aversion to company. There may be dreams of violence and arguments, irritability accompanied by sadness, feelings of self-doubt, mistakes and awkwardness.

Dreams of aliens and danger, and a pervading sense of fear upon waking.

Sharp stabbing pains, dull headache, and numbness also present.

The most striking of all the skin symptoms was the intolerable itch, like fleabites, but no amount of superficial scratching relieved it.

Peculiar symptoms include sneezing after bath, sensation of the scalp being pulled up, and pain upon smiling.

Dose: 30 C. Provings were done by Catherine Anne Morris in South Africa on thirty people in 2002. The C4 trituration trials were conducted on six people in Brisbane, Australia, and ten people in Stockholm, Sweden.

— VERMEULEN

Essential Oil

The bracket fungus from poplar, *Trametes suaveolens,* yields an essential oil from steam distillation that contains amanitol, which is also present in *Amanita muscaria.* It contains anisal-

dehyde and 78 percent methyl anisate, which gives a licorice fragrance.

The related *T. odorata* is slightly anise-like, but also scented like rose, honey, and fruit. It contains methyl phenylacetate, geraniol, nerol, and citronellol.

Fungi Essences

Turkey tail *(Trametes versicolor)* essence helps bring you face to face with love and nurturing all parts of yourself, all parts of you belong. A part of you is to be discovered and given face, helping you find a greater whole.

— CANADIAN FOREST

Turkey tail essence is for the eternal worrier, for those who need to ground their energies into the physical world and for those who work with nature. It is for low energy, immune problems, vision, diabetes, rheumatism and lungs.

— SILVERCORD

Trametes versicolor essence increases our capacity for self-awareness, helping us through difficult crises and at key transition points in our life. It helps us recognize outside influences for what they are, protecting us against parasitic energies when we are vulnerable.

— KORTE PHI

Turkey tail essence works through the energy circuits that influence the chemical structures holding the imprint of childhood abuse or trauma at the cellular level. Use it when you are ready to break down and release the patterns and memories of childhood abuse or trauma. Holding onto these energies can lead to physical symptoms such as fibromyalgia or autoimmune disorders, or emotional symptoms such as fear, powerlessness or disassociation.

— TREE FROG

Cinnamon red polypore is for inner transformations, and for creating a synergy between the many aspects of your being and personality. The essence will aid your work with guides and teachers, as you are able to translate the information more easily and directly in the conscious mind.

— CANADIAN FOREST

Red polypore *(P. sanguineus)* essence has a strong grounding effect as it stimulates the root chakra. It strengthens our connection to the earth and promotes better circulation in the lower extremities especially the feet.

— KORTE PHI

Turkey tail essence supports necessary demarcation against foreign influence and prevents seizure of social personality. It prevents spread of negative mood in social fabric and for those who think we should all do exactly the same thing. It is anti-bullying essence.

— MARIANA

Cinnabar polypore essence promotes inner transformation and changes. The essence helps bring things from the subconscious to surface to get into conscious mind and help integrate into everyday life.

— MARIANA

Mycoremediation

For *T. pubescens,* laccase production is best stimulated by xylidine. It also tests very high in lipase activity, suggesting application in a variety of oleochemical, petrochemical, and biodiesel applications (Goud et al. 2009).

Turkey tail was identified as far back as 1963 as a lignin degrader. One study found this fungus to be the most powerful degrader of 3,4-dichloroaniline, dieldrin, and phenanthrene.

Another study found that the dose of PCP per mycelium mass, rather than a concentration in the medium, regulated the growth and myco-degradation. *T. versicolor* was found to be the best at both PCP resistance and its degradation.

Turkey tail produces peroxidase enzymes, which quickly break down wood lignins. It has been studied for the pulping of wood and the degradation of aromatic hydrocarbons. Black and Reddy isolated six genes responsible for lignin peroxidase production.

It is still considered the most effective fungi to combat lignin and chlorine-containing effluent.

Kwang Soo Shin and Yeo Jin Lee (2000) identified an extracellular peroxidase that works optimally at pH 3 and between fifty and sixty-five degrees Celsius (122 and 149 degrees Fahrenheit).

Various researchers have shown that secondary metabolites from the mycelium break down polycyclic aromatic hydrocarbons including antracines, pyrenes, flourene, methoxybenzene, and styrene. One study found heat-sterilized mycelium absorb mercury ions from water systems.

It absorbs chromium from wastewater.

One study found both *T. versicolor* and *Tyromyces palustrin* metabolize dibenzyl sulphide to benzyl alcohol and benzyl mercaptan.

Chlorophenols up to two thousand parts

per million can be effectively remediated with turkey tail. One study found immobilizing the white rot basidiomycete in nylon mesh created far greater efficiency. The idea is worth investigating for pulp and paper, as well as pharmaceutical wastes. The nylon mesh is fixed to a metal frame around the perimeter of bioreactor and replaced at intervals, and so on. Brilliant.

Fragoeiro and Magan (2008) suggest that the mushroom has the ability to degrade different groups of pesticides. Complete degradation of dieldrin and trifluralin, as well as 80 percent of simazine, were observed.

One study found free cell cultures of the mushroom in nylon mesh helped remove PCP and 2,4-dichlorophenol, via laccase and manganese peroxidase.

Black liquors from a soda pulping mill were treated with the fungus in the form of pellets in aerated reactors, and showed reductions of 70 to 80 percent in color and aromatic compounds, and 60 percent in chemical oxygen demand.

Soil contaminated with PCP responded well to inoculation by the fungus (Tuomela et al. 1998).

Turkey tail laccase was able to oxidize 35 percent of anthracene in only seventy-two hours.

Itmura et al. (1997) identified two genes induced by exposure to PCP.

Work by Zorn et al. (2003) found beta-ionone to be the main metabolite from submerged culture with beta, beta-carotene.

Turkey tail has great promise in mycoremediation, with burlap sacks filled with sawdust or wood chips and mycelium, able to filter heavy metals, organophosphates, PAHs, pesticides, and various microbes including *E. coli*, *Listeria monocytogenes*, and *Candida albicans*.

Hairy turkey tail shows promise in conversion of dioxins, enzymatic decolorization of melanoidins, and oxidation of phenols, like its more famous cousin. Co-cultivation with *Cerrena maxima* showed oxidation of the phenolic component of lignins from birch sawdust.

Various *Trametes* species, including *T. hirsutus* and *T. villosa,* can help mycofilter chemical and color dyes.

One study found laccase from this species has some superior characteristics such as high stability, high activity, and low carbohydrate content.

Hairy turkey tail, in liquid cultures, shows potential to degrade DDT, aldrin, dieldrin, lindane, and heptachlor.

It breaks down waste from wool clothing production.

Earlier work found a purified laccase-degraded triarylmethane, indigoid, azo, and anthraquinonic dyes.

Van Hamme et al. (2003) identified *T. hirsuta* and *Funalia trogii* mycelicum as helping to metabolize dibenzyl sulphide.

Cinnabar polypore has been studied for its ability to hydroxylate biphenyl and diphenyl ether.

Purified laccase broke down the chromophore of Chicago Sky Blue dye in the presence of oxygen.

This laccase transforms benzo[a]pyrene in the presence of ABTS.

Increasing apramycin sulfate concentrations enhanced laccase production. Pointing et al. (2000) found increased laccase production in submerged liquid culture fifty-fold from *P. sanguineus* in the presence of twenty micromoles xylidine.

Red polypore *(T. sanguineus)* absorbs heavy metals from water solution using a fixed-bed column, removing more than 90 percent of lead, copper, and cadmium.

Both *T. pubescens* and *T. sanguineus* are useful for breaking down lignins for industry.

Cosmetics

Turkey tail is prized in the Far East for cosmetic purposes as well as treating areas of weak connective tissue, massage formulations, acne, and irritated erythema due to excessive ultraviolet sun radiation. Suggested applications include sunscreen or after-sun products as well as acne and anti-cellulite creams.

Food Industry

Cinnabar polypore is rich in protease enzymes, suggesting not just anti-inflammatory application but use in detergents, cheese making, meat tenderizers, flavor development, and the leather industry (Goud et al. 2009).

Cinnabar polypore and sugar beets have an unusual relationship. Beet pulp is rich in the precursors rhamnose and ferulic acid that through microbial bioconversion form vanillin. Ferulic acid is first released by enzymes and specific ferulic acid esterases, and then biotransformed into vanillin by the selected fungi, or a two-step process first using *Aspergillus niger* to transform ferulic acid into vanillic acid, and then cinnabar polypore to obtain vanillin from vanillic acid. Vanillin, of course, can be easily converted into vanilla, the world's most popular food flavor. It also has uses in the pharmaceutical and perfume industries.

The biological transformation of high-value food flavors from agricultural by-products is an ongoing and interesting area of study. This natural biotech vanillin has high economic potential, with utilization of approximately fifty to one hundred tons per year for high quality chocolates, ice cream, and pastries.

One study looked at laccase from this fungus for food preparation. An infusion of green tea for a beverage drink was improved significantly by incubating with *Pycnoporus* laccase.

Both *P. cinnabarinus* and *P. sanguineus* produce tryrosinase, which has applications for the food additive industry.

It has been found to increase maximum resistance of wheat flour dough.

The addition of ethanol increases laccase activity from the culture medium as compared with ferulic acid induced cultures. High quality flax pulp can be bleached in a totally chlorine-free method using this laccase. Vanillic acid is transformed by the fungus and produces crystalline vanillin from autoclaved corn bran without any purification step.

Textile Industry

The multicolored fans of various *Trametes* have been used worldwide in art, earrings, necklaces, ancient weapons, and articles of clothing.

The dried fungus is used to dye wool a grayish yellow color, without mordant.

Recipes and Dosage

Up to twenty grams of turkey tail three times per day brewed as a tea.

In powdered form (in capsules), take up to five grams PSK per day before or between meals. Some patients experience a darkening of the fingernails as a side effect of PSK.

Take one-gram PSP capsules three times per day.

Optimal extraction of polysaccharides is best accomplished by crushing into a powder and then boiling at one hundred degrees Celsius (212 degrees Fahrenheit) for eighty minutes and extracting three times from the same marc.

Star jelly is named for the one-time belief that it was the remains of a meteor shot from the stars. In fact, the first fifteenth-century English encyclopedia, by William Caxton, mentions this link.

The Mirror of the World, translated from a French manuscript of 1464 and, in turn, from a copy of the Latin dated 1245 AD, discusses shooting stars . . . "and when they come where it is fallen, they find none other things but a litl asshes or like thing some leef of a tree roten, that were weet."

Tremella mesenterica

T. lutescens
(YELLOW WITCH'S BUTTER)
(FAIRY BUTTER)
(STAR JELLY)
(YELLOW BRAIN JELLY)
T. foliacea
(BROWN WITCH'S BUTTER)
(LEAFY JELLY FUNGUS)
T. glandulosa
Exidia glandulosa
E. intumescens
E. spiculosa
(BLACK WITCH'S BUTTER)
(BLACK JELLY ROLL)
Dacrymyces palmatus
D. chrysospermus
(ORANGE JELLY FUNGUS)
T. helvelloides
Phlogiotis helvelloides
Guepinia helvelloides
(APRICOT JELLY)
(SALMON SALAD)

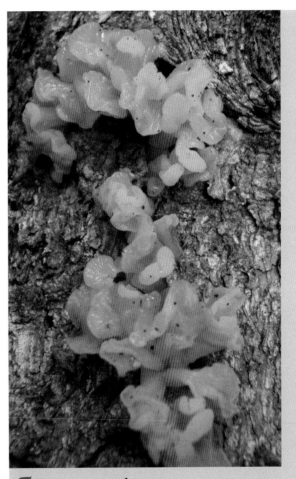

Dacrymyces palmatus

415

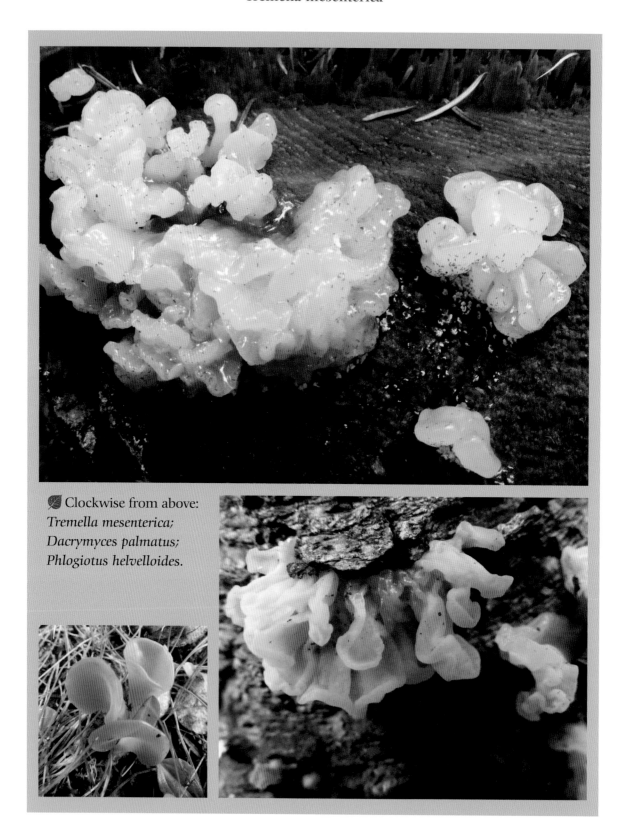

Clockwise from above:
Tremella mesenterica;
Dacrymyces palmatus;
Phlogiotus helvelloides.

John Donne wrote, in a seventeenth-century poem:

> As he that sees a starre fall, runs apace.
> And finds a gellie in the place,
> So doth the bridegroom hast as much
> Being told this starre is faine, and finds
>   her such. . . .

Ernst Chaldni, at the turn of the eighteenth century, was even bolder, suggesting jelly mushrooms were extra-terrestrial.

Yellow witch's butter looks like bright yellow-orange, brain-like lobes thrown onto dead poplar and other hardwoods and sticks. Thompson natives of British Columbia call this fungus "product of tree coming to be split open." It is edible, once you get over the idea that something that bright and unusual looking can be eaten. It is jelly-like when wet, and small and hard when dry.

Brown witch's butter is brown, flabby, and gelatinous, often found on fallen white spruce. It is not recommended for eating but is used medicinally.

Orange jelly *(Dacrymyces palmatus)* looks similar and is found on spruce trees. As the name suggests, it is more orange in color and has Y-shaped basidia and two long narrow spores that develop cross walls. *Tremella* species have four spored, longitudinally septate basidia.

The related *D. stillatus (D. deliquescens)* is somewhat smaller. This species, along with *Piptoporus betulina, Panellus stipticus,* and *Auricularia auricula* immediately re-adjusted their spore discharge periods when light and dark cycles were reversed. Artist's conk *(Ganoderma applanatum),* in contrast, took forty-eight hours to readjust.

Black witch's butter is found on hardwoods including poplar and birch, but I have also seen it on decaying pine in late fall.

The mycelium of the related *T. aurantia,* harvested from liquid culture, is added to walnut cakes, biscuits, noodles, and breads in China.

The related silver ears or white jelly fungus *(T. fuciformis)* is the only mushroom in the world that is considered a dessert food. It is known as *yin er* in China, *hakumokuji* in Japan, and *baekmoki* in Korea.

Traditional Uses

Tremella is used in traditional Chinese medicine to relieve inflammation of the upper respiratory tract and is soothing, demulcent, and slightly expectorant.

Yellow witch's butter was rubbed on chilblains in parts of England.

The related silver ears or white jelly fungus *(T. fuciformis)* has been used medicinally since the sixteenth century, as a tonic for vigor and longevity. In Japan, the fungus is eaten to prevent atherosclerosis, by lowering total blood

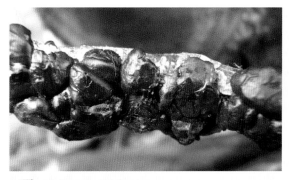

Exidia glandulosa

cholesterol levels, and maintaining levels in the linings of cells, where it is most needed. The powder is used in cholesterol-controlling functional foods and drinks.

It moistens the lungs and helps generate fluids, making it useful for treating a dry, nonproductive cough due to lung *yin* deficiency.

Culture and Folklore

During Midsummer's Eve in Sweden, bonfires with nine different woods are lit. Witch's butter, known as *trollsmor* or "troll's butter," is tossed into the flames to thwart evil spirits.

When the fungus was found near animals, it was customary to burn it in fires, to force a troll to appear and beg for mercy from thirst created by the heat of the flames.

Medicinal Use

Chemical Constituents

- *T. mesenterica*: **glucurmomannan 1,3-alpha-glucan; epitope (beta-D-glucuronosyl), 1,3-beta-1,6-beta glucan, chitin, xylose, mannose, glucurmic acid, and a trace of galactose.**

Mice trials of *T. aurantia* indicate benefit in lowering cholesterol and treating coronary disease.

Tremella is an expectorant for the lungs, widely used in medicine for bronchial inflammation and asthma. It has a comparative immunological profile to type II anti-pneumococcal serum.

It contains a pheromone mating scent, tremerogen A-10, which is of interest.

Yellow witch's butter *(T. mesenterica)* has a wide range of medicinal value, including immune stimulation, radiation protection, and anti-diabetic, anti-inflammatory, hypocholesterolemic, hepato-protective, and anti-allergenic activity.

Vinogradov et al. (2004) at the National Research Council in Ottawa, along with colleagues in Israel and Denmark, helped develop a new strain CBS 101939, in submerged culture.

One study looked at the culture requirements and found a two-stage technology for the development of acidic glucuronoxylomannan.

A crude product obtained by alcohol precipitation of the culture broth contained 40 percent of the desired constituent.

Med Myco Ltd, an Israeli company, has developed a submerged fermentation method to produce tremellastin with 50 percent glucuronoxylomannan in only a few days.

Tremellastin, containing 40 to 45 percent acidic heteropolysaccharide glucuronoxylomannan was tested on lab animals and was found to produce a statistically significant effect on blood sugar levels after fifteen days, as well as triglyceride-lowering activity (Elisashvili et al. 2002a). They also found it induced interferon production and immune-modulating effect. This places it in the class of a biological-response modifier, which means it supports all the major systems of the body, including hormonal, nervous, and immune.

Recent studies suggest that the fungus suppressed hCG-treated steroidogenesis in MA-10 cells without any toxic effect. This followed a previous study by the authors that showed it reduced plasma testosterone production in normal rats without any positive effect in dia-

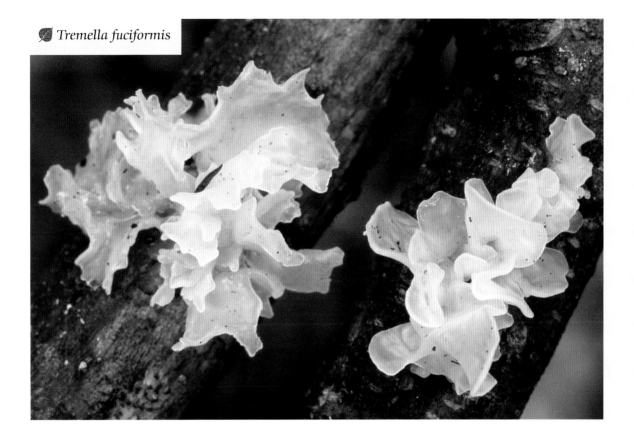

Tremella fuciformis

betic models. This temporary suppression of progesterone production needs further study (Lo, H. C. et al. 2005).

Ethanol extracts of the fruiting body induce apoptosis in lung carcinoma cell line A549 (Chen, N. Y. et al. 2008).

It increases production of interferon and interleukin-2, as well as macrophages; increases natural killer cells and effectiveness of antibodies; and reduces the rate at which cancers spread, by angiogenesis.

The fungus has been shown in clinical trials to benefit patients with hepatitis B. After thirty-six months, the cure rate was better than 90 percent, and between 50 to 75 percent after only three months of treatment.

Extracts kill cervical cancer cells and sensitize the uterus and cervix to radiation treatment, increasing the effectiveness of the therapy. It also prevents leukopenia, a common side effect of radiation and chemotherapy.

Various *Tremella* species contain glucuronoxylomannan acids that stimulate vascular endothelial cells; have anti-radiation effects; stimulate hematogenesis; and possess anti-diabetic, anti-inflammatory, anti-allergenic, hypocholesterolemic, and liver-protectant qualities.

Tremella aurantia, for example, decreases glycemia in insulin-dependent diabetes, due to an active compound TAP, or *Tremella* acidic polysaccharide (Kiho et al. 2000).

Studies indicate their use in immune-deficient conditions, as well as prevention of senile degeneration of micro blood vessels. A recent study found a 70 percent ethanol extract to be active against prostate cancer cell lines LNCaP and PC-3, through G2/M phase cell cycle arrest (Kiho et al. 2010).

One study found mushroom extracts of benefit in chickens infected with *Eimeria tenella.*

Black witch's butter shows 90 percent inhibition of sarcoma 180 cancer cell lines (Ohtsuka et al. 1973).

Dacrymenone, an extract from the *Dacrymyces* species, is weakly antifungal and antibacterial. Another compound, VM 3298-2, is cytotoxic and antifungal (Mierau et al. 2003). VM 3298-2 is cytotoxic against human colon adenocarcinoma cells lines, with IC$_{50}$ of ten micrograms per milliliter and five micrograms per milliliter against HL-60 and L1210 cells respectively.

Apricot jelly *(T. hevelloides)* shows 100 percent inhibition of both sarcoma 180 and Ehrlich carcinoma cancer cell lines (Ohtsuka et al. 1973).

Fungi Essences

Black witch's butter essence supports the spiritual confrontation with negative experience to the blockage of their own spirituality.

— MARIANA

Yellow witch's butter essence is for young people who react defiantly. It helps dissolve rigid attitudes and opens up the possibility partner is also opening.

— MARIANA

Spiritual Properties

Tremella nostoc, or *T. coelifolium,* is green-like and grows in wet areas. It was known as sky fall by Linnaeus, and thought to originate from fallen stars.

Tremella Nestoe. A curious gelatinous plant, once celebrated among alchemists, who used it in their search for the philosopher's stone and the universal panacea, had defied all botanical research even up to a century ago. The botanists could not analyze it or classify it; it was variously assumed that it was not a plant at all but the droppings of herons which had fed upon frogs, or even, by the old alchemists, that it was an emanation from the stars.

— CLAIRE POWELL

Cosmetics

Glucuronoxylomannan is a high molecular substance useful for skin cosmetics, helping to retain skin moisture and giving skin protection, flexibility, and flattening effect. It is free of pH dependence and forms a film when dried in a state attached to skin or hair. It has application for cleansing and massage creams, facial washes, *eau de toilette,* and hair preparations.

Recipes and Dosage

Three to six grams: Soak the dried fungi in water to hydrate, or use fresh. Simmer in water for six to eight hours, until pasty, and then add honey. Drink for ten days, then take three days off. It is good for colds, flu, asthma, bronchitis, and general debility, as it is an immunomodulator.

Be careful using *Tremella* for coughs resulting from cold wind, due to the mushroom's cooling nature.

Tremellodon gelatinosum

Pseudohydnum gelatinosum
(JELLY TONGUE)
(TOOTHED JELLY FUNGUS)

Jelly tongue is a gelatinous, hydnum-like toothed fungus common to coniferous forests in colder climates. It can be eaten raw or cooked. David Arora says this mushroom is one of his fifty-five favorite fleshy fungal fructifications. He says in *Mushrooms Demystified* that "they are unique, and look funnier than they do fungal—in fact, it is hard to take them seriously!"

Medicinal Use

The inhibition rate against sarcoma 180 and Ehrlich carcinoma cell lines is 90 percent (Ohtsuka et al. 1973).

Fungi Essence

Jelly tongue (*P. gelatinosum*) essence helps us center ourselves and to concentrate, keeping us in balance. It strengthens our cellular structure, preserving our power (and our body heat) at the center of our being rather than allowing it to dissipate and be wasted.

— KORTE PHI

Trichaptum biforme

Polyporus biformis
Hirshioporus biformis
H. pargamenus
P. pargamenus
(PURPLE TOOTHED POLYPORE)
(PARCHMENT BRACKET)
T. abietinum
H. abietinus
Polyporus abietinea
(VIOLET PORED BRACKET FUNGUS)
(VIOLET FIR BRACKET FUNGUS)
(FIR POLYPORE)
T. fuscoviolaceum
T. hollii
H. fusco-violaceus
P. abietinus var. irpiciformis

Both bracket fungi are common, the former growing mainly on deciduous trees, and the latter on conifers.

Purple toothed polypore has a pore surface that is violet to bluish, becoming more tooth-like with age.

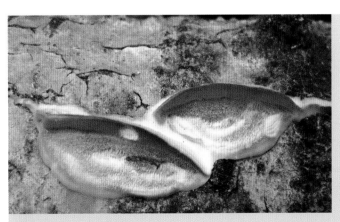

Trichaptum biforme

T. abietinum is similar, but smaller and thinner, with a whitish, hairy cap and purple underside.

Traditional Uses

The Thompson First Nation of B.C. used this fungus, called owl wood, or *kalulaa'iuk,* and its spore powder as a rub to give strength to young men.

Medicinal Use

Violet pored bracket fungus shows activity against *E. coli* and *Staphylococcus aureus* bacteria (Ohtsuka et al. 1973).

Purple toothed polypore has been studied and found to possess antitumor activity. It has been found in clinical studies to possess antineoplastic activity (Jong and Gantt 1987).

The closely related *T. fuscoviolaceum* has been shown to inhibit tumors, with an inhibition rate against sarcoma 180 of 45 percent (Ohtsuka et al. 1973).

Mycoremediation

Bruno Boulet, in his beautiful book on polypores of Quebec, mentions the use of purple toothed fungi as a cold-weather mycoremediator of PCPs, which are organochlorine toxics. He also mentions the use of *Irpex lactius* and *Diplomitoporus* species. This is an area of great interest, helping clean up our environment by using mycelium power in cold climates.

Tricholoma magnivelare

T. ponderosum
Armillaria ponderosa
(PINE MUSHROOM)
(WHITE MATSUTAKE)

It is no dream!
Matsutake are growing
On the belly of the mountain
　　— SHIGETAKA

Matsutake:
From the depth of the pine forest,
The voice of the hawk
　　— KOYA

Tricholoma is Greek meaning "with hair on the edge or lump." *Magnivelare* is Latin meaning "with big veil."

This is the highly prized pine mushroom, very closely related to the matsutake *(A. matsutake)* of Japan.

Today, in Tokyo, a perfect specimen of the fresh T. matsutake mushroom (a variety that grows natively in Japan) can fetch up to $113 per pound. It has a sweet smell, reminiscent of garden cress *(Lepidium sativum)*.

Every year, mushroom pickers in Alberta rush to the beds of reindeer moss under older jack pine for our related delicacy. It fetches a good price, especially for fresh, when it has good taste, and a pleasant fresh, spicy odor. Some compare the scent to cinnamon and others to fresh watercress. Arora suggests calls it reminiscent of dirty socks with a hint of cinnamon. It is, however, a mycoaccumulator of arsenic at rates of twenty-two times concentration, so care must be taken as to where it is picked.

It is sometimes mistaken for *A. caligata*, which has a cinnamon odor, crossed with alpha thujone (think wormwood or sage).

It is responsible for the fifth flavor (in addition to bitter, sweet, salty, and sour) which the Japanese call *umami* or, roughly translated, "deliciousness."

This mushroom represents a sizable income for some residents, and others who travel to the pine forests for the annual harvest, with prices in the range of $10 to $15 per pound for prime specimens.

The wild mushroom is picked in China, where it is known as *songron* or *songkuomo*, and exported to Japan.

More than six thousand tons of raw mushrooms, worth more than $82 million, were exported from North America in 1996 alone. The worldwide trade is now believed to be worth at least several billion dollars annually, but that is dependent on worldwide economy and availability from Asian sources.

Retail prices of up to $113 per pound have been obtained in Japan, but not in recent years. Note that there are seven different grades, ranging from grade one, with tight buttons more than six centimeters long and with no partial veil evident, to grade seven, which are wormy but still firm.

It is a culinary waste to sauté these mushrooms, as the unique aroma is lost. Instead, slice thinly, salt lightly, and then grill them until very slightly brown. They will be chewy and most aromatic.

I. H. Cho et al. (2006) have characterized the aroma active compound in raw and cooked pine mushrooms.

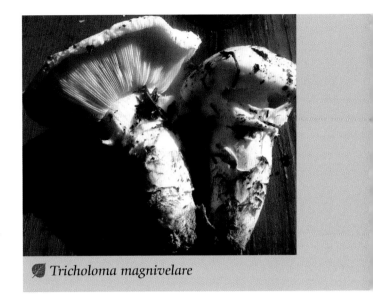

Tricholoma magnivelare

A Japanese company has developed a synthetic essence of matsutake that can be poured over ordinary mushrooms to allow the diner to imagine he is eating the real thing. Methyl cinnamate is a major constituent of this essence.

Medicinal Use

Pine mushroom has been used as a remedy for difficult labor, acute gastritis, fevers, and convulsions. It is also used to treat tonsillitis and as a vermifuge.

Scientists have been studying the mushroom for its antitumor properties. One study found matsutake had a sarcoma 180 tumor-inhibition rate of 91.8 percent, and a cure rate in mice of 55 percent, very similar to shiitake. The inhibition rate for Ehrlich carcinoma is 100 percent.

Matsunaga et al. (2003) found mycelium active against colon cancer cells.

A novel immune-modulating alpha-glucan has been identified from the mycelium (Hoshi et al. 2005).

423

One study identified a polysaccharide fraction that is immune stimulating and increases production of NO and TNF-alpha. Another found a novel antitumor protein specific to inhibition of SV-40 and the human papilloma virus, believed to contribute to increased risk for cervical cancer.

Research found an alpha-glucan fraction inhibited growth of both primary and metastatic tumors.

Earlier work by same author suggests benefit against fibrosarcoma.

Another study found that the mycelium enhanced recovery of natural killer cell activity in mice.

The mycelium has been found to exert immune-modulating effect (Hoshi et al. 2005). They cultured *T. matsutake* in tanks, and found that the mycelial preparation, named CM6271, given orally, recovered natural killer cell activity and serum 1L-12 levels that had been reduced by stress. It showed antitumor activity against fibrosarcoma and prevented formation of precancerous lesions induced in the colon. The molecule was found distributed in M cells of intestinal Peyer's patches one hour after ingestion.

A more recent article by same author confirmed localization of a single peak fraction, MPG-1, in Peyer's patches, mesenteric lymph nodes, and the spleen, as well as promotion of iL-12 p70 production and natural killer cell activity (Hoshi et al. 2008).

Not only was the immune system stimulated through Peyer's patches, the fraction was also taken into the blood and stimulated the systemic immune system. The mode of action is different than that of beta-D-glucans, on enhancement of antitumor or anti-infectious activities.

Hyun-Woo Lim et al. (2007) identified anti-inflammatory properties due to inhibition of nitric oxide production, as well as antioxidant activity.

Jong Hyun Kim et al. (2008) found cultured beta-glucan stimulates the immune system due to NF-kappaB activation.

Earlier work found the fruiting bodies show antitumor activity against fibrosarcoma.

Ryong et al. (1989) found anti-atherogenic and anti-atherosclerotic properties in *A. matsutake* extracts.

Tricholomic acid is a flavor enhancer that excites the central nervous system. In larger doses, it is lethal to flies. Jonathan Ott, in his wonderful book *Pharmacotheon,* mentions a "single fly even squeezed through the tiny opening of the screw-cap vial in which the small amount of tricholomic acid solution was kept, and there met his death!"

The structural analog, glutamic acid, in the form of monosodium glutamate (MSG), is a neurotoxin. It is associated with headaches, numbness and tingling, nausea, dizziness, and other symptoms, especially in those people deficient in B6.

The compound is used in many foods for flavor enhancement, and although considered safe for humans, it was voluntarily removed from baby food in 1970, when it was found that the amount of glutamate in a jar of baby food was enough to induce damage in an immature brain.

Cosmetics

Matsutake *(A. matsutake)* owes its pine-like fragrance to alpha- and beta-pinene, cembrene, and S-matsutake alcohols. It also contains amino acids and methyl cis-a-methyl cinnamate, which aids in moisture retention and 2-octen-1-ol, found in many mushrooms, which stimulates peripheral circulation. Matsutake is believed to be an important dietary item for the musk deer, which is the source of the rare and expensive natural musk. This is identical in structure and chemistry to the pheromones secreted by the human male, and used in a number of cosmetic and perfumery items. Various Song Yi mushroom extracts, from water to ethanol to ceramide blends, are available in Asia.

The fungus was used traditionally in Korea in a decoction, steeped overnight, and then applied as a facial wash to remove dark skin spots from sun damage and to tighten skin wrinkles. An alcohol extract rich in songyic acid is of great interest in Korea as a skin whitening agent and alternative to kojic acid.

Matsutake is recommended for facial creams and lotions for sensitive skin, moisturizing products, and for stimulating bath and shower products. It can be found in products like Amore Pacific Treatment Cleansing Lotion.

Food Industry

Matsunaga et al. (2003) have developed a method to mass-produce mycelium of matsutake for functional food application.

Cultivation

In parts of Japan, the mushroom is threatened with extinction due to nematodes attacking the root hairs of pine trees, and attempts at cultivation have met with limited success.

One study successfully inoculated pine trees with *T. matsutake.* This technique may be of value to creation of a sustainable pine mushroom industry in the Pacific Northwest.

Tricholoma portentosum

(STREAKED TRICHOLOMA)
(PRETENTIOUS TRICHOLOMA)
(STICKY GRAY TRICH)
T. populinum
(THE SANDY)
(COTTONWOOD MUSHROOM)

Streaked *Tricholoma* is known in Japan as *shimo-furishimeji,* in Poland as *siwki,* and in Sweden as *streckmusseron.*

The gills and stalks are tinged a greenish yellow. It is commonly found under pine.

It is a perfectly edible fungi if you manage to find it before the insects do.

Tricolomic acid, as previously mentioned, is a flavor enhancer that excites brain neurons.

The monoterpene volatiles responsible for streaked Tricholoma's aroma have been identified in work by Breheret et al. (1997) and include alpha-pinene, and beta-phellandrene.

Cottonwood mushroom is also called "the sandy" in reference to its common home of sandy soil beneath cottonwood trees near a source of water. The Shuswap call it *smetl' aka,* the Thompson *meaqi,* the Okanagan-Colville, *petl'kin,* and the Lillooet, *meix qin.*

It grows in clumps under various hardwood trees and has a sweet, mealy scent similar to sweet bedstraw or cucumber. It is a popular edible mushroom of First Nations in the interior of British Columbia. The fungi were traditionally strung and dried for winter use, but also eaten raw or cooked.

Traditional Uses

The First Nations people of British Columbia used the juice from cooking cottonwood or pine mushrooms to wash infants, which was believed to help them grow up strong and independent, like a mushroom that can push through rocks and logs as it grows.

Medicinal Use

Chemical Constituents

- Tricholidic acid and tricolomic acid.

- The mushrooms are 94 percent water, but contain significant content of iron 0.67 percent, copper 0.51 percent, zinc 0.45 percent, magnesium, chromium, and manganese.

These mushrooms have been found to contain ergosterol and the recently discovered and novel steroid portensterol.

This sterol is found in the toxic *Clitocbye nebularis* and choice edible blewit *(C. nuda).*

They contain a number of other sterols and the triterpenoid tricholidic acid.

Methanol extracts indicate antioxidant and free radical-quenching activity.

An extract derived from dimethyl sulfoxide (DMSO) shows activity against *Bacillus subtilis* and *B. cereus,* as well as *Cryptococcus neoformans* associated with cryptococcosis (Barros et al. 2007a).

It shows inhibition of sarcoma 180 and Ehrlich carcinoma cancer cell lines by 70 percent and 60 percent respectively.

Pine mushrooms are a source of polyprenols, not usually associated with mushrooms. Kukina et al. found what they called "fungoprenols" in *T. populinum, Armillaria mellea,* and *Lycoperdon perlatum* (Kukina et al. 2005). They all contain predominately acetylated polyprenols. Their use and function is undetermined.

Eating the mushroom led to the regression of severe allergic symptoms in one patient with thromboangitis obliterans and in another with urticaria.

Various ergosterol peroxides have been identified.

Tricholoma ustale
(BURNT TRICHOLOMA)
(BITTER TRICHOLOMA)
T. vaccinum
(SCALY TRICHOLOMA)
(RUSSET SCALY TRICH)
T. virgatum
(FIBRIL TRICHOLOMA)
T. flavovirens
T. equestre
T. auratum
Agaricus equestre
A. flavovirens
(MAN ON HORSEBACK)

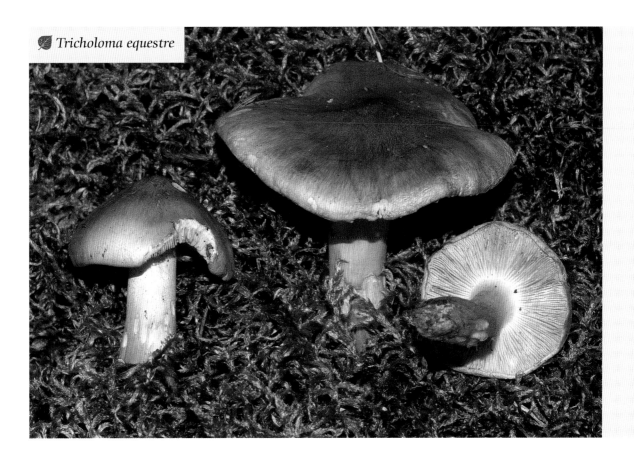

Tricholoma equestre

(SADDLE SHAPE TRICH)
(CANARY TRICH)
(YELLOW KNIGHT)
T. aurantium
(SLIMY ORANGE TRICH)
(VEILED TRICH)
T. aggregatum (see *Lyophyllum decastes*)
T. nudum (see *Lepista nuda*)

Ustale is Latin meaning "burnt cinnabar," a pigment. *Vaccinum* is related to "cow-like color." *Aurantium* means "orange." *Virgatum* means "streaked." *Flavovirens* suggests "golden yellow spring," and *equestre* pertains to "a horse."

Burnt *Tricholma* has the odor of wild licorice, and is found under deciduous trees.

The largest specimen in the world is located in Mushroom Park in the tiny village of Vilna, Alberta. Weighing more than seventeen thousand pounds and standing nearly twenty feet high, this replica sculpture of three burnt *Tricholoma* was built in 1993 and is a popular destination for tourists and mycophiles. Unfortunately, its name is misspelled as *T. uspale,* and it is wrongly suggested that the mushroom was a choice edible enjoyed by the Ukrainian settlers of the area. In fact, burnt *Tricholoma* is a gastric irritant, containing the toxin ustalic acid.

It has a high protein content, from 30 to 50 percent.

Fibril *Tricholoma* has a grayish cap, with distinctive pointed knob. It is found under spruce and jack pine in late summer.

These two *Tricholoma* species are not recommended for eating, as they may cause diarrhea and vomiting.

Man on horseback, known to my Polish in-laws as *gaski,* is, on the other hand, considered by some to be a delicious edible mushroom. In the Middle Ages, it is said that French knights reserved pride of place for this mushroom at their tables, and left the less desired bovine bolete for the peasants. It is widely sold in European markets. Man on horseback is believed by some authors to relate to General Ernest Berlanger, a dictator of France, who almost always appeared in public on horseback.

One study suggests avoiding this mushroom, as it may cause fatal rhabdomyolysis. This is a breaking down of skeletal muscles that may lead to kidney failure. It is a good thing I never enjoyed the flavor.

The poisoning was the result of a rather large quantity of mushrooms. One found the same effect in rats using *Boletus edulis,* so something is amiss. Later work by the same researchers reported myocardio and hepatoxic effects from *T. equestre* when consumed by mice for long periods of time. The mushrooms were freshly frozen and not cooked. Cook all mushrooms, even for your pet rodents!

Slimy orange *Tricholoma* is not considered an edible mushroom, which is too bad because the odor is cucumber-like. Helene Schalkwijk-Barendsen wrote that they smell like bulrush hearts, a rather apt description of the odor. They contain physcion, a nasty toxin. Personally, I don't bother picking them, as to me the taste is rather rancid.

The related *T. pardinum,* or tiger *Tricholoma,* is found occasionally, but is poisonous! It can be mistaken for a white *Tricholoma,* but will cause severe gastroenteritis. Badalyan et al. (2001) found in laboratory studies that the fungus produced ill effects on the central nervous system of mice.

Dirty or earthy *Tricholoma (T. terreum)* is edible, not choice, but certainly worth picking and cooking. It has an earthy flavor and odor that is unpleasant to some, and favored by others. Optimal storage is obtained by submerging it in boiling water for six minutes and then putting it quickly into cold storage.

Medicinal Use

Chemical Constituents

- *T. equestre:* **tryptophan, serotonin, tryptamine, and flavomannin-6,6'-dimethyl ether.**

Traditional Uses

Tricholoma gambosum, also known as *T. georgii* and *Calocybe gambosa,* is used in China to treat measles and sick children feeling agitated and upset.

Inhibition rate against both sarcoma 180 and Ehrlich carcinoma is 90 percent.

Tricholoma ustale, T. vaccinum, and *T. virgatum* have shown inhibition rates against sarcoma 180 and Ehrlich carcinoma of 70 to 90 percent.

The related *T. robustum* shows 100 percent inhibition of both; *T. sejunctum* shows 90 percent inhibition of both, and *T. fulvum* 80 percent and 70 percent respectively (Ohtsuka et al. 1973).

Methanol extracts of *T. equestre* contain a

sterol that stimulates the enzyme alkaline phosphatase in mouse osteoblasts, or bone cells. High levels of this enzyme activity are associated with increased proliferation and differentiation of osteoblasts and prevention of osteoporosis. This sterol protected osteoblasts from apoptosis that normally occurs in serum starvation.

The novel compound flavomannin-6,6'-dimethyl ether shows potent inhibition of human adenocarcinoma colorectal Caco-2 cells, with arrest in the G0/G1 phase.

Chloroform extracts of *T. aurantium* fruiting body show weak antibacterial activity against *E. coli, Staphylococcus aureus,* and *S. epidermidis,* but strong activity against *Bacillus subtilis.* An ethyl acetate extract showed weak activity against *Pseudomonas aeruginosa.* Mycelium extracts were active against *E. coli* and *S. aureus* (Yamac and Bilgili 2006).

A novel polysaccharide-bound protein (PSPC) has been isolated from *T. mongolicum* and shown to activate both lymphocytes and macrophages from BALB/c mice, and yet it shows no direct cytotoxic activity against fibroblasts, hepatoma, or choriocarcinoma cells.

Le Li et al. (2005) found a lectin from these edible mushrooms stimulates gene expression of immunomodulating cytokines in mice.

Another PSPC purified from *T. lobayense* inhibits growth of sarcoma 180, with no signs of in vivo toxicity.

It appears that immune cells are responding to PSPC through gene expression and production of immune-modulating cytokines that may mediate immunopotentiation of this agent in vivo.

White *Tricholoma (T. album)* myco-accumulates titanium.

The mycelium of the related *T. panaeolum (Clitocybe fasiculata),* grown in fermentation tanks, shows inhibition of malignant adenoma 755 in mice (Espenshade and Griffith 1966; Gregory et al. 1966).

Tricholomalides A-C identified by Tsukamoto et al. (2003) show significant induction of neurite growth.

Sulphur knight *(T. sulphureum)* is a poisonous species that nonetheless inhibits sarcoma 180 and Ehrlich carcinoma cells by 90 percent and 80 percent respectively (Ohtsuka et al. 1973).

Tricholomopsis rutilans

Tricholoma rutilans
(PLUMS AND CUSTARD)
(VARIEGATED MOP)
T. platyphylla
Megacollybia platyphylla
Oudemansiella platyphylla
(BROAD GILL)

Plums and custard mushroom is edible, but not highly recommended, unless you like the taste of rotten wood. With its reddish hairs on yellow caps, and bright yellow gills, plums and custard mushroom is a striking mushroom. It has a musty smell and is often found on rotting pine or spruce stumps and deadfall in the boreal forest. It is sold in markets in central Europe.

Broad gill is widespread and common on logs and underground wood. It has a white spore print. It is not edible, and can cause

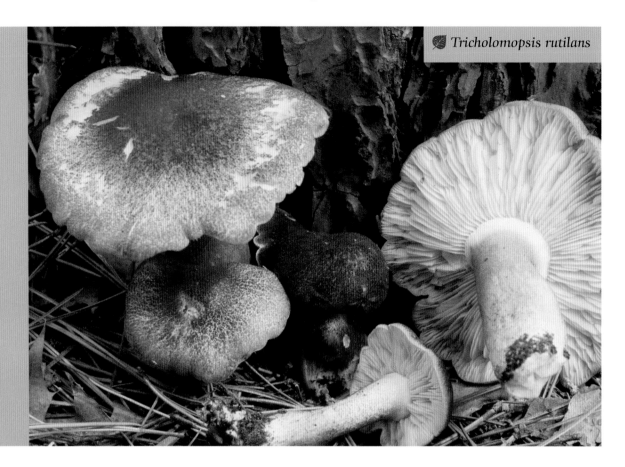

Tricholomopsis rutilans

abdominal pain, vomiting, diarrhea, and muscle spasms.

Medicinal Use

Chemical Constituents

- **Fomecin B, steryl esters with a polyhydroxylated ergostane-type nucleus, and two hexynoic and hexenoic acids.**

Fomecin B has been found to be antagonistic to various cancer cell lines.

Koch et al. (1998) looked at ethanol extracts of both the fruiting bodies and mycelium of plums and custard mushroom. They found the extract reduced the binding of lipopolysaccharide and the release of mediators. At a concentration of one hundred micrograms per milliliter, the extract inhibited more than half of the LPS binding. It also decreased LPS-induced release of interleukin 1 and tumor necrosis factor alpha.

New steryl esters with a polyhydroxylated ergostane-type nucleus have been identified (Wang, F. and J. K. Liu 2005).

Two hexynoic and hexenoic acids have been identified in the fruiting body (Hatanaka and Niimura 1972).

One study found this species to possess the highest antioxidant levels of several species tested.

Pujol et al. (1990) found fungal extracts of

broad gill to be active against *Candida albicans,* *C. tropicalis,* and *Aspergillus fumigatus.*

Inhibition rates of 80 percent against sarcoma 180 and 90 percent against Ehrlich carcinoma have been noted in mice studies (Ohtsuka et al. 1973).

Tubaria furfuracea
(TOTALLY TEDIOUS TUBARIA)

David Arora says that this species is "your quintessential 'LBM [little brown mushroom],' as boring as it is ubiquitous and innocuous as it is inconspicuous.... To say more about it would do the more interesting mushrooms in this book an injustice." It is found in woodchips and lawns.

Medicinal Use

It shows inhibition of sarcoma 180 at 80 percent and Ehrlich carcinoma 90 percent (Ohtsuka et al. 1973).

Tulostoma simulans
(BURIED STALKED PUFFBALL)

Tulos is Greek meaning "tumor." *Stoma* means "stomach." *Simulans* is Latin meaning "imitating" or "simulating." Hence, "imitating stomach tumor."

This fungus and desert drumstick *(Battarraea stevenii)* are the only two local species of the *Tulostemataceae* family in my part of the world.

It is fairly common across western North America, found on sandy soil. The mature mushroom is inedible.

Culture and Folklore

Tulostoma simulans was used by various native tribes for its symbolism, in ceremonies and displays of art.

Medicinal Use

The related *T. obesum* exhibits significant antibacterial activity (Al-Fatimi et al. 2005).

Tylopilus felleus

T. alutarius
Boletus alutarius
B. felleus
(BITTER BOLETE)
T. plumbeoviolaceus
(GRAY VIOLET BOLETE)

This mushroom looks similar to the king bolete and is found under mixed or coniferous woods. It has a pink spore print and pink billowed tubes. Unlike the king bolete, however, the taste is very bitter, like gall.

The related *T. plumbeoviolaceus* is a bitter tasting violet-brown species.

Medicinal Use
Chemical Constituents

- *T. felleus:* **2-butyl-1-azacyclohexane iminium salt, N-y-Glutamul boletine, and tylopilan.**

- *T. plumbeoviolaceus:* **two seco-ergosterols, tylopiol A and B, allitol, and ergosta-7,22-dien-3beta-ol uridine.**

Slane et al. (2004) found the fungus inhibited pancreatic lipase by 96 percent, and was the second highest of 110 macrofungi they tested.

A toxic principle, 2-butyl-1-azacyclohexane

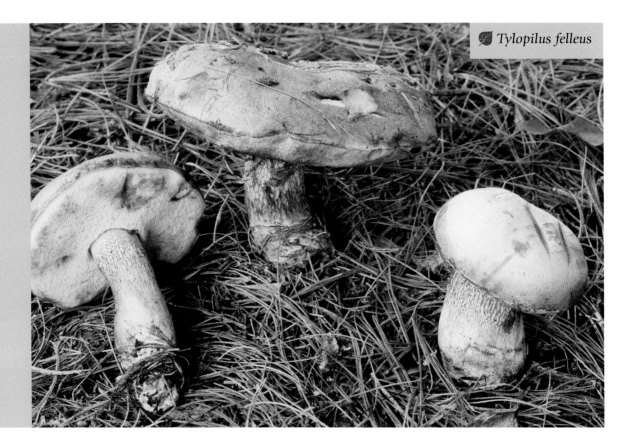

Tylopilus felleus

iminium salt, was extracted from *Tylopilus* species and found to exhibit moderate acute toxicity against ddY mice (Watanabe, R. et al. 2002).

The compound N-y-glutamyl boletine exhibits moderate antibacterial activity.

Subcutaneous administration of a lycophilized preparation inhibited inflammation, but oral dosage did not produce significant results in work by Kohlmunzer et al. It is said to possess anticancer activity, due to its content of mucilage. This chemical is believed to stimulate the immune system and fight infection (Kohlmunzer et al. 1977).

The initial research was conducted in Po-land and is now being followed up by a Japanese laboratory.

One study identified tylopilan, a beta-glucan chain cytotoxic to 180-TG Crocker tumor cells in vitro. A combination of tylopilan and *Propionibacterium acnes* injected in mice suggests that immune stimulation enhances the antitumor activity.

Early work by Ohtsuka et al. (1973) found an extract of the fruiting body inhibited both sarcoma 180 and Ehrlich carcinoma cell lines in mice by 100 percent.

The related *T. plumbeoviolaceus* contains two seco-ergosterols, tylopiol A and B, as well as allitol and ergosta-7,22-dien-3beta-ol uridine.

Tyromyces chioneus

T. albellus
Leptoporus albellus
L. chioneus
Polystictus chioneus
Ungularia chionea
(WHITE CHEESE POLYPORE)
T. caesius
Postia caesia
Oligoporus caesius
(BLUE CHEESE POLYPORE)
T. fragilis
Postia fragilis
Oligoporus fragilis
(RUSTY CHEESE POLYPORE)

White cheese polypore is widespread on hardwood trees and is occasionally found on dead conifers. It is reminiscent of the oyster mushroom, except that it has pores instead of gills and the color is pure white.

Medicinal Use

Cadinane sesquiterpenes isolated from these fungi have been found to possess anti-HIV-1 activity. The potency is significant with an EC_{50} equal to three micrograms per milliliter (Liu, D.-Z. et al. 2007).

Early work by Hervey (1947) found that blue and rusty cheese polypore both show activity against *Staphylococcus aureus*. Earlier work by Robbins et al. (1945) found the same activity in white cheese polypore.

The related *Irpex mollis (Spongipellis pachydon)* also grows on conifers and has pores that become tooth-like with age. It exhibits activity against *Staphylococcus aureus*, cited above.

The related *S. delectans (Polporus delectans)*, *T. fumidiceps, T. guttulatus, T. balsameus,* and *T. galactinus* showed moderate activity in the same study. The related *T. stipticus*, also known as *T. immitis*, shows significant activity.

Tyromyces subvermispora, now known as *Ceriporiopsis subvermispora*, is a white rot fungus that degrades lignin without significant damage to cellulose. Ceriporic acid is believed to be the important compound.

Mycoremediation

White cheese polypore was shown by Sasek et al. (1998) to be useful as a myco-degrader of synthetic dyes.

Ustilago maydis

U. zeae
(CORN SMUT)

Corn smut is occasionally found on corn ears. In Mexico, it is known as *huitlacoche,* which is derived from the original Nahuatl name for the fungus, *cuitlacoche,* which translates literally as "sleeping excrement," referring either to the hidden nature of the fungi within the husks, or the state of mind in sleep.

Early ethnobotanists may have been mistaken and this may refer to corn ergot, or *Claviceps gigantea*. Often referred to as *diente de caballo,* or horse's tooth fungus, this ergot is hard, dry, and smelly and cannot be mistaken for food. Of course, it would have effects similar to rye ergot (see *Claviceps*).

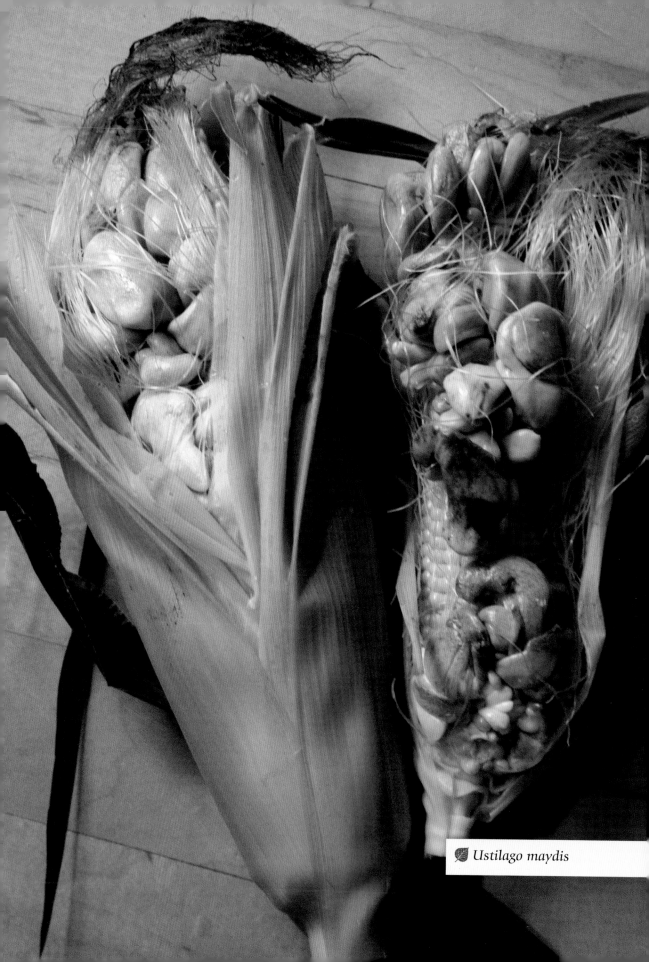

Ustilago maydis

In Mexico, corn smut is eaten in tacos and other stir-fried dishes. It is ready to eat when it feels like a pear starting to ripen.

Medicinal Use

Chemical Constituents

- **Proteinase pumA and pumB, aminopeptidase pumAPE, and dipeptidylaminopeptidase pumDAP.**

The fungus is believed to prevent or cure hepatic or gastroenteric ulcers and relieve constipation. The spore powder is combined with brown sugar and used in cases of neurasthenia and infantile malnutrition.

A tincture is used to treat poor circulation to the brain, dizziness, impaired vision, and dull headaches at the top of the head. It is made with one part fresh fungus to ten parts 40 percent alcohol.

Ustilagic acid has been found to inhibit *Candida albicans.* The fungus inhibited the growth of sarcoma 180 in mice trials (Gregory et al. 1966).

Water extracts inhibit sarcoma 180 in white mice (Ohtsuka et al. 1973).

Homeopathy

Ustilago maydis, or corn smut, is indicated in atonic (passive) uterine hemorrhages and threatened or habitual miscarriage. Nervous headaches from menstrual irregularity are common.

It is also indicated in heavy menstrual bleeding, in spotting and bleeding between menstrual periods, and in retroversion of the uterus. There may be ovarian pain during hemorrhage, or the cervix may bleed easily, with dark clotted blood that forms long black strings.

It can be used to treat alopecia or dry skin, small boils, eczema, and crusta lactea.

It can be specific to psoriasis, used internally and externally.

In the male, there is an uncontrollable desire to masturbate, with erotic fancies and amorous dreams. This is accompanied by a dull pain in the lumbar region, great despondency, and mental irritability.

Muscular debility with the sensation of boiling water along the back should be looked for. Muscular contractions, especially of the lower limbs, are another indication worth noting.

Dose: 3C tincture. The attenuation is prepared from the spores of the fungus, *Ustilago zeae,* which lives parasitically on the stalk, flower, and grains of the maize. The powdered spores are then tinctured at a ratio of one to ten in 90 percent alcohol.

Ustilago crameri
(MILLET SMUT)

Ustilago crameri is a fungus that infects the spikelets of *Setaria italica* and other members of the genus. The spores have a thin, grayish membrane that later breaks open with buff-brown to olive-brown powder.

Traditional Uses

The fungus is used in traditional Chinese medicine for curing indigestion related to fidgeting and agitation.

Recipes and Dosage

Three grams of spores are mixed with honey and taken with water twice daily.

Ustilago esculenta

(WILD RICE SMUT)

This fungus is found growing on the shoots of wild rice.

The sori, or clusters of spores, grow within the young stems, causing the stem to swell with infection. In an early stage, it can be eaten as a delicious and tasty vegetable. To prepare it, slice the wild rice shoots and dry the slices in the sun. Cook the dried shoots as a soup, adding salt and vinegar.

Traditional Uses

It has been found useful as a diuretic and laxative. It is used to treat redness of the eyes, alcohol intoxication, and carbuncles.

Ustilago nuda

(WHEAT SMUT)

Like rye, wheat spikes are susceptible to ergot infestation. *Ustilago nuda* is a common spore mass on wheat and barley. It is mild in nature and tasteless.

Traditional Uses

In traditional Chinese medicine, it is noted for its diaphoretic and analgesic properties.

Pills made by collecting the sori are used to cure febrile and sensorial diseases, headaches, high fever with lack of perspiration, annoyance, and trismus, or grinding and gnashing of the teeth.

It is used to cure metrorrhagia, or in-between-period bleeding from the uterus.

Xerula furfuracea

X. radicata

Oudemansiella radicata

(ROOTED OUDEMANSIELLA)

This edible is found in mixed forests in summer and early fall. It is rarely found on the Pacific coast but has been identified in the midwestern plains.

Medicinal Use

Chemical Constituents
- **Oudenone and oudemansin X.**

Oudenone strongly inhibits biosynthesis of enzymes associated with phenylalanine and tyrosine. One study found that this compound significantly lowers blood pressure. It appears to inhibit tyrosine hydroxylase in adrenal glands and reduce catecholamine levels in these glands as well as in the hearts of hypertensive animals.

Oudemansin X has been shown to possess antifungal properties (Anke, T. et al. 1990; Umezawa et al. 1995).

The inhibition rate against sarcoma 180 and Ehrlich carcinoma cell lines is 100 percent and 90 percent respectively (Ohtsuka et al. 1973).

Fermentation yields production of exo-polysaccharides (Zou et al. 2005).

Xylaria polymorpha

Xylosphaera polymorpha
X. obovata
Hypoxylon polymorphum
Sphaeria polymorpha
(DEAD MAN'S FINGERS)
X. hypoxylon
Xylosphaera hypoxylon
(CANDLE SNUFF FUNGUS)
(STAGHORN FUNGUS)

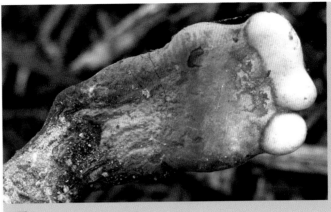

Xylaria polymorpha

The genus name starts with an X, but is pronounced Zylaria as in "sigh."

Dead man's finger is common and widespread near the base of rotting tree stumps.

Candle snuff is named for its shape, which is similar to the tool used for putting out candle flames. Other authors suggest the name is related to the manner in which spores are carried away in wind currents. This fungus is common year-round in the Pacific Northwest and has been reported to possess luminous mycelia.

Another name, staghorn, is related to its antler shape.

X. longipes is slimmer than *X. polymorpha* and is found on hardwood trees across North America.

Traditional Uses

In Ayurvedic folk medicine from India—where it is known as *phoot doodh,* literally "to gush milk"—dead man's finger is used to promote milk flow after birth. The fruiting body is ground into a powder, blended with equal parts of sugar, and formed into pea-sized pills. These are taken twice daily before meals with cow's milk for five days.

The closely related *X. nigripes* sclerotia is used in traditional Chinese medicine for eliminating dampness, easing infant convulsions, and stopping heart palpitations. It is diuretic and sedative, promotes lactation, and stops blood loss related to the lungs or nose and after childbirth.

Medicinal Use

Chemical Constituents

- *X. polymorpha:* **piliformic acid, mannitol, globoscinic acid, globoscin and two cytotoxic cytochalasins, xyloketals A-E, xylarinic acids A and B.**

- *X. hypoxylon:* **cyochalasins, 19,20-epoxy-cytochalasin D, xylarone, and 8,9-dehydroxylarone.**

- *X. longipes:* **xylaramide.**

437

Piliformic acid in the fruiting body shows moderate activity against KB and BC-1 cancer cell lines (Chinworrungsee et al. 2001).

The mushroom shows cytotoxic activity against human cancer cell line HL-60 through induction of apoptosis.

It also contains about 6 percent mannitol, a known diuretic compound.

Xyloketals A-E are potent acetylcholinesterase inhibitors, suggesting they may be useful in treating various brain memory conditions (Lin 2001).

Xylarinic acids A and B, isolated from the fruiting body, show significant antifungal effect against pathogenic fungi species including *Fusarium oxysporium* (Jan et al. 2007).

Xylaria species contain peptides that inhibit angiotensin-converting enzyme (ACE) (Vecchi et al. 2009).

Osmanova et al. (2010) found 170 azaphilone compounds in twenty-three genera that form vinylogous y-pyridines. They are particularly plentiful in *Xylariaceae* and *Trichocomaceae* members, and exhibit a wide range of natural antibacterial, antiviral, antifungal, anti-inflammatory, and antioxidant activity, as well as cytotoxic properties.

The mycelium of *Xylaria* species has been well studied and is marketed as a medicinal product. Studies show Wu Ling powder has a tranquilizing effect on the central nervous system. It contributes to the brain's uptake of glutamic acid and GABA, and reinforces activity of glutamate decarboxylase. Sleep is improved and the abnormal stimulation of dopamine is reduced. A clinical trial of 2,372 patients with insomnia was carried out at more than fifty

hospitals throughout China with a success rate of 91.1 percent.

It helps increase DNA synthesis of lymphocytes, improves macrophage activity to kill tumor cells, and stimulates production of cytokine IL-1. In this manner it helps restore body strength after chemotherapy, surgery, or radiation treatments.

The mycelium restores normal levels of erythrocytes and hemoglobin, and helps improve iron deficient anemia.

Hormonal imbalance is restored, including symptoms associated with menopause, prostate hypertrophy, and abnormal menstruation.

Both acute and chronic toxicity tests were negative.

Candle snuff contains cyochalasin, a compound that binds to actin, which is a protein found in muscle tissue. Espada et al. (1997) have identified several of these compounds.

Lin-Mei Shi and Zha-Jun Zhang (2007) identified 19,20-epoxycytochalasin D and its antitumor activity against P388 cancer cell lines.

Qinghong Liu et al. (2006) identified a lectin from the fresh fruiting body that possesses highly potent hemagglutinating, anti-proliferative, and anti-mitogenic activities. The lectin showed potent inhibition of tumor cell lines M1 and HepG2 with an IC_{50} of less than one micrometer. It is stable to thirty-five degrees Celsius (ninety-five degrees Fahrenheit). Earlier work by Liu found polysaccharides in the fruiting body that inhibit HIV reverse transcriptase.

Xylarone and 8,9-dehydroxylarone, a-pyrone derivatives, isolated from submerged culture of the mushroom, show cytotoxic activity.

Culture fluids from the related *X. longipes* contain xylaramide, a potent antifungal with activity against *Nematospora coryli* and *Saccharomyces cerevisiae.*

The related *X. multiplex* exhibits activity against *Candida albicans* (Boonphong 2001).

Xylaria species contain benzoquinone metabolites that show in vitro activity against *Plasmodium falciparum* (Tansuwan et al. 2007).

Follow-up work by Jimenez-Romero et al. (2008) found activity against chloroquinone-resistant strains of the organism associated with malaria. The compounds phomalactone and 5-hydroxymellein are involved.

Fungi Essence

Candle snuff essence is for those who hear what you say, but do not want to be involved. It will help you say NO! It is for those who have lost a loved one and are grieving. From death comes life. For nasal and digestive problems, inflammation and swelling.

— Silvercord

Mycoremediation

The fungi produce laccase in a complex medium based on tomato juice, while peroxidase activity is only detected when grown in soybean meal.

Xylaria is a one of the few ascomycetes species that decompose Manitoba maple.

Music

A Swiss researcher, Francis Schwarze, made a replica of a Stradivari violin using maple wood treated with *X. longipes.* The mushroom nibbles away at the wood's surface and thus reduces the density and improves the sound. Another musical use for fungi! Perhaps he should get together with the Czech composer Halek and make a true symfungy.

Xylobolus frustulatus

X. frustulosus
Stereum frustulatum
Thelephora frustulata
T. sinuans
Xerocarpus frustulosus
(CERAMIC FUNGUS)
(CERAMIC PARCHMENT)

Ceramic fungus is a flat-crusted fungus common to older, de-barked oak and other hardwoods. It creates localized pockets, known as partridge rot or honeycomb rot, that resemble broken pieces of tile.

Medicinal Use

Chemical Constituents

- **Frustulosin, frustulosinol, and torreyol.**

Nair and Anchel (1977) identified the antibiotic-like compounds frustulosin and frustulosinol. Activity against *Bacillus subtilis, B. mycoides,* and *Staphylococcus aureus* was noted in their work. Weak activity against *Vibrio cholerae* and *Mycobacterium smegmatis* was noted.

The sesquiterpene torreyol, also known as d-cadinol, has also been found in the wings of the male northern blue butterfly, *Lycaeides argyrognomon,* and may act as a pheromone (Lundgren 1975).

Part Two
The Lichens

Or to swamps where the usnea lichen hangs in festoons from the white spruce trees.

— HENRY DAVID THOREAU

Did you hear the one about the fungus and the algae? They took a lichen to each other.

Lichen is from the Greek *leiko* meaning "to lick" or "lick up," in reference to the way the algae appears to lap its tongues all over the host. Lichen may also come from the Greek for "leprous, wart, or eruption," because Dioscorides thought they resembled the skin of afflicted people and used the Doctrine of Signatures as an attempted cure. The French scientist Tournefort named them back in 1700 AD.

Usnea is from the Arabic *ushna* for "moss." *Bryoria* is derived from *Bryopogon* and *Alectoria,* two classifications to which lichens were formerly assigned.

Lichens are a slow growing symbiotic combination of fungi and algae. As such, they do not completely resemble either group, but have their own beautiful and distinctive look. One lichenologist called lichens "fungi that have

discovered agriculture" in reference to their supposed symbiotic relationship.

There are 42 percent lichenized, and 58 percent non-lichenized fungal species within *Ascomycota* (Lutzoni et al. 2001).

Lichen fossils have been discovered dating back to the Devonian period some four hundred million years ago.

For a long time, it was believed that the relationship was symbiotic. Many scientists now believe, following laboratory study, that the fungus is really a parasite. When lichens were experimentally separated in labs and grown apart, the algae grew more quickly and the fungus more slowly. However, when the two join forces, they can survive where neither would make it on its own. In fact, scientists could get them to rejoin only when conditions would not support them separately. Strange bedfellows indeed!

When this idea of two organisms living together was first proposed, it was considered quite radical.

Mordecai Cooke denounced this dualism as

"unqualified romance, which a future generation will contemplate as fairy tales."

The German Simon Schwendener wrote in 1869, "This fungus['s]…slaves are green algae, which it has sought out or indeed caught hold of, and compelled into its service. It surrounds them, as a spider its prey, with a fibrous net of narrow meshes, which is gradually converted into an impenetrable covering, but while the spider sucks its prey and leaves it dead, the fungus incites the algae found in its net to more rapid activity, even to more vigorous increase."

The term helotism, suggesting a master-slave relationship, may best describe lichens, according to this ancient dictum. They are what they are, and we need to see them as whole organisms instead of succumbing to reductionist redundancy.

They have the ability to grow in the coldest, snow-free alpine and boreal forests, often growing less than a millimeter a year. Lichens have been found growing on rocks just 264 miles from the South Pole!

It is estimated that from thirteen thousand to fourteen thousand lichen species inhabit our planet.

Lichenographs, or printed illustrations, were first published in 1480. Linnaeus was not keen on lichens and called them *rustici pauperrimi,* or "the poor trash of vegetation."

Medicinal use of *Evernia furfuracea* has been traced back to 1800 BC.

A thriving brandy-making industry in Sweden and Russia went bankrupt in the nineteenth century when the lichen supply was exhausted. One kilogram of lichen was needed to produce one-half liter of alcohol.

In France, today, lichens are used in the production of chocolates, using the lichen as a filler and substitute for starch.

After all, lichen fiber is composed mainly of mannose, galactose, and glucose, with each species having different make-ups. *Cetraria* and *Alectoria* species, for example, contain significantly more glucose than *Cladina* and *Stereocaulon* species, which in turn contain much more mannose and galactose.

This higher glucose level is reflected in higher lichenan content, making these species more than 50 percent soluble in water, while *Cladina* fiber is less than 5 percent soluble.

Aspicilia esculenta, which is closely related to *A. cinerea* and *A. caesiocinerea,* is believed by some scholars to be the manna mentioned in Exodus 16:31 of the Bible. The lichen forms small, round, pebble-like growths that are easily disturbed and blown around by the wind. They swell in morning dew, and they are edible.

Iwatake *(Umbilicaria esculenta* or *Gyrophora esculenta),* also known as stone mushroom, is collected in the mountains of Japan and exported to China as a luxury item. Properly prepared, it resembles tripe. The bitter constituents are neutralized by soda ash to lessen stomach irritation. The blacker the lichen, the lower the concentration of usnic acid, which causes irritation.

With two notable exceptions, lichens are not poisonous. You must be wary of the bright yellow big, bad wolf lichen *(Letharia vulpina)* and the lemon-yellow powdered sunshine lichen *(Vulpicida pinastri).* These lichens contain pinastric and vulpinic acid, both extremely poisonous. These compounds, combined with ground glass, nails, and *Nux vomica,* have been used to kill wolves. The Achomawai of northern California soaked their arrowheads in the wet lichen for an entire year, sometimes combined with rattlesnake venom, to make the tips poisonous to game.

Be careful when collecting *L. vulpina* as it can cause severe respiratory irritation and nosebleeds in closed environments.

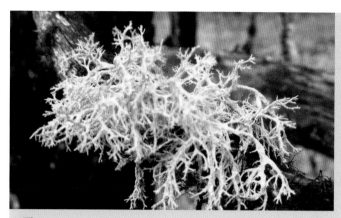

🍃 *Letharia vulpina*

Traditional Uses

The lichens were often assigned medicinal properties based on the ancient doctrine of signatures. A lichen resembling lungs was used for respiratory complaints, for example.

Unidentified black lichen known to the Paiute as *kawa siin,* or "packrat urine," was scraped off rocks and boiled as liquor for treating venereal disease.

Highly prized as a treatment for epilepsy in medieval Europe were lichens that grew on human skulls. The demand was so heavy and profitable for this "heady" medicine *(mucus cranii humani)* that collectors devised methods to paste the skull and cultivate lichens.

The Okanagan Colville boiled it on occasions with Oregon grape bark as a yellow dye. Both the Okanagan Colville and neighboring Blackfoot used *Letharia vulpina* and *Vulpicida pinastri* externally to treat skin problems; the latter for warts and eczema after blackened in fire.

The Paiute of western Nevada recognized the yellow and orange lichens for their anti-bacterial and antifungal properties. They called them lizard semen, in reference to the little pushups that western fence lizards do on rocks.

The Pima and Maricopa of the southwestern United States sprinkled gray colored lichen on cuts and sores, such as rattlesnake bites.

The Waorani of Ecuador use a species of *Dictyonema* as a hallucinogen.

One as yet unidentified lichen that grows like thick, yellow-green paint on boulders of the Rockies is used by natives as a narcotic. Wild bighorn sheep, especially young ewes, also enjoy a nibble, grinding their teeth to the gums to scrape it off the rocks. It grows slowly, taking more than a century to spread over one square inch of rock. It is a pioneer plant, growing where other plants offer no competition. I suspect it is a *Lecanora* species. Sheep in the deserts of Libya chew the lichen *L. esculenta* to the point of tooth loss from abrasion.

The Pima and Maricopa of the southwestern United States used gray colored lichen on rocks and dead wood with a strong violet odor.

They called it earth flower, and mixed it with tobacco as a hallucinogen, as well as to attract women and luck.

Caution: all lichens have the tendency to mold if not handled properly. The resulting mold can cause bronchial or dermal irritation or allergies.

Medicinal Use

During World War II, both the Germans and Americans investigated lichens for antibiotic potential, and found that more than 50 percent of the species tested showed such activity. More than seven hundred secondary lichen substances have been identified, with new compounds being discovered all the time.

Aromatic compounds such as depsides, depsidones, and unusual carotenoids are unique to the lichens.

Studies out of India have shown species of *Lepraria* to exhibit hypotensive, analgesic, anti-inflammatory, anti-spasmodic, and neuro-muscular-junction-blocking activity. Further studies could be carried out on *Lepraria* species in our region of the world.

Moo Sung Kim et al. (2006) found that lichens possess anti-thrombotic properties due to anti-platelet activity. The same author identified the ability to reduce melanin in human melanoma cells and inhibit tyrosinase glycosylation (Kim, M. S. et al. 2007).

Two of the very few organic chlorine-containing substances occurring in nature—gangaleoidin and diploiein—have been isolated from lichens.

Rhizocarpic acid and various depsidones found in various lichens are active against methicillin resistant strains of *Staphylococcus aureus*. Kokubun et al. (2007a) found hybocarpine the most active compound.

Essential Oils

All lichens will give up a certain percentage of essential oils. Certain varieties like the oakmoss lichen *(Evernia prunastri)* have been used in Europe for centuries by the perfume industry as fixatives and bass notes. It was shipped from Cyprus and Greece to Egypt for packing embalmed mummies.

Solvent extractions of spruce moss have been used for perfume since the sixteenth century.

West of the Rockies, *E. prunastri* is quite prominent, and a good source of perfume fixatives. I have also seen it in Nova Scotia. About nine thousand tons are still shipped from Macedonia to France today to produce oakmoss absolute. It is often mixed with *Pseudoevernia furfuracea,* which is more aromatic but inferior as a perfume fixative. This lichen is not found in North America.

Dr. Schweinfurth, traveling through the Nile Valley in 1864, found a scrap of *Evernia furfuracea* in a vase of the eighteenth Dynasty (1700 BC). It does not grow in that country, so it was procured through trade.

Over the centuries, certain lichens have been dried and powdered for the white powdered wigs of aristocrats and to repel lice. Lichen extracts are also found in soups and deodorants, due in part to their antibacterial activity, which, in turn, helps reduce underarm odor.

It has been used to dye wool a violet color when treated with urine or ammonia. It is slow

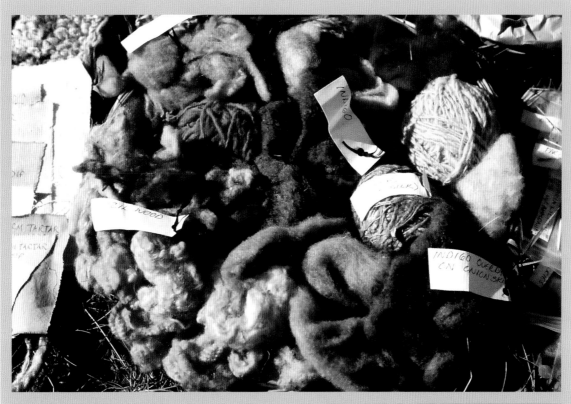

🌿 Lichen dyes: wool (above and below) and horse hair (right).

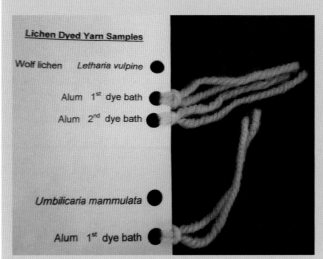

Lichen Dyed Yarn Samples

Wolf lichen   *Letharia vulpine* ●

     Alum   1st dye bath ●

     Alum   2nd dye bath ●

Umbilicaria mammulata ●

     Alum   1st dye bath ●

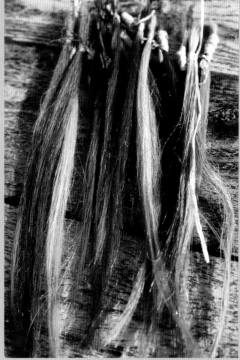

growing, only about two millimeters a year, so do not over-harvest.

Iceland moss has been distilled and yields 0.051 percent of a brownish oil from which unidentified crystals separate upon standing. It contains cetrarine, a phenol-ketone.

Lungwort *(Lobaria pulmonaria)* makes a fine perfume by alcohol extraction.

Diluted lichen absolutes can be rubbed into the forehead and over sinus area for pain relief.

Some lichens such as *Sticta fulgininosa* have an oceanic or fishy smell, not appreciated by all, but prized by perfumists and aromatherapists.

Considering the vast expanses of raw material available, there are great possibilities for creating viable business opportunities.

Lichens possess the ability to retain scent, and are used extensively in potpourri for this purpose.

Spiritual Properties

I have always felt lichens spoke to the essence of unconditional love. They consist of two unrelated living entities, a fungus and an algae, dependent on each other for nourishment, protection and habitat.... Their biological systems become so intermingled that they act as a single living entity we call a lichen. When speaking botanically this is pure symbiosis, in human terms could it not be unconditional love?

— K. Keane

Usnea's keyword is clairvoyance. *Usnea* gives one trust in their higher consciousness. *Usnea* supports all the extrasensory perceptions and heightens any kind of clairvoyance.

— Mulders

Myco-Indicators

Lichens, especially usnea, are more susceptible to damage from sulphur dioxide than other plants and are, therefore, good monitors of air quality. Researchers from Italy, in a 1997 article in *Nature,* suggest a strong inverse correlation between lichen biodiversity and lung cancer.

The lichen, *Hypogymnia physodes,* is the most tolerant macro-lichen to sulphur dioxide pollution, and will incorporate it into cellular tissue, as a measure of toxicity in the area.

Lichens are resistant to radiation, and in one experiment they survived a thousand rads per day for nearly two years from a distance of eight meters—and they continued to grow. To put that fact into context, a single exposure of four hundred rads will kill a human. The potential use of lichens as bio-indicators of radionuclides is very high.

Cosmetics

Tanning, perfumery, and even powdered wigs relied on lichens.

Aromatic lichen acids, such as atranorin, absorb ultra-violet rays and several are able to protect photosensitive human skin. Atranorin is the most frequently involved.

Other Uses

The Cree of northern Canada used *Dicranum* lichen for lamp wicks. Other lichens, such as the snow bed Iceland, were simply used as hot burning tinder.

Natives of northern Canada incorporated both *Alectoria* and *Bryoria* into clothing. They were interwoven with cedar or silverberry bark to make vests, leggings, and moccasins. Although not very durable in wet weather, this material was used by those who could not obtain furs, or as part of ceremonies.

Architects and model railroad buffs use glycerin-soaked lichens for model trees. Lichens are used for "sizing," or giving firmness, in bookbinding and for applying gold leaf and color; they are also used in fabric industries for filling pores in the surface of paper and fiber.

Lichens are used in funeral decorations, as they will last for several weeks at the grave.

Natives throughout Canada produced rock pictures, pictographs of real and grotesque animals, by scraping the lichen off large vertical rock faces. These have lasted centuries, due to the slow growth of lichens.

Lichens have been used for natural dyes, including in the tartans of Scotland. A few crofters still produce Harris Tweed using the lichen *Parmelia omphalodes.* An added advantage over synthetic dye is that bitter lichen acids repel moths. The related *P. chlorochroa,* which grows on calcareous rocks on the prairie grassland, was used by the Navaho to produce nice warm brown dyes for their wools and blankets.

Brilliant blues, pinks, and purples are possible, something highly unusual in the plant kingdom, by using the ammonia of urine and fermenting for several weeks. It is said the smell of urine disappears in time and finally exudes a violet-like scent. If not fixed by mordant, the colors quickly dull to a pale brown in sunlight.

Ochrolechia oregonensis, which grows with little pink discs on the rough bark of conifers, makes a violet-purple dye and is somewhat plentiful.

Both *Letharia vulpina* and *Vulpicida pinastri* have been used for the brilliant yellow dyes they produce. The coastal Tlingit and Haida traded fish oils for the lichen, which they used to color their spruce root baskets and dancing blankets. Interior people used the lichen to dye buckskins, horsehair, porcupine quills, or mountain goat's wool. The Cheyenne of Montana used the yellow dye for quills as well. The Apache used the lichen to paint crosses on their feet to pass through enemy territory unseen. The Huna of northern California used it to dye bear grass (*Xerophyllum tenax*).

Natives of the southwest used *Physcia* mixed with pine resin for a yellow paint.

The Yuki of California used it in bedding.

The related brown eyed sunshine lichen (*V. canadensis*) is used to dye mountain goat's wool.

Various constituents of lichens decompose to produce orcin, that in the presence of ammonia and oxygen produce orecein, and a purple color.

Bits and Pieces

The novel *Trouble with Lichen,* by John Wyndham, is a sci-fi novel about their long life span, as it relates to humans. One species, *Acarospora chlorophana,* a bright yellow crustose lichen found in western Alberta, grows so slowly on rocks it is almost un-measurable.

The great mystery in the chemistry of lichens is their "secondary compounds," which are not by-products of normal plant metabolism. Because of the energy required to produce them, scientists speculate they must have

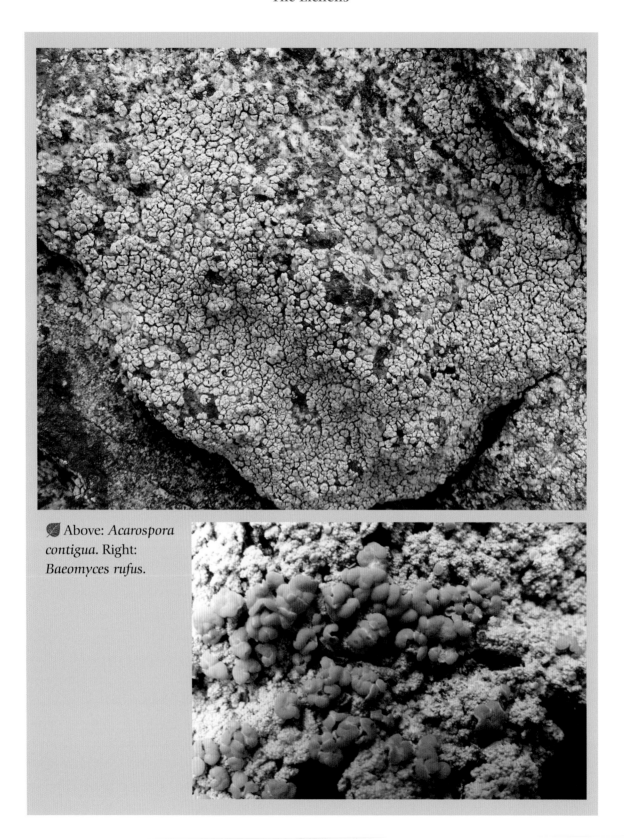

Above: *Acarospora contigua*. Right: *Baeomyces rufus*.

important value. Lichens produce over five hundred biochemicals that help control UV exposure, repel herbivores, attack microbes, and discourage competition, according to Vermeulen.

A number of lichens are presently being genetically engineered in Japan to produce medical and industrial compounds.

Personality Traits

Lichens are an amazing partnership between fungi and algae, the one providing support and structure, the other nutrients and sustenance.

Lichens can live several hundred years on trees and in harsh habitats such as wind-ravaged mountain rocks. They even adapt happily to life on graveyard tombstones. They draw nutrients from dew and rainfall, and store the food in their bodies for very long periods, releasing nourishment gradually as needed. The lichen can thus sustain itself almost indefinitely in a tough environment.

What provisions do you need to sustain you tomorrow? A certain amount of food, money, clothing, and household goods are only a start. What about the sustenance that comes from family, friendships, and sound values? It's never too soon to stock your storehouse with these treasures that nourish over a lifetime.

— GINA MOHAMMED

Many people are familiar with litmus papers, those little pH indicator strips that turn either red or blue when dipped in acid or alkali. Litmus papers are imbued with special dyes derived from several species of lichen. In modern times, the *litmus test* has been used in a philosophical sense as well. We may say something is a litmus test of success, or love, or commitment, meaning that it is a discriminating test that will produce a definitive answer.

I wonder how many of us would be willing to subject our priorities to a litmus test. What if we chose peace of mind as our litmus, and held it against each of the priorities, large and small, that we hold at this very moment. Take a few moments to run the test, and see what doesn't pass. Perhaps these are burdens we shouldn't be carrying.

— GINA MOHAMMED

In certain districts of Scotland, as Aberdeenshire, almost every farm or cotter had its tank or barrel (litpig) of putrid urine (graith) wherein the mistress of the household macerated from lichens (crotals or crottles) to prepare dyes for homespun stockings, nightcaps, or other garments. The usual practice was to boil the lichen and woolen clothes together in water or in the urine-treated lichen mass until the desired color, usually brown, was obtained.

This took several hours, or less on the addition of acetic acid, producing fast dyes without the benefit of a mordant or fixing agent. The color was intensified by adding salt or saltpeter. This method was prevalent in Iceland as well as Scotland for those homespuns best known to the trade as Harris Tweed.

— G.A. LLANO, 1951

Actinogyra muhlenbergii

Gyrophora muhlenbergii
Umbilicaria muhlenbergii
(PLATED ROCK TRIPE)
U. vellea
G. vellea
U. americana
(FROSTED ROCKTRIPE)
Dermatocarpon miniatum
(LEATHER LICHEN)

There is some confusion as to the exact identity of the lichen, with *Dermatocarpon miniatum* sometimes identified as the same lichen.

Rock tripe is flat, brown, circular lichen that attaches to rocks with a cord.

The Woods Cree of Saskatchewan called it *asiniwakon* and used it to thicken fish soups. They broke it into very small pieces and poured very hot water over it, letting it soak for five to ten minutes until the pieces were softened and the broth was thickened. It was considered good nourishment for those who were sick, because it does not upset the stomach.

The Chipewyan also used this "rock dirt," or *tthe tsi,* as a food source. The dried flakes were boiled in soup, imparting a sour, mushroom flavor. This soup was used to fatten up sled dogs.

Usually the lichen is first added to boiling water that is discarded to remove some of the more irritating and bitter acids. Ashes are sometimes added to the water to neutralize the acidity; even baking soda will make rock tripe more digestible.

It is considered a delicacy in Japan, where it is sold under the name *iwatake* and taken as part of a special tea ceremony or natural food in mountain inns. It is either boiled until tender and then seasoned with rice vinegar or sesame paste, eaten as a vegetable in soybean soup, or deep fried as a tempura.

The lichens *U. vellea* and *U. americana* have recently been separated into two distinct species. The latter is found in a sweeping arc from Lake Winnipeg to Great Slave Lake in the Northwest territories.

Leather lichen, or stippleback lichen *(D. miniatum),* is found on limestone rock.

Traditional Uses

The Chipewyan burned it to ash, and then boiled it to make syrup for the treatment of tapeworms.

The Inuit, who know rock tripe as *quajautit,* a word associated with slippery underfoot, use them to absorb blood for cleaning a wound and to ripen boils. A spoonful of the boiled lichen water is considered good for any illness, but the lichen is not eaten.

Decoctions can be used as a gargle for soothing canker sores and bleeding gums.

Medicinal Use

Chemical Constituents

- **Gyrophoric acid.**

In Japan, a sulfate isolate from rock tripe showed an inhibitory effect on the replication of HIV-1 in vitro. The compound (GE-3-S) appears to work in a manner similar to dextran sulphate and heparin, preventing attachment of HIV to the surface of T4 cells. This partially acetylated pustulan sulphate is only one of four polysaccharides that show weak animal toxicity, with GE-3-S showing no acute toxicity in mice at very high doses.

The lichen is active against gram-positive bacteria. A substance similar to pustulan, an acylated B-1-6 glucan, has shown antitumor activity against sarcoma 180 (Narui 1999).

Work by Swanson and Fahselt (1997) found that UVA exposure increased and UVB exposure decreased their content of secondary compounds.

Textile Industry

In Scotland, rock tripe was used to make *corkir,* a brilliant red dye used to color tartans. When treated with urine, it yielded purple.

Leather lichen, or stippleback lichen *(D. miniatum)* is used as a source of ash green dye for wool in some parts of Europe.

U. vellea, which contains gyrohoric acid, was used in Sweden to dye wool a violet color.

Alectoria sarmentosa

(WITCH'S HAIR)

A. ochroleuca

(GREEN WITCH'S HAIR)

This lichen looks at first glance like *Usnea,* but it lacks the central spongy cord. It is found in the same boreal forests, hanging from conifers that are at least a century old.

The Bella Coola of British Columbia called it *ipts-aak* or "limb moss" and used the long hair for their dance masks.

The Haida call it crow's mountain goat wool or crow's blanket.

The Inuit call it greenbeard, caribou moss, or *tinqaujait* meaning "what looks like pubic hair." It is a handy fire starter.

Traditional Uses

In Scandinavia, different colored *Alectoria* and *Usnea* lichens are used to make figures of trolls to warn children to be good. (Legends told of trolls carrying off naughty children into the woods.)

When found on alder, it was used as a poultice for sores and boils.

In western Canada, it was mainly used as a fiber for mattresses, baby diapers, and sanitary napkins. It was woven with *Bryoria fremontii,* below, for poor quality clothing, when skins were unavailable. It was often interwoven with wolf willow bark to make it more durable.

It was used traditionally to make false whiskers and hair for decorative dance masks by variety of coastal natives.

It contains a yellow dye.

Medicinal Use

Chemical Constituents

- *A. sarmentosa:* **dibenzofuranoid lactol, usnic acid, physodic acid, 8'-0-ethyl-beta-alectoronic acid, alectosarmentin, a-collatolic acid, squamatic acid, mannitol, arabitol, and physocid acid.**

- *A. ochroleuca:* **diffractaic, thamnolic, barbatic, alectoronic, chloroatranorin, and usnic acids.**

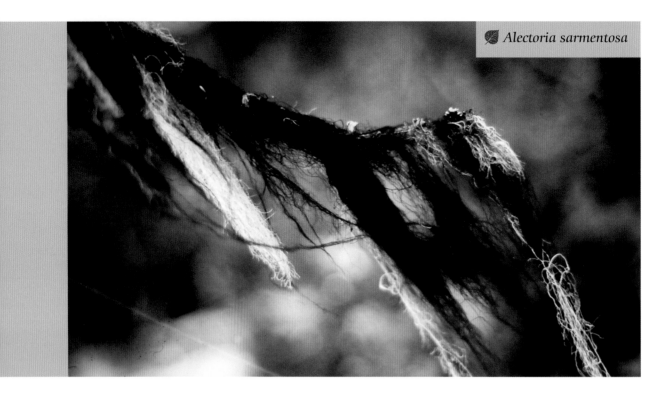

Alectoria sarmentosa

Recent studies indicate that a new antimicrobial dibenzofuranoid lactol called alectosarmentin has been isolated from witch's hair. The compound exhibits activity against *Staphylococcus aureus* and *Mycobacterium smegmatis*.

Usnic and physocid acids in this lichen were found effective against these two bacteria as well as *Candida albicans*.

One study showed four antimicrobial compounds including usnic acid, physodic acid, 8'-0-ethyl-beta-alectoronic acid, and alectosarmentin, the newly discovered dibenzofuranoid lactol.

Previous studies have indicated the presence of mannitol and arabitol, active antitumor polysaccharides.

The closely related gray witch's hair *(A. nigricans)* lacks usnic acid, but does contain alectorialic acid. An extract was found to exhibit notable inhibition of ODC activity induced by 12-0-tetradecanoylphorbol-13-acetate in cultured mouse epidermal 308 cells. The IC50 value was only 2.6 micrograms per milliliter. Ingólfsdóttir et al. (2000) found this lichen active against leukemia cell lines and to exhibit quinone reductase activity.

Green witch's hair *(A. ochroleuca)* shows strong activity against *S. aureus*.

Food Industry

Green witch's hair *(A. ochroleuca)* was used during the 1930s in Russia to make a type of molasses. It yielded 82 percent of its dry weight to glucose and produced light yellow syrup.

At one time, it was used by distillers to make alcohol.

Bryoria fremontii

(BLACK TREE LICHEN)
(EDIBLE HORSEHAIR)
B. trichodes
(HORSE HAIR LICHEN)

Horsehair lichen *(B. trichodes)* is found isolated in central Saskatchewan, but it is common eastern North America. The related subspecies *americana* is found in British Columbia and in parts of southern Alaska.

Black tree lichen can be collected at any time of year, and the flavor is definitely influenced by the tree it grows on.

The Northern Okanagan preferred specimens growing on ponderosa or lodge pole pines; whereas the Southern Okanagan preferred the douglas fir or western larch specimens. These preferences were probably based on availability.

This lichen has been used by native tribes for food. Some aboriginals say it tastes like candy, if properly prepared; others maintain it is strictly a survival food. In the Okanagan, young natives would bring back lichen from various areas to their grandmother to taste. If sweet, the family would claim the area where it was growing.

Long poles were utilized to pull the lichen from branches or youngsters would climb into the trees to throw it down. In a good site, five or six trees would yield sufficient harvest for one family for the year!

The fresh lichen is light and bulky and was soaked in water, then cooked in a steam pit created by putting hot rocks at the bottom and covering with green leaves and masses of lichens. It was left for the night, removed after cooling in the morning, and cut into jelly-like loaves. It can be eaten then or stored for several years, and soaked before eating.

It compacts when cooked; a twenty-centimeter-thick layer reduces to four centimeters after steaming. It is rather bland, so it was often cooked with layers of onions, mixed with Saskatoon berries, or dipped in berry juice after cooking. The Okanagan would also cook it with the false solomon seal rhizomes, while others would sweeten it with douglas fir sugar.

The Carrier mixed it with flour and baked it like fruitcake.

The Okanagan would roast it until dry and crumbly, and then boil it until molasses-like. Further south, the Coeur D'Alêne also ate the lichen, which they call *skola'pken.*

The Nlaka'pamux still prepare it to this day in modern ovens, and serve it as a form of taffy, called *we'ia,* with the texture and flavor of licorice. The dried cakes were used for long journeys. Pregnant women did not eat this, as they believed it would make their babies dark.

One related lichen, inedible horsehair *(B. tortuosa),* which looks somewhat like black tree lichen, contains high concentrations of the poisonous vulpinic acid and is a potential toxin. This is mainly a coastal species and not present east of the Rockies.

The related *Bryoria fremontii* is said to taste like acorns. It was called *wa kamwa* by the native peoples of Oregon, who dried it, powdered it, and added it to soups.

Traditional Uses

The Okanagan Colville mixed the dry lichen with grease and rubbed it on the navels of newborns to prevent infection. They also gave a mixture of Saskatoon berry juice and syrup of *B. fremontii* to babies after weaning.

Natives of the northern Boreal forest heat the various horsehair lichens into a powder for burns. Further south, the Nez Perce used it for treating diarrhea and indigestion.

Horsehair lichen *(B. trichodes)* was gathered and piled on a sick person in steam baths to help hold in heat, and used to staunch bleeding wounds by various native groups.

Medicinal Use

Chemical Constituents

- *B. fremontii*: **vulpinic acid, atranorin, thamnolic acid, and alectorialic acid. It is incredibly rich in iron containing 8.3 milligrams per hundred grams.**
- **Horsehair lichen: fumar-protocetraric acid and atranorin.**

Spiritual Properties

The coyote is the trickster and transformer of all things in their present state. The black tree lichen was originally derived from coyote's hair braid which became tangled on a tree branch he was climbing.

He cut himself loose and fell to the ground, without his braid. Looking up he said, "You shall not be wasted, my valuable hair. After this, you shall be gathered by the people. The old women will make you into food."

It was changed into lichen and has been used as food ever since.

— MOURNING DOVE

Other Uses

Horsehair lichen was also gathered by First Nations people of Canada and burned into a black powder for wood paint, as was shiny horsehair lichen *(B. glabra)*.

Caloplaca spp.
(FIREDOT LICHENS)

Various *Caloplaca* species grow on arctic alpine soil, and others on the bark of aspen poplar trees. They appear as orangey, rusty dots on the bark or on granite rocks and sidewalks.

A species occurring in the genus has been found to produce physcion. This is identical to the monomethyl ester of emodine.

Medicinal Use

Work by Manojlovic et al. (2005b) on various *Caloplaca* species suggest both antimicrobial and antifungal activity. They contain anthraquinones.

Gray rimmed firedot lichen *(C. cerina)* contains parietin, found by same author to possess antifungal activity (Manojlovic et al. 2005a).

Lichen Essence

Sulphur firedot lichen *(C. flavescens)* leaf lichen essence acts as an energy support for the skin. It helps us change or redefine our contact with the outside world. The essence is people who are too thin-skinned in their relationships.

— KORTE PHI

Candelaria concolor

(CANDLE FLAME LICHEN)
(LEMON LICHEN)

Candle flame or lemon lichen *(Candelaria concolor)* contains callopismic acid, also known as ethylpulvic acid; stictaurin or dipulvic acid, barbatic acid, and dipulvic dilactone; and tetronic acid derivatives, vulpinic acid, calycin and 5-chloroatranorin.

Candelariella vitellina

(COMMON GOLDSPECK)

The fungus from this lichen, an egg-yolk-colored species with scattered and flattened growth on acid and calcareous rocks and tree bark, contains stictaurin. They all contain calycin, a yellow pigment, formerly used in Sweden for dyes.

Cetraria islandica

(ICELAND MOSS)
C. ericetorum
(ICELAND LICHEN)
C. laevigata
(STRIPED ICELAND LICHEN)
C. nivalis
Flavocetraria nivalis
(CRINKLED SNOW LICHEN)
C. palustris
(MARSH LICHEN)
C. cucullata
F. cucullata
(CURLED SNOW LICHEN)

Although called a moss, this brown lichen attaches to rocks in open sub-alpine forests. It is best collected when green and fully grown between May and September. An average yield of seven hundred kilograms (1,540 pounds) per acre of air-dried Iceland moss could be expected if solidly covered.

The lichen is symbolic of health, and associated symbolically with the birth date January sixteenth. Other lichen, such as *Ramalina* and *Cladonia* species, symbolize dejection, and relate to January fourteenth.

It is associated with the second rune, UR, of Norse mysticism.

In Iceland it is called *fjallagros,* and the first written laws of that country, from as far back as 1280 AD, banned people from picking it on another's land.

Bread moss, or *brodmose,* is a Scandinavian name due to its use in extending wheat flour or potatoes in times of famine. It is also known as *matmasa* or "food moss" and *svinmasa* meaning "swine moss."

In Europe, it was traditionally soaked in birch ash (2 percent) to decrease the lichen acids before ingestion. The flour was used for porridge, jellies, and bread. It was mixed with mashed potatoes, rye, or oatmeal at about 25 percent.

The Chipewyan called it *tsanju* and used it as a source of both food and medicine.

The closely related Iceland lichen *(C. ericetorum)* is also common, and although similar, does not contain fumarprotocetraric acid, but lichenesterinic acid. Yup'ik of Alaska used it to flavor and thicken soups.

Striped Iceland lichen *(C. laevigata)* in the

extreme north contains fumarprotocetraric, protolichesterinic, and lichesterinic acids.

Crinkled snow lichen (formerly *C. nivalis* and now *Flavocetraria nivalis*) is found near the tree line or tundra.

The related *C. palustris* is a bright yellow species that favors buffalo berry *(Shepherdia canadensis)*, alder *(A. crispus)*, willow, and labrador tea *(Ledum groenlandicum)*, as well as the base of pine.

Curled snow lichen (formerly *C. cucullata* and now *F. cucullata*) is found at higher elevations of coniferous woods and on tundra. Natives of Alaska use it to flavor their fish or duck soups.

Medicinal Use
Chemical Constituents

- *C. islandica:* **lobaric acid; glucans lichenin (polysaccharides 30 to 40 percent); isolichenin (10 percent); lichenan (17 percent); galactomannan (7.6 percent); various usnic, salicylic, cetraric, physodalic, and fumaric acids; estrosterol peroxide; protolichesterinic acid (0.1 to 0.5 percent); lichesterinic; protocetraric acid (0.2 to 0.3 percent); fumarprotocetraric acids (2 to 11 percent); aromatic lichen acids (2 to 3 percent); aliphatic lichen acids (1 to 1.5 percent); cetrarin; picrolichenin; oxalic acid; furan derivatives; iodine; vitamin A; trace minerals including iron, iodide, and calcium salts; fatty acid lactones; terpenes; mucilage; fiber; and gums.**

Crinkled snow lichen (formerly *C. nivalis* and now *Flavocetraria nivalis*) is brewed into a tea in parts of the high Andes and used as a tonic for heart conditions and to relieve altitude sickness.

In Switzerland, Iceland moss is used for sore throat pastilles.

Iceland moss is a nutritious and soothing tonic, with slight laxative effect. It helps improve the appetite and digestion of the elderly and those recovering from a debilitating illness. The bitter principles benefit the stomach in both tincture and infusion form, stimulating a poor appetite, through increasing the production of saliva and gastric juices. It therefore can be used for both hyper and hypo-acidic stomach conditions.

However, Iceland moss may aggravate gastric or duodenal ulcers, and is contraindicated in cases of excessive catarrh or mucus congestion.

Decoctions are used for chronic diarrhea and respiratory problems. Like lungwort, it increases the flow of breast milk, but not with inflamed or sore breasts. Low thyroid and anemia are helped by trace levels of iodine and iron and other nutritive properties.

Dr. King's American Dispensatory is a classic of eclectic herbal medicine. He writes that the lichen is "used as a demulcent in chronic catarrhs, chronic dysentery, and diarrhoea, and as a tonic in dyspepsia, convalescence, and exhausting diseases. Boiled with milk it forms an excellent nutritive and tonic in phthisis and general debility. It relieves the cough of chronic bronchitis."

It soothes nausea from gastritis and vomiting, and combines well with borage and chickweed for peptic ulcers, hiatus hernia, and esophageal reflux. In fact, for those individuals with a yin or fluid deficiency, it would work better than a straight astringent herb.

Mild infusions of Iceland moss can be used as a vaginal douche for its soothing, demulcent properties.

Tincture form is best for whooping cough, asthma, tuberculosis, and kidney and bladder complaints; especially those related to a dry, irritating condition. Here, the sweet, moist, and astringent nature of Iceland moss helps address the underlying concern.

It may be used for night sweats or fevers, but is taken during the day to prevent recurrence. Do not use Iceland moss when a fever is present.

When untreated lichen was fed to mice as 50 percent of their diet, the mice died in four to five days. When the lichen was first ash-soaked and boiled, survival times increased to twenty to twenty-two days, and when lichen was only 25 percent of their diet it was well tolerated for six weeks (Airaksinen et al. 1986).

Early work by Burkholder and Evans (1945) found activity against *Bacillus subtilis, B. mycoides,* and *Sarcina lutea.* Stoll et al. found strong activity against *S. aureus.*

The related *C. palustris* contains + l-usnic acid and vulpinic acid, and shows strong activity against *S. aureus* in work by Stoll above.

Burkholder and Evans (1945) found the curled snow lichen to exhibit activity against *Bacillus subtilis, B. mycoides,* and *Sarcina lutea* as well as *Streptococcus species* such as *S. pneumoniae, S. pyogenes, S. viridans, Staphylococcus aureus,* and *S. albus* (hemolytic).

Iceland moss has been used in the manufacture of antibiotics to treat tuberculosis.

In Finland, an antifungal cream called USNO is made, for treating athlete's foot and ringworm. The lichen entered the Finnish Pharmacopoeia in 1915.

Lichenin is soluble in hot water, and upon cooling forms a gel; while isolichenin, present in smaller amounts, is soluble in both hot and cold water.

Lichenan is a polysaccharide similar to beta-glucan, found in oats and barley. One study found lichenan exhibited strong antiviral activity.

In an open clinical trial, one hundred patients with pharyngitis, laryngitis, or bronchial ailments were given lozenges containing 160 milligrams of an aqueous extract of the lichen. There was an 86 percent positive response with good gastric tolerance and lack of side effects.

In vitro studies have shown protolichesterinic acid to be a potent inhibitor of HIV, as well as 5-lipoxygenase (Pengsuparp et al. 1995).

Other components, such as polysaccharides, have been found by Ingólfsdóttir et al. (1994) to stimulate the immune system. Later, the same author found the polysaccharides comparable to the fungal polysaccharide lentinan (shiitake) used for clinical cancer therapy in Japan. The author found extracts of Iceland moss to suppress the growth of *Helicobacter pylori,* which contributes to gastric and duodenal ulcers (Ingólfsdóttir et al. 1997b).

Protolicheresterinic acid has been found to be significantly anti-carcinogenic with regards to two breast carcinoma and erythro-leukemia cell lines, and to possess anti-inflammatory properties. The ED50 for lobaric acid is between fourteen and forty-four micrograms per milliliter for these three cancer cell lines.

Haraldsdottir et al. (2004) found lobaric acid

very effective against a number of human cancer cell lines in vitro.

One study determined that Iceland moss has significant potential as a natural antioxidant. Just fifty micrograms of water extract showed higher antioxidant activity than five hundred micrograms of alpha tocopherol.

Eight secondary compounds in *C. islandica* decreased by 52 percent when screened from natural UVA and UVB radiation.

The closely related snow bed Iceland lichen (*C. delisei*) contains gyrophoric acid and shows significant activity on estrogen through inhibition of aromatase. Extracts at a concentration of forty micrograms per milliliter showed 82 percent inhibition. Aromatase inhibition is one approach to preventing overgrowth of hormone-sensitive cancer cells.

The genus contains caperatic acid and atranorin. The related *C. halei* contains alectoronic acid.

The common spiny heath lichen (*C. aculeata*), also known as *Coelocaulon aculeatum*, has significant effect on various bacterial systems, but not mammalian cells.

The lichen extract and its active constituent protolichesterinic acid exhibit activity against *Aeromonas hydrophilia*, *Proteus vulgaris*, *Streptococcus faecalis*, *Bacillus cereus*, *B. subtilis*, *Pseudomonas aeruginosa*, and *Listeria monocytogenes*.

Homeopathy

Iceland moss (*Cetraria islandica*) is used for acute and chronic bronchitis, asthma, and pains in the chest while coughing.

Dose: ten to twenty drops of tincture as needed. The mother tincture is prepared from the dried lichen, 1:10 at 40 percent alcohol.

Essential Oil

Iceland moss is steam distilled and yields brownish oil (0.051 percent). It has a saponification value of ninety-eight and an acid value of seventy-two.

The bulk of aliphatic acids are saturated (66.8 percent), composed mainly of palmitic, stearic, and behenic acids. Unsaturated acids compose the rest, with oleic and linoleic acids the most common.

Spiritual Properties

Iceland moss and its spiritual properties are related to the signature of this lichen. Individuals struggling with their personal evolving of spiritual issues, or those in difficult environments, physically and emotionally, will benefit from this plant.

When an individual comes close to achieving deeper awareness of God, there is often great fear and unwillingness to continue. This is often related to the incorrect belief that nothing will remain to be done on earth.

Those working toward spiritual goals based in Eastern philosophies will also be helped. In the martial arts, one seeks to let go of the mind, and yet be ready for full physical response. Iceland moss will help develop this trust, as well as help an individual discover and feel comfortable with their own level of spiritual purpose.

— GURUDAS

Cosmetics

Iceland moss is used as a source of glycerol in the soap industry, and because of its lack of odor, in cold cream manufacture.

Europe's best selling natural tooth whitener, BlanX, contains silica and Arctic moss.

Food Industry

In Russia, during World War II, Iceland moss, *Alectoria ochroleuca,* and various *Cladina* species were used to make a type of molasses, with the glucose yield from Iceland moss at 78 percent of dry weight.

A patent issued in 1951 suggested the use of Iceland moss as a preservative for luncheon meats, or cream filled pastries. It is both antibiotic and heat stable, and safe for human consumption.

In Switzerland, Iceland moss is used as an additive to luncheon meats and pastries to retard spoilage.

Textile Industry

Iceland moss has been used for tanning hides and dyeing wool.

Ragbag or varied rag lichen *(Platismatia glauca),* formerly classified as *Cetraria glauca,* yields a chamois-colored dye for wool.

Agriculture

Water extracts of the lichen have been found to inhibit development of the tobacco mosaic virus. Even at one part to five hundred, it reduced the number of brown lesions on leaves by 80 percent, due to an enzyme called ribonuclease.

Personality Traits

The moistened *Cetraria* gives off an aroma that suggests still other mammals or things mammalian—a blended whiff of suede worn by an equestrian, and of the horse, sweating.

It is a good-bad-intriguing scent, probably with pheromonal powers, and of the sort that is used as ballast in the making of a perfume. I would not be at all surprised if an essence of this plant is eventually stirred into some concoction with a name like The Devil's Dew, to be dabbed on by would be Dionysians.

— George Schenk

Cladina rangiferina

(GRAY REINDEER LICHEN)
(TRUE REINDEER LICHEN)
C. mitis
(GREEN REINDEER LICHEN)
C. arbuscula
(TREE REINDEER LICHEN)
C. alpestris
C. stellaris
C. aberrans
(REINDEER LICHEN)
(STAR TIPPED REINDEER LICHEN)
(NORTHERN REINDEER LICHEN)
(CAULIFLOWER LICHEN)
(CARIBOU LICHEN)
C. stygia
(BLACK FOOTED REINDEER LICHEN)

The Woods Cree of Saskatchewan call it *wapiskastaskamih* or sometimes *atikomiciwin.*

Rangifer is the scientific grouping for both reindeer and caribou.

True reindeer lichen is very common across northern Canada, where it is used as a food source by caribou. It is very fragile and slow growing; averaging 3.4 millimeters of growth

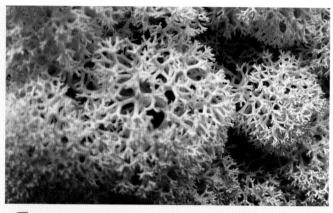

🌿 *Cladina stellaris*

In Denmark, the popularity of a whiskey made from the caribou or reindeer moss so endangered the lichen that production was shut down by the government. A similar brandy venture in Sweden also closed down in 1883.

In Russia, *C. mitis* syrup was too bitter for human consumption, and used to produce alcohol, or medium for food yeast, with a glucose yield of 75 percent dry weight.

In Alaska, the lichen is added for flavoring to duck or fish soup.

Traditional Uses

Decoctions of the dried powder were taken by the Woods Cree of Saskatchewan to rid the body of intestinal worms.

Inuit ate the undigested stomach contents of caribou as a source of vitamin C.

The Aleuts of Alaska used infusions of this lichen for chest pains while the Tanaina boiled and ate it for diarrhea.

Cladina species, separated from grass in caribou stomachs, was stirred with oil while the word *teniyash,* meaning "increase," was sung repeatedly so the mixture would rise and become light.

The Chipewyan call it *tsanju.* The use of partially digested reindeer lichen from caribou digestive tracts has long been a traditional part of their diet. The contents of the rumen, *eburti,* were boiled by placing heated rocks into the cut out rumen or large intestine, with added meat, fat, and blood. This is known to the Chipewyan as *ebie hechelh* or "bowel soup."

per year. After grazing by caribou, it takes up to fifteen years to recover. Although *C. rangifera* is the true reindeer lichen, the equally slow-growing star tipped lichen is a more important food, and preferred by caribou.

Caribou and reindeer produce lichenase in their stomachs, which, along with bacteria and protozoa in the rumen, help them survive extreme conditions. The enzyme, lichenase, is also found in snail livers.

Black footed reindeer lichen has a pinkish jelly; as opposed to the clear, colorless jelly from the true reindeer lichen.

The Gwich'in of the Mackenzie delta call it *uhdeezhu* or "white moss." It makes a stimulating tea that is good for stomach and chest pain. It can also be boiled for an hour and then fried for a crispy treat.

When removed from freshly killed caribou rumen, it is known as *it'rik.* It is eaten in soup, or placed on other meat to tenderize and enhance its flavor. It is sometimes hung for up to a week to age, and then mixed with fat, marrow, and berries.

The Ojibwa decocted *C. rangiferina* to bathe newborns and give them strength. They call the lichen *asa'gunink*.

The Inuit of Baffin Island make a broth of *niriat (C. stellaris)* for sickness and eye infections.

Traditionally, the lichen was used in Russia in the form of powder for treating wounds.

In Finland, the lichen was traditionally boiled in water as a laxative, or boiled in milk for respiratory afflictions.

Medicinal Use

Chemical Constituents

- *C. stellaris:* usnic, fumarprotocetraric, perlatolic acids; atronorin; various polysaccharides including nigeran, galactomannan, arabinitol, and mannitol; and small amounts of rangiformic, psoromic, pseudonor-rangiformic, and ventoric acids; proteins; and sterols.

- *C. rangiferina:* fumaroprotocetraric acid, atranorin, trace amounts of vitamin D, some ergosterol, arabitol, mannitol, volemitol, alpha trehalose, sucrose, umbilicin, and 54 to 63 percent lichenin acid.

- *C. arbuscula:* fumarprotocetraric and usnic acids.

- *C. mitis:* usnic and rangiformic acids.

- *C. squamosa:* squamatic acid.

- Usnic acid is significantly higher in young lichen tissue, with the first few millimeters containing up to twelve times that of the older growth just four to eight millimeters back.

- *Cladina* species are 94 percent carbohydrate, 2.7 percent protein, 2 percent fat, and 1.3 percent minerals.

C. alpestris water extracts have been demonstrated to have strong effect against *Trichomonas vaginalis* in vitro. No significant difference has been found between the effect of usnic acid and metronidazole at concentrations of 0.4 and 0.6 milligrams per milliliter.

Reindeer lichen *(C. rangiferina)* has been shown to be more effective in chronic inflammation than acute conditions. Compared to indomethacin, the lichen extract showed 43 percent inhibition, as compared to the drug at 72 percent.

Atranorin appears to be stimulated by UVA sunlight.

Recent work identified new compounds, hangokenols A and B. These and other previously identified compounds were tested for activity against MRSA (methicillin-resistant *Staphylococcus aureus*) and VRE (vancomycin-resistant *Enterococci* species) (Yoshikawa, K. et al. 2008).

Both *C. mitis* and *C. stellaris* show activity against *Staphylococcus aureus* and *Bacillus subtilis*.

One study showed strong activity against *S. aureus* by d-usnic acid in the former species.

Early work by Burkholder and Evans (1945) indicated *C. mitis* showed activity against *S. albus, Diplococcus pneumoniae, Streptococcus hemolyticus, S. viridans, Bacillus mycoides,* and *Sarcina lutea.*

Cladina alpestris shows activity against *Bacillus subtilis.*

Northern reindeer lichen *(C. arbuscula)* shows activity against *Mycobacterium tuberculosis.*

Homeopathy

Reindeer lichen *(C. rangiferina)* was proved at 30C potency by Misha Norland in 2002.

Mental symptoms include jealousy, suspicion, and delusion. Dreams of crime, evil, guns, murder, war, fights, and robbery are prevalent.

Physically, there is vertigo, throat huskiness or loss of voice, and head and eye pain. Nasal congestion, burning tongue, stomach nausea, and abdominal flatulence are present. A dry cough, thick expectoration, stitching pain in the chest, cold extremities, and itching skin are also common. A more complete description can be found in *Fungi* by Frans Vermeulen.

Lichen Essence

Reindeer lichen *(C. mitis)* is for transformation. It revitalizes the lifeblood congestion or over-stimulation of the etheric heart that impedes the free circulation of life force.

— FINDHORN

Textile Industry

In Europe, true reindeer lichen has been used to produce an iron red dye for wool.

Agriculture

Star tipped reindeer lichen is harvested commercially for flower arrangements and wreaths and architects and model railway hobbyists use it for miniature trees and shrubs. In Finland and Sweden, this is a million dollar export business, with some three thousand tons harvested per year.

Cladonia

Numerous texts have mixed up *Cladina* and *Cladonia,* but unlike the former, the latter has a squamulose primary thallose that makes for accurate identification. *Cladonia* now refers to pixie cup lichens and their relatives, but previously represented all reindeer lichens.

Cladonia species contain usnic and isusnic acids, especially in the cortex, as well as beta-orcinol depsides and depsidones such as barbatic and squamatic acids; atranorin, fumarprotocetraric, and proto-cetraric acids; and norstitic, psoromic, rhodocladonic, and thamnolic acids. They also contain ursolic acid, found in apples and various medicinal herb species.

Medicinal Use

Usnic acid from *Cladonia* species has shown high cytotoxic activity against cancer cells (Bezivin et al. 2004).

Various *Cladonia* species have been found effective in the treatment of tuberculosis. This confirms the traditional use in Finland of hot water lichen infusions for this dreadful disease.

Didymic acid, found in many *Cladonia* species, inhibits the mycobacterium at twenty-five micrograms per milliliter.

Species inhibiting *Bacillus subtilis* include *C. gracilis, C. deformis C. amaurocraea, C. bacillaris, C. coniocrae, C. fimbriata, C. pleurota,* and *C. uncialis.*

Species inhibiting *Staphylococcus aureus* are *C. gonechu,* also known as *C. sulphurina, C. deformis,* and *C. amaurocraea.*

Cladonia cristatella
(BRITISH SOLDIERS)

This lichen is so named due to its green body and red head, reminiscent of the early British red coats.

The red-tipped *C. bellidiflora* is common. Other *Cladonia* species worth mentioning are gritty British soldiers *(C. floerkeana)* containing cocellic acid; and *C. macilenta* with thamnolic acid. Both are eastern species.

Dragon *Cladonia,* or dragon funnel *(C. squamosa),* contains atranorin.

Traditional Uses

Mealy pixie cup *(C. chlorophaea)* was boiled by the Okanagan-Colville of British Columbia, who knew it as Liver on Rock or *pen' pen'emekxixxn',* and used it to wash sores that were slow to heal.

This lichen is an old whooping cough remedy mentioned in early European herbals. It is boiled in milk and used today in Wales under the name *cwpanau pas.*

The Haida dipped the red tip into human breast milk and applied it to sore eyes.

Medicinal Use
Chemical Constituents
- **Research in Michigan found four different chemical populations of** *Cladonia cristatella,* **with each race occupying a different habitat, leading to significant differences in constituents, from grayanic acid to cryptochlorophaeic acid to merochlorophaeic acid, to the more common fumar-procetraric acid strain.**

- *Cladonia cristatella:* **usnic, didymic, barbatic, and rhodocladonic acids.**
- *C. bacillaris:* **barbatic acid.**
- *C. coccifera:* **zeorin and usnic acid.**
- *C. convoluta:* **usnic, fumarprotocetraric, and 9'-(O-methyl) protocetraric acids.**

Mealy pixie cup is active against *Staphylococcus albus, Diplococcus pneumoniae, Bacillus subtilis, B. mycoides,* and *Sarcina lutea* (Burkholder and Evans 1945).

The same authors found both *C. pleurota* and *C. uncialis* active against the above bacteria as well as several *Streptococcus* species, including *S. pneumoniae, S. pyogenes,* and *S. viridans.* The latter contains usnic acid and sometimes squamatic acid.

9'-(O-methyl) protocetraric acid, contained in *C. convoluta,* has been shown to induce apoptosis of murine leukemia cells (Bezivin et al. 2004).

Cladonia deformis
(LESSER SULPHUR CUP)

Medicinal Use

Cladonia deformis has been investigated for an unusual iron substance. Work by Alagna et al. in Italy indicates that the iron is present as high-spin Fe(III), and coordinates in an oxygen containing environment arising graciliformin ligands. It also contains zeorin.

It is strongly inhibitory against *S. aureus.*

Cladonia fimbriata

C. major
(TRUMPET LICHEN)

Medicinal Use

Chemical Constituents

- **Trumpet lichen** *(C. fimbriata)* **contains only 12.9 micrograms per gram of carotenoids, while some** *Caloplaca* **ssp. contain up to 151 micrograms per gram of various carotenoids.**

Work from Poland published a list of carotenoids from thirty-four lichen species. The lichen also contains atranoric acid, fimbriatic acid, and fumaroprotocetraric acid.

Textile Industry

It has been used in the past as a red dye for wool.

Cladonia furcata

C. subrangiformis
(MANY FORKED CLADONIA)

Medicinal Use

C. furcata has been shown to weakly inhibit the *Staphylococcus aureus* bacteria, and contains fumarprotocetraric acid.

One study identified a polysaccharide in the lichen that induced apoptosis in human leukemia K562 cells.

Cladonia gracilis

(BLACK FOOT CLADONIA)
(SMOOTH CLADONIA)

Gracilis means slender, referring to the slender cup shape. It may be the most common lichen in dry lodge pole pine forests, where it grows in huge mats in some places.

Medicinal Use

This lichen shows significant inhibitory effect on estrogen formation from the estrogen precursor sulfatase.

Extracts at a concentration of forty micrograms per milliliter showed an 83 percent inhibition rate.

It contains fumarprotocetraric acid, and shows activity against *C. subtilis* (Huneck 1999).

Textile Industry

The lichen has been used to produce an ash green dye for wool.

Cladonia pyxidata

(BROWN PIXIE CUP)
(CUP MOSS)
(CHIN CUPS)

Pyxidata is from the Latin *pyxis,* meaning a box. A pyx is now a term applied at the Canadian mint for a box containing sample coins. "Chin cup" comes from its former use in whooping cough or chin cough, as it was known.

It grows mainly on soil that is high in mineral content.

Its cup-like shape can identify it.

Medicinal Use

Chemical Constituents

- **Abundant atranorin and fumaroproto-cetraric, barbatic, and psoromic acids; mucilage; parellic acid, protofumarcetraric acid, and an enzyme emulsin.**

Brown pixie cup shows activity against both *S. aureus* and *B. subtilis* (Burkholder and Evans 1945).

This lichen is fairly widespread throughout the area and exhibits demulcent, anti-tussive, and expectorant properties.

The lichen has been shown effective against bronchitis and coughs (including whooping cough), combining well with coltsfoot and sundew.

Textile Industry

It was used traditionally in Europe to dye wool red, purple, or ash green.

Homeopathy

Symptoms include hurried feeling, but less anxious and nervous; bloated abdomen, disorientation, uncertainty, and dryness of tongue, lips, throat, skin, and rectum.

Tired and yet sleepless, desire for open air; difficulty breathing in a hot room.

Dose: 6C to 30C potency, proved by Izzie Azgad and Rosalind Floyd on nine provers in 1994. See Vermeulen's excellent book for greater detail.

Collema flaccidum
(FLACCID JELLY LICHEN)

Flaccid jelly lichen *(Collema flaccidum),* found on the east coast of North America, has been found to possess antitumor activity.

Lichen Essences

Smooth *Cladonia* lichen essence is the mirror— for helping open new doors into consciousness. It is like a spotlight focusing deep within, reflecting up into awareness, an unacknowledged part of oneself.

It helps to discover and understand the patterns developed and enacted today. It allows one to reclaim power through awareness.

— CANADIAN FOREST

Arctic alpine *Cladonia* lichen releases deep-seated patterns and worn-out old issues by transmuting negative karma, which is ripe for resolution. Destructive emotions are then purified, self-punishment, anger, and low self-esteem relinquished.

— FINDHORN

Dermatocarpon moulinsii
(STIPPLEBACK LICHEN)
D. miniatum
(LEATHER LICHEN)

This fairly common lichen is found on gravel. When wet the upper part turns green and becomes translucent. It can be soaked in water and then chewed slowly as a food source. When boiled for about fifteen minutes with a little salt, it has a flavor reminiscent of mushroom. It is a good addition to help thicken and flavor rock soup.

Medicinal Use

Crude extracts inhibit the growth of *Staphylococcus aureus* (Burkholder and Evans 1945).

Dermatocarpon miniatum contains a powerful antioxidant.

Textile Industry

Leather lichen has been used as an ash-green dye for wool in Europe.

Diploschistes scruposus

(CRATER LICHEN)

Crater lichen *(Diploschistes scruposus)* has a zinc content up to 9.34 percent of its dry weight, showing unusual ability to absorb ions from the soil. It makes a red-brown dye after treatment with urine or ammonia. It contains atranorin, lecanoric and diploschistesic acid.

Evernia mesomorpha

(SPRUCE MOSS LICHEN)
(BOREAL OAKMOSS LICHEN)
(BIRCH LICHEN)

From the northern boreal muskegs, spruce moss lichen, or boreal oakmoss lichen *(E. mesomorpha),* grows on the branches and bark of black spruce, larch, and birch. Chipewyan natives call it *k'tsa"ju* or birch lichen. They use a cooled decoction of the lichen from birch trees to treat snow-blindness.

Oakmoss lichen has been used in Egypt as a bread additive, and by the Turks to make a type of jelly.

Oakmoss is used today in aromatherapy for its grounding nature, and to create a sense of security and personal prosperity. It helps one work with nature spirits and prevents slipping of secrets.

Evernia prunastri

Evernia prunastri contains evernic acid. This compound shows activity against mycobacterium at rates similar to usnic acid. It was used traditionally to leaven bread and as a hops substitute for beer. It shows moderate activity against *S. aureus*.

Flavocetraria cucullata

(CURLED SNOW LICHEN)
F. nivalis
(CRINKLED SNOW LICHEN)

Other interesting lichens include the snow lichens, such as curled *(Flavocetraria cucullata)* and crinkled *(F. nivalis).*

The former, previously classified as *Cetraria cucullata,* has been used in northern Canada as a condiment for fish or duck soup. The Yup'ik call it *ninguujug* meaning "would like to be stretched," perhaps in reference to its filling nature.

Traditional Uses

Crinkled snow lichen is infused in hot water as a cardio-pulmonary tonic for heart attack and altitude sickness.

Medicinal Use

Chemical Constituents
- **Usnic and protolichesterinic acids.**

Crinkled snow lichen is weakly active against *Staphylococcus aureus* (Burkholder and Evans 1945).

According to the *Pharmacopoeia Universalis* of 1846, the medicinal uses are similar to Iceland moss.

Food Industry

Curled snow lichen has been used as a food, and was used in Russia during World War II to produce glucose molasses, yielding 71 percent by dry weight.

Textile Industry

It produces a violet dye with the addition of ammonia or urine.

Flavoparmelia caperata
(COMMON GREEN SHIELD LICHEN)

Common green shield lichen *(Flavoparmelia caperata)* is throughout northeastern Canada and United States, as well as the southwest.

Powder-edged speckled greenshield *(Flavopunctelia soredica)* is found on bark in open woods.

Green starburst lichen *(Parmeliopsis ambigua)* is widespread.

Traditional Uses

It was made into a dry powder and applied on burns by the Tarahumara of Mexico.

Medicinal Use

Chemical Constituents
- *Flavoparmelia caperata:* **usnic, protocetraric, and caperatic acids, as well as atranorin.**
- *Flavopunctelia soredica:* **usnic and lecanoric acids.**
- *Parmeliopsis ambigua:* **divaricatic acid.**

Ethanol extracts were found to be active against the virulent strain of *M. tuberculosis* $H_{37}Rv$ (Gupta et al. 1997).

Burkholder and Evans (1945) found activity against *Staphylococcus aureus, Diplococcus pneumoniae, Streptococcus hemolyticus, S. viridans, Bacillus subtilis, B. mycoides,* and *Sarcina lutea.*

Textile Industry

It has been used as an orange-brown to yellow dye on the Isle of Man.

The Navaho of New Mexico use it to produce a flesh colored dye.

Graphis

G. scripta
(COMMON SCRIPT LICHEN)

Common script lichen *(Graphis scripta)* is found scribbled on birch and other hardwood trees, mainly in eastern North America, but occasionally on the West Coast. It has been found to contain antioxidant ability and inhibit tyrosinase and xanthine oxidase (Yamamoto, Y. et al. 1993).

Behera et al. (2004) looked at the tyrosinase and xanthine oxidase activity of various *Graphis* species in India. Tyrosinase plays a role in melanin production and may play a role in some human cataracts. Xanthine oxidase is found in those individuals suffering gout due to excess uric acid and observed in patients with hepatitis and brain tumors. More study is needed.

Haematomma lapponicum
(BLOOD SPOT LICHEN)
H. coccineum

Blood spot lichen *(Haematomma lapponicum)* and other species of this genus contain porphyrillic acid, which shows antibiotic activity, as well as divaricatic and usnic acids. The related *H. coccineum* contains 20 percent usnic acid dry weight, a phenomenal amount.

Heterodermia species

Elegant centipede or elegant fringe lichen *(Heterodermia leucomela)* is found in New England, Appalachia, Florida, and along the west coast of North America.

Gupta et al. (2007) found an ethanol extract quite active against the virulent strain of tuberculosis $H_{37}Rv$. More work should follow. It contains a number of interesting compounds of which hydroxy-4-methoxybenzoic acid, which shows mosquito larvicidal activity, is most interesting (Kathirgamanathar et al. 2006).

Orange tinted fringe lichen *(H. obscurata)* was researched by Peter Cohen for a PhD thesis at the University of British Columbia in 1995. It contains a number of interesting compounds, including blastenin, zeorin, atra-

norin, 7-chloro-emodin, emodin, flavoobscurin A-B, 7,7'-dichlorohypericin, and 5,7-dichloro-emodin. The latter compound has antiviral activities that respond in the presence of light. Emodin and 7-chloro-emodin both show activity against the herpes simplex virus at two micrograms per milliliter.

Cupped fringe lichen *(H. diademata)* is confined to southern Arizona and New Mexico. In Nepal, it is known as *dhungo ku seto jhau*. The lichen is mixed with leaves of *Ageratina adenophora* and made into a poultice for cuts and wounds to protect against infection. It contains atranorin and zeorin.

Hypotrachyna revoluta
(POWDERED LOOP LICHEN)

Powdered loop lichen *(Hypotrachyna revoluta)*, found in small, scattered areas of North America, contains beta-orcinol metabolites hypotrachynic acid, deoxystictic acid, cryptostictinolide, and 8'-methyl-constictic acid.

Hypogymnia physodes
Parmelia physodes
(HOODED BONE)
(HOODED TUBE LICHEN)
(MONK'S HOOD LICHEN)
(PUFFED LICHEN)
H. tubulosa
(POWDER HEADED TUBE LICHEN)

This pale gray-green lichen is commonly found on coniferous and birch trees in the boreal forest. Research shows it is more tolerant of pollution from sulphur dioxide than most macro-lichens, but is still used as an indicator of pollution.

Traditional Uses

The Potawatomi used it in soup and as a treatment for constipation.

In fifteenth-century Europe, it was combined with *Evernia prunastri* and *Evernia furfuracea* to create the mixture *lichen quercinus virides*.

Medicinal Use

Chemical Constituents

- *H. physodes*: **atranorin, physodic acid, orcinol, and beta- orcinol depsidones including protocetraric and physodalic acids.**
- *H. tubulosa*: **3-hydroxyphysodic acid.**
- **Varnished tube lichen** (*H. austerodes*) **contains oxyphysodic acid, physodic acid, and sometimes 3-hydroxyphysodic acid, in addition to above constituents.**

Physodic acid at six to twelve micrograms per milliliter inhibits mycobacterium tuberculosis.

Early work by Burkholder and Evans (1945) found the lichen active against *Staphylococcus aureus*, *S. albus*, *Bacillus subtilis*, and *Sarcina lutea*.

Powder headed tube lichen contains 3-hydroxyphysodic acid. One study found this compound active against *Aeromonas hydrophila*, *Bacillus cereus*, *B. subtilis*, *E. coli*, *Klebsiella pneumoniae*, *Listeria monocytogenes*, *Proteus vulgaris*, *Salmonella typhimurium*, *Staphylococcus aureus*, *Streptococcus faecalis*, and *Candida albicans*.

Gyrophoric acid and stenosporic acid from *Hypogymnia* genus show antimicrobial potential (Candan et al. 2006).

Mycoremediation

Hooded bone appears to be able to bio-remediate arsenic, both by arsenite excretion and methylation of the toxic mineral.

Textile Industry

In Sweden and Scotland, the lichen is used to yield a brown dye for wool.

Fungicide

One research group studied the effect of water extracts of the lichen. They found it to inhibit many of the common wood-destroying fungi such as *Heterobasidon annosum*, *Laxitextum bicolor*, *Schizophyllum commune*, *Stereum hirsutum*, and *S. rugosum*.

This work could lead to some innovative inoculants or antifungal treatments for woodlot management.

The tube lichens contain atranorin, physodic acid, and often orcinol, as well as beta- orcinol depsidones including protocetraric and physodalic acids.

Lecanora cenisia

(SMOKY RIM LICHEN)
L. polytropa
(GRANITE SPECK RIM LICHEN)
L. rupicola
(WHITE RIM LICHEN)
L. sordida

Smoky rim lichen is found commonly throughout North America.

Granite speck rim lichen (*L. polytropa*) is found worldwide, including at twenty-four thousand feet on the south side of Makalu.

The related *L. esculenta* has a naturally sweet flavor and is edible, hence the species name. In Alexandria, it is called the "fat of the earth," and it is sometimes flavored with anise and honey into *panakarpian,* a type of bread popular there.

In 1829, during the war between Persia and Russia, a Caspian town was covered with lichen, which literally fell from the skies. This was made into bread and helped stave off starvation.

Culture and Folklore

The related *L. esculenta* grows on cliffs of the Middle East, and is believed to be the manna that fed the Hebrew people fleeing from Egypt, as told in the Bible.

Moses told everyone to gather it up because "this is the bread which the Lord hath given you to eat"... tasting "like wafers made with honey." High desert winds sometimes scatter it, even to this day, falling on Bedouin settlements like rain.

Traditional Uses

Three parts lichen and one part meal are made into a bread called *schirsad,* which can be bought today in the bazaars of Tehran and is used to encourage breast milk production.

Medicinal Use

Chemical Constituents

- *Lecanora cenisia:* **atranorin and fatty acids, especially roccellic acid. It sometimes contains gangaleoidin.**

- *L. polytropa:* **usnic acid, zeorin and fatty acids.**

- **The related** *L. californica* **contains norgangaleoidin and a fatty acid known as nephrosteranic acid.**

- *Lecanora rupicola:* **atranoric acid, rocellic acid, and thiophanic acid, as well as sordidone, eugenetin, and eugenitol, mycobionts not found in the thallus.**

The related *L. sordida* contains roccellic acid. Barry and McNally (1945) found the isolated acid had low activity against *Mycobacterium phlei* and *M. tuberculosis,* but its monoesters and mono amides inhibit growth at very high dilutions. Some of these compounds inhibited *M. phlei, M. smegmatis,* and *M. rabinowitz* at one part in twenty thousand to one part in forty thousand, and the bovine type of *M. tuberculosis* at one part in two hundred thousand to one part in four hundred thousand. Activity against *S. aureus* and *C. diphtheriae* was found.

The related *L. muralis* shows activity against *Bacillus subtilis.*

Lepraria latebranum
(DUST LICHEN)
L. lobificans
(FLUFFY DUST LICHEN)

The dust lichen (*Lepraria latebranum*) contains lepraric acid and fuciformic acid, while fluffy dust lichen (*L. lobificans*) contains atranorin, stictic, and constictic acids as well as zeorin.

Lobaria pulmonaria

Sticta pulmonaria
(LUNGWORT)
(LUNGMOSS)
(HAZELCROTTLE)
(HAZELRAW)

Note how *Lobaria pulmonaria* is a rhyming couplet, a taxonomic rarity. Another two are *Chrysanthemum leucanthemum,* the ox-eye daisy, and *Humulus lupulus,* or hops.

Sticta is from the Greek *stiktos* meaning "spotted."

Lungwort grows in the old-growth boreal forests, where its nitrogen fixing accumulation is very important.

It is distinguished by large thalli that cover the branches, trunks, and fallen logs of spruce and poplar. It looks like flaccid lungs, and was used for respiratory distress by native tribes. Like some other lichens, it is fairly luxuriant, with an average annual growth of 4.8 millimeters.

Traditionally, lungwort is boiled in milk to make a "cough tea" or "lichen chocolate."

It was also used before hops for beer making in European and Siberian monasteries during the seventeenth and eighteenth centuries.

The closely related lettuce lichen, *Lobaria oregana,* is most commonly found in the mountains, on the top of hundred-year-old douglas firs. Here, the lichen capture nitrogen, fall to the ground, and decompose, releasing the nutrient to nitrogen-deficient soils.

Textured lungwort *(L. scrobiculata),* called *qelquaq* by the Yup'ik of Alaska, is found west of the continental divide, as well as from northern Saskatchewan to the Great Slave and Great Bear Lakes. It is edible, and can be eaten right from the tree.

The Haida refer to it as tree blanket, forest cloud, or cloud leaves medicine, alluding to its health properties.

Traditional Uses

The Gitksan and other First Nations of British Columbia, who associated this lichen with frogs and called it *nagaganaw* or "frog dress," decocted it as a treatment for sore throats.

The Hesquiat used it for sunburned faces.

Lungwort is very useful for all sorts of upper respiratory complaints, including what was formerly called lymphatic tuberculosis.

It is useful in formulas for hay fever, head colds, and flu, as well as for intermittent fevers or night sweats.

Its nourishing and blood-building nutrients are useful for those suffering chronic internal dryness. It also restores moisture to the tissue that produces breast milk.

It combines well with borage or herbal lungwort for gastric ulcers, and should be given consideration in treating ulcerative colitis and allergies associated with the gastrointestinal tract. Tannins, quercetin, mucilage, and other constituents help repair and regenerate mucosal membranes, and calm mast cell reactivity.

Its traditional use in Ireland for treating hemorrhoids probably has basis in fact.

It acts on the base of the brain and the vagus nerve, relieving fevers and irritative coughs, both acute and chronic.

The lungwort cough is wheezing, rasping dry, and persistent, often worse in the dry, dusty months of summer.

Lungwort possesses anti-rheumatic and analgesic activity, useful in pain occurring between the scapula, shoulders, and occipital bone of the head. Sometimes the pain extends into the chest and shoulders. Myalgia and arthralgia of the small joints may also benefit.

Medicinal Use

Chemical Constituents

- *L. pulmonaria:* **mucilage, including 30 to 40 percent lichenin; lichen acids, including stictic, norstictic, sticinic, constictic, peristictic, cryptostictic, methyl stictic, thelophoric, and gyrophoric acids; fumaric and oxalic acids; fatty acids such as palmitic, oleic, and linolenic acids; trace minerals; ergosterol; fucosterol; protein; and tannins.**

- *L. oregana:* **stictic, constitic, cryptostictic, and norstictic acids.**

- *L. scrobiculata:* **stictic, constitic, norstitic, and usnic acids and scrobiculin.**

- **The related peppered moon lichen *(S. fuliginosa)* contains trimethylamine.**

- **Cabbage lungwort *(L. linita)* contains tenuiorin.**

Studies conducted at the Institute of Radiation Medicine in Tianjin, China, have shown lungwort to be protective of bone marrow stromal and hematopoietic stem cells when exposed to radiation. This may be due, in part, to its anti-oxidant properties (Odabasoglu et al. 2004).

Stictic, constictic, and norstictic acids from this lichen show significant inhibition of *Salmonella gallinarum.*

Lungwort shows moderate activity against *Staphylococcus aureus.*

Polyporic acid, derived from *Sticta coronata,* was shown to double the life expectancy of mice infected with acute leukemia and other cancers.

Melanic acid compounds in lungwort are induced by UVB radiation.

Homeopathy

Lungwort is for a general feeling of dullness and malaise, when a cold is coming on. The patient may feel as if floating in air, and have a great desire to talk. This is accompanied by dull pressure in the forehead and root of nose, with an unsuccessful, constant desire to blow. There may be a dry, hacking cough during the night that is worse on inhalation. The extremities may be red and inflamed. Changes of weather affect the symptoms.

Dose: 6C tincture. The mother tincture is prepared from the fresh thallus of the lichen (Boericke).

Essential Oil

An essential oil is steam-distilled from this lichen and used in perfumery.

Cosmetics

In India and Sikkim, lungwort has been used as a cleansing hair powder.

Lungwort was used in France for perfume, but was not plentiful. In Germany it was used for perfume as well and called *lungenfletche.*

Textile Industry

In India and Sikkim, lungwort has been used to tan hides and woolens an orange brown color.

In Scotland, *L. scrobiculata* has been used to dye wool a brown color.

Nephroma arcticum
(GREEN LIGHT)
(ARCTIC KIDNEY LICHEN)
N. parile
(POWDERY KIDNEY LICHEN)
N. laevigatum
(MUSTARD KIDNEY LICHEN)

Green light is found in the extreme north following the Canadian Shield, and on the extreme tops of the Rocky Mountains. The Yup'ik of Alaska call it *kusskoak*. The lichen is collected and stored until winter and then boiled with fish eggs.

Powdery kidney lichen is found in the sub-alpine region and mountains. Natives of Alaska also cooked this lichen with crushed fish eggs. The lichen was picked in summer and then stored until needed.

Mustard kidney lichen *(N. laevigatum)* is found on the west coast of North America.

Traditional Uses
The Yup'ik of Alaska give a hot water infusion to people with weakened constitutions or after a lengthy illness.

Medicinal Use
Chemical Constituents
- *N. arcticum:* **emodin, 7-chloro-emodin, 1-O-methyl-emodin, 7,7'-dichlorohypericin, and 2,2',7,7'-tetrachlorohypericin.**

- *7-chloroemodin and 7,7'dichlorohypericin:* **various anthroquinones, nephromin, nephrin, usnic acid, and fatty acids.**

It contains emodin and 7-choro-emodin, which show activity against herpes simplex virus at low concentrations. Peter Cohen wrote his PhD thesis at UBC in 1995 on this lichen and *Hetereodermia obscurata.* He identified hypericin compounds in both that possess antiviral activity. It also contains usnic acid, zeorin, and phenarctin.

Powdery kidney lichen shows mild activity against *Staphylococcus aureus.* Rankovic et al. (2010) found it weak against various bacteria and fungi tested.

Textile Industry
Powdery kidney lichen has been used in Scotland as a blue dye for wool.

Parmelia saxatilis
(ROCK SHIELD)
(SALTED SHIELD)
(CROTTLE)
P. omphalodes
(SMOKY CROTTLE)

Parmelia was divided into a number of different genera starting in 1974. Research conducted before that year referring to *Parmelia ssp.* can be extremely confusing.

Saxatilis is from the Latin *saxum* meaning "a rock."

Parmelia saxatilis is found abundantly on acidic rocks and outcroppings in boreal forests. It increases in size by an average of 3.4 millimeters per year.

In Sweden, country people call this dye lichen or stone moss. It is collected from rocks easily after a rain with a table knife.

This lichen accumulates the rare mineral beryllium.

Traditional Uses

Various *Parmelia* species have been used traditionally in both India and China for medicinal purposes.

In traditional Chinese medicine *P. saxatilis* is known as *shih hua.*

The dried lichen was sprinkled in stockings in parts of the Highlands to prevent foot inflammation and pain from long journeys.

In parts of Ireland it was applied to bad sores under the chin, as well as burns and cuts.

During the fifteenth century, the lichen was known in parts of Europe as *Muscus cranii humanii* when found growing on a human skull and was much prized for treating epilepsy. It sold for its weight in gold.

The Nishinam of California call it *wa'-hat-tak* and use it, infused as a tea, to treat colic.

Medicinal Use

Chemical Constituents

- **Smoky crottle: salazinic acid, sometimes accompanied by lobaric acid.**

- **Rock shield: altranoric acid (0.5 percent) and salazinic acid (3.1 percent).**

- **Ingólfsdóttir et al. in Iceland found salazinic acid to contain MIC values of 125 micrograms per milliliter (Ingólfsdóttir et al. 2000).**

Textile Industry

It yields various shades of brown, depended on the quantity used, and does not require a mordant. In Scotland it is used to dye wool for Harris Tweed. The scent of Harris Tweed is that of the lichen itself; it is especially pronounced when wet.

Smoky crottle *(P. omphalodes),* more often found in the northern territories, was also used traditionally for dyeing the deep red browns and rusty oranges prized by weavers. The brown shades produced are known as crottle and the red shades as corkir. Studies have shown that the dye is produced by a reaction between the free amino groups of the wool with aldehyde groups on the lichen acids.

Concentric ring lichen *(Arctoparmelia centrifuga)* has been used traditionally in the north as a red brown dye for wool.

There is no correlation between the color of the lichen and the color obtained by boiling with wool. Lichen substances such as gyrophoric, evernic and lecanoric acid, and erythrin convert to a purple compound in the presence of oxygen and ammonia. August picking yields the richest dye material.

Bits and Pieces

The lichen was used in the early nineteenth century in England in a ritual in which plant and fungi materials were used to create miniature scenes up to ten feet long. These were leaned up against wells during summer festivals.

Parmelia sulcata

(WAXPAPER LICHEN)
(HAMMERED SHIELD LICHEN)
P. molliuscula
(GROUND LICHEN)
P. olivacea
Melanelia olivacea
(SPOTTED CAMOUFLAGE LICHEN)

Sulcata is from the Latin *sulcus,* meaning "a furrow or groove."

Also known as powdered shield lichen, it is common on dead spruce branches throughout the north. Rufus hummingbirds use it to decorate and hide their nests.

Ground lichen *(P. molliuscula)* is a flat species that grows from Nebraska to South Dakota and west to the Rockies. It causes severe paralysis and death to range cattle and sheep when forage is scarce.

Traditional Uses

The lichen was rubbed on the gums of teething babies to help make them less restless and sleep.

In Italy, various species of *Parmelia* are used as a cholagogue.

Medicinal Use

Chemical Constituents

■ **Lecanoric, fumarprotocetraric, stictic, perlatolic, salazinic, lobaric, echinocarpic, and galbinic acids.**

■ *Parmelia entotheiochria* **contains secalonic acid A, related to the ergochromes from ergot.**

Salazinic and lobaric acids are antiseptic.

Waxpaper lichen shows activity against *Aeromonas hydrophila, Bacillus cereus, B. subtilis, Listeria monocytogenes, Proteus vulgaris, Yersinia enterocolitica, Staphylococcus aureus, Streptococcus faecalis, Candida albicans, C. glabrata, Aspergillus funigatus, A. niger,* and *Penicillium notatum* (Candan et al. 2007; Rankovic et al. 2007).

Parmelia species exhibit astringent, resolvent, aperient, and diuretic properties.

Ethanol extracts of *Parmelia* species are potentiated by colloidal silver in the treatment of *Staphylococcus aureus.*

Textile Industry

Because it contains salizinic acid, it can be used for dyeing wool.

Spotted camouflage lichen *(M. olivacea)* has been used in Great Britain to produce a brown dye.

Parmotrema

P. stuppeum
(POWDER EDGED RUFFLE LICHEN)
P. reticulatum
Rimelia reticulata
(CRACKED RUFFLE LICHEN)
P. performatum
(PERFORATED RUFFLE LICHEN)

Parmotrema species containing atranonin and chloroatranonin exhibit COX 1 and 2 inhibition, suggesting anti-inflammatory activity (Bugni et al. 2009).

Powder edged ruffle lichen *(P. stuppeum)* is found in the Appalachians and on the west coast of California. It contains methyl orsenillate, orsenillic acid, atranorin, and lecanoric acid that show moderate antioxidant activity.

Parmotrema reticulatum (Rimelia reticulata), a cracked ruffle lichen, has been found to have moderate activity against the virulent Mycobacterium tuberculosis strains H37Rv and Ra (Gupta et al. 1997).

Perforated ruffle lichen *(Parmotrema performatum)* is found mainly in the southeastern

United States. It is used in India for food and medicine under the name chharila. It is used for a wide variety of conditions including dyspepsia, spermatorrhea, amenorrhea, kidney stones, enlarged spleen, bronchitis, hemorrhoids, sore throat, and pain in general. It is mentioned in various Indian materia medicas, under both *P. performatum* and *P. chinense*.

The smoke is used to relieve headaches. It is powdered and used as snuff or applied to bleeding wounds. It is commonly adulterated with other lichens. It contains atranorin and norstictic acid.

Peltigera aphthosa

(STUDDED LEATHER LICHEN)
(FAIRY PELT)
(LEMON LICHEN)
(FRECKLE PELT)
(SEA GREEN LICHEN)
P. praextator
(SCALY DOG LICHEN)
P. leucophlebia
(RUFFLED FRECKLE PELT LICHEN)

Peltigera is from the Greek and Latin meaning "shield bearing." *Pelta* means "a light shield."

Aphthosa is from the Latin meaning "thrush," referring to the disease of the throat, for which it was once a specific. Or perhaps, originally, it is from the Greek *aphthai* meaning "pustule" or "eruption."

When moist, this lichen turns a brilliant green, later dulling to a gray-green. It is commonly found growing over true mosses in coniferous forests.

Traditional Uses

Peltigera is a strong purgative and anthelmintic that combines well with other plants for cleansing worms and other parasites.

The Swedes boil the lichen in milk for treating thrush in children. Back in the 1800s, it was believed that white spots inside the cheeks of feverish children were caused by elves and fairy pelt was the treatment of choice. This is another example of matching a plant's signature to the symptoms to be treated. The cephaloida was thought to be similar to the eruptions caused in children's mouths by thrush.

Given the prevalence of chronic thrush and yeast infections today, it is a plant worthy of further attention.

When cooked, the lichen becomes a thick and glue-like paste, which, applied to the skin and left to dry, is a great remedy for diaper rash or chapped skin.

The Nitinaht of Vancouver Island chewed both *P. aphthosa* and closely related *P. britannica* for tuberculosis. The Tlingit sprinkled the dry, powdered lichen on scalds and burns, and the Nitinaht used the fresh poultice on leg sores.

Membranacous dog lichen (*P. membranacea*) was used by the Kwakiutl of British Columbia as a love charm, as well as by Nitinaht men who could not easily urinate. I noted in my clinical practice that difficulty with urination sometimes followed using love charms, if you know what I mean.

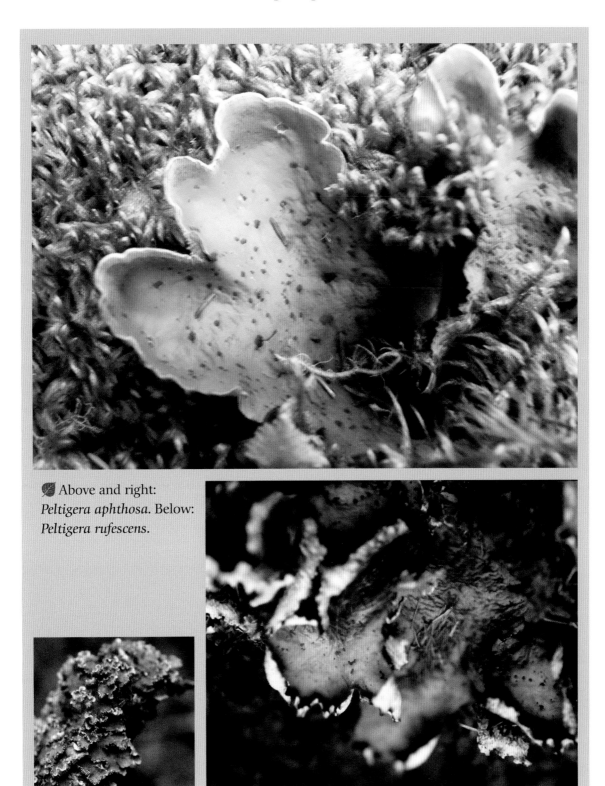

Above and right: *Peltigera aphthosa.* Below: *Peltigera rufescens.*

Medicinal Use

Chemical Constituents

- *P. aphthosa:* **various phenolics including aphtosin and tenuiorin; methyl gyrophorate; gyrophoric acid; triterpenoids; and phlebic acid A and B.**

- *P. polydactylon:* **peltigerin (2 to 3 percent), tenuiorin, methyl gyrophorate, gyrophoric acid, and triterpenes.**

The antimicrobial active compounds in *Peltigera* were found to be effective against fungi and both gram-positive and gram-negative bacteria.

It contains several laccases that may have application in biological reactions.

The closely related ruffled freckle pelt *(P. leucophlebia)* was at one time considered to be the same species, but is now thought to be distinct. Both are extremely widespread and common.

Ingólfsdóttir et al. (2000) showed the lichen to possess moderate inhibition of HL-60 human leukemia cells. Early work by same author found petroleum and chloroform extracts show activity against *Pseudomonas aeruginosa.*

The phycobiont of this lichen, *Coccomyxa* sp., excretes sixteen times more biotin in a culture medium than free-living *Chlorella.*

The related frog pelt, or many fruited pelt *(P. polydactylon),* is used medicinally in Sikkim as a paste to stop bleeding and as an antiseptic. It contains 2 to 3 percent peltigerin, a derivative of orcinol; as well as tenuiorin, methyl gyrophorate, gyrophoric acid, and triterpenes.

Water extracts show activity against various bacteria including *Bacillus subtilis, E. coli,* and *Staphylococcus aureus.*

Peltigera rufescens shows remarkably high antioxidant activity despite low levels of phenolics (Odabasoglu et al. 2005).

Scaly dog lichen, or born again pelt *(P. praetextata),* has been observed to exhibit activity against *Bacillus subtilis, E. coli,* and *S. aureus.*

Food Industry

Fairy pelt, or lemon lichen, contains a mixture of methyl and ethyl orsellinates that have been shown to be superior to commonly used preservative agents like methyl and proply p-hydroxybenzoates.

Textile Industry

All *Peltigera* are used for boiling water dyes, usually brown in nature.

Agriculture

Studies in Wales indicate that the lichen inhibits the germination of grass seeds, as well as root production and elongation in grass seeds.

This suggests the use of this and other lichens in organic farming and weed control. Water extracts of dog pelt inhibit various bent, meadow, and rye grasses, as well as fescue.

Peltigera canina
(GROUND LIVERWORT)
(DOG PELT)

The species name *canina* was based on its traditional use as protection against dog bites and that the fruiting bodies resemble dog teeth or ears.

The Kwakiult call it *tl'extl'ekw'es* meaning "seaweed of the ground" and used it as a love charm.

Traditional Uses

Peltigera canina is a safe, reliable laxative if used in moderate amounts and a mild but effective liver tonic.

Early German settlers to North America used the plant for strengthening a weak liver or cooling one that was inflamed.

It was ground into a powder, mixed with white wine, and given to little boys suffering hernia.

In parts of Wales during the nineteenth century it was powdered and mixed with black pepper as a treatment for dog bites.

The Nitanaht of Vancouver Island used *P. canina* (or *P. aphthosa*) as an infusion for those suffering anuria, or the inability to urinate.

Boiled in water and gargled, the lichen soothes the swelling of tonsils and the uvula.

A few tablespoons of the distilled water, taken several times daily, is excellent for an inflamed liver or for treating jaundice. The high concentration of methionine may be responsible, in part, for its high curative rate.

Flaky freckle pelt *(P. britannica)* was chewed by the Nitinaht of British Columbia to treat tuberculosis.

Medicinal Use

Chemical Constituents

- **Ergosterol, emulsin, mannitol-like substances, free methionine, and all of the essential amino acids save histidine.**

- **Concentric pelt** (*P. elisabethae*), **ruffled freckle pelt** (*P. leucophlebia*), **veinless pelt** (*P. malacea*), **black saddle lichen** (*P. neckeri*), **carpet pelt** (*P. neopolydactyla),* **and flat fruited pelt** (*P. horizontalis*) **contain tenuiorin, methyl gyrophorate, gyrophoric acid, peltigerin, and various triterpenes.**

- *P. Britannica* **contains tenuiorin, methyl gyrophate, gyrophoric acid, and triterpenes.**

Tenuiorion showed moderate activity against human breast, pancreatic, and colon cancer cell lines (Ingólfsdóttir et al. 2002).

Homeopathy

Ground liverwort is used whenever there is lots of throat congestion, with profuse expectoration and hoarseness. The throat is tickling and irritating, with a scraping and rough sensation.

Liverwort induces free and easy expectoration, relieving that continual feeling of something caught in the epiglottis.

Dose: 2C. One to two pellets under the tongue, as needed (Boericke).

Textile Industry

P. canina was a dye source in Europe as an iron red color for wool.

Personality Traits

The noble liverwort does not appear,
Without a speck, like the unclouded air,
A plant of noble use and endless fame,
The liver's great preserver, hence its name.
— ABRAHAM COWLEY

Pertusaria amara

(BITTER WART LICHEN)

P. communis

P. pertusa

Bitter wart lichen *(Pertusaria amara)* is found on the west coast and eastern seaboard of North America. It is extremely bitter, as the name suggests. It contains arabitol, mannitol, and emulsin, as well as picrolichenic acid and is used to treat high fever. The genus contains a variety of depsides, depsidones, and xanthones. Decoction of *Pertusaria amara* was said to be a quinine replacement. The related *P. communis (P. pertusa)* was said more useful for men than women.

Physcia

P. caesia

(BLUE GRAY ROSETTE LICHEN)

(POWDERBACK LICHEN)

P. stellaris

(STAR ROSETTE LICHEN)

Blue gray rosette lichen, or powderback lichen *(Physcia caesia),* contains atranoric acid, haematommic acid, and zeorin.

Star rosette lichen *(P. stellaris)* contains atranorin.

Physcia species have been combined with pine resins to produce a yellow-staining paint.

Platismatia glauca

(VARIED RAG LICHEN)

Varied rag lichen or *Platismatia glauca,* found on lodgepole pine and white spruce, was studied for cytotoxic activity along with seven other lichens. All demonstrated activity on human cancer cell lines (Bezivin et al. 2003a).

Platismatia glauca contains proto-lichesterinic acid.

Elders of Haida refer to *Platismatia glauca* as "red cedar goat wool" or "light clouds."

Pseudephebe pubescens

(FINE ROCK WOOL)

Fine rock wool *(Pseudephebe pubescens)* derives its common name for its appearance of black steel wool. The Haisla of British Columbia used it to make a black wood paint. It is used in Nepal for its antiseptic properties, and in China as a medicated tea.

Ramalina farinacea

(DOTTED RAMALINA)

R. intermedia

(ROCK RAMALINA)

R. celastri

(PALMETTO LICHEN)

R. pollinaria

(DUSTY RAMALINA)

There are a number of interesting *Ramalina* species.

Rock *Ramalina (R. intermedia),* which resembles the dotted species in some respects, contains sekikaic acid.

Palmetto lichen *(R. celastri)* is confined to southern Texas. It contains parietin that shows antiviral activity against arenaviruses.

Dusty or chalky *Ramalina (Ramalina pollinaria)* is common.

Traditional Uses

The related *R. bourgeana* is used in Europe to dissolve kidney stones.

The Manchurian drug *shih hua,* which translates as "stone-flower" and is known to the Japanese as *seki ka,* consists of a mixture of *Ramalina* species.

Medicinal Use

Chemical Constituents

- *Ramalina farinacea:* **ramalinolic acid, sekikaic acid, arabitol, mannitol, and d-usnic acid.**

- *Ramalina pollinaria:* **usnic, obtusatic, evernic, and sekikaic acids.**

Tay et al. (2004) found (+)-usnic acid from this lichen active against *Bacillus subtilis, Listeria monocytogenes, Proteus vulgaris, Staphylococcus aureus, Streptococcus faecalis, Yersinia enterocolitica, Candida albicans,* and *C. glabrata.*

One study found methanol lichen extracts active against *B. subtilis, S. aureus, S. epidermidis,* and *E. coli.*

Norstictic acid showed activity against all the above, except for *Y. enterocolitica,* as well as against *Aeromonas hydriphila.* Protocetraric acid showed activity against the yeasts.

Ethyl acetate fractions have shown the ability to inhibit lentiviral and adenoviral as well as HIV-1.

One study tested against herpes simplex virus type 1 and the respiratory syncytial virus. Both were potently inhibited (IC_{50} + 6.09 and 3.65 micrograms per milliliter, respectively). It also inhibited HIV-1 reverse transcriptase with an IC_{50} of only 0.022 micrograms per milliliter.

Cosmetics

Dotted *Ramalina,* or the dotted line *(R. farinacea),* and *Ramalina pollinaria* have long histories of use in cosmetics and perfumes throughout Europe.

Textile Industry

It has been used traditionally as a light brown dye for wool.

Rhizocarpon geographicum
(YELLOW MAP LICHEN)

Yellow map lichen *(Rhizocarpon geographicum)* is used in Scandinavia to produce a brown dye for woolens. It contains the pigment rhizocarpic acid, as well as parellic, psoromic and rhizonic acid, and tetronic acid derivatives.

Rhizoplaca melanophthalma
(GREEN ROCK POSY)

Green rock posy *(Rhizoplaca melanophthalma)* is widespread from the northernmost points of Canada down to New Mexico. It shows activity against both *Bacillus subtilis* and *S. aureus* bacteria.

Rinodina oreina

Dimelaena oreina

(PEPPER SPORE LICHEN)

The poetically named pepper spore lichen, *Rinodina oreina (Dimelaena oreina),* contains gyrophoric and fumarprotocetraric acids.

Solorinia crocea

(ORANGE CHOCOLATE CHIP LICHEN)

Orange chocolate chip lichen *(Solorinia crocea)* contains solorinic and norsolorinic acid, as well as methyl gyrophorate and gyrophoric acid. Solorinic acid is an anthraquinone. It was used for coloring woolens in Scotland at one time. As its common name suggests, *S. crocea* is unmistakable with its bright orange medulla and red born apothecia. Common throughout the mountains, it contains at least two lacasses.

Sphaerophorus fragilis

(FRAGILE SPHAEROPHORUS)
(FRAGILE CORAL LICHEN)
S. globosus var. gracilis
S. globosus var. globosus
(ALPINE SPHAEROPHORUS)
(CORAL LICHEN)

Fragile *Sphaerophorus* is an Arctic species that grows in dense cushions and has very fragile branches. Alpine *Sphaerophorus* has two variations: *gracilis,* which grows on coniferous forest west of the continental divide and *globosus,* a rare type that grows on the ground or in rock crevices. They both contain hypothamnolic acid, with the latter sometimes containing squamatic acid.

Medicinal Use

Both lichens exhibit significant inhibition against the estrogen precursor sulfatase. When tested at forty micrograms per milliliter, the former showed inhibition of 95 percent, and the latter 90 percent.

Alpine *Sphaerophorus* exhibits inhibition against aromatase, another estrogen precursor. While only at 74 percent, the combined inhibition of both precursors makes this a potentially exciting prospect for the future.

Stereocaulon alpinum

(ALPINE CORAL)
S. paschale
(EASTER LICHEN)
S. vesuvianum
(VARIEGATED FOAM LICHEN)

Stereocaulon is from the Greek *stereos* meaning "hard" or "firm"; and *kaulos,* meaning "stem," referring to its firm brittle texture when dry.

Stereocaulon alpinum is a rose-white, grayish lichen common to sub-alpine forest floors. It is often confused with the closely related *S. tomentosum,* which is silvery-gray.

Variegated foam lichen *(S. vesuvianum)* is found on newly exposed rock in the Rocky Mountains as well as throughout the northern territories.

Medicinal Use

Chemical Constituents

- *S. alpinum:* **methyl beta-orsellinate, lobaric acid, atranorin, and 9-cis-octadecenamide.**

- *S. paschale:* **dextro mannose, dextro galactose, atranorin, and lobaric acid.**

- **The related rock foam lichen** (*S. saxatile*), **grand foam** (*S. grande*), **and Easter lichen** (*S. paschale*) **contain lobaric acid, while woolly foam lichen** (*S. tomentosum*) **contains stictic acid.**

- **Snow foam lichen** (*S. rivulorum*) **usually contains lobaric acid, with some areas containing perlatolic and anzaic acid, and others only atranorin.**

- **The related variegated foam lichen** (*S. vesuvianum*) **contains stictic and norstictic acids.**

Easter lichen is used in traditional Chinese medicine for various skin and respiratory conditions.

The active ingredient of *S. alpinum* (methyl beta-orsellinate) is antifungal and shows signs of gram-positive and gram-negative bactericidal activity.

Early work by Ingólfsdóttir et al. (1985) found chloroform and acetone extracts active against *Staphylococcus aureus,* petroleum and acetate extracts active against *Bacillus subtilis,* chloroform against *E. coli,* and acetone against *Pseudomonas aeruginosa.* Petroleum, chloroform, and acetone extracts all inhibited the fungi *Candida albicans.*

Lobaric acid isolated from this lichen has shown in vitro inhibitory effects on arachidonate 5-lipoxygenase, similar to the flavone baicalein, found in skullcap.

Studies conducted in Iceland, a mecca of polar lichens, show some exciting results. On cultured human cells, three malignant cell lines from breast carcinomas and erythro-leukemia (K-562) were tested. At concentrations of twenty milligrams per milliliter, significant cancer cell death was detected. In contrast, the proliferation and survival of normal skin fibroblasts and DNA synthesis was not affected. These results open up the opportunity for future studies of protolichesterinic acid with regards to antitumor and anti-inflammatory properties.

Atranorin and lobaric acids, isolated from the lichen, also showed activity against *Mycobacterium avian,* a non-pathogenic organism with sensitivity similar to the *Tuberculinum mycobacterium.*

Ingólfsdóttir et al. (1997) showed the presence of an alkamide called 9-cis-octadecenamide. This compound showed moderate inhibitory activity against cyclooxygenase from sheep seminal vesicle microsomes with an IC50 of 64.3 micromoles, indicating anti-inflammatory properties.

Early work by Burkholder and Evans (1945) showed activity against *Staphylococcus aureus, Bacillus subtilis, B. mycoides,* and *Sarcina lutea.*

Petroleum extracts show activity against *Pseudomonas aeruginosa,* water extracts against *Candida albicans,* and chloroform extracts against *Staphylococcus aureus* and *Bacillus subtilis* (Ingólfsdóttir et al. 1985).

Lichen Essence

Variegated foam lichen essence is like the lichen, the first plant to grow on cooled lava.

It gives us the power to begin over again. It strengthens our resolve to move forward even in small steps.

— Korte Phi

Food Industry

Several studies indicate that the active ingredient of *S. alpinum* (methyl beta-orsellinate) is a superior food preserving agent to commonly used methyl and propyl p-hydroxybenzoates.

Textile Industry

Easter lichen, like other flat lichens, was used by the Barrens-Keewatin Inuit as a filler in caribou skins to make rafts for crossing rivers and streams.

It was used in parts of Europe as an ash-green dye for wool.

Teloschistes chrysophthalmus
(GOLD EYE LICHEN)

Gold eye lichen *(Teloschistes chrysophthalmus)* contains usnic acid that shows activity against the arenaviruses Junin and Tacaribe.

Thamnolia vermicularis
(WHITEWORM LICHEN)

Whiteworm lichen *(Thamnolia vermicularis* var. *subuliformis)* is frequently found on tundra and arctic alpine areas. Birds like the golden plover use the lichen for nesting material. There are two distinct strains, one containing thamnolic acid and another with squamatic and baeomy-

cic acid, the former found more on the West Coast and the latter in the Rocky Mountains.

The distinct shiny bluish-gray appearance of this genus is due to a thin layer of calcium oxalate crystals that deflect light and help lichens survive extreme conditions.

Medicinal Use

Whiteworm contains baeomycesic acid, a beta-orcinol depside, which shows weak inhibition of platelet type 12 (S) lipoxygenase (Ingólfsdóttir et al. 1997a).

One study identified thamnolan as one of the immuno-modulating polysaccharides.

Another study found strong activity against *S. aureus.*

Ingólfsdóttir et al. (1985) found petroleum extracts active against *S. aureus, B. subtilis, E. coli,* and *Candida albicans.*

Usnea hirta
(SHAGGY OLD MAN'S BEARD)
(SUGARY BEARD)
U. lapponica
(POWDERY BEARD)
U. cavernosa
(PITTED BEARD)
U. scabrata
(SCRUFFY BEARD)
(STRAW BEARD)
U. filipendula
U. dasypoga
(FISHBONE BEARD LICHEN)
U. longissima
(METHUSALA'S BEARD LICHEN)

The Dakota call it *chan wiziye,* translating as either "on the north side of the tree," or "spirit of the north wind." The northern Chipewyan know it as *k'i tsaju,* while the Dena'ina call it *ch'vala andazi* or spruce hair.

Usnea, or old man's beard, hangs in gray-green strands from larch and spruce of the boreal forest. Look for the central white, elastic thread inside *Usnea* for correct identification.

As noted, lichens are quite slow growing, but *U. longissima* has been found to double in length annually.

Usnea species are used as catalysts for making fermented corn beverages by the Tarahumara of northern Mexico.

Traditional Uses

Usnea was recommended in the *Formulary of Al-Kindi* around 850 AD. It was suggested for a swollen spleen, a part of the immune system. Earlier in ancient Greece, both Hippocrates and Dioscorides recommended *Usnea barbata* for uterine problems.

The Chinese have used various *Usnea* species *(Sung-Luo)* for thousands of years. It is prized for its broad-spectrum antibacterial and immune stimulating properties in various respiratory and urinary infections. *Usnea diffracta* has been called Lao Tzu's beard. Chinese herbalists will only gather this lichen during the fifth lunar month for maximum benefit. Overuse of *Usnea* for colds, flu, and infections can damage spleen *qi.*

Usnea is very effective in trichomoniasis, giardia, and candida infections; and particularly effective in cervical erosion, or dysplasia, as a douche.

The Malaysians use *Usnea* species as a general tonic and tea for colds, and the neighboring Indonesians used *U. thallus,* or *kayu angin* meaning "windy wood," as an astringent and anti-spasmodic for intestinal problems.

It was traditionally burned in homes to combat evil spirits and wind borne diseases.

In my region of Canada, it is used as a bitter stomachic, for coughs, and to relieve menstrual pain.

The Blackfoot, who call it *e-simatch-sis,* and the Cree by *mithapakwan,* use *Usnea* for stopping nosebleeds and bleeding wounds. A decoction was also used to wash sore or infected eyes.

The Nitinaht, who call it P'u7up, used *Usnea* species for diapers, sanitary napkins, and dressing wounds.

Fishbone beard lichen *(U. filipendula)* has been used on Sakhalin Island, now belonging to Russia, as a powder to treat wounds. Modern research indicates it has antibacterial activity.

Warty beard lichen *(U. ceratina)* was known by the Pomo of California as *kôchih* and used for diapers and toilet paper.

The lichen *U. longissima* has long been used in Ayurvedic and Unani medicine for arthritis, edema, eczema, cardiac tonics, and massage oils for rheumatism, gout, and sciatica.

Usnea longissima has been used in China and India as an expectorant, while First Nations people used it for feminine hygiene products and bedding.

Ayurvedic scholars equate its medicinal use with another lichen, *Parmelia perlata.*

In Argentina, usnea is used for washing warts. It is a constituent of the Chinese drug *shi-koa* and the Japanese medicinal drug *seki-ka*. The Maori of New Zealand utilize *Usnea* to increase resistance to infection and stimulate the appetite.

Medicinal Use

Chemical Constituents

- *U. hirta:* (+) usnic acid (3 percent); alectoric, hirtic, thamnolic, diffractaic (rare), hertillic, and usnaric acids; anthraquinones; hirtusneanoside; and various fatty acids.

- *U. filipendula:* salazinic acid, usnaric acid, barbatic acid, d-usinic acid, and emulsin.

- *U. cavernosa:* salazinic acid and/or usnic acid.

- *U. lapponica:* usnic and/or salazinic acid and sometimes barbatic acid.

- *U. scabrata:* usnic acid.

- *C. longissima:* various B-orcinol depsides including evernic, barbatic, and diffractaic acids; glutinol; and longissimione A and B.

- *U. ceratina:* diffractiaic acids.

Dr. William Mitchell Jr. considers *Usnea* a valuable diuretic that combines well with parsley. He recommends up to ninety drops of tincture three times daily.

It combines well with Oregon grape root, dandelion root, and uva ursi for damp heat strangury; and with scullcap and elecampane root for phlegm heat in the lungs.

For giardia infection, or amoebic dysentery, combine with Oregon grape root and elecampane root.

The active parts of *Usnea* are poorly water soluble, slightly better in alcohol and most soluble in oil.

Usnic acid is influenced by the solvent used, pH value, and with what powders or ointments it is mixed.

Energetically, *Usnea* clears heat and resolves toxins due to its bitter and cold nature.

This makes it very valuable in traditional Chinese medicine theory for damp heat in the lower burner, as well as lung conditions when qi is disrupted due to dampness, phlegm, or heat.

The outer, green-grey cortex contains the antibiotic substances, while the white inner core contains immune-stimulating polysaccharides. Recently, the polysaccharides have been found to possess antitumor activity, confirming their traditional use in cancer treatment. For example, in the case of sarcoma-180 in mice, daily injections for ten days after implantation led to complete regression of tumors compared to controls. Although researchers are not certain of the mechanism, it is thought that an outpouring of lymphoid and plasma cells, as well as macrophages to the area of the grafted tumor is responsible. Similar active constituents are found in *Umbilicaria, Lobaria,* and *Sticta* species.

Other constituents have been found to be nonsteroidal and anti-inflammatory.

In a 1993 Romanian study of *Usnea hirta,* it was demonstrated that the anti-inflammatory activity was comparable or superior to phenylbutazone and hydrocortisone. The analgesic activity is close to noraminophenazone, and the antipyretic activity equal or superior to aminophenazone.

One study found usnic acid significantly reduced inflammation in both acute and chronic conditions.

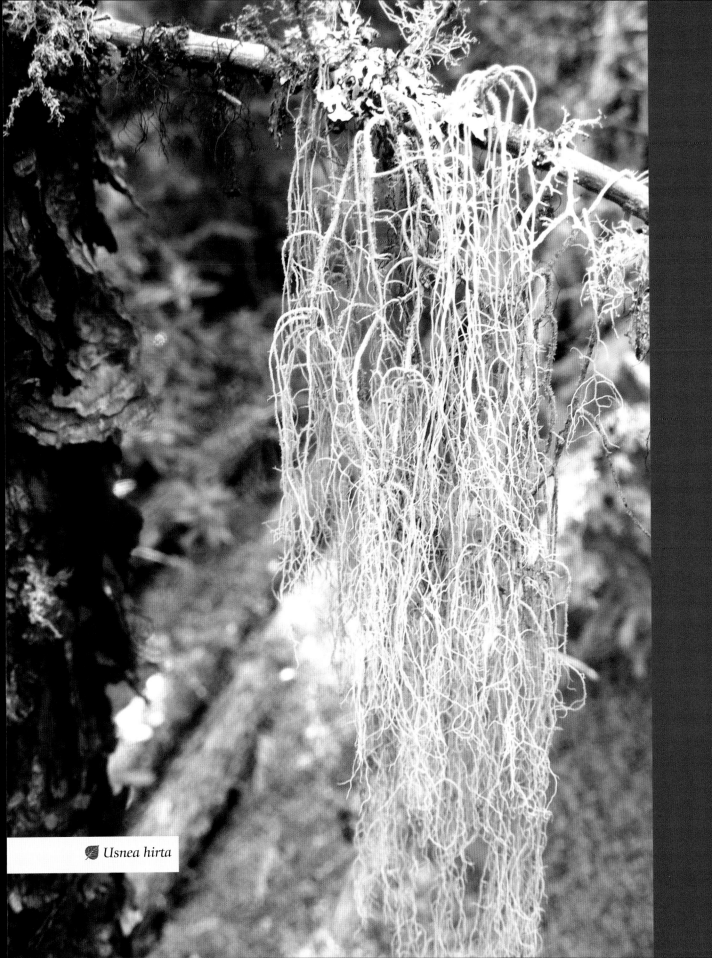

Usnea hirta

Hirtusneanoside, isolated from *U. hirta,* shows activity against gram-positive bacteria.

Similar studies in Japan showed *Usnea diffracta* with similar analgesic and anti-pyretic effect (Okuyama 1995).

In northern Europe, the medicinal values of *Usnea* and other lichens have long been recognized.

Studies show effectiveness against gram-positive bacteria such as *Streptococcus* (strep throat), *Staphylococcus* (impetigo), and *Mycobacterium tuberculosis* (Ingólfsdóttir 2002).

Usnic acid is more effective against some bacterial strains than penicillin. And it is able to completely inhibit the growth of different strains of human tuberculosis in dilutions of one part to twenty thousand.

Other studies cite effectiveness at one part per million, similar to streptomycin.

Microbes like the tubercle bacterium form heavily waxed coats and stiff cell walls that allow them to persist and even divide inside macrophages. They are able to prevent the host's lyosomes from taking in the hydrogen ions needed to create an acidic environment, thus neutralizing their effect.

Usnea also has a different mode of action. Synthetic antibiotics resemble the cell walls of bacteria, and are incorporated into the cell. This results in a weak cell structure as the bacteria swell and burst. Scientists believe usnic acid disrupts cellular metabolism, either by preventing ATP formation or by un-coupling oxidative phosphorization. Thus, the cells run out of energy and die.

Honda, N. K. et al. (2010) looked at a variety of lichen constituents and their activity against tuberculosis, drug-resistant strains of which are currently undergoing a worldwide resurgence. Usnic acid ranked third, behind norstictic acid and the most powerful, diffractaic acid.

Weckesser et al. (2007) found *Usnea* species active against *Propionibacterium acnes, Corynebacterium* species, and most importantly, against MRSA, or methicillin-resistant *Staphylococcus aureus.*

Usnea may be superior to Flagyl (metronidazole) against *Trichomonas,* a parasite that causes serious uterine and cervical infection and tissue destruction.

It is effective against candidiasis, giardiasis (or beaver fever, as it is known), and bowel inflammation in general. *Usnea* is a relaxant of the smooth muscles of the body, including the colon and lungs.

In Russia, a sodium salt of usnic acid called binan is used for second and third degree burns to prevent infection; it is also used for varicose ulcers, furuncolosis, impetigo, trichomonas, and lupus erythematosus. Binan is a vigorous antibiotic, effective against microbes and protozoa in concentrations of one part in three hundred thousand to one part per million when applied externally.

In Germany, a product called Evosin, a mixture of usnic and evernic acids, is used for impetigo, furunculosis, and lupus vulgaris, as well as mastitis in cows. Usniplant, containing 0.2 percent usnic acid, is used for skin conditions.

Likewise, sodium usnate is used in China for pulmonary tuberculosis. In thirty cases treated, twenty-four were cured and six were improved after seventy-one days.

Mastitis in cows, athlete's foot, ringworm, and acute bacterial infections can be treated internally and externally.

Usnic acid shows activity against *Streptococcus mutans,* which creates dental plaque and caries without disrupting normal oral flora.

Usnic acid is not only antifungal and antibactcrial, but also effective against viruses and protozoa.

Usnic acid was tested in one study in Saudi Arabia for the possibility of use for cancer and leprosy. It was found to have no adverse effect on testicular nucleic acids or epididymis spermatozoa in laboratory mice, unlike most anticancer drugs.

Usnic acid has been found to inhibit Ehrlich ascitic cells in laboratory studies. It has a vasodilating effect, and helps relax the muscles of the uterus, bronchi, and intestine.

Other studies indicate usnic acid has antiproliferative, anti-inflammatory, analgesic, anti-growth, anti-herbivore, and anti-insect properties.

Both (+)-usnic acid and (-)-usnic acid, especially the former, show high cytotoxic activity against cancerous cells.

Nine usnic acid amine conjugates were tested for cancer on L1210 cell lines. Bazin et al. found significant toxicity and induction of apoptosis (Bazin et al. 2008).

Usnic acid inhibits both HIV-1 and 2 integrase and mammalian topoisomerases I.

Usnea hirta has an LD50 of 21.02 grams vegetal material per kilogram of body weight.

The compound (+)-usnic acid shows protection against hyper proliferative skin wound healing, and when combined with gyrophoric acid increased wound closure most effectively (Burlando 2009).

Hirtuseanoside shows activity against gram-positive bacteria.

The coastal species *Usnea longissima* has been studied for its anti-platelet and anti-thrombotic activity (Lee, K.-A. and M. S. Kim 2005).

Diffractaic acid in this species has been found to enhance the antioxidant defense system as well as reduce effects on neutrophil infiltration. One study identified anti-inflammatory compounds.

Methanol extracts show in vitro melanogenesis inhibition. Tyrosinase glycosylation is believed to be involved (Kim, M. S. et al. 2007).

Odabasoglu et al. (2006) found usnic acid from this species both antioxidant and protective of indomethacin-induced gastric ulcers. Noted herbalists Christopher Hobbs and Chanchal Cabrera mention its use to treat tuberculosis lymphadenitis.

Other lichens are richer in usnic acid. In one *Haematomma* species *(H. coccineum),* it makes up nearly 20 percent of its content. The closely related blood spot lichen *(H. lapponicum)* has not been studied.

A fungal strain, *Corynespora* species, has been found on *Usnea cavernosa*. One study found extracts of this strain cytotoxic to breast and prostate cancer cell lines.

Usnic and salazinic acid from *U. filipendula* show activity against *Serratia marcescens.*

Usnic acid, evernic acid, and vulpinic acid inhibit the growth of gram-positive bacteria such as *Staphylococcus aureus, Bacillus subtilis,* and *B. megaterium,* but has no effect on gram-negative bacteria such as *Escherichia coli* and *Pseudomonas aeruginosa.*

Homeopathy

Usnea barbata is the remedy to remember for all forms of congestive headaches, especially sunstroke. The head can feel ready to burst at the temples, or the eyes feel like bursting from their sockets. The face is reddish.

Dose: mother tincture in drop doses. 1C potency is used for the elimination of heavy metals.

Essential Oil

Usnea barbata and others are extracted with ethanol to produce a tree moss concrete and absolute.

The semi-solid mass is greenish-brown, and contains methyl beta-orcinol carboxylate, and olivetonide. It is used largely in soap perfumery, although it does supply the requisite "mossy" notes in Fougere and related perfumes.

It should be restricted to 3 percent of any fragrance compound for best effect.

Lichen Essence

Usnea lichen essence is for individuals in the helping or healing professions. At times, due to the desperate situations and energies of patients, there is danger of empathizing too strongly, and beginning to take on their "illness."

Usnea essence helps retain boundaries, so that effective work can be carried out without endangering their own health. This can be subtle, but once observed, which the essence helps reveal, it will be recognized and dealt with.

— Prairie Deva

Spiritual Properties

Usnea represents the north, the place of gray hairs. It maintains the lung system of the planet. When *Usnea* came to me, personified as a young man, and spoke to me of its uses, it told me that its healing qualities are specific for the lung system of the planet—the trees.

Its use for people was secondary to its primary function. This was the first time I realized that the plants provided medicinal actions with the ecosystem, that they evolved and developed to help the Earth ecosystem, Gaia, maintain a healthy balance within itself. I realized at that time that it was only because we are a part of the ecosystem that the plants also work for us as healing agents.

There is an ancient compact between *Usnea* and the trees, and coming into contact with the deeper spiritual aspects of *Usnea,* one makes contact with ancient powers that existed long before humans.

— Stephen Harrod Buhner

Cosmetics

In Sudan, the closely related *U. molliuscula,* known as *sheiba,* is used in perfumery and as an aphrodisiac.

The related *U. subfloridana* is a boreal forest lichen that was mixed with tobacco and butter, and then boiled and cooled as a lotion for skin in Europe.

Recent work suggests that lichens may produce more usnic acid when levels of UVB are high. This suggests a biomonitor for increased radiation levels, and potential for development of more effective sunscreens.

Usnic acid absorbs ultraviolet light and may be used in sunscreen products with good results.

Textile Industry

Usnea species are used in Peru to produce a dark blue dye.

Pitted beard lichen *(U. cavernosa)* was used by the Wylackie of California to tan leather. Animal brains were wrapped in the lichen to hold together, and then rubbed vigorously into the hide.

Agriculture

Usnea has been fed to cows in the alpine regions of Europe to help them get through cold winters and fight mastitis. Sodium usnate is used as a spray for fighting mildew and other plant diseases.

Sodium usnate has been found effective against the tomato canker *(Corynebacterium michiganensis);* usnic acid shows a moderate degree of inhibition of the blue-staining wood fungus *Trichosporium* and tobacco mosaic virus.

It is used in a spray at one hundred to five hundred parts per million for bean rusts, mildews, and brown rot on some stone fruits.

Recent work has found usnic acid strongly inhibits the red bread mold *Neurospora crassa*.

Tree fellers in western Canada are susceptible to skin rashes, and usnic acid has been identified as a potential photo-sensitizer and respiratory irritant.

Kahlee Keane, or Root Woman, in her enjoyable new book *The Standing People,* suggests *Usnea* as a heartworm medicine for wolves. Interesting!

Recipes and Dosage

Stuff a glass jar tightly full of *Usnea* and cover with canola or olive oil. Cover with cheesecloth and set in a warm, sunny window for several months. This may be used internally, taken in gelatin capsules, or used externally as a healing salve with beeswax for infected boils, carbuncles, impetigo, and even vaginal boluses for trichomonas.

Dose: twenty to thirty drops of tincture as needed. For serious infection, like trichomonas and tuberculosis, it is taken long-term up to six times daily. When collecting and making tinctures use only living lichens. *Usnea* tincture is contraindicated during pregnancy.

Prepare at an equal weight-to-volume (i.e. one pound to sixteen ounces) ratio in 95 percent alcohol.

Xanthoparmelia chlorchroa
(TUMBLEWEED SHIELD LICHEN)
X. conspersa
(PEPPERED ROCK SHIELD LICHEN)

Tumbleweed shield lichen gets its name from its tendency to detach from rock and tumble around with the wind. It is common to the Great Western Basin and down through the Midwest and is an indicator of good antelope grazing territory. Up to 126 kilograms per hectare communities have been found in parts of Montana.

Peppered rock shield lichen is present in eastern and western North America.

The related *X. taractica* is common throughout the boreal forest, on exposed rock associated with gravel and slides.

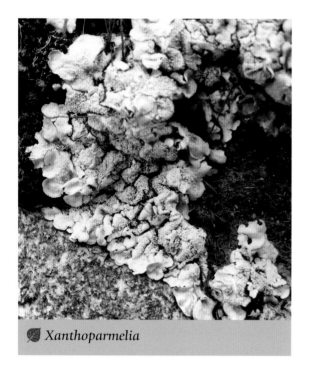

🍃 *Xanthoparmelia*

Traditional Uses

The Navajo used it medicinally to treat impetigo, possibly due to its content of salazinic and norstitic acid. It contains 2 percent usnic acid, compared to 1.5 percent in *Usnea barbata*.

Peppered rock shield lichen is used in southeastern Africa for medicine, both internally and applied as a powder to treat snakebites and venereal disease, especially syphilis.

Medicinal Use

It contains a sticitic acid complex including cryptostictic acid, and variable amounts of norstitic acid.

A crude extract inhibits *Bacillus subtilis* (Burkholder and Evans 1945).

One test showed weak activity against *S. aureus*.

The related *X. scabrosa* has been found to

induce smooth muscle relaxation, which promotes arterial dilation and increases blood flow. It is a main ingredient in a novel sexual stamina formula, a sort of natural Viagra approach to arousal.

Textile Industry

The entire plant, called ground lichen by the Navajo, was boiled for a red, brown, or orange dye for leather, baskets, and wool.

Peppered rock shield lichen has been used in England for dye, producing a red-brown color for wool.

Mining Industry

X. taractica is a hyper-accumulator of zinc, and may be a prospecting tool for mining companies.

Xanthoria elegans

(ROCK ORANGE LICHEN)
(ELEGANT SUNBURST LICHEN)
X. chlorochroa
(TUMBLEWEED SHIELD LICHEN)
X. parientina
Teloschistes parientinus
(MARITIME SUNBURST LICHEN)
(WALL LICHEN)
X. candelaria
(SHRUBBY SUNBURST LICHEN)

These rock lichens are easy to spot against limestone-type rocks with their flat fan shape and bright orange color. Occasionally they may be found on old wood or bones, but they seem to prefer the carbonic environment.

Nitrogen from bird or mammal waste encourages its growth, so Inuit hunters use it to locate the burrows of animals such as the hoary marmot.

The rock orange lichen was found growing on the graves of crewmembers of Franklin's last expedition. The lichens are slow growers, and after more than a hundred years only grew 4.4 centimeters in diameter.

It is quite hardy and has been found on Himalayan mountain rocks at seven thousand meters.

The related wall lichen *(X. parietina)* is sometimes called maritime sunburst lichen. It is bright yellow in sunny regions, and gray in the shade, suggesting a protective mechanism from UV radiation.

The related hooded sunburst lichen *(X. fallax),* commonly found on elm and poplar, contains fallacinal.

Traditional Uses

In fifteenth-century Europe, the wall lichen *(X. parietina)* was erroneously thought, due to its orange color, to be a treatment for jaundice, based on the doctrine of signatures.

Wall lichen is decocted in wine in Spain to treat menstrual problems, and simply decocted for kidney disorders, toothache, and as part of a cough syrup. Throughout Spain it is known as *flor de piedra* ("stone flower") or *rompiedra* ("stone breaker").

Medicinal Use

Chemical Constituents
- *X. elegans:* **salazinic and norstictic acids.**

Ingólfsdóttir et al. (2000) found rock orange lichen showed significant induction of quinone reductase against hepatoma cells. The concentration to double activity was determined to be only 4.8 micrograms per milliliter. This is significant because many plant constituents with cytotoxic activity are also harmful to healthy cells. One study found significant induction of quinone reductase activity in an assay using cultured Hepa 1c1c7 hepatoma cells.

Xanthoric acid, besides possessing cytoxicity, is anti-convulsive, antibacterial, and antifungal (Malhotra 2008).

Activity against *Bacillus subtilis, E. coli,* and *S. aureus* has been shown.

All *Xanthoria* species contain various anthraquinone pigments such as parietin, and xanthroin.

It contains bromoperoxidase and significant amounts of beryllium and vanadium as well as parietinic and atranoric acids. Parietin pigment levels are strongly influenced by UVB radiation. It shows activity against *S. aureus,* and is antiviral.

Lichen Essence

Xanthoria parietina essence facilitates an awakening, bringing wisdom and understanding. It can help to relieve fears, nervousness, and confusion. It is for those who walk around in circles. It helps balance the solar plexus, CNS, liver, skin, lungs and nerves.
— SILVERCORD

Cosmetics

The lichen is used as part of hair powder in India. In England, it is known as gold moss or gold lichen to be more accurate.

493

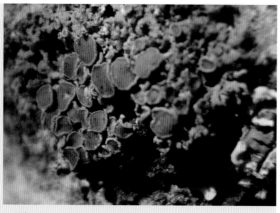

Xanthoria polycarpa

Textile Industry

Tumbleweed shield lichen is prepared as a warm brown dye by Navajo weavers.

Shrubby sunburst lichen *(X. candelaria)*, also called candle lichen in Sweden, is used to color animal fat to make candles. Other shield lichens would work just as well.

The Fung-Alchemical Process

Kingdom Fungi is more than a metaphor for mystery, fear, and the unknown. Similar to *Homo sapiens* searching for the philosopher's stone, mushrooms and lichens recycle, transmute, and transform.

Harmful matter is turned into something of value. Many alchemists use a seven-step process when referring to the cycle of changing lead to gold or, with human characteristics, something flawed becoming precious.

The first step of alchemy is calcination, where a substance is burned until only ash remains. Thunder and lightning are present, promoting visitation with intuition and imagination.

Morel mushrooms are a good example, rising like a phoenix from the ashes of the previous year's forest fire.

Dissolution soon follows as the ash dissolves in fluid, including water and rain. It is a step of cultivating detachment, but it is also related to creativity and a catalyst of sexuality.

The split gill mushroom, for example, exhibits over 28,000 various sexual expressions. Minerals are dissolved to an ionic phase and exchanged via root hairs of neighboring plants for sweet molecules of life.

The third stage, separation, is about coming apart. For fungi this represents gaining new territory and advancing into unknown space. Arguably the largest organism on earth, the honey mushroom is mainly underground. It thrives with awareness of time but retains a sense of boundary. Adversity sharpens the process of separation and encourages movement from under to upper. As above, so below.

The fourth stage is conjunction, where opposite elements reunite. Separation is two minus one. This is one plus one equals three. Lichens are a perfect example of fungi and algae coming together to create what each could not achieve on their own. They represent respiration and the lungs of the planet. Territory is transmuted to integrity. The process that translates intention is hard-won and persistent.

Fungi require protein—the building blocks of life—and lasso nematodes and paralyze springtails for nourishment. The growing mycelial fibers transmit intelligence, and the rhythm or heartbeat of the earth. This process illustrates the complex and fragile, strong, and united qualities of this kingdom. Conjunction develops empathy, compassion, and a reuniting of intention.

The fifth stage, fermentation, although often the most difficult for humans, seems natural for fungi.

Fermentation requires darkness and solitude. While most humans tend to fight this often uncomfortable state of depression and depth, fungi, born of the dark, seem to thrive in it. Unlike traditional alchemy, in which the goal is to transform lead into gold, the fung-alchemical process turns lead, mercury, and other heavy metals and hydrocarbon toxins into carbon, nitrogen, hydrogen, and oxygen. Fungi transmute the periodic table into building blocks of life.

Humans, at this stage of transition, experience the dark night of the soul and spirit. They require an adjustment of will, as in "thy will be done." Individuals attracted to the healing arts may experience their own health challenge. The ego, or "I am the healer," is re-examined and replaced with empathy and compassion. Carl Jung suggested that only the wounded physician heals and can only heal others to the extent they have healed themselves.

Appreciation for silence, stillness and changing deeply from within can help make this process more tolerable to the human ego, which feels safer in conditions of light and expansion. This lunar stage instead requires depth, dark, and acceptance. It has its own rhythm and is set back by intolerance and impatience.

Unique vibrational essences prepared from fungi and lichens address many of the negative moods and emotions, as well as the lunar traumas of the psyche.

The sixth stage is sublimation, where the essence rises to the top. Symptoms associated with this stage are confusion, hyperactivity, and feeling out of control. Fruiting bodies of *Psilocybe* and related species represent conscious awareness and magical intuition. This is the culmination of the previous five steps and a collective source of wisdom and change.

Magic and mushrooms impact those around them with shared visions and dreams. Rituals are introduced to help aid concentration and intention. Various fungi contain volatile oils that represent essence. These help to soothe the skin and protect the layer that creates sense of self and attracts like-minded individuals. It initiates mastery of the natural laws of cause and effect.

The final stage is coagulation or illumination, the forming of the philosopher's stone. This solid landscape is a place of sacred magic and surrender. Various fungi, especially of the *Mycena* genus, exhibit luminescence, representing enlightenment. They shine because they do. They express because they know. The fung-alchemical process is complete.

Medicinal Properties

	Analgesic	Antibacterial	Antifungal	Anti-inflammatory	Antioxidant	Anti-tumor	Antiviral	Bloodsugar	Cardiovascular	Cholesterol	Hypertension	Immune Tonic	Kidney Tonic	Liver Tonic	Nerve Tonic	Respiratory Tonic	Sexual Tonic	Stress	Vision
Agaricus arvensis		■				■													
A. bisporus		■		■				■		■	■		■						
A. brasiliensis		■		■		■	■	■	■	■		■							
A. campestris		■				■	■	■											
Agrocybe dura		■	■			■													
A. aegerita		■	■	■	■	■	■	■						■	■				
Albatrellus spp.	■	■			■	■				■						■			
Armillaria mellea		■	■		■	■	■		■		■	■	■		■			■	■
Auricularia auricula					■	■	■	■	■	■	■	■				■			
Bjerkandera spp.			■			■						■							
Boletus edulis			■			■			■										
Boschniaka rossica					■						■					■			
Calocybe spp.						■		■											
Calvatia spp.		■	■			■	■												
Cantharellus spp.						■	■		■							■			■
Cerrena unicolor									■										
Clitocybe gibba		■				■			■										
C. inversa						■													

	Analgesic	Antibacterial	Antifungal	Anti-inflammatory	Antioxidant	Anti-tumor	Antiviral	Bloodsugar	Cardiovascular	Cholesterol	Hypertension	Immune Tonic	Kidney Tonic	Liver Tonic	Nerve Tonic	Respiratory Tonic	Sexual Tonic	Stress	Vision
Collybia maculata			■			■	■												
Coprinus spp.		■	■			■	■	■	■	■									
Cordyceps spp.		■	■		■	■	■	■	■		■	■	■	■	■	■	■	■	
Cortinarius spp.						■	■												
Craterellus spp.						■													
Crucibulum spp.																			■
Cryptoporus volvatus				■	■	■										■			
Cyathus striatus		■																	
Daedaleopsis confragos	■																		
Dictyphora spp.																	■		
Fistulina hepatica						■													
Flammulina velutipes			■	■		■	■			■		■							
Fomes fomentarius		■				■	■												
Fomitopsis officinalis			■			■	■	■								■			
F. pinicola	■		■			■						■			■				
Ganderma applanatum	■	■		■		■	■	■				■					■		■
G. lucidum		■	■	■	■	■	■	■	■	■	■	■	■	■	■	■	■		
G. resinaceum						■													
G. tsugae			■	■		■		■				■		■					
Gleophyllum separium					■														
Grifola frondosa		■	■	■	■	■	■	■	■		■	■			■		■	■	

	Analgesic	Antibacterial	Antifungal	Anti-inflammatory	Antioxidant	Anti-tumor	Antiviral	Bloodsugar	Cardiovascular	Cholesterol	Hypertension	Immune Tonic	Kidney Tonic	Liver Tonic	Nerve Tonic	Respiratory Tonic	Sexual Tonic	Stress	Vision
Gymnopilus spp.						■													
Hericium spp.	■	■	■	■		■						■			■	■		■	
Heterobasidium annosum	■			■															
Hydnum spp.						■			■	■									
Hypholoma fasiculare									■										
Hypsizygus spp.		■	■			■													
Inonotus obliquus		■		■	■	■	■	■				■	■						
Ischoderma resinosum						■													
Laccaria spp.						■													
Lactarius spp.		■	■			■	■		■										
Laetiporus sulphureus		■	■			■		■											
Lentinula edodes		■	■	■		■	■	■		■	■	■	■				■	■	
Lentinus lepideus						■						■							
Lenzites betulina						■			■			■							
Lepista nuda		■						■											
Lyophyllum decastes								■		■	■	■							
Marasmius androsaceus	■	■		■								■			■				
Merulius spp.		■				■													
Morchella esculenta						■						■				■			
Mycena spp.		■				■													
Omphalotus spp.		■				■	■												

The Fungal Pharmacy

	Analgesic	Antibacterial	Antifungal	Anti-inflammatory	Antioxidant	Anti-tumor	Antiviral	Bloodsugar	Cardiovascular	Cholesterol	Hypertension	Immune Tonic	Kidney Tonic	Liver Tonic	Nerve Tonic	Respiratory Tonic	Sexual Tonic	Stress	Vision
Paxillus spp.	■	■			■														
Peziza spp.		■			■							■							
Phallus spp.		■		■	■							■			■				
Phellinus spp.			■		■	■													
Pholiota mutabilis		■			■	■	■		■	■									
Piptoporus betulinus	■	■	■	■	■	■						■			■			■	
Pleurotus ostreatus		■			■	■	■		■	■	■				■	■			
Polyporus tuberaster										■									
P. umbellatus	■		■		■	■					■		■		■				
Ramaria spp.					■														
Sarcodon spp.			■			■			■										
Schizophyllum commune		■	■	■	■		■					■		■					
Sparassis crispa		■	■			■		■			■	■							
Suillus spp.					■	■													
Trametes sanguinea				■															
T. versicolor		■		■	■	■	■		■	■		■	■	■					
Tremella mesentericum								■		■		■		■					
Trichaptum biforme					■														
Tricholoma spp.					■							■							
Tricholomopsis spp.		■	■		■														

500

Appendix C

Anticancer Activity

	Bladder	Breast	Cervical	Esophagus	Gastric	Leukemia	Liver	Lung	Lymphoma	Melanoma	Ovarian	Pancreas	Prostate	Rectal/Colon	Skin
Agaricus bisporus		■											■		
A. brasiliensis		■	■				■	■			■		■	■	
Albatrellus spp.										■					
Bjerkandera adusta			■												
Boletopsis leucomelas						■									
Bondarzewia Montana						■									
Clitocybe inversa														■	
Coprinus comatus													■		
Cordyceps sinensis		■				■		■		■					
Cryptoporus volvatus														■	
Flammulina velutipes								■	■	■			■		
Fomes fomentarius			■	■	■										
Fomitopsis officinalis		■											■		
Ganoderma applanatum				■											
G. lucidum		■	■			■	■	■					■		
G. resinaceum		■											■		
Grifola frondosa	■	■	■			■	■	■					■	■	
Hericium spp.				■	■		■		■	■					■

501

	Bladder	Breast	Cervical	Esophagus	Gastric	Leukemia	Liver	Lung	Lymphoma	Melanoma	Ovarian	Pancreas	Prostate	Rectal/Colon	Skin
Hypsizygus spp.				■		■		■							
Inonotus obliquus		■	■					■							
Laetiporus sulphureus						■									
Lentinula edodes		■	■		■	■	■			■			■		■
Lepiota Americana		■											■		
Omphalotus spp.		■						■			■	■			
Phallus impudicus		■	■								■				
Phellinus igniarius							■	■							
Piptoporus betulinus			■							■	■				
Pisolithus tinctorius						■				■					
Pleurotus ostreatus	■														
Polyporus umbellatus	■		■		■	■	■	■						■	
Russula spp.						■									
Schizophyllum commune			■		■									■	
Sparassis		■													
Suillus spp.						■		■							
Tremella spp.			■												
Trametes versicolor		■	■	■	■	■	■	■	■	■				■	■

Antiviral Activity

	Hepatitis B	Herpes simplex	Influenza	Poliomyelitis	Rabies	Respiratory syncytial	Rous sarcoma	Tobacco mosaic	Vaccinia	Varicella zoster	Vesicular stomatitis	HIV
Agaricus campestris	■											
Agrocybe aegerita								■				
Calvatia bovista			■	■								
C. gigantea			■	■								
Chlorophyllum molydites				■								
Collybia confluens										■	■	
C. maculata											■	
Coprinus micaeus				■								
Cordyceps sinensis	■											■
Flammulina velutipes												■
Fomes fomentarius		■						■				
Fomitopsis officinalis									■			■
Ganoderma applanatum									■		■	
G. lucidum	■	■	■								■	■
Grifola frondosa												■
Inonotus hispidus			■									
I. obliquus			■									■

	Hepatitis B	Herpes simplex	Influenza	Poliomyelitis	Rabies	Respiratory syncytial	Rous sarcoma	Tobacco mosaic	Vaccinia	Varicella zoster	Vesicular stomatitis	HIV
Laetiporus sulphureus												■
Lentinula edodes		■	■								■	■
Panaeolus subbalteatus				■					■			
Piptoporus betulinus				■			■					■
Pleurotus ostreatus												■
Polyporus umbellatus	■											
Rozites caperata		■					■	■		■		
Schizophyllum commune	■											■
Suillus luteus			■									
Trametes sanguinea					■							
T. versicolor												■
Tremella spp.	■											

Antimicrobial Activity

	Aspergillus spp	Bacillus spp	Candida albicans	Escherichia coli	Helicobacter pylori	Klebsiella pneumoniae	Micrococcus spp	Mycobacterium tuberculosis	Plasmodium spp	Proteus spp	Pseudomonas spp	Salmonella spp	Serratia marcescens	Shigella paradysenteras	Staphylococcus spp	Streptococcus spp
Agaricus bisporus					■							■				
A. brasiliensis				■								■				■
Agrocybe aegerita		■		■								■				■
A. dura	■		■													
Albatrellus confluens		■		■								■				
Armillaria mellea		■													■	
Auricularia spp.					■											
Calvatia bovista											■				■	■
C. candida	■		■													
Chlorophyllum rachodes															■	
Clavaria zollingeri								■								
Clitocybe candida								■								
C. gibba		■														
C. nebularis		■		■				■				■				■
Coprinus comatus	■	■	■	■							■				■	

	Aspergillus spp	Bacillus spp	Candida albicans	Escherichia coli	Helicobacter pylori	Klebsiella pneumoniae	Micrococcus spp	Mycobacterium tuberculosis	Plasmodium spp	Proteus spp	Pseudomonas spp	Salmonella spp	Serratia marcescens	Shigella paradysenteras	Staphylococcus spp	Streptococcus spp
C. plicatilis		■														
Cortinarius spp.									■							
Cyathus striatus	■	■	■												■	
Fistulina hepatica		■		■											■	
Flammulina velutipes					■										■	
Fomes fomentarius			■								■		■			
Fomitopsis officinalis								■			■					
Ganoderma applanatum		■		■							■				■	■
G. lucidum	■	■	■	■			■		■						■	■
Grifola frondosa			■					■								
Hericium spp.	■	■	■													
Hydnum spp.					■											
Hypholoma fasiculare		■														
Hypoxylon multiforme	■		■	■		■					■	■			■	
Hypsizygus spp.																■
Lactarius spp.			■	■											■	
Laetiporus sulphureus		■		■					■				■		■	
Lepista nuda		■	■												■	
Macrolepiota procera															■	
Merulius spp.		■													■	

	Aspergillus spp	Bacillus spp	Candida albicans	Escherichia coli	Helicobacter pylori	Klebsiella pneumoniae	Micrococcus spp	Mycobacterium tuberculosis	Plasmodium spp	Proteus spp	Pseudomonas spp	Salmonella spp	Serratia marcescens	Shigella paradysenteras	Staphylococcus spp	Streptococcus spp
Mutinus elegans		■	■	■								■			■	
Mycena leaiana												■				
Omphalotus spp.									■		■				■	
Phaelous schweinitzii				■								■			■	
Phallus spp.		■		■								■			■	
Pholiota spp.		■						■				■			■	
Piptoporus betulinus		■					■				■				■	
Plectania nigrella																■
Pleurotus ostreatus	■	■		■					■		■					
Polyporus umbellatus				■					■						■	
Psilocybe spp.															■	
Rhizopogon spp.									■							
Schizophyllum commune			■	■			■				■				■	
Sparassis crispa		■														
Stereum hirsutum		■		■				■					■		■	
Stropharia rugoso-annulata				■												
Trametes sanguinea				■			■		■		■	■		■	■	■
T. versicolor	■		■	■					■							
Tricholomopsis spp.	■		■													
Ustilago spp.			■													

Abraham, Wolf Rainer. 2001. Bioactive sesquiterpenes produced by fungi: Are they useful for humans as well? *Current Medical Chemistry* 8 (6): 583–606.

Abraham, Wolf Rainer and Grigor Spassov. 1991. 4–Hydroxymethyl–quinoline from *Polyporus* species. *Phytochemistry* 30 (1): 371–372.

Acharya, Krishnendu et al. 2004. Antioxidant and nitric oxide synthase activation properties of *Auricularia auricula*. *Indian Journal of Experimental Biology* 42 (5): 538–540.

Adams, Lynn S. et al. 2008. White button mushroom *(Agaricus bisporus)* exhibits antiproliferative and proapoptotic properties and inhibits prostate tumor growth in athymic mice. *Nutrition and Cancer* 60 (6): 744–756.

Ahn, W.–S. et al. 2004. Natural killer cell activity and quality of life were improved by consumption of a mushroom extract, *Agaricus blazei* Murill Kyowa, in gynecological cancer patients undergoing chemotherapy. *International Journal of Gynecological Cancer* 14 (4): 589–594.

Ajith, Thekkuttuparambil A. and Kainoor K. Janardhanan. 2002. Antioxidant and antihepatotoxic activities of *Phellinus rimosus* (Berk) Pilat. *Journal of Ethnopharmacology* 81 (3): 387–391.

Ajith, Thekkuttuparambil A. and Kainoor K. Janardhanan. 2003. Cytotoxic and antitumor activities of a polypore macrofungus, *Phellinus rimosus* (Berk) Pilat. *Journal of Ethnopharmacology* 84 (2–3): 157–162.

Akamatsu, Y. 1998. Reutilization of culture wastes of *Pleurotus ostreatus* and *Phollota nameko* for cultivation of *Lyophyllum decastes*. *Journal of Wood Science* 44 (5): 417–420.

Akin, D. E. et al. 1993. Microbial delignification with white rot fungi improves forage digestibility. *Applied and Environmental Microbiology* 59 (12): 4274–4282.

Al–Fatimi, M. A. A. et al. 2005. Antimicrobial, cytotoxic and antioxidant activity of selected Basidiomycetes from Yemen. *Die Pharmazie* 60 (10): 776–780.

Al–Fatimi, M. A. A. et al. 2006. Bioactive components of the traditionally used mushroom *Podaxis pistillaris*. *Evidence–Based Complementary and Alternative Medicine* 3 (1): 87–92.

Al–Kassim, Loola et al. 1994. Optimization of phenol removal by a fungal peroxidase from *Coprinus macrorhizus* using batch, continuous, and discontinuous semibatch reactors. *Enzyme and Microbial Technology* 16 (2): 120–124.

Ali, N. A. et al. 1996. Inhibition of chemiluminescence response of human mononuclear cells and suppression of mitogen–induced proliferation of spleen lymphocytes of mice by hispolon and hispidin. *Pharmazie.* 51 (9): 667–670.

Amoros, M. et al. 1997. Antiviral activity of Homobasidiomycetes: Evaluation of 121 Basidiomycetes extracts on four viruses. *International Journal of Pharmacognosy* 35 (4): 255–260.

Anke, H. et al. 1995. Secondary metabolites with nematicidal and antimicrobial activity from nematophagous fungi and Ascomycetes. *Canadian Journal of Botany* 73 (S1): S932–S939.

Anke, Timm and F. Oberwinkler. 1977. The striatins: New antibiotics from the Basidiomycete *Cyanthus striatus* (Huds. ex Pers.) Willd. *The Journal of Antibiotics* 30 (3): 221–225.

Anke, Timm et al. 1980. Antibiotics from Basidiomycetes. X. Scordinin, a new antibacterial and antifungal metabolite from *Marasmius scorononius* (Fr.) Fr. *The Journal of Antibiotics* 33 (3): 463–467.

Anke, Timm et al. 1987. Antibiotics from Basidiomycetes. XXVI. Phlebiakauranol aldehyde an antifungal and cytotoxic metabolite from *Punctularia atropurpurascens*. *The Journal of Antibiotics* 40 (4): 443–449.

Anke, Timm et al. 1990. Antibiotics from Basidiomycetes. XXXIII. Oudemansin X, a new antifungal (E)–b–methoxyacrylate from *Oudemansiella radicata* (Relhan ex Fr.) Sing. *The Journal of Antibiotics* 43 (8): 1010–1011.

Anke, Timm et al. 2002. Studies on the biosynthesis of striatal–type diterpenoids and the biological activity of herical. *Zeitschrift für Naturforschung C* 57 (3–4): 263.

Aoki, Michiko et al. 1993. Antiviral substances with systemic effects produced by Basidiomycetes such as *Fomes fomentarius*. *Bioscience, Biotechnology, and Biochemistry* 57 (2): 278–282.

Appleton, R. E. et al. 1988. *Laetiporus sulphureus* causing visual hallucinations and ataxia in a child. *Canadian Medical Association Journal* 139 (1): 48–49.

Arnone, Alberto et al. 1993. Two cinnamic allenic ethers from the fungus *Clitocybe eucalyptorum*. *Phytochemistry* 32 (5): 1279–1281.

Arnone, Alberto et al. 1994. Secondary mould metabolites. Part 47. Isolation and structure elucidation of clavilactones A–C, new metabolites from the fungus *Clitocybe clavipes*. *Journal of the Chemical Society, Perkins Transactions* 1 (15): 2165–2168.

Arora, David. 2008. Xiao ren ren: The "little people" of Yunnan. *Economic Botany* 62 (3): 540–544.

Asakawa, Yoshinori et al. 1992. Cryptoporic acids A–G, drimane–type sesquiterpenoid ethers of isocitric acid from the fungus *Cryptoporus volvatus*. *Phytochemistry* 31 (2): 579–592.

Asatiani, Mikheil D. et al. 2007. Antioxidant activity of submerged cultured mycelium extracts of higher Basidiomycetes mushrooms. *International Journal of Medicinal Mushrooms* 9 (2): 151–158.

Atkinson, N. 1946. Antibacterial activity in members of the higher fungi. *Australian Journal of Experimental Biology and Medicinal Science* 24 (3): 169–174.

Atsumi, S. et al. 1990. Production, isolation and structure determination of a novel beta–glucosidase inhibitor, cyclophellitol, from *Phellinus* sp. *Journal of Antibiotics* 43 (1): 49–53.

Auer, Nadja et al. 2005. Degradation of nitrocellulose by fungi. *Biodegradation* 16 (3): 229–236.

Awadh Ali, Nasser A. et al. 2003. Antiviral activity of *Inonotus hispidus*. *Fitoterapia*. 74 (5): 483–485.

Ayer, William A. and Peter A. Craw. 1989. Metabolites of the fairy ring fungus, *Marasmius oreades*. Part 2. Norsesquiterpenes, further sesquiterpenes, and agrocybin. *Canadian Journal of Chemistry* 67 (9): 1371–1380.

Ayer, William A. and Hubert Taube. 1973. Metabolites of *Cyathus helenae*. A new class of diterpenoids. *The Canadian Journal of Chemistry* 51 (23): 3842–3854.

Ayer, William A. et al. 1992. Chemical investigation of the metabolites from the Canadian tuckahoe, *Polyporus tuberaster*. *Journal of Natural Products* 55 (5): 649–653.

Ayoub, Nahla et al. 2009. Volatile constituents of the medicinal fungus chaga *Inonotus obliquus* (Pers.: Fr.) Pilat (Aphyllophoromycetideae). *International Journal of Medicinal Mushrooms*. 11 (1): 55–60.

Backen, S. et al. 1984. Antibiotics from basidiomycetes, XIX and Naematolin and Naematolon. *Liebigs Annalen der Chemie* 7: 1332–1342.

Badalyan, Susanna. 2003. Edible and medicinal higher Basidiomycetes mushrooms as a source of natural antioxidants. *International Journal of Medicinal Mushrooms* 5 (2): 161–170.

Badalyan, Susanna and A. V. Gasparyan. 2007. Antioxidant activity of several Basidiomycete mushrooms cultures. *Seventh International Mycological Congress Book of Abstracts* #304.

Badalyan, Susanna and S. H. Sisakyan. 2007. Antiprotozoal activity and mitogen effect of edible medicinal mushroom *Lentinus edodes* (Berk.) Sing. (shiitake). *Seventh International Mycological Congress Book of Abstracts* #364.

Badalyan, Susanna et al. 2001. Pharmacological activity of the mushrooms *Flammulina velutipes* (Curt.: Fr.) Sing., *Paxillus involutus* (Batsch: Fr.) Fr., and *Tricholoma pardinum* Quel. (Basidiomycota). *International Journal of Medicinal Mushrooms* 3 (1): 25–31.

Badalyan, Susanna et al. 2003. Edible and medicinal higher Basidiomycetes mushrooms as a source of natural antioxidants. *Mikologiya i Fitopatologiya* 37 (5): 63–68.

Badole, Sachin L. et al. 2006. Hypoglycemic activity of aqueous extract of *Pleurotus pulmonarius* in alloxan–induced diabetic mice. *Pharmaceutical Biology* 44 (6): 421–425.

Badole, Sachin L. et al. 2008. Interaction of aqueous extract of *Pleurotus pulmonarius* (Fr.) Quel–Champ. with glyburide in alloxan–induced diabetic mice. *Evidence–Based Complementary and Alternative Medicine* 5 (2): 159–164.

Bae, Eun–Ah et al. 1997. Effect of *Lentinus edodes* on the growth of intestinal lactic acid bacteria. *Archives of Pharmacal Research* 20 (5): 443–447.

Baggio, Cristiane Hatsuko et al. 2010. Antinociceptive effects of ((1 3),(1 6)–linked –glucan isolated from *Pleurotus pulmonarius* in models of acute and neuropathic pain in mice: Evidence for a role for glutamatergic receptors and cytokine pathways. *The Journal of Pain* 11 (10): 965–971

Bailey, C. J. et al. 1984. Effect of *Coprinus comatus* on plasma glucose concentrations in mice. *Planta Medica* 50 (6): 525–526.

Baldrian, Petr and Jiri Gabriel. 2002. Intraspecific variability in growth response to cadmium of the wood–rotting fungus *Piptoporus betulinus*. *Mycologia* 94 (3): 428–436.

Barker, Duane and John C. Holliday. 2010. Blood lymphocyte and neutrophil response of cultured rainbow trout, *Oncorhynchus mykiss,* administered varying dosages of an oral medicinal mushroom–based immunomodulator—"FinImmune™." *International Journal of Medicinal Mushrooms* 12 (2): 185–192.

Barros, Lillian et al. 2007a. Antimicrobial activity and bioactive compounds of Portugese wild edible mushrooms methanolic extracts. *European Food Research and Technology* 2007 225(2): 151–156.

Barros, Lillian et al. 2007b. Effect of fruiting body maturity stage on chemical composition and antimicrobial activity of *Lactarius* sp. mushrooms. *Journal of Agricultural and Food Chemistry* 55 (21): 8766–8771.

Barros, Lillian et al. 2007c. Fatty acid and sugar compositions, and nutritional value of five wild edible mushrooms from northeast Portugal. *Food Chemistry* 105 (1): 140–145.

Barry, Jean. 1968. General and comparative study of the psychokinetic effect on a fungus culture. *Journal of Parapsychology* 32 (4): 237–243.

Barry, V. C. and McNally, P. A. 1945. Inhibitory action of dialkyl succinic acid Derivatives on the Growth in vitro of Acid-fast Bacteria. *Nature* 156: 48–49.

Batterbury, M. et al. 2002. *Agaricus bisporus* (edible mushroom lectin) inhibits ocular fibroblast proliferation and collagen lattice contraction. *Experimental Eye Research* 74 (3): 361–370.

Bazin, Marc–Antoine et al. 2008. Synthesis and cytotoxic activities of usnic acid derivatives. *Bioorganic and Medicinal Chemistry* 16 (14): 5860–6866.

Beaudette, Lee A. et al. 1998. Comparison of gas chromatography and mineralization experiments for measuring loss of selected polychlorinated biphenyl congeners in cultures of white rot fungi. *Applied Environmental Microbiology* 64 (6): 2020–2025.

Becker, Uta et al. 1994. A novel bioactive illudalane sesquiterpene from the fungus *Pholiota destruens*. *Natural Product Research* 5 (3): 171–174.

Becker, Uta et al. 1997. Puraquinonic acid, a novel inducer of differentiation of human hl–60 promyelocytic leukemia cells from *Mycena pura* (Pers. Ex Fr.). *Natural Product Research* 9 (3): 229 –236.

Beelman, Robert B. and Daniel J. Royse. 2005. Selenium enrichment of *Grifola frondosa* (Dicks.: Fr.) S.F. Gray (maitake) mushrooms. *International Journal of Medicinal Mushrooms* 7 (3): 340.

Beelman, Robert B. et al. 2003. Bioactive components in button mushroom *Agaricus bisporus* (J. Lge) Imbach (Agaricomycetideae) of nutritional, medicinal, and biological importance (review). *International Journal of Medicinal Mushrooms* 5 (4): 345–362.

Behera, B. C. et al. 2004. Capacity of some graphidaceous lichens to scavenge superoxide and inhibition of tyrosinase and xanthine oxidase activities. *Current Science* 87 (1): 83–86.

Belcarz, A. et al. 2005. Extracellular enzyme activities of *Bjerkandera adusta* R59 soil strain, capable of daunomycin and humic acids degradation. *Applied Microbiology and Biotechnology* 68 (5): 686–694.

Bellini, M. F. et al. 2006. Antigenotoxicity of *Agaricus blazei* mushroom organic and aqueous extracts in chromosomal aberration and cytokinesis block micronucleus assays in CHO–k1 and HTC cells. *Toxicology in Vitro* 20 (3): 355–360.

Belsare, D.K. and D. Y. Prasad. 1988. Decolorization of effluent from the bagasse–based pulp mills by white–rot fungus, *Schizophyllum commune*. *Applied Microbiology and Biotechnology* 28 (3): 301–304.

Benie, Tanon et al. 2008. Estrogen effects of *Daldinia concentrica* and *Psathyrella efflorescens* extracts in vitro. *Journal of Ethnopharmacology* 116 (1): 152–160.

Bernardshaw, Soosaipillai et al. 2005. An extract of the mushroom *Agaricus blazei* Murill administered orally protects against systemic *Streptococcus pneumoniae* infection in mice. *Scandinavian Journal of Immunology* 62 (4): 393–398.

Bernardshaw, Soosaipillai et al. 2006. An extract of the mushroom *Agaricus blazei* Murill protects against lethal septicemia in a mouse model of fecal peritonitis. *Shock* 25 (4): 420–425.

Berne, Sabina et al. 2007. Ostreolysin enhances fruiting initiation in the oyster mushroom *(Pleurotus ostreatus)*. *Mycological Research* 111 (2): 1431–1436.

Bernicchia, A. et al. 2006. DNA recovered and sequenced from an almost 7000 year–old neolithic polypore, *Daedaleopsis tricolor*. *Mycological Research* 110 (1): 14–17.

Bernillon, J. et al. 1989. First isolation of (+)-epipentenomycin 1 from Peziza sp. Carpophores. *Journal of Antibiotics* (Tokyo) 42 (9): 1430–1432.

Bezivin, Carine et al. 2002. Cytotoxic activity of tricholomatales determined with murine and human cancer cell lines. *Pharmaceutical Biology* 40 (3): 196–199.

Bezivin, Carine et al. 2003a. Cytotoxic activity of some lichen extracts on murine and human cancer cell lines. *Phytomedicine* 10 (6): 499–503.

Bezivin, Carine et al. 2003b. Toxicity and antitumor activity of a crude extract from *Lepista inversa* (Scop.: Fr.) Pat. (Agaricomycetideae): A preliminary study. *International Journal of Medicinal Mushrooms* 5 (1): 25–30.

Bezivin, Carine et al. 2004. Cytotoxic activity of compounds from the lichen: *Cladonia convoluta*. *Planta Medica* 70 (9): 874–877.

Bianco C. M. A. and L. Giardino. 1996. Antibiotic activity in Basidiomycetes. X. Antibiotic activity of mycelia and cultural filtrates of 25 new strains. *Allionia* 34 (1): 39–43.

Birnbacher, J. et al. 2008. Isolation and biological activity of new norhirsutanes from *Creolophus cirrhatus*. *Zeitschrift für Naturforschung C* 63 (1–2): 203–206.

Bisakowski, Barbara et al. 2000. Characterization of lipoxyase activity from a partially purified enzyme extract from *Morchella esculenta*. *Process Biochemistry* 36 (1–2): 1–7.

Bisko, Nina A. et al. 2005. Antioxidant and gene protective effects of medicinal mushrooms *Inonotus obliquus* (Pers.: Fr.) Pilát and *Phellinus robustus* (P. Karst.) Bourd. et Galz. *International Journal of Medicinal Mushrooms* 7 (3): 388.

Blanchette, Robert. 2001. Fungus ashes and tobacco: The use of *Phellinus igniarius* by the indigenous people of North America. *Mycologist* 15 (1): 4–9.

Bobek, P. and S. Galbavy. 1999. Hypocholesterolemic and antiatherogenic effect of oyster mushroom *(Pleurotus ostreatus)* in rabbits. *Die Nahrung* 43 (5): 339–342.

Bobek, P. et al. 1993. The mushroom *Pleurotus ostreatus* reduces secretion and accelerates the fractional turnover rate of very–low–density lipoproteins in the rat. *Annals of Nutrition and Metabolism* 37 (3): 142–145

Bobek, P. et al. 1995. Dietary oyster mushroom *(Pleurotus ostreatus)* accelerates plasma cholesterol turnover in hypercholesterolaemic rat. *Physiological Research* 44 (5): 287–291.

Boh, Bojana et al. 2004. *Ganoderma lucidum* (W.Curt.: Fr.) Lloyd and *G. applanatum* (Pers.) Pat. (Aphyllophoromycetideae) from Slovenian habitats: Cultivation, isolation, and testing of active compounds. *International Journal of Medicinal Mushrooms* 6 (1): 18.

Böker, Andreas et al. 2001. Raspberry ketone from submerged cultured cells of the Basidiomycete *Nidula niveo–tomentosa*. *Biotechnology Progress* 17 (3): 568–572.

Bois, G. et al. 2005. Mycorrhizal inoculum potentials of pure reclamation materials and revegetated tailing sands from the Canadian oil sand industry. *Mycorrhiza* 15 (3): 149–58.

Bonnen, Alice M. et al. 1994. Lignin–degrading enzymes of the commercial button mushroom, *Agaricus bisporus*. *Applied and Environmental Microbiology* 60 (3): 960–965.

Boustie J. et al. 2005. Chemotaxonomic interest of volatile components in *Lepista inversa* and *Lepista flaccida* distinction. *Cryptogamie Mycologie* 26 (1): 27–35.

Brachvogel, R. 1986. Reduction of blood sugar by *Calocybe gambosa* Fr. Donk. *Zeitschrift für Mykologie* 52 (2): 445.

Braun–Lullemann, A. et al. 1997. Degradation of styrene by white–rot fungi. *Applied Microbiology and Biotechnology* 47 (2): 150–155.

Braun–Lullemann, A. et al. 1999. Screening of ectomycorrhizal fungi for degradation of polycyclic aromatic hydrocarbons. *Applied Microbiology and Biotechnology* 43 (1): 127–132.

Breheret, Sophie et al. 1997. Monoterpenes in the aromas of fresh wild mushrooms (Basidiomycetes). *Journal of Agricultural and Food Chemistry* 45 (3): 831–836.

Bressa, Giuliano et al. 1988. Bioaccumulation of mercury in the mushroom *Pleurotus ostreatus*. *Ecotoxicology and Environmental Safety* 16 (2): 85–89.

Brunner, Ivano et al. 1996. Influence of ectomycorrhization and cesium/potassium ratio on uptake and localization of cesium in Norway spruce seedlings. *Tree Physiology* 16 (8): 705–711.

Bu'lock, John D. and John Darbyshire. 1976. Lagopodin metabolites and artefacts in cultures of *Coprinus*. *Phytochemistry* 15 (12): 2004.

Buchanan, Malcolm et al. 1995. Five 10–phenyl–[11]–cytochalasans from a *Daldinia* fungal species. *Phytochemistry* 40 (1): 135–140.

Buchanan, Malcolm et al. 1996a. Cytochalasins from a *Daldinia* sp. of fungus. *Phytochemistry* 41 (3): 821–828.

Buchanan, Malcolm et al. 1996b. A 10–phenyl–[11]–cytochalasan from a species of *Daldinia*. *Phytochemistry* 42 (1): 173–176.

Buchanan, Malcolm et al. 1999. Strobilurin N and two metabolites related to chorismic acid from the fruit bodies of *Mycena crocata* (Agaricales). *Zeitschrift für Naturforschung C* 54 (7–8): 463–468.

513

Budde, Cheryl L. et al. 2001. Enzymatic nitration of phenols. *Journal of Molecular Catalysis B* 15 (1–3): 55–64.

Bugni, Tim S. et al. 2009. Biologically active components of a Papua New Guinea analgesic and anti–inflammatory lichen preparation. *Fitoterapia* 80 (5): 270–273.

Bumpus John A. and S. D. Aust. 1987. Biodegradation of DDT [1,1,1–trichloro–2,2–bis(4–chlorophenyl)ethane] by the white rot fungus *Phanerochaete chrysosporium. Applied Environmental Microbiology* 53 (9): 2001–2008.

Bumpus John A. and Matthew Tatarko. 1994. Biodegradation of 2,4,6–trinitrotoluene by *Phanerochaete chrysosporium:* Identification of initial degradation products and the discovery of a TNT metabolite that inhibits lignin peroxidases. *Current Microbiology* 28 (3): 185–190.

Bumpus, John A. et al. 1985. Oxidation of persistent environmental pollutants via white rot fungus. *Science* 228 (4706): 1434–1436.

Burczyk, J. et al. 1996. Antimitotic activity of aqueous extracts of *Inonotus obliquus. Bollettino Chimico Farmaceutico* 135 (5): 306–309.

Burkholder, Paul R. and Alexander W. Evans. 1945. Further studies of the antibiotic activity of lichens. *Bulletin of the Torrey Botanical Club* 72 (2): 157–164.

Buzina, Walter et al. 2005. The polypore mushroom *Irpex lacteus,* a new causative agent of fungal infections. *Journal of Clinical Microbiolog,* 43 (4): 2009–1011.

Cabrera, Gabriela M. et al. 2002. Cryptoporic and isocryptoporic acids from the fungal cultures of *Polyporus arcularius* and *P. ciliatus. Phytochemistry,* 61 (2): 189–193.

Cali, Valeria et al. 2004. Sarcodonins and sarcoviolins, bioactive polyhydroxy–*p*–terphenyl pyrazinediol dioxide conjugates from fruiting bodies of the Basidiomycete. *European Journal of Organic Chemistry* 2004 (3): 592–599.

Calvino, Eva et al. 2010. *Ganoderma lucidum* induced apoptosis in NB4 human leukemia cells:

Involvement of AKT and ERK. *Journal of Ethnopharmacology* 128 (1): 71–78.

Candan, Mehmet et al. 2006. Antimicrobial activity of extracts of the lichen *Xanthoparmelia pokornyi* and its gyrophoric and stenosporic acid constituents. *Zeitschrift für Naturforschung C* 61 (5–6): 319–323.

Candan, Mehmet et al. 2007. Antimicrobial activity of extracts of the lichen *Parmelia sulcata* and its salazinic acid constituent. *Zeitschrift für Naturforschung C* 62 (7–8): 619–622.

Chairul Sofni M. and Yuji Hayashi. 1994. Lanostanoid triterpenes from *Ganoderma applanatum. Phytochemistry* 35 (5): 1305–1308.

Chang, Chia–Yu et al. 2008. The adjuvant effects of *Antrodia camphorata* extracts combined with anti–tumor agents on multidrug resistant human hepatoma cells. *Journal of Ethnopharmacology* 118 (3): 387–395.

Chang, Heng–Yuan et al. 2011. Analgesic effects and the mechanisms of anti–inflammation of hispolon in mice. *Evidence–Based Complementary and Alternative Medicine* 2011.

Chang, Hson–Mou and Paul Pui–Hay But, editors. 1986. *Pharmacology and Applications of Chinese Materia Medica,* Vol. 1. Singapore: Mainland Press.

Chang, Hson–Mou and Paul Pui–Hay But, editors. 1987. *Pharmacology and Applications of Chinese Materia Medica,* Vol. 2. Singapore: Mainland Press.

Chang, Ii–Moo and Yoshio Yamaura. 1993. Aucubin: A new antidote for poisonous *Amanita* mushrooms. *Phytotherapy Research* 7 (1): 53–56.

Chang, Mun Seog et al. 2009. Treatment with astragali radix and angelicae radix enhances erythropoietin gene expression in the cyclophosphamide–induced anemic rat. *Journal of Medicinal Food* 12 (3): 637–642.

Chang, Zhia Qiang et al. 2008. Comparative immunomodulating activities of polysaccharides isolated from *Phellinus* spp. on cell–mediated immunity. *Phytotherapy Research* 22 (10): 1396–1399.

Chen, Caifa et al. 2007. Aqueous extract of *Inonotus bliquus* (Fr.) Pilat (Hymenochaetaceae) significantly inhibits the growth of sarcoma 180 by inducing apoptosis. *American Journal of Pharmacology and Toxicology* 2 (1): 10–17.

Chen, Haixia et al. 2010. Glycosidase inhibitory activity and antioxidant properties of a polysaccharide from the mushroom *Inonotus obliquus*. *Journal of Food Biochemistry* 34 (1): 178–191.

Chen, J. T. and J. W. Huang. 2004. Identification of *Gliocladium roseum,* the causal agent of brown spot of the king oyster mushroom *Pleurotus eryngii*. *Plant Pathology Bulletin* 13: 17–26.

Chen, Jih–Jung et al. 2007. Anti–inflammatory benzenoids from *Antrodia camphorata*. *Journal of Natural Products* 70 (6): 989–992.

Chen, Jiun–Lang et al. 2009. Immunological alterations in lupus–prone autoimmune (NZB/NZW) F1 mice by mycelia Chinese medicinal fungus *Cordyceps sinensis*–induced redistributions of peripheral mononuclear T lymphocytes. *Clinical and Experimental Medicine* 9 (4): 277–284.

Chen, Liang and HanJuan Shao. 2006. Extract from *Agaricus blazei* Murill can enhance immune responses elicited by DNA vaccine against foot–and–mouth disease. *Veterinary Immunology and Immunopathology* 109 (1–2): 177–182.

Chen, Nan–Yin et al. 2008. Induction of apoptosis in human lung carcinoma A549 epithelial cells with an ethanol extract of *Tremella mesenterica*. *Bioscience, Biotechnology, and Biochemistry* 72 (5): 1283–1289.

Chen, Shih Chung et al. 2005. Antiangiogenic activities of polysaccharides isolated from medicinal fungi. FEMS *Microbiology Letters* 249 (2): 247–254.

Chen, Shiuan et al. 2005. Chemopreventive properties of mushrooms against breast cancer and prostate cancer. *International Journal of Medicinal Mushrooms* 2005 7 (3): 342–343.

Chen, Shiuan et al. 2006. Anti–aromatase activity of phytochemicals in white button mushrooms (*Agaricus bisporus*). *Cancer Research* 66 (24): 12026–12034.

Chen, Wei et al. 2006. The apoptosis effect of hispolon from *Phellinus linteus* (Berkeley & Curtis) Teng on human epidermoid KB cells. *Journal of Ethnopharmacology* 105 (1–2): 280–285.

Chen, Yu–Jen et al. 1997. Effect of *Cordyceps sinensis* on the proliferation and differentiation of human leukemic U937 cells. *Life Sciences* 60 (25): 2349–2359.

Cheng, Jing–Jy et al. 2008. Properties and biological functions of polysaccharides and ethanolic extracts isolated from medicinal fungus, *Fomitopsis pinicola*. *Process Biochemistry* 43 (8): 829–834.

Chien, Shih–Chang et al. 2008. Anti–inflammatory activities of new succinic and maleic derivatives from the fruiting body of *Antrodia camphorata*. *Journal of Agricultural and Food Chemistry* 56 (16): 7017–7022.

Chihara, G. 1983. Preclinical evaluation of lentinan in animal models. *Advances in Experimental Medicine and Biology* 166: 189–197.

Chinworrungsee, Maneekarn et al. 2001. Antimalarial halorosellinic acid from the marine fungus *Halorosellinia oceanica*. *Bioorganic & Medicinal Chemistry Letters* 11 (15): 1965–1969.

Chiu, Siu Wai et al. 2005. Artificial hybridizaton of *Ganoderma lucidum* and *G. tsugae* Murrill by protoplast fusion for sustainability. *International Journal of Medicinal Mushrooms* 7 (1): 263–280.

Chiu, Siu Wai et al. 2009. Role of two species of medicinal mushrooms from genus *Ganoderma* P. Karst. (*G. lucidum* and *G. tsugae;* Aphyllophoromycetideae) in selective estrogen–receptor modulations. *International Journal of Medicinal Mushrooms* 11 (1): 39–54.

Cho, I. H. et al. 2006. Difference in the volatile composition of pine–mushrooms (*Tricholoma matsutake* Sing.) according to their grades. *Journal of Agricultural and Food Chemistry* 54 (13): 4820–4825.

Cho, S. M. et al. 2006. Effect of a *Pholiota adiposa* extract on fat mass in hyperlipidemic mice. *Mycobiology* 34 (4): 236–239.

Choi, Hye–Seon and Yu–Seon Sa. 2000. Fibrinolytic and antithrombotic protease from *Ganoderma lucidum*. *Mycologia* 92 (3): 545–552.

Choi, Joon–Seok et al. 2007. Cyclin–dependent protein kinase 2 activity is required for mitochondrial translocation of Bax and disruption of mitochondrial transmembrane potential during etoposide–induced apoptosis. *Apoptosis* 12 (7): 1229–1241.

Choi, Won–Sik et al. 2005. Inhibitory effect on proliferation of vascular smooth muscle cells and protective effect on CCl_4–induced hepatic damage of HEAI extract. *Journal of Ethnopharmacology* 100 (1–2): 176–179.

Choi, Yun Ho et al. 2006. Inhibitory effects of *Agaricus blazei* on mast cell–mediated anaphylaxis–like reactions. *Biological and Pharmaceutical Bulletin* 29 (7): 1366–1371.

Chung, Ill–Min et al. 2005. Cytotoxic chemical constituents from the mushroom of *Pholiota adiposa*. *Food Science and Biotechnology* 14 (2): 255–258.

Clericuzio, Marco et al. 2004. Cucurbitane triterpenoids from *Leucopaxillus gentianeus*. *Journal of Natural Products* 67 (11): 1823–1828.

Clericuzio, Marco et al. 2006. Cucurbitane triterpenes from the fruiting bodies and cultivated mycelia of *Leucopaxillus gentianeus*. *Journal of Natural Products* 69 (12): 1796–1799.

Clericuzio, Marco et al. 2007. Non–phenolic dicinnamamides from *Pholiota spumosa*: Isolation, synthesis and antitumour activity. *European Journal of Organic Chemistry* 33: 5551–5559.

Coatney, G. R. et al. 1953. Survey of antimalarial agents. *Public Health Monogram* 9, Federal Security Agency, Washington D.C.

Coetzee, Johannes C. and Abraham E. van Wyk. 2009. The genus *Calvatia* ('Gasteromycetes', Lycoperdaceae): A review of its ethnomycology and biotechnological potential. *African Journal of Biotechnology* 8 (22): 6007–6015.

Colak et al. 2009. Nutritional composition of some wild edible mushrooms. *Turkish Journal of Biochemistry* 34 (1): 25–31.

Colauto et al. 2002. Genetic characterization of isolates of the Basidiomycete *Agaricus blazei* by RAPD. *Brazilian Journal of Microbiology* 33 (2): 131–133.

Coletto, Bianco et al. 1981. Basidiomycetes in relation to antibiosis. II. Antibiotic activity of mycelia and culture liquids. *Giornale di Batteriologia Virologia ed Immunologia* 74 (7–12): 267–274.

Colleto, Bianco et al. 1992. Antibiotic activity in Basidiomycetes. VI. Antibiotic activity of mycelia and cultural filtrates of thirty–three new strains. *Allionia* 31: 87–90.

Collins, Graham P. 2006. Computing with quantum knots. *Scientific American* 294 (4): 56–63.

Collins, L. et al. 2006. *Phellinus linteus* sensitises apoptosis induced by doxorubicin in prostate cancer. *British Journal of Cancer* 95: 282–288.

Collins, R. P. and A. F. Halim. 1972. An analysis of the odorous constituents produced by various species of *Phellinus*. *Canadian Journal of Microbiology* 18: 57–64.

Colpaert, Jan V. and Jozef A. Assche. 1992. Zinc toxicity in ectomycorrhizal *Pinus sylvestris*. *Plant and Soil Journal* 143 (2): 201–211.

Cui, F. J. et al. 2007. Structural analysis of anti–tumor heteropolysaccharide GFPS1B from the cultured mycelia of *Grifola frondosa* GF9801. *Bioresource Technology* 98 (2): 395–401.

Cui, Yong et al. 2005. Antioxidant effect of *Inonotus obliquus*. *Journal of Ethnopharmacology* 96 (1–2): 79–85.

Czarnecki, R. and J. Grzybek. 1995. Antiinflammatory and vasoprotective activities of polysaccharides isolated from fruit bodies of higher fungi P.1. polysaccharides from *Trametes gibbosa* (Pers.: Fr)Fr. (Polyporaceae). *Phytotherapy Research* 9 (2): 163–167.

Czederpiltz, Daniel L. Lindner et al. 2001. Field observations and inoculation experiments to determine the nature of the carpophoroids associated with *Entoloma abortivum* and *Armillaria*. *Mycologia* 93 (5): 841–851.

D'Annibale, Alessandro et al. 1999. Characterization of immobilized laccase from *Lentinula edodes* and its use in olive–mill wastewater treatment. *Process Biochemistry* 34 (6–7): 697–706.

Da Eira, Augusto Ferreira et al. 2002. Is a widely cultivated culinary–medicinal royal sun *Agaricus* (the himematsutake mushroom) indeed *Agaricus blazei* Murrill? *International Journal of Medicinal Mushrooms* 4 (4): 281–304.

Dai, Y. C. 2003. New Knowledge on the medicinal basidiomycetes *Phellinus baumii*. *Zhong Cao Yao* 34: 94–95.

Damjan et al. 2007. Antibacterial activity in higher fungi (mushrooms) and endophytic fungi from Slovenia. *Pharmaceutical Biology* 45 (9): 700–706.

Danai et al. 2008. Introduction of new exotic mushroom species into cultivation in Israel. *Israeli Journal of Plant Sciences* 56 (4): 295–301.

Davitashvili, E. et al. 2008. Evaluation of higher Basidiomycetes mushroom lectin activity in submerged and solid–state fermentation of agro–industrial residues. *International Journal of Medicinal Mushrooms* 10 (2): 171–179.

De Jong, Ed and Jim A. Field. 1997. Sulfur tuft and turkey tail: Biosynthesis and biodegradation of organohalogens by Basidiomycetes. *Annual Review of Microbiology* 51: 375–414.

Ding, Guang–Sheng. 1987. Anti–arrhythmia agents in traditional Chinese medicines. *Abstracts of Chinese Medicine* 1 (2): 287–308.

Ding, Guang–Sheng and You–Yi Liang. 1991. Antidotal effects of dimercaptosuccinic acid. *Journal of Applied Toxicology* 11 (1): 7–14.

Ding, Zhongyang et al. 2010. Hypoglycaemic effect of comatin, an antidiabetic substance separated from *Coprinus comatus* broth, on alloxan–induced–diabetic rats. *Food Chemistry* 121 (1): 39–43.

Diyabalanage et al. 2009. Liperoxidation and cyclo-oxygenase enzyme inhibitory compounds from the lipophilic extracts of some culinary–medicinal higher Basidiomycetes mushrooms. *International Journal of Medicinal Mushrooms* 11 (4): 375–382.

Doljak et al. 2001. Screening for selective thrombin inhibitors in mushrooms. *Blood Coagulation and Fibrinolysis* 12 (2): 123–128.

Dombrovska et al. 1998. Biotransformation of lignocellulose by the fungi *Pleurotus floridae* (Fried) Kummer and *Phelinus igniarius* (Linnaeus: Fries) Quelet – the pathogens of white rot in trees. *Ukrainskii Biokhimicheskii Zhurnal* 70 (1): 68–74.

Domondon et al. 2004. –Adenosine, a bioactive compound in grass chaff stimulating mushroom production. *Phytochemistry,* 65 (2): 181–187.

Donatini, B. and I. Le Blaye. 2007. Mushrooms and weight loss: A randomised, double-blind study. *Seventh International Mycological Congress Book of Abstracts #305.*

Dong, C. H. and Y.–J. Yao. 2005. Nutritional requirements of mycelial growth of *Cordyceps sinensis* in submerged culture. *Journal of Applied Microbiology* 99 (3): 483–492.

Donnelly, Dervilla M. X. et al. 1986. New sesquiterpene aryl esters from *Armillaria mellea*. *Journal of Natural Products* 49 (1): 111–116.

Donnelly, P. K. et al. 1993. Degradation of atrazine and 2,4–dichlorophenoxyacetic acid by mycorrhizal fungi at three nitrogen concentrations in vitro. *Applied and Environmental Microbiology* 59 (8): 2642–2647.

Dornberger, K. et al. 1986. Antibiotics from Basidiomycetes evidence for the occurrence of the 4–hydroxybenzenediazonium ion in the extracts of *Agaricus xanthodermus* Genevier (Agaricales). *Tetrahedron Letters* 27 (5): 559–560.

Dufresne et al. 1997. Illudinic acid, a novel illudane sesquiterpene antibiotic. *Journal of Natural Products* 60 (3): 188–190.

Dulger, Basaran. 2005. Antimicrobial activity of ten Lycoperdaceae. *Fitoterapia* 76 (3): 352–354.

Dulger, Basaran el al., 2002a. Antimicrobial activity

of some *Lactarius* species. *Pharmaceutical Biology* 40 (4): 304–306.

Dulger, Basaran et al. 2002b. Antimicrobial activity of the macrofungus *Lepista nuda*. *Fitoterapia* 73 (7–8): 695–697.

Duncan, Christine J. G. et al. 2002. Isolation of a galactomannan that enhances macrophage activation from the edible fungus *Morchella esculenta*. *Journal of Agricultural and Food Chemistry* 50 (20): 5683–5685.

Duncan, Christine J. G. et al. 2003. Chemical and biological investigation of the fungus *Pulveroboletus ravenelii*. *Journal of Natural Products* 66 (1): 103–107.

Duran et al. 1994. A new alternative process for Kraft E1 effluent treatment. *Biodegradation* 5 (1): 13–19.

Ehrenberg, L. et al. 1946. Antibiotic effect of agarics on tubercle bacilli. *Svensk Kemisk Tidskrift* 58: 269–270.

Elisashvili, Vladimir I. et al. 2002a. Hypoglycemic, interferonogenous, and immunomodulatory activity of tremellastin from the submerged culture of *Tremella mesenterica* Retz.: Fr. (Heterobasidiomycetes). *International Journal of Medicinal Mushrooms* 4 (3): 215–227.

Elisashvili, Vladimir I. et al. 2002b. Some approaches to the evaluation of the white rot Basidiomycetes ligninolytic activity. *Seventh International Mycological Congress Book of Abstracts* #202.

Endo et al. 2010. Agaritine purified from *Agaricus blazei* Murrill exerts anti–tumor activity against leukemic cells. *Biochimica et Biophysica Acta* 1800 (7): 669–673.

Engler, M. et al. 1998. Production of antibiotics by *Collybia nivalis, Omphalotus olearis,* a *Favolaschia* and a *Pterula* species on natural substrates. *Zeitschrift für Naturforschung C* 53 (5–6): 318–324.

Enman, Josefine et al. 2007. Quantification of the bioactive compound eritadenine in selected strains of shiitake mushroom *(Lentinus edodes).*

Journal of Agricultural and Food Chemistry 55 (4): 1177–1180.

Enman, Josefine et al. 2008. Production of the bioactive compound eritadenine by submerged cultivation of shiitake *(Lentinus edodes)* mycelia. *Journal of Agricultural and Food Chemistry* 56 (8): 2609–2612.

Erkel, G. et al. 1996. Nidulal, a novel inducer of differentiation of human promyelocytic leukemia cells from *Nidula candida*. *Journal of Antibiotics* 49 (12): 1189–1195.

Ersel, Fadime Yilmaz and Levent Cavas. 2008. Enzyme–based scavengers and lipid peroxidation in some wild edible Agaricales s.l. mushrooms from Mug La (Turkey). *International Journal of Medicinal Mushrooms* 10 (3): 269–277.

Ershova et al. 2003. Antimicrobial activity of *Laetiporus sulphureus* strains grown in submerged culture. *Antibiotiki i Khimioterapiia* 48 (1): 18–22.

Espada et al. 1997. New cytochalasins from the fungus *Xyylaria hypoxylon*. *Tetrahedron* 53 (18): 6485–6492.

Espenshade, M. A. and E. W. Griffith. 1966. Tumor–inhibiting Basidiomycetes: Isolation and cultivation in the laboratory. *Mycologia* 58 (4): 511–517.

Evans, Larry. 2010. Fire morels part II: Morels, fire, and nontimber forest products management. *Fungi* 3 (2): 45–47.

Falandysz et al. 1994. Silver content of wild–grown mushrooms from northern Poland. *Zeitschrift fur Lebensmitteluntersuchung und–Forschung A* 199 (3): 222–224.

Fäldt, Jenny et al. 1999. Volatiles of bracket fungi *Fomitopsis pinicola* and *Fomes fomentarius* and their functions as insect attractants. *Journal of Chemical Ecology* 25 (3): 567-590.

Farrell, I. W. et al. 1973 Natural acetylenes. Part 41. Polyacetylenes from fungal fruiting bodies. *Journal of the Chemical Society: Perkins Transactions I* 22 :2642–2643.

Fatmawati, Sri et al. 2009. The inhibitory effect

on aldose reductase by an extract of *Ganoderma lucidum*. *Phytotherapy Research* 23(1): 28–32.

Feng et al. 2006. Isolation and characterization of a novel lectin from the mushroom *Armillaria luteo–virens*. *Biochemical and Biophysical Research Communications* 345 (4): 1573–1578.

Ferrey et al. 1994. Nodulation efficiency of *Bradyrhizobium japonicum* strains with genotypes of soybean varying in the ability to restrict nodulation. *Canadian Journal of Microbiology* 40 (6): 456–460.

Field, Jim A. et al. 1992. Biodegradation of polycyclic aromatic hydrocarbons by new isolates of white rot fungi. *Applied Environmental Microbiology* 58 (7): 2219–2226.

Field, Jim A. et al. 1996. Biological elimination of polycyclic aromatic hydrocarbons in solvent extracts of polluted soil by the white rot fungus, *Bjerkandera* sp. strain BOS55. *Environmental Technology* 17 (3): 317–323.

Figlas et al. 2007. Cultivation of culinary–medicinal Lion's Mane mushroom *Hericium erinaceus* (Bull.: Fr.) Pers. (Aphyllophoromycetideae) on substrate containing sunflower seed hulls. *International Journal of Medicinal Mushrooms* 9 (1): 67–73.

Fleck et al. 1996. Isolation of isodrimenediol, a possible intermediate of drimane biosynthesis from *Polyporus arcularius*. *Journal of Natural Products* 59 (8): 780–781.

Florey, Howard Lord et al. 1949. *Antibiotics: A survey of penicillin, streptomycin and other antimicrobial substances from fungi, actinomycetes, bacteria and plants.* London: Oxford University Press.

Fortes et al. 2008. Effects of dietary supplementation with medicinal fungus in fasting glycemia levels of patients with colorectal cancer: A randomized, double–blind, placebo–controlled clinical study. *Nutricion Hospitalaria* 23 (6): 591–598.

Fragoeiro, S. and Magan, N. 2008. Impact of *Trametes versicolor & Phanerochaete chrysosporium*. *International Biodeterioration & Biodegradation* 62 (4): 376–383.

Francois et al. 1999. Vismione H and structurally related anthranoid compounds of natural and synthetic origin as promising drugs against the human malaria parasite *Plasmodium falciparum*: Structure–activity relationships. *Parasitology Research* 85 (7): 582–588.

Friman, V. et al. 2006. A fatal case of severe immunodeficiency associated with disseminated *Merulius tremellosus* infection. *Scandinavian Journal of Infectious Disease* 38 (1): 76–78.

Fu, H. D. and Z. Y. Wang. 1982. The clinical effects of *Ganoderma lucidum* spore preparations in 10 cases of atrophic myotonia. *Journal of Traditional Chinese Medicine* 2 (1): 63-65.

Fujimoto et al. 1994. Isolation and characterization of immunosuppressive components of three mushrooms, *Pisolithus tinctorius, Microporus flabelliformis* and *Lenzites betulina*. *Chemical & Pharmaceutical Bulletin* 42 (3): 694–697.

Fujita et al. 2005. Anti–androgenic activities of *Ganoderma lucidum*. *Journal of Ethnopharmacology* 102 (1): 107–112.

Furukawa, K. et al. 1995. Hemagglutinins in fungus extracts and their blood group specificity. *Experimental and Clinical Immunogenetics* 12 (4): 223–231.

Furukawa, Mai et al. 2006. Effect of *Agaricus brasiliensis* S. Wasser et al. (Agaricomycetideae) on murine diabetic model C57BL / KSJ–DB / DB. *International Journal of Medicinal Mushrooms* 8 (2): 115–128.

Furuya, Tsutomu et al. 1983. N^6–(2–hydroxyethyl) adenosine, a biologically active compound from cultured mycelia of *Cordyceps* and *Isaria* species. *Phytochemistry* 22 (11): 2509–2512.

Gan, K. H. et al. 1998. Mediation of the cytotoxicity of lanostanoids and steroids of *Ganoderma tsugae* through apoptosis and cell cycle. *Journal of Natural Products* 61 (4): 485–487.

Gao, Bin and Gui–Zhen Yang. 1991. Effects of *Ganoderma applanatum* polysaccharide on cellular and humoral immunity in normal and sarcoma

180 transplanted mice. *Phytotherapy Research* 5 (3): 134–138.

Gao, J. M. et al. 2001. New glycosphingolipid containing an unusual sphingoid base from the Basidiomycete *Polyporus ellisii*. *Lipids* 36 (5): 521–527.

Gao, J. M. et al. 2004. Paxillamide: A novel phytosphingosine derivative from the fruiting bodies of *Paxillus panuoides*. *Helvetica Chimica Acta* 87 (6): 1483–1487.

Gao, X. X. et al. 2000a. Effects of polysaccharides (FI0-b) from mycelium of *Ganoderma tsugae* on proinflammatory cytokine production by THP-1 cells and human PBMC (I). *Acta Pharmacologica Sinica* 21 (12): 1179-1185.

Gao, X. X. et al. 2000b. Effects of polysaccharides (FI0-b) from mycelium of *Ganoderma tsugae* on proinflammatory cytokine production by THP-1 cells and human PBMC (II). *Acta Pharmacologica Sinica* 21 (12): 1186-1192.

Gao, Yihuai et al. 2002. A phase I/II study of a *Ganoderma lucidum* (Curt.: Fr.) P. Karst.(ling zhi, reishi mushroom) extract in patients with chronic hepatitis B. *International Journal of Medicinal Mushrooms* 4 (4): 333–339.

Gao, Yihuai et al. 2003. Antibacterial and antiviral value of the genus *Ganoderma* P. Karst. species (Aphyllophoromycetideae): A review. *International Journal of Medicinal Mushrooms* 5 (3): 251–262.

Gao, Yihuai et al. 2004a. Chemopreventive and tumoricidal properties of ling zhi mushroom *Ganoderma lucidum* (W. Curt.: Fr.) Lloyd (Aphyllophoromycetideae). Part I. Preclinical and clinical studies. *International Journal of Medicinal Mushrooms* 6 (2): 99–110.

Gao, Yihuai et al. 2004b. Chemopreventive and tumoricidal properties of ling zhi mushroom *Ganoderma lucidum* (W. Curt.: Fr.) Lloyd (Aphyllophoromycetideae). Part II. Mechanism considerations. *International Journal of Medicinal Mushrooms* 6 (3): 227–238.

Gao, Yihuai et al. 2004c. *Ganoderma lucidum* polysaccharide fractions accelerate healing of acetic acid–induced ulcers in rats. *Journal of Medicinal Food* 7 (4): 417–421.

Gao, Yihuai et al. 2004d. A phase I/II study of ling zhi mushroom *Ganoderma lucidum* (W.Curt.: Fr.) Lloyd (Aphyllophoromycetideae) extract in patients with type II diabetes mellitus. *International Journal of Medicinal Mushrooms* 6 (1): 33–40.

Garaudee, Sandrine et al. 2002. Allosteric effects in norbadione A. A clue for the accumulation process of 137Cs in mushrooms? *Chemical Communications* 9 (8): 944–945.

Gartz, Jochen. 1989. Analysis of aeruginascin in fruit bodies of the mushroom *Inocybe aeruginascens*. *Pharmaceutical Biology* 27 (3): 141–144.

Gartz, Jochen and G. Drewitz. 1985. Der erste Nachweis von *Psilocybin* in Risspilzen. *Zeitschrift fur Mykologie* 51 (2): 199–203.

Gau et al. 1990. The lack of antiplatelet effect of crude extracts from *Ganoderma lucidum* on HIV–positive hemophiliacs *American Journal of Chinese Medicine* 18 (3–4): 175–179.

Gbolagade, Jonathan S. and Ishola O. Fasidi. 2005. Antimicrobial activities of some selected Nigerian mushrooms. *African Journal of Biomedical Research* 8 (2): 83–87.

Geethangili et al. 2009. Review of pharmacological effects of *Antrodia camphorata* and its bioactive compounds. *Evidence–Based Complementary and Alternative Medicine* 2011 http://ecam.oxfordjournals.org/cgi/content/abstract/nep108.

Geissler, Torsten et al. 2010. Acetylcholinesterase inhibitors from the toadstool *Cortinarius infractus*. *Bioorganic and Medicinal Chemistry* 18 (6): 2173–2177.

Geml, Jozsef et al. 2008. Evidence for strong inter– and intracontinental phylogeographic structure in *Amanita muscaria,* a wind–dispersed ectomycorrhizal Basidiomycete. *Molecular Phylogenetics and Evolution* 48 (2): 694–701.

Geraci, Corrada et al. 1992. Cytotoxic activity of tetraprenylphenols related to suillin, an antitumor principle from *Suillus granulatus*. *Journal of Natural Products* 55 (12): 1772–1775.

Geraci, Corrada et al. 2000. An unusual nitrogenous terphenyl derivative from fruiting bodies of the Basidiomycete *Sarcodon leucopus*. *Journal of Natural Products* 63 (3): 347–351.

Gerasimenya, Valeriy P. et al. 2001. Antimicrobial and antitoxic action of *Pleurotus ostreatus* (Jacq.: Fr.) Kumm extracts. *International Journal of Medicinal Mushrooms* 3 (2–3): 148.

Giannetti, B. M. et al. 1978. Antibiotics from Basidiomycetes, VI. Merulinic acids A, B, and C, new antibiotics from *Merulius tremellosus* and *Phlebia radiata*. *Zeitschrift für Naturforschung* 33 (11–12): 807–816.

Gorbunova et al. 2005. Medicinal mushrooms of southwest Siberia. *International Journal of Medicinal Mushrooms* 7 (3): 403–404.

Goud et al. 2009. Extracellular hydrolytic enzyme profiles of certain South Indian Basidiomycetes. *African Journal of Biotechnology* 8 (3): 354–360.

Graf, E. and H. J. J. Winckelmann. 1960. Versuche zum umbau der Hydroxy–Triterpencarbonsäuren von Fungus *Laricis* zu 11–Keto–Cortigosteroiden. *Planta Medica* 8 (4): 403–410.

Gray, A. M. and P. R. Flatt. 1998. Insulin–releasing and insulin–like activity of *Agaricus campestris* (mushroom). *Journal of Endocrinology* 157 (2): 259–266.

Gregory, F. J. et al. 1966. Studies on antitumor substances produced by Basidiomycetes. *Mycologia* 58 (1): 80–90.

Griessmayr, P. C. et al. 2007. Mushroom–derived maitake PETfraction as single agent for the treatment of lymphoma in dogs. *Journal of Veterinary Internal Medicine* 21 (6): 1409–1412.

Grinde et al. 2006. Effects on gene expression and viral load of a medicinal extract from *Agaricus blazei* in patients with chronic hepatitis C infection. *International Immunopharmacology* 6 (8): 1311–1314.

Grodzinskaya et al. 1999. Testing of biologically active compounds in Stropharia rugosoannulata. *International Journal of Medicinal Mushrooms* 1 (3): 229–234

Grube et al. 2001. White button mushroom phytochemicals inhibit aromatase activity and breast cancer cell proliferation. *The Journal of Nutrition* 131 (12): 3288–3293.

Gruhn, C. M. and O. K. Miller Jr. 1991. Effect of copper on tyrosinase activity and polyamine content of some ectomycorrhizal fungi. *Mycological Research* 95 (3): 268–272.

Gruhn, N. et al. 2007. Biologically active etabolites from the Basidiomycete *Limacella illinita* (Fr.) Urr. *Zeitschrift für Naturforschung C* 62 (11–12): 808–812.

Gruter, A. et al. 1990. Antimutagenic effects of mushrooms. *Mutation Research / Fundamental and Molecular Mechanisms of Mutagenesis* 231 (2): 243–249.

Grzybek, J. et al. 1992. Evaluation of anti–inflammatory and vasoprotective actions of the polysaccharides isolated from fruit bodies of *Boletus edulis*. *Planta Medica* 58 (S1): 641.

Grzywnowicz, Krzysztof. 2001. Medicinal mushrooms in Polish folk medicine. *International Journal of Medicinal Mushrooms*. 3 (2–3): 156.

Gu, Y. H. and M. A. Belury. 2005. Selective induction of apoptosis in murine skin carcinoma cells (CH72) by an ethanol extract of *Lentinula edodes*. *Cancer Letters* 220 (1): 21–28.

Gu, Y. H. and J. Leonard. 2006. In vitro effects on proliferation, apoptosis and colony inhibition in ER–dependent and ER–independent human breast cancer cells by selected mushroom species. *Oncology Reports* 15 (2): 417–424.

Gu, Y. H. and G. Sivam. 2006. Cytotoxic effect of oyster mushroom *Pleurotus ostreatus* on human androgen–independent prostate cancer PC–3 cells. *Journal of Medicinal Food* 9 (2): 196–204.

Gu, Yeunhwa et al. 2005. Immunostimulating and antitumor effects by *Inonotus obliquus* (Ach.:Pers.) Pilat. *International Journal of Medicinal Mushrooms* 7 (3): 406.

Guler, P. et al. 2009. Antifungal activities of *Fomitopsis pinicola* (Sw.: Fr) Karst and *Lactarius vellereus* (Pers.) Fr. *African Journal of Biotechnology* 8 (16): 3811–3813.

Gunde–Cimerman et al. 1995. *Pleurotus* fruiting bodies contain the inhibitor of 3–hydroxy–3–methylglutaryl–coenzyme A reductase–lovastatin. *Experimental Mycology* 19 (1): 1–6.

Gupta et al. 2007. Antimycobacterial activity of lichens. *Pharmaceutical Biology* 45 (3): 200–204.

Gzogian et al. 2005. Trypsin–like proteinases and trypsin inhibitors in fruiting bodies of higher fungi. *Prikladnaya Biokhimicheskii i Mikrobiologiy* 41 (6): 612–615.

Hallen, H. E. et al. 2003. Taxonomy and toxicity of *Conocybe lactea* and related species. *Mycological Research* 107 (8): 969–979.

Hamlyn and Schmidt. 1994. Potential therapeutic application of fungal filaments in wound management. *Mycologist* 8 (4): 147–152.

Hammel and Tardone. 1988. The oxidative 4–dechlorination of polychlorinated phenols is catalyzed by extracellular fungal lignin peroxidases. *Biochemistry* 27 (17): 6563–6568.

Hammerschmidt. 1980. Szechwan *Purpura*. *The New England Journal of Medicine* 302 (21): 1191–1193.

Hammond et al. 2000. Enhanced antitumour activity of 6–hydroxymethylacylfulvene in combination with topotecan or paclitaxel in the MV522 lung carcinoma xenograft model. *European Journal of Cancer* 36 (18): 2430–2436.

Han, B et al. 1999. Induction of apoptosis by *Coprinus disseminatus* mycelial culture broth extract in human cervical carcinoma cells. *Cell Structure and Function* 24 (4): 209–215.

Han, C. et al. 2006. Hypoglycemic activity of fermented mushroom of *Coprinus comatus* rich in vanadium. *Journal of Trace Elements in Medicine and Biology* 20 (3): 191–196.

Han, C. et al. 2003. A study on the co–effect of *Coprinus comatus* fermentation liquid and sodium vanadate on the process of inhibiting ascension of blood glucose in mice. *Edible Fungi of China* 22 (1): 39–40.

Han, C. H. et al. 2005. A novel homodimeric lactose–binding lectin from the edible split gill medicinal mushroom *Schizophyllum commune*. *Biochemical and Biophysical Research Communications* 336 (1): 252–257.

Hanson, Amy et al. 2003. Mycophagy among primates. *Mycologist* 17 (1): 6–10.

Harada, Toshie et al. 2002a. Effect of SCG, 1,3––D–glucan from *Sparassis crispa* on the hematopoietic response in cyclophosphamide induced leukopenic mice. *Biological & Pharmaceutical Bulletin* 25 (7): 931–939.

Harada, Toshie et al. 2002b. IFN– Induction by SCG, 1,3––D–glucan from *Sparassis crispa*, in DBA/2 mice in vitro. *Journal of Interferon and Cytokine Research* 22 (12): 1227–1239.

Harada, Toshie et al. 2004. Granulocyte–macrophage colony–stimulating factor (GM–CSF) regulates cytokine induction by 1,3––D–glucan SCG in DBA/2 mice in vitro. *Journal of Interferon and Cytokine Research* 24 (8): 478–479.

Harada, Toshie et al. 2005. Soy isoflavone aglycone modulates a hematopoietic response in combination with soluble –glucan: SCG. *Biological & Pharmaceutical Bulletin* 28 (12): 2342–2345.

Harada, Toshie et al. 2006a. Cell to cell contact through ICAM–1–LFA–1 and TNF– synergistically contributes to GM–CSF and subsequent cytokine synthesis in DBA/2 mice induced by 1,3––D–glucan SCG. *Journal of Interferon and Cytokine Research* 26 (4): 235–247.

Harada, Toshie et al. 2006b. Comparison of the immunomodulating activities of 1,3––glucan fractions from the culinary–medicinal mushroom *Sparassis crispa* Wulf.: Fr. (Aphyllophoromycetideae). *International Journal of Medicinal Mushrooms* 8 (3): 231–244.

Harada, Toshie et al. 2006c. Mechanism of enhanced hematopoietic response by soluble –

glucan SCG in cyclophosphamide–treated mice. *Microbiology and Immunology* 50 (9): 687–700.

Harada, Toshie et al. 2008. Dectin–1 and GM–CSF on immunomodulating activities of fungal 6–branched 1,3– –glucans. *International Journal of Medicinal Mushrooms* 10 (2): 101–114.

Haraldsdottir et al. 2004. Anti–proliferative effects of lichen–derived lipoxygenase inhibitors on twelve human cancer cell lines of different tissue origin in vitro. *Planta Medica* 70 (11): 1098–1100.

Harttig et al. 1990. Leaianafulvene, a sesquiterpenoid fulvene derivative from cultures of *Mycena leaiana*. *Phytochemistry* 29 (12): 3942–3944.

Hashimoto T. and Y. Asakawa. 1998. Biologically active substances of Japanese inedible mushrooms. *Heterocycles* 47 (2): 1067–1110.

Hashimoto, T. et al. 2006. Hydnellins A and B, nitrogen–containing terphenyls from the mushrooms *Hydnellum suaveolens* and *Hydnellum geogerirum*. *Chemical and Pharmaceutical Bulletin* 54 (6): 912.

Hatanaka and Niimura. 1972. L–2–Aminohex–4–ynoic acid: A new amino acid from *Tricholomopsis rutilans*. *Phytochemistry* 11 (11): 3327–3329.

Hatvani, Nora. 2001. Antibacterial effect of the culture fluid of *Lentinus edodes* mycelium grown in submerged liquid culture. *International Journal of Antimicrobial Agents* 17(1): 71–74.

Hatvani, Nora and Imre Mecs. 2003. Effects of certain heavy metals on the growth, dye decolorization, and enzyme activity of *Lentinula edodes*. *Ecotoxicity and Environmental Safety* 55 (2): 199–203.

He, Jian et al. 2003. Fomlactones A−C, novel triterpene lactones from *Fomes cajanderi*. *Journal of Natural Products* 66 (9): 1249–1251.

Hearst et al. 2009. An examination of antibacterial and antifungal properties of constituents of shiitake *(Lentinula edodes)* and oyster *(Pleurotus ostreatus)* mushrooms. *Complementary Therapies in Clinical Practice* 15 (1): 5–7.

Heim, R. 1972. Mushroom madness in the Kuma. *Human Biology in Oceania* 1 (1): 170–178.

Heinfling et al. 1997. Biodegradation of azo and phthalocyanine dyes by *Trametes versicolor* and *Bjerkandera adusta*. *Applied Microbiology and Biotechnology* 48 (2): 261–266.

Hellsten et al. 2008. Galiellalactone is a novel therapeutic candidate against hormone–refractory prostate cancer expressive activated Stat3. *The Prostate* 68 (3): 269–280.

Hellwig, Veronika et al. 1998. New triquinane–type sesquiterpenoids from *Macrocystidia cucumis* (Basidiomycetes). *European Journal of Organic Chemistry* 1998 (1): 73–79.

Hellwig, Veronika et al. 2002. Calopins and cyclocalopins—bitter principles from *Boletus calopus* and related mushrooms. *European Journal of Organic Chemistry* 2002 (17): 2895–2904.

Hellwig, Veronika et al. 2003. Activities of prenylphenol derivatives from fruitbodies of *Albatrellus* spp. on the human and rat vanilloid receptor 1 (VR1) and characterisation of the novel natural product, confluentin. *Archiv der Pharmazie* 336 (2): 119–126.

Hendrix et al. 1985. Relationship between the ectomycorrhizal fungus *Pisolithus tinctorius* associated with loblolly pine and acid–generating *Thiobacillus* spp. on an acidic strip mine site. *Canadian Journal of Microbiology* 31 (9): 878–879.

Hervey, A. H. 1947. A survey of 500 Basidiomycetes for antibacterial activity. *Bulletin of the Torrey Botanical Club* 74 (6): 476–503.

Hideno et al. 2007. Utilization of spent sawdust matrix after cultivation of *Grifola frondosa* as substrate for ethanol production by simultaneous saccharification and fermentation. *Food Science and Technology Research* 13 (2): 111–117.

Hikino, H. et al. 1985. Isolation and hypoglycemic activity of ganoderans A and B, glycans of *Ganoderma lucidum* fruit bodies. *Planta Medica* 51 (4): 339–340.

Hikino, H. et al. 1989. Mechanisms of hypoglycemic activity of ganoderan B: A glycan of

523

Ganoderma lucidum fruit bodies. *Planta Medica* 55 (5): 423–428.

Hilton, R. N. 1987. Podiatric polypore. *Mycologist* 1 (3): 121.

Hirata et al. 1950. Grifolin, an antibiotic from a Basidiomycete. *The Journal of Biological Chemistry* 184 (1): 135–144.

Hiyoshi, T. et al. 1996. *Cordyceps sinensis* effects on cardiopulmonary function of long–distance runners. *Japanese Journal of Physical Fitness and Sports Medicine* 45: 474.

Honda N. K. et al. 2010. Antimycobacterial activity of lichen substances. *Phytomedicine* 17 (5): 328–332.

Hong, Lei et al. 2007. Anti–diabetic effect of an alpha–glucan from fruit body of maitake *(Grifola frondosa)* on KK–AY mice. *Journal of Pharmacy and Pharmacology* 59(4): 575–582.

Hong, Seo Ah et al. 2008. A case–control study on the dietary intake of mushrooms and breast cancer risk among Korean women. *International Journal of Cancer* 122 (4): 919–923.

Hong, Soon Gyu and Hack Sung Jung. 2004. Phylogenetic analysis of *Ganoderma* based on nearly complete mitochondrial small–subunit ribosomal DNA sequences. *Mycologia* 96(4): 742–755.

Horner et al. 1993. Basidiospore allergen release: Elution from intact spores. *Journal of Allergy and Clinical Immunology* 92 (2): 306–312.

Hoshi, Hirotaka et al. 2005. Isolation and characterization of a novel immunomodulatory-d-glucan–protein complex from the mycelium of *Tricholoma matsutake* in Basidiomycetes. *Journal of Agricultural and Food Chemistry* 53 (23): 8948–8956.

Hoshi, Hirotaka et al. 2005. Absorption and tissue distribution of an immunomodulatory –d–glucan after oral administration of *Tricholoma matsutake*. *Journal of Agricultural and Food Chemistry* 56 (17): 7715–7720.

Hosoe, Tomoo et al. 2007. Lepidepyrone, a new gamma–pyrone derivative, from *Neolentinus lepideus,* inhibits hyaluronidase. *Journal of Antibiotics* 60 (6): 388–390.

Hseu, You–Cheng et al. 2006. Inhibition of cyclo-oxygenase–2 and induction of apoptosis in estrogen–nonresponsive breast cancer cells by *Antrodia camphorata*. *Food and Chemical Toxicology* 45 (7): 1107–1115.

Hseu, You–Cheng et al. 2008. *Antrodia camphorata* inhibits proliferation of human breast cancer cells in vitro and in vivo. *Food and Chemical Toxicology* 46 (8): 2680–2688.

Hsieh, K.–Y. et al. 2003. Oral administration of an edible–mushroom–derived protein inhibits the development of food–allergic reactions in mice. *Clinical and Experimental Allergy* 33 (11): 1595–1602.

Hsieh, T. C. and J. M. Wu. 2001. Cell growth and gene modulatory activities of yunzhi (Windsor wunxi) from mushroom *Trametes versicolor* in androgen–dependent and androgen–insensitive human prostate cancer cells. *International Journal of Oncology* 18 (1): 81–89.

Hsu, Chi–Chao et al. 2003. In vivo and in vitro stimulatory effects of *Cordyceps sinensis* on testosterone production in mouse Leydig cells. *Life Sciences* 73 (16): 2127–2136.

Hsu, Shi–Chung et al. 1998. *Ganoderma tsugae* extracts inhibit colorectal cancer cell growth via G(2)/M cell cycle arrest. *Journal of Ethnopharmacology* 120 (3): 394–401.

Hu, Honghai et al. 2009. Comparative study of antioxidant activity and antiproliferative effect of hot water and ethanol extracts from the mushroom *Inonotus obliquus*. *Journal of Bioscience and Bioengineering* 107 (1): 42–48.

Hua, Q et al. 1991. Biological characteristics of *Cryptoporus volvatus* (Peck) Hubb., a medicinal fungus. *Zhongguo Zhong Yao Za Zhi* 16 (12): 719–722.

Huang, Bu–Miin et al. 2004. Upregulation of steroidogenic enzymes and ovarian 17 –estradiol in human granulosa–lutein cells by *Cordyceps sinensis* mycelium. *Biology of Reproduction* 70 (5): 1358–1364.

Huang, Jin and W. S. Winston Ho. 2008. Effects

of system parameters on the performance of CO_2–selective WGS membrane reactor for fuel cells. *Journal of the Chinese Institute of Chemical Engineers* 39 (2): 129–136.

Huang, Yu–Ting et al. 2009. In vitro inhibitory effects of pulvinic acid derivatives isolated from chinese edible mushrooms, *Boletus calopus* and *Suillus bovinus,* on cytochrome P450 activity. *Bioscience, Biotechnology, and Biochemistry* 73 (4): 855–860.

Hung, W. S. et al. 2001. Cytotoxicity and immunogenicity of sacchachitin and its mechanism of action on skin wound healing. *Journal of Biomedical Materials Research* 56 (1): 93-100.

Hutchison et al. 1996. The presence and antifeedant function of toxin–producing secretory cells on hyphae of the lawn–inhabiting agaric *Conocybe lactea. Canadian Journal of Botany* 74 (3): 431–434.

Hwang, Eui Il et al. 2000. Phellinsin A, a novel chitin synthases inhibitor produced by *Phellinus* sp. PL3. *Journal of Antibiotics* 53 (9): 903–911.

Hwang, Eui Il et al. 2006. Phellinsin A from *Phellinus* sp. PL3 exhibits antioxidant activities. *Planta Medica* 76 (6): 572–575.

Hwang, Hye–Jin et al. 2005. Hypoglycemic effect of crude exopolysaccharides produced by a medicinal mushroom *Phellinus baumii* in streptozotocin–induced diabetic rats. *Life Sciences* 76 (26): 3069–3080.

Hyun, Jin Won et al. 1996. Antitumor components of *Agrocybe cylindracea. Archives of Pharmacal Research* 19 (3): 207–212.

Hyun, Kwang Wook et al. 2006. Isolation and characterization of a novel platelet aggregation inhibitory peptide from the medicinal mushroom, *Inonotus obliquus. Peptides* 27 (6): 1173–1178.

Ichikawa et al. 2001. Novel cytokine production inhibitors produced by a Basidiomycete, *Marasmeiellus* sp. *Journal of Antibiotics* 54 (9): 703–709.

Ichimura et al. 1998. Inhibition of HIV–1 protease by water–soluble lignin–like substance from an edible mushroom, *Fuscoporia oblique. Bioscience, Biotechnology, and Biochemistry* 62 (3): 575–577.

Iimura Y, et al. 1997. Isolation of mRNAs induced by a hazardous chemical in white-rot fungi *Coriolus versicolor* by differential display. *FEBS Letters* 412 (2) 370–374.

Ikehata, Keisuke et al. 2004. Optimization of extracellular fungal peroxidase production by 2 *Coprinus* species. *Canadian Journal of Microbiology* 50 (12): 1033–1040.

Ikehata, Keisuke et al. 2005. Purification, characterization and evaluation of extracellular peroxidase from two *Coprinus* species for aqueous phenol treatment. *Bioresource Technology* 96 (16): 1758–1770.

Ikekawa, Tetsuro. 2005. Cancer risk reduction by intake of mushrooms and clinical studies on eem. *International Journal of Medicinal Mushrooms* 7 (3): 347.

Ikekawa, Tetsuro et al. 1968. Antitumor action of some Basidiomycetes, especially *Phellinus litenus. GANN: Japanese Journal of Cancer Research* 59 (2): 155–157.

Ikekawa, Tetsuro et al. 1969. Antitumor activity of aqueous extracts of edible mushrooms. *Cancer Research* 29: 734–735.

Inamori et al. 2008. Antibacterial activity of two chalcones, xanthoangelol and 4–hydroxyderricin, isolated from the root of *Angelica keiskei* (koidzumi). *Chemical & Pharmaceutical Bulletin* 39 (6): 1604–1605.

Inaoka et al. 1994. Studies on active substances in herbs used for hair treatment. I. Effects of herb extracts on hair growth and isolation of an active substance from *Polyporus umbellatus* F. *Chemical and Pharmaceutical Bulletin* 42 (3): 530–533.

Inchausti et al. 1997. Leishmanicidal and trypanocidal activity of extracts and secondary metabolites and Basidiomycetes. *Phytotherapy Research* 11 (3): 193–197.

Ingólfsdóttir, Kristín et al. 1985. In vitro evaluation of the antimicrobial activity of lichen metabolites as potential preservatives. *Antimicrobial Agents and Chemotherapy* 28 (2): 289–292.

Ingólfsdóttir, Kristín et al. 1994. Immunologically active polysaccharide from *Cetraria islandica*. *Planta Medica* 60 (6): 527–531.

Ingólfsdóttir, Kristín et al. 1997a. Biologically active alkamide from the lichen *Stereocaulon alpinum*. *Phytomedicine* 4 (4): 327–330.

Ingólfsdóttir, Kristín et al. 1997b. In vitro susceptibility of *Helicobacter pylori* to protolichesterinic acid from the lichen *Cetraria islandica*. *Antimicrobial Agents and Chemotherapy* 41 (1): 215–217.

Ingólfsdóttir, Kristín et al. 2000. Evaluation of selected lichens from Iceland for cancer chemopreventive and cytotoxic activity. *Pharmaceutical Biology* 38 (4): 313–317.

Ingólfsdóttir, Kristín et al. 2002. Effects of tenuiorin and methyl orsellinate from the lichen *Peltigera leucophlebia* on 5–/15–lipoxygenases and proliferation of malignant cell lines in vitro. *Phytomedicine* 9 (7): 654–658.

Inuzuka et al. 2002. Clinical utility of ABCL (*Agalicus* mushroom extract) treatment for C–type hepatitis. *Japanese Pharmacology and Therapeutics* 30 (2): 103–107.

Isaka et al. 2007. A xanthocillin–like alkaloid from the insect pathogenic fungus *Cordyceps brunnearubra* BCC 1395. *Journal of Natural Products* 70 (4): 656–658.

Ishida, H. et al. 1999. Studies of the active substrates in herbs used for hair treatment. III. Isolation of hair–regrowth substances from *Polygara senega* Var. Latifolia Torr. et Gray. *Biological and Pharmaceutical Bulletin* 22 (11): 12499–1250.

Ishida, M and H. Shinozaki. 1988. Excitatory action of a plant extract, stizolobic acid, in the isolated spinal cord of the rat. *Brain Research* 473 (1): 193–197.

Ishikawa et al. 2001. Antimicrobial cuparene–type sesquiterpenes, enokipodins C and D, from a mycelial culture of *Flammulina velutipes*. *Journal of Natural Products* 64 (7): 932–934.

Ito, H. et al. 1973. Antitumor activity of Basidiomycete polysaccharides. I. Antiumor effect of wild and cultured Basidiomycetes on sarcoma 180 subcutaneously implanted in mice. *Mie Medical Journal* 22 (103–113).

Ito, H. et al. 1976. Antitumor polysaccharide fraction from the culture of *Fomes fomentarius*. *Chemical and Pharmaceutical Bulletin* 24 (10): 2575.

Izawa, Hanako and Yasuo Aoyagi. 2006. Inhibition of angiotensin converting enzyme by mushroom. *Journmal of the Japanese Society for Food Science and Technology* 53 (9): 459–465.

Jang et al. 2007. Xlarinic acids A and B, new antifungal polypropionates from the fruiting body of *Xylaria polymorpha*. *Journal of Antibiotics* 60 (11): 696–699.

Jarosz et al. 1990. Effect of the extracts from fungus *Inonotus obliquus* on catalase level in HeLa and nocardia cells. *Acta Biochimica Polonica* 37 (1) 149–151.

Jasinghe et al. 2006. Vitamin D2 from irradiated mushrooms significantly increases femur bone mineral density in rats. *Journal of Toxicology and Environmental Health A* 69 (21): 1979–1985.

Jauregui et al. 2003. Microsomal transformation of organophosphorus pesticides by white rot fungi. *Biodegradation* 14 (6): 397–406.

Jayasuriya et al. 1998. Clavaric acid: A triterpenoid inhibitor of farnesyl–protein transferase from *Clavariadelphus truncates*. *Journal of Natural Products* 61 (12): 1568–1570.

Jensen et al. 2006. Aeruginascin, a trimethyl-ammnium analogue of psilocybin from the hallucinogenic mushroom *Incocybe aeruginascens*. *Planta Medica* 72 (7): 665–666.

Jeong, Sang–Chul et al. 2004. Production of an anti–complement exo–polymer produced by *Auricularia auricula–judae* in submerged culture. *Biotechnology Letters* 26 (11): 923–927.

Jeong, Sang–Chul et al. 2006. Macrophage–stimulating activity of polysaccharides extracted from fruiting bodies of *Coriolus versicolor* (turkey tail mushroom). *Journal of Medicinal Food* 9 (2): 175–181.

Jeong, W. et al. 2002. Phylogenetic relationships of *Phellinus* and allied taxa based on ITS1–5.8S–ITS2 sequences. *Seventh International Mycological Congress Book of Abstracts* #361.

Jeong, Yong–Tae et al. 2008. *Ganoderma applanatum:* A promising mushroom for antitumor and immunomodulating activity. *Phytotherapy Research* 22 (5): 614–619.

Ji, Deng–Bo et al. 2010. Antiaging effect of *Cordyceps sinensis* extract. *Phytotherapy Research* 23 (1): 116–122.

Jimenez–Romero et al. 2008. Activity against *Plasmodium falciparum* of lactones isolated from the endophytic fungus *Xylaria* sp. *Pharmaceutical Biology* 46 (10–11): 700–703.

Jin, C. Y. et al. 2006. Induction of G2/M arrest and apoptosis in human gastric epithelial AGS cells by aqueous extract of *Agaricus blazei*. *Oncology Reports* 16 (6): 1349–1356.

Jin, H. et al. 1996. Treatment of hypertension by ling zhi combined with hypotensor and its effects on arterial, arteriolar and capillary pressure and microcirculation. *Microcirculatory Approach to Asian Traditional Medicine.* New York: Elsevier Science, 131–138.

Jin, L. et al. 1990. Mineralization of the methoxyl carbon of isolated ligninby brown–rot fungi under solid substrate conditions. *Wood Science and Technology* 24 (3): 263–276.

Jin, Mirim et al. 1996. Induction of B cell proliferation and NF– B activation by a water–soluble glycan from *Lentinus lepideus*. *International Journal of Immunopharmacology* 18(8–9): 439–448.

Jin, Mirim et al. 2003. Activation of selective transcription factors and cytokines by water–soluble extract from *Lentinus lepideus*. *Experimental Biology and Medicine* 228 (6): 749–758.

Jin, S. H. et al. 2003. Effect of *Cryptoporous volvatus* (Peck) Schear on leukotriene production from polymorphonuclear leukocytes in rats. *Zhongguo Zhong Yao Za Zhi* 28 (7): 650–653.

Jin, W. et al. 2006. 5–Alkylresorcinols from *Merulius incarnates. Journal of Natural Products* 69 (4): 704–706.

Jo et al. 2009. Changes in quality of *Phellinus gilvus* mushroom by different drying methods. *Mycoscience* 50 (1): 70–73.

Job, Daniel and Isabelle Schiff–Giovannini. 2004. Influence of strain and substrate formulation of culinary–medicinal maitake mushroom *Grifola frondosa* (Dicks.: Fr.) S.F. Gray (Aphyllophoromycetideae). *International Journal of Medicinal Mushrooms* 6 (1): 73–82.

Johansson et al. 2001. Coprinol, a new antibiotic cuparane from a *Coprinus* species. *Zeitschrift für Naturforschung C* 56 (1): 31–34.

Jonathan et al. 2003. Antimicrobial activities of two Nigerian edible macro–fungi (*Lycoperdon pusilum* (Bat. Ex) and *Lycoperdon giganteum* (Pers.)) *African Journal of Biomedical Research* 6 (1): 85–90.

Jones, Susan and Kainoor K. Janardhanan. 2000. Antioxidant and antitumor activity of *Ganoderma lucidum* (Curt.: Fr.) P. Karst.—reishi (Aphyllophoromycetideae) from south India. *International Journal of Medicinal Mushrooms* 2 (3): 215–220.

Jong, S.C. and M. J. Gantt. 1987. *Catalogue of fuingi and yeasts.* American Type Culture Collection: Rockville, MD.

Jose, Nayana et al. 2002. Antioxidant, anti–inflammatory, and antitumor activities of culinary–medicinal mushroom *Pleurotus pufmonanus* (Fr.) Quel. (Agaricomycetideae). *International Journal of Medicinal Mushrooms* 4 (4): 340–346.

Ju, H. K. et al. 2010. Effect of steam treatment on soluble phenolic content and antioxidant activity of the chaga mushroom *(Inonotus obliquus)*. *Food Chemistry* 119 (2): 619–625.

Jung et al. 2005. Inhibitory effects of *Ganoderma applanatum* on rat lens aldose reductase and sorbitol accumulation in streptozotocin–induced diabetic rat tissues. *Phytotherapy Research* 19 (6): 477–480.

Kahlos, K. et al. 1989. Antitumour activity of some extracts and compounds from *Inonotus radiatus*. *Fitoterapia* 60 (2): 166–168.

Kahlos, K. et al. 1996. Preliminary test of antiviral activity of two *Inonotus obliquus* strains. *Fitoterapia* 67 (4): 344–347.

Kamasuka et al. 1968. Antitumor activity of polysaccharide fractions prepared from some strains of Basidiomycetes. *GANN: Japanese Journal of Cancer Research* 59 (5): 443–445.

Kameda, Y. et al. 1978. Antitumor activity of *Bacillus natto*. VI. Analysis of cytolytic activity on Ehrlich ascites carcinoma cells in the culture medium of *Bacillus natto* KMD 1126. *Yakugaku Zasshi* 98 (10): 1432–1435.

Kamo, Tsunashi et al. 2003. Anti–inflammatory lanostane–type triterpene acids from *Piptoporus betulinus*. *Journal of Natural Products* 66 (8): 1104–1106.

Kamo, Tsunashi et al. 2004a. Anti–inflammatory cyathane diterpenoids from *Sarcodon scabrosus*. *Bioscience, Biotechnology, and Biochemistry* 68 (6): 1362–1365.

Kamo, Tsunashi et al. 2004b. Geranylgeraniol–type diterpenoids, boletinins A–J, from *Boletinus cavipes* as inhibitors of superoxide anion generation in macrophage cells. *Journal of Natural Products* 67 (6): 958–963.

Kanamoto et al. 2001. Anti–human immunodeficiency virus activity of YK–FH312 (a betulinic acid derivative), a novel compound blocking viral maturation. *Antimicrobial Agents and Chemotherapy* 45 (4): 1225–1230.

Kandefer–Szerszen et al. 1974. Ether extracts from the fruiting body of *Piptoporus betulinus* as interference inducers. *Acta Microbiologia Polonica* 6 (2): 197–200.

Kandefer–Szerszen et al. 1979. Fungal nucleic acids as interferon inducers. *Acta Microbiologia Polonica* 28 (4): 277–291.

Kang, Hahk–Soo et al. 2007. Cyathusals A, B, and C, antioxidants from the fermented mushroom *Cyathus stercoreus*. *Journal of Natural Products* 70 (6): 1043–1045.

Kang, Tai Hyun et al. 1999. Protective effects of the water extracts of herbal medicine on BNL CL.2 cells. *Korean Journal of Pharmacognosy* 30 (2): 222–225.

Kanmatsuse, K. et al. 1985. Studies on *Ganoderma lucidum*. I. Efficacy against hypertension and side effects. *Yakugaku Zasshi*. 105 (10): 942–947.

Kantola et al. 2009. Early molecular adsorbents recirculating system treatment of *Amanita* mushroom poisoning. *Therapeutic Apheresis and Dialysis* 13 (5): 399–403.

Karaman, Maja et al. 2009a. Antibacterial properties of selected lignicolous mushrooms and fungi from northern Serbia. *International Journal of Medicinal Mushrooms*. 11 (3): 269–279.

Karaman, Maja et al. 2009b. Biological activities of the lignicolous fungus *Meripulus giganteus* (Pers.: Pers.) Karst. *Archives of Biological Sciences* 61 (4): 853–861.

Kasatkina, T. B. et al. 1980. Development of higher fungi under weightlessness. *Life Sciences and Space Research* 18: 205–211.

Kathirgamanathar et al. 2006. Chemistry and bioactivity of Physciaceae lichens *Pyxine consocians* and *Heterodermia leucomelos*. *Pharmaceutical Biology* 44 (3): 217–220.

Kawabe, Tatsuya and Hideo Morita. 1994. Production of benzaldehyde and benzyl alcohol by the mushroom *Polyporus tuberaster* K2606. *Journal of Agricultural and Food Chemistry* 42 (11): 2556–2560.

Kawagishi, Hirokazu et al. 1988. Isolation and properties of a lectin from the fruiting bodies of *Agaricus blazei*. *Carbohydrate Research* 183 (1): 150–154.

Kawagishi, Hirokazu et al. 1991. Hericenones C, D and E, stimulators of nerve growth factor (NGF)–synthesis, from the mushroom *Hericium erinaceum*. *Tetahedron Letters* 32 (35): 4561–4564.

Kawagishi, Hirokazu et al. 1994. Erinacines A, B

and C, strong stimulators of nerve growth factor (NGF)–synthesis, from the mycelia of *Hericium erinaceum. Tetahedron Letters* 35 (10): 1569–1572.

Kawagishi, Hirokazu et al. 1995. Mushroom lectins. *Food Reviews International* 11 (1): 63–68.

Kawagishi, Hirokazu et al. 1996. A pyradine–derivative from the mushroom *Albatrellus confluens. Phytochemistry* 42 (2): 547–548.

Kawagishi, Hirokazu et al. 2002. Novel hydroquinone as a matrix metallo–proteninase inhibitor from the mushroom *Piptoporus betulinus. Bioscience, Biotechnology, Biochemistry* 66(12): 2748–2750.

Kawagishi, Hirokazu et al. 2004a. The anti–dementia effect of lion's mane mushroom and its clinical application – *Hericium erinaceum* – lion's mane. *Townsend Letter for Doctors & Patients* 249: 54–56.

Kawagishi, Hirokazu et al. 2004b. Estrogenic substances from the mycelia of medicinal fungus *Cordyceps ophioglossoides* (Ehrh.) Fr. (Ascomycetes). *International Journal of Medicinal Mushrooms* 6 (3): 255–259.

Kawagishi, Hirokazu et al. 2007. Novel bioactive compound from the *Sparassis crispa* mushroom. *Bioscience, Biotechnology, and Biochemistry* 71(7): 1804–1806.

Kawakami et al. 2002. TNF– and NO production from macrophages is enhanced through up–regulation of NF– B by polysaccharides purified from *Agaricus blazei* Murrill. *Seventh International Mycological Congress Book of Abstracts* #172.

Kawecki et al. 1978. Studies of RNA isolated from *Piptoporus betulinus* as interferon inducer. *Archivum Immunologiae et Therapiae Experimentalis* 26 (1–6): 517–522.

Keller, C. et al. 2002. Screening of European fungi for antibacterial, antifungal, larvicidal, molluscicidal, antioxidant and free–radical scavenging activities and subsequent isolation of bioactive compounds. *Pharmaceutical Biology* 40 (7): 518–525.

Keller, F. A. et al. 2003. Microbial pretreatment of biomass: Potential for reducing severity of ther-mochemical biomass pretreatment. *Applied Biochemistry and Biotechnology* 105 (1–3): 27–41.

Keller, S. et al. 1996. Structure elucidation of auxofuran, a metabolite involved in stimulating growth of fly agaric, produced by the mycorrhiza helper bacterium *Streptomyces* AcH 505. *Journal of Antibiotics* 59 (12): 801–803.

Kelner, Michael J. et al. 2002. Enhanced antitumor activity of irofulven in combination with thiotepa or mitomycin C. *Cancer Chemotherapy and Pharmacology* 49 (5): 412–418.

Kennedy et al. 1990. Comparative biodegradation of alkyl halide insecticides by the white rot fungus, *Phanerochaete chrysosporium. American Society for Microbiology* 56 (8): 2347–2353.

Kent et al. 2003. Edible mushroom (*Agaricus bisporus*) lectin modulates human retinal pigment epithelial cell behaviour in vitro. *Experimental Eye Research* 76 (2): 213–219.

Kerrigan, Richard W. 2005. *Agaricus subrufescens,* a cultivated edible and medicinal mushroom, and its synonyms. *Mycologia* 97 (1): 12–14.

Khadrani, A. et al. 1999. Degradation of three phenylurea herbicides (chlortoluron, isoproturon and diuron) by Micromycetes isolated from soil. *Chemosphere* 38 (13): 3041–3050.

Khanna et al. 1965. Atromentin, anticoagulant from *Hydnelum diabolus. Journal of Pharmaceutical Sciences* 54 (7): 1016–1020.

Khoo K.–M. and Y.–P. Ting. 2001. Biosorption of gold by immobilized fungal biomass. *Biochemical Engineering Journal* 8 (1): 51–59.

Kiho, Tasashi et al. 1994. Structural features and hypoglycemic activities of two polysaccharides from a hot–water extract of *Agrocybe cylindracea. Carbohydrate Research* 251 (1): 81–87.

Kiho, Tasashi et al. 2000. Structural features of an anti–diabetic polysaccharide (TAP) from *Tremella aurantia. Chemical Pharmaceutical Bulletin* 48 (11): 1793–1795.

Kiho, Tasashi et al. 2010. Effect of polysaccharides and 70% ethanol extracts from medicinal mushrooms on growth of human prostate cancer LNCaP and PC–3 cells. *International Journal of Medicinal Mushrooms* 12 (2): 205–211.

Killermann, S. 1938. Ehemalige Apotheke Pilze. *Zeitschrift für Pilzkunde* 22 (1): 11–13

Kim, Chun Sung et al. 2008. *Cordyceps militaris* induces the IL–18 expression via its promoter activation for IFN– production. *Journal of Ethnopharmacology* 120 (3): 266–371.

Kim, Dong Hyun et al. 1996. Anti–*Helicobacter pylori* activity of mushrooms. *Archives of Pharmacal Research* 19 (6): 447–449.

Kim, Dong Hyun et al. 2001. Production of a hypoglycemic, extracellular polysaccharide from the submerged culture of the mushroom, *Phellinus linteus. Biotechnology Letters* 23 (7): 513–517.

Kim, Eun Mi et al. 2001. Purification, structure determination and biological activities of 20(29)–lupin–3–one from *Daedaleopsis tricolor* (Bull. ex Fr.) Bond. et Sing. *Bulletin of the Korean Chemical Society* 22 (1): 59–62.

Kim, Gi Young et al. 2005. Effect of water–soluble proteoglycan isolated from *Agaricus blazei* on the maturation of murine bone marrow–derived dendritic cells. *International Immunopharmacology* 5 (10): 1523–1532.

Kim, Ha Won et al. 2000. *Ganoderma lucidum* (Curt.: Fr.) P. Karst. (Aphyllophoromycetideae) inhibits proliferation of human peripheral blood lymphocytes by blocking interleukin–2 secretion. *International Journal of Medicinal Mushrooms* 2 (4): 313–321.

Kim, Ho Gyoung et al. 2006. Cordycepin inhibits lipopolysaccharide–induced inflammation by the suppression of NF– B through AKT and P38 inhibition in RAW 264.7 macrophage cells. *European Journal of Pharmacology* 545 (2–3): 192–199.

Kim, Ho Gyoung et al. 2007. Ethanol extract of *Inonotus obliquus* inhibits lipopolysaccharide–induced inflammation in RAW 264.7 macrophage cells. *Journal of Medicinal Food.* 10 (1): 80–89.

Kim, Hwan Mook et al. 1996. Stimulation of humoral and cell mediated immunity by polysaccharide from mushroom *Phellinus linteus. International Journal of Immunopharmacology* 18 (5): 295–303.

Kim, Hyun–Jeong amd Kap–Rang Lee. 2003. Effect of *Ramaria botrytis* methanol extract on antioxidant enzyme activities in benzopyrene–treated mice. *Korean Journal of Food Science Technology* 354: 286–290.

Kim, Hyung Sook et al. 2010. Cordlan polysaccharide isolated from mushroom *Cordyceps militaris* induces dendritic cell maturation through toll–like receptor 4 signalings. *Food and Chemical Toxicology* 48 (7): 1926–1933.

Kim, Jeong Ah et al. 2008. NF– B inhibitory activity of compounds isolated from *Cantharellus cibarius. Phytotherapy Research* 22 (8): 1104–1106.

Kim, Jeong Hyun et al. 2004. Polyozellin isolated from *Polyozellus multiplex* induces phase 2 enzymes in mouse hepatoma cells and differentiation in human myeloid Leukaemic cell lines. *Journal of Agricultural and Food Chemistry* 52 (3): 451–455.

Kim, Jin Woo et al. 2006. Free radical–scavenging delta–lactones from *Boletus calopus. Planta Medica* 72 (15): 1431–1432.

Kim, Jong Hyun et al. 2008. Molecular characterization of regulatory genes associated with biofilm variation in a *Staphylococcus aureus* strain. *Journal of Microbial Biotechnology* 18 (1): 28–34.

Kim, Min Young et al. 2008. Phenolic compound concentration and antioxidant activities of edible and medicinal mushrooms from Korea. *Journal of Agricultural and Food Chemistry* 56 (16): 7265–7270.

Kim, Moo Sung et al. 2006. Antithrombotic activity of methanolic extract of *Umbilicaria esculenta. Journal of Ethnopharmacology* 105 (3): 342–345.

Kim, Moo Sung et al. 2007. Melanogenesis inhibitory effects of methanolic extracts *of Umbilicaria esculenta* and *Usnea longissima. Journal of Microbiology* 45 (6): 578–582.

Kim, Sun Kyung et al. 2008. *Armillariella mellea* induces maturation of human dendritic cells without induction of cytokine expression. *Journal of Ethnopharmacology* 119 (1): 153–159.

Kim, Sung In et al. 2009. Cooperative effect of the lipopolysaccharide and culinary–medicinal cauliflower mushroom *Sparassis crispa* (Wulf.) Fr. (Aphyllophoromycetideae)–derived –glucan on inflammatory cytokine secretion by the murine macrophage cell line. *International Journal of Medicinal Mushrooms* 11 (1): 9–20.

Kim, Won Gon et al. 1997. New indole derivatives with free radical scavenging activity from *Agrocybe cylindracea*. *Journal of Natural Products* (60) 7: 721–723.

Kim, Yea Woon et al. 2005. Anti–diabetic activity of –glucans and their enzymatically hydrolyzed oligosaccharides from *Agaricus blazei*. *Biotechnology Letters* 27 (7): 483–487.

Kim, Yong Ook et al. 2005. Immuno–stimulating effect of the endo–polysaccharide produced by submerged culture of *Inonotus obliquus*. *Life Sciences* 77 (19): 2438–2456.

Kim, Young–So et al. Antiherpetic activities of acidic protein bound polysacchride isolated from *Ganoderma lucidum* alone and in combinations with interferons. *Journal of Ethnopharmacology* 72 (3): 451–458.

Kim, Young Sook et al. 2010. Induction of ICAM–1 by *Armillariella mellea* is mediated through generation of reactive oxygen species and JNK activation. *Journal of Ethnopharmacology* 128 (1): 198–205.

Kimura, C. et al. 2005. –hydroxyergothioneine, a new ergothioneine derivative from the mushroom *Lyophyllum connatum,* and its protective activity against carbon tetrachloride–induced injury in primary culture hepatocytes. *Bioscience, Biotechnology, and Biochemistry* 69 (2): 357–363.

Kimura, Yo et al. 1994. Clinical evaluation of sizofilan as assistant immunotherapy in treatment of head and neck cancer. *Acta Oto–Laryngologica* 114 (S511):

Kimura, Yoshiyuki and Kimiye Baba. 2003. Antitumor and antimetastatic activities of *Angelica keiskei* roots, part 1: Isolation of an active substance, xanthoangelol. *International Journal of Cancer* 106 (3): 429–437.

King, Anna and Roy Watling. 1997. Paper made from bracket fungi. *Mycologist* 11 (2): 52–54.

Kitamura et al. 1994. An antitumor, branched (13)– –d–glucan from a water extract of fruiting bodies of *Cryptoporus volvatus*. *Carbohydrate Research* 263 (1): 111–121.

Kneifel et al. 1977. Ophiocordin, an antifungal antibiotic of *Cordyceps ophioglossoides*. *Archives of Microbiology* 113 (1–2): 121–130.

Ko, Han Gyu et al. 2005a. Comparative study of mycelial growth and basidiomata formation in seven different species of the edible mushroom genus *Hericium*. *Bioresource Technology* 96 (13): 1439–1444.

Ko, Han Gyu et al. 2005b. Detection and recovery of hydrolytic enzymes from spent compost of four mushroom species. *Folia Microbiology* 50 (2): 103–6.

Ko, Horng–Huey et al. 2008. Antiinflammatory triterpenoids and steroids from *Ganoderma lucidum* and *G. tsugae*. *Phytochemistry* 69 (1): 234–239.

Ko, Jiunn–Liang et al. 1995. A new fungal immunomodulatory protein, FIP–five isolated from the edible mushroom, *Flammulina velutipes* and its complete amino acid sequence. *European Journal of Biochemistry* 228 (2): 244–249.

Kobayashi, H. et al. 1983. Substrate specificity of a carboxyl proteinase from *Irpex lacteus*. *Agricultural and Biological Chemistry* 47 (8): 1921–1923.

Kobayashi, Yuuki et al. 1994a. Oxidative stress relief for cancer–bearing hosts by the protein–bound polysaccharide of *Coriolus versicolor* QUEL with SOD mimicking activity. *Cancer Biotherapy* 9 (1): 55–62.

Kobayashi, Yuuki et al. 1994b. Suppression of cancer cell growth in vitro by the protein–bound polysaccharide of *Coriolus versicolor* QUEL (PS–K) with SOD mimicking activity. *Cancer Biotherapy* 9 (1): 63–69.

Kobayashi, Yuuki et al. 1994c. Suppressive effects on cancer cell proliferation of the enhancement of superoxide dismutase (SOD) activity associated with the protein–bound polysaccharide of *Coriolus versicolor* QUEL. *Cancer Biotherapy* 9 (2): 171–178.

Kobayashi, Yuuki et al. 1994d. Enhancement of anti–cancer activity of cisdiaminedichloroplatinum by the protein–bound polysaccharide of *Coriolus versicolor* QUEL (PS–K) in vitro. *Cancer Biotherapy* 9 (4): 351–358.

Kobori et al. 2007. Ergosterol peroxide from an edible mushroom suppresses inflammatory responses in RAW264.7 macrophages and growth of HT29 colon adenocarcinoma cells. *British Journal of Pharmacology* 150 (2): 209–219.

Koch, Jacqueline et al. 1998. The influence of extracts of *Tricholomopsis rutilans* (Schff. ex Fr.) Sing. on the binding of LPS to CD14+–cells and on the release of inflammatory mediators. *Phytotherapy Research* 12 (S1): S27–S29.

Koch, Jacqueline et al. 2002. The influence of selected higher Basidiomycetes on the binding of lipopolysaccharide to CD14+–cells and on the release of cytokines. *International Journal of Medicinal Mushrooms* 4 (3): 228–234.

Kodama, Eiichi N. et al. 2000. Antileukemic activity and mechanism of action of cordycepin against terminal deoxynucleotidyl transferase–positive (TdT+) leukemic cells. *Biochemical Pharmacology* 59 (3): 273–281.

Kodama, Noriko et al. 2002. Effects of D–fraction, a polysaccharide from *Grifola frondosa,* on tumor growth involve activation of NK cells. *Biological & Pharmaceutical Bulletin* 25 (12): 1647–1650.

Kodama, Noriko et al. 2010. Effect of a hot water soluble extraction from *Grifola frondosa* on the viability of a human monocyte cell line exposed to mitomycin C. *Myoscience* 51 (2): 134–138.

Kodani et al. 2008. Occurrence and identification of chalcones from the culinary–medicinal cauliflower mushroom *Sparassis crispa* (Wulf.) Fr. (Aphyllophoromycetideae). *International Journal of Medicinal Mushrooms* 10 (4): 331–336.

Kohda, Hiroshi et al. 1985. The biologically active constituents of *Ganoderma lucidum* (Fr.) Karst. Histamine release-inhibitory triterpenes. *Chemical & Pharmaceutical Bulletin* 33 (4): 1367-1374.

Kohlmunzer, S. et al. 1977. Antiinflammatory activity of *Tylopilus felleus* (Bull. ex Fr.) P. Karst. *Polish Journal of Pharmacology* 29 (5): 539–541.

Kohlmunzer, S. et al. 2000. Indole metabolites in mycelial culture of higher fungi. *Herba Polonica* 46 (2): 98–104.

Kokubun, Tetsuo et al. 2007a. Inhibitory activities of lichen–derived compounds against methicillin– and multidrug–resistant *Staphylococcus aureus. Planta Medica* 73 (2): 176–179.

Kokubun, Tetsuo et al. 2007b. Serialynic acid, a new phenol with an isopentenyne side chain from *Antrodia serialis. Journal of Antibiotics* 60 (4): 285–288.

Kolter and Sandhoff 1999. Sphingolipids—their metabolic pathways and the pathobiochemistry of neurodegenerative diseases. *Angewandte Chemie International Edition* 38 (11): 1532–1568.

Komarek et al. 2007. Metal/metalloid contamination and isotopic composition of lead in edible mushrooms and forest soils originating from a smelting area. *Environment International* 33 (5): 677–684.

Komatsu, N. et al. 1963. Flammulin, a basic protein of *Flammulina velutipes* with antitumor activities. *The Journal of Antibiotics* 16: 139–143.

Komatsu, N. et al. 1969. Host–mediated antitumor action of schizophyllan, a glucan produced by *Schizophyllum commune. GANN: Japanese Journal of Cancer Research* 60 (2): 137–144.

Konno, Sensuke et al. 2002. Anticancer and hypoglycemic effects of polysaccharides in edible and medicinal maitake mushroom [*Grifola frondosa*

(Dicks.: Fr.) S. F. Gray]. *International Journal of Medicinal Mushrooms* 4 (3): 187–197.

Koo, Kyo–Chui et al. 2006. Production and characterization of antihypertensive angiotensin I–converting enzyme inhibitor from *Pholiota adiposa*. *Journal of Microbiology and Biotechnology* 16 (5): 757–763.

Kopp et al. 2009. Systemic allergic contact dermatitis due to consumption of raw shiitake mushroom. *Clinical and Experimental Dermatology* 34 (8): 910–913.

Kornillowicz–Kowalska et al. 2005. Extracellular enzyme activities of *Bjerkandera adusta* R59 soil strain, capable of daunomycin and humic acids degradation. *Applied Microbiology and Biotechnology* 68 (5): 686–694.

Kotterman et al. 1998. Polycyclic aromatic hydrocarbon oxidation by the white–rot fungus *Bjerkandera* sp. strain BOS55 in the presence of nonionic surfactants. *Biotechnology and Bioengineering* 57 (2): 220–227.

Koyama, K. et al. 1997. Antinociceptive components of *Ganoderma lucidum*. *Planta Medica* 63: 224–227.

Koyama, Yu et al. 2002. Apoptosis induction by lectin isolated from the mushroom *Boletopsis leucomelas* in U937 cells. *Bioscience, Biotechnology, and Biochemistry* 66 (4): 784–789.

Koyama, Yu et al. 2005. Involvement of G2/M cell cycle arrest and the mitochondrial pathway in *Boletopsis leucomelaena* (Pers.) Fayod (Agaricomycetideae) lectin–induced apoptosis of human leukemia U937 cells. *International Journal of Medicinal Mushrooms* 7 (1–2): 201–212.

Koyyalamudi et al. 2009. Vitamin B12 is the active corrinoid produced in cultivated white button mushrooms *(Agaricus bisporus)*. *Journal of Agricultural and Food Chemistry* 57 (14): 6327–6333.

Krasnopolskaya, Larissa M. et al. 2005. Screening systems for medicinal Basidiomycetes antitumor extracts. *International Journal of Medicinal Mushrooms* 7 (3): 423–425.

Krasnopolskaya, Larissa M. et al. 2008. Antitumor properties of submerged cultivated biomass and extracts of medicinal mushrooms of genus *Hypsizygus* Singer (Agaricomycetideae). *International Journal of Medicinal Mushrooms* 10 (1): 25–35.

Krishna, K. Rama and Ligy Phillip. 2005. Bioremediatiton of CR(VI) in contaminated soils. *Journal of Hazardous Materials* 121 (1–3): 109–117.

Kronberger et al. 1964. Pilzrunde im Bayreuther Raum–Rückblick auf das Jahr. *Festschrift der Naturwissenschaftlichen Gesellschaft Bayreuth* 11 (1): 71–72.

Kruger and Pfeil. 1976. Purification and characterization of peroxidase from *Phellinus igniarius*. *Archives of Microbiology* 109 (1–2): 175–179.

Kubo, M. et al. 1983. *Ganoderma lucidum*. (4) Effects on disseminated intravascular coagulation. *Yakugaku Zasshi* 103 (8): 871-877.

Kukina, Tatyana P. et al. 2005. Mushrooms as a source of polyprenols. *International Journal of Medicinal Mushrooms* 7 (3): 425–426.

Kuo, Michael. 2005. *Inocybe rimosa*. MushroomExpert.com. Accessed May 2, 2011. http://www.mushroomexpert.com/inocybe_rimosa.html

Kuo, Yuh–Chi et al. 1994. Growth inhibitors against tumor cells in *Cordyceps sinensis* other than cordycepin and polysaccharides. *Cancer Investigation* 12 (6): 611–615.

Kurashige, S. et al. 1997. Effects of *Lentinus edodes, Grifola frondosa* and *Pleurotus ostreatus* administration on cancer outbreak, and activities of macrophages and lymphocytes in mice treated with a carcinogen, N-butyl-N-butanolnitrosoamine. *Immunopharmacology and Immunotoxicology* 19 (2): 175–183

Kuvibidila, Solo et al. 2010. Extracts from culinary–medicinal mushrooms increase intracellular –defensins 1–3 concentration in HL60 cells. *International Journal of Medicinal Mushrooms* 12 (1): 33–41.

Kweon et al. 2002. Lowering effects in plasma cholesterol and body weight by mycelial extracts of two mushrooms: *Agaricus blazei* and *Lentinus* edodes. *Korean Journal of Microbiology and Biotechnology* 30 (4): 402–409

Kwok, O. C. H. et al. 1992. A nematicidal toxin from *Pleurotus ostreatus* NRRL 3526. *Journal of Chemical Ecology* 18 (2): 127–136.

Lagaron et al. 2007. Using ATR–FTIR spectroscopy to design active antimicrobial food packaging structures based on high molecular weight chitosan polysaccharide. *Journal of Agricultural and Food Chemistry* 55 (7): 2554–2562.

Lai, Li Kuan et al. 2010. Anti–human papillomavirus (HPV) 16 E6 activity of ling zhi or reishi medicinal mushroom, *Ganoderma lucidum* (W. Curt.: Fr.) P. Karst. (Aphyllophoromycetideae) extracts. *International Journal of Medicinal Mushrooms* 12 (3): 279–286.

Lakkireddy et al. 2006. Comparative studies on the influence of higher–Basidiomycetes polysaccharide fractions on reactive oxidizing species production. *International Journal of Medicinal Mushrooms* 8 (2): 135–148.

Lakshmi et al. 2004. Evaluation of antioxidant activity of selected Indian mushrooms. *Pharmaceutical Biology* 42 (3): 179–185.

Lam, S. K. and Tzi Bun Ng. 2001. Hypsin, a novel thermostable ribosome–inactivating protein with antifungal and antiproliferative activities from fruiting bodies of the edible mushroom *Hypsizigus marmoreus*. *Biochemical and Biophysical Research Communications* 285 (4): 1071–5.

Lau, C. B. S. et al. 2004. Cytotoxic activities of *Coriolus versicolor* (yunzhi) extract on human leukemia and lymphoma cells by induction of apoptosis. *Life Sciences* 75 (7): 797–808.

Laufer, Berthold. 1912. *Jade: A study in Chinese archaeology and religion*. Chicago: Field Museum of Natural History.

Lavi et al. 2006. An aqueous polysaccharide extract from the edible mushroom *Pleurotus ostreatus* induces anti–proliferative and pro–apoptotic effects of HT–29 colon cancer cells. *Cancer Letters* 244 (1): 61–70.

Law, W. M. et al. 2003. Removal of biocide pentachlorophenol in water system by the spent mushroom compost of *Pleurotus pulmonarius*. *Chemosphere* 52 (9): 1531–7.

Lee, Charles C. 2005. Cloning and characterization of the Xyn11A gene from *Lentinula edodes*. *Protein Journal* 24 (1): 21–26.

Lee, Daekyun et al. 2010. HMGB2 stabilizes P53 by interfering with E6/E6AP–mediated p53 degradation in human papillomavirus–positive HeLa cells. *Cancer Letters* 292 (1): 125–132.

Lee, Eun Woo et al. 2000. Suppression of D–galactosamine–induced liver injury by mushrooms in rats. *Bioscience, Biotechnology, and Biochemistry* 64 (9): 2001–2004.

Lee, Haemi et al. 2006. Induction of apoptosis by *Cordyceps militaris* through activation of caspase–3 in leukemia HL–60 cells. *Biological and Pharmaceutical Bulletin* 29 (4): 670–674.

Lee, Hyun Jin et al. 2000. Kynapcin–12, a new P–terphenyl derivative from *Polyozellus multiplex* inhibits prolyl endopeptidase. *Journal of Antibiotics* 53 (7): 714–719.

Lee, In–Kyoung et al. 2002. Dictyoquinazols A, B, and C, new neuroprotective compounds from the mushroom *Dictyophora indusiata*. *Journal of Natural Products* 65 (12): 1769–1772.

Lee, In–Kyoung et al. 2003. Neuroprotective activity of P–terphenyl leucomentins from the mushroom *Paxillus panuoides*. *Bioscience, Biotechnology, and Biochemistry* 67 (8): 1813–1816.

Lee, In–Kyoung et al. 2007. New antioxidant polyphenols from the medicinal mushroom *Inonotus obliquus*. *Bioorganic and Medicinal Chemistry Letters* 17 (24): 6678–6681.

Lee, In–Seon and Akiyoshi Nishikawa. 2003. *Polyozellus multiplex*, a Korean wild mushroom, as a potent chemopreventive agent against stomach cancer. *Life Sciences* 73 (25): 3225–3234.

Lee, Jong–Suk et al. 2008. *Grifola frondosa* (maitake mushroom) water extract inhibits vascular endothelial growth factor–induced angiogenesis through inhibition of reactive oxygen species and extracellular signal–regulated kinase phosphorylation. *Journal of Medicinal Food* 11 (4): 643–651.

Lee, Kyung–Ae and Moo–sung Kim. 2005. Antiplatelet and antithrombotic activities of methanol extract of *Usnea longissima*. *Phytotherapy Research* 19 (12): 1061–1064.

Lee, Kyung–Ae et al. 2005. Hepatoprotective effects of waxy brown rice cultured with *Agrocybe cylindracea* (DC.) Gillet. *International Journal of Medicinal Mushrooms* 7 (3): 351–352.

Lee, Sanghyun et al. 2005. Aldose reductase inhibitors from the fruiting bodies of *Ganoderma applanatum*. *Biological & Pharmaceutical Bulletin* 28 (6): 1103.

Lee, Sang–Il et al. 2008. Antihyperglycemic effect of *Fomitopsis pinicola* extracts in Streptozotocin–induced diabetic rats. *Journal of Medicinal Food* 11 (3): 518–524.

Lee, Shiuh–Sheng et al. 2003. Antitumor effects of polysaccharides *of Ganoderma lucidum* (Curt.: Fr.) P. Karst. (ling zhi, reishi mushroom) (Aphyllophoromycetideae). *International Journal of Medicinal Mushrooms* 5 (1): 1–16.

Lee, Soo–Min et al. 2005. Degradation of bisphenol A by white rot fungi, *Stereum hirsutum* and *Heterobasidium insulare,* and reduction of its estrogenic activity. *Biological & Pharmaceutical Bulletin* 28 (2): 201–207.

Lee, Suan Li et al. 2010. Comparative cytotoxicity and hemagglutination activities of crude protein extracts from culinary–medicinal mushrooms. *International Journal of Medicinal Mushrooms* 12 (2): 213–222.

Lee, Tzong–Huei et al. 2007. A new cytotoxic agent from solid–state fermented mycelium of *Antrodia camphorata*. *Planta Medica* 73 (13): 1412–1414.

Lehmann et al. 2003. Illudin S, the sole antiviral compound in mature fruiting bodies of *Omphalotus illudens*. *Journal of Natural Products* 66 (9): 1257–1258.

Lemieszek, Marta Kinga et al. 2009. Anticancer effect of fraction isolated from medicinal birch polypore mushroom, *Piptoporus betulinus* (Bull.: Fr.) P. Karst. (Aphyllophoromycetideae): In vitro studies. *International Journal of Medicinal Mushrooms* 11 (4): 351–364.

Leon, Francisco et al. 2004. Lanostanoid triterpenes from *Laetiporus sulphureus* and *Apoptosis induction* on HL–60 human myeloid leukemia cells. *Journal of Natural Products* 67 (12): 2008–2011.

Leon, Francisco et al. 2006. Isolation, structure elucidation, total synthesis, and evaluation of new natural and synthetic ceramides on human SK–MEL–1 melanoma cells. *Journal of Medical Chemistry* 49 (19): 5830–5839.

Leon, Francisco et al. 2008. A new ceramide from *Suillus luteus* and its cytotoxic activity against human melanoma cells. *Chemistry & Biodiversity* 5 (1): 120–125.

Leu, Sew–Fen et al. 2005. The in vivo effect of *Cordyceps seninsis* mycelium on plasma corticosterone level in male mouse. *Biological and Pharmaceutical Bulletin* 28 (9): 1722–1725.

Li, J. J. et al. 2000. Inhibitory activity of *Dianthus superbus* L. and 11 kinds of diuretic traditional Chinese medicines for urogenital *Chlamydia trachomatis* in vitro. *Zhongguo Zhong Yao Za Zhi* 25 (10): 628–630.

Li, L. S. et al. 1996. Experimental study on effect of *Cordyceps sinensis* in ameliorating aminoglycoside induced nephrotoxicity. *Zhongguo Zhong Xi Yi Jie He Za Zhi* 16 (12): 733–737.

Li, Le et al. 2005. Correlation of antioxidant activity with content of phenolics in extracts from the culinary–medicinal abalone mushroom *Pleurotus abalones* Han, Chen et Cheng (Agaricomycetideae). *International Journal of Medicinal Mushrooms* 7 (1–2): 237–242.

Li, Peng et al. 2007. Biosynthesis of theobroxide and its related compounds, metabolites of *Lasiodiplodia theobromae*. *Phytochemistry* 68 (6): 819–823.

535

Li, Yan–Ping et al. 2005. Protective effect of *Armillaria mellea* polysaccharide on mice bone marrow cell damage caused by cyclophosphamide. *Zhongguo Zhong Yao Za Zhi* 30 (4): 283–286.

Liang, Yi et al. 2010. A nuclear ligand MRG15 involved in the proapoptotic activity of medicinal fungal galectin AAL (*Agrocybe aegerita* lectin). *Biochimica et Biophysica Acta* 1800 (4): 474–480.

Lim, Hyun–Woo et al. 2007. Free radical–scavenging and inhibition of nitric oxide production by four grades of pine mushroom (*Tricholoma matsutake* Sing.). *Food Chemistry* 103 (4): 1337–1342.

Lim, Jong–Min and Jong–Won Yun. 2006. Enhanced production of exopolysaccharides by supplementation of toluene in submerged culture of an edible mushroom *Collybia maculata* TG–1. *Process Biochemistry* 41 (7): 1620–1626.

Lin, Ronghui et al. 2009. Synthesis and evaluation of 2,7–diamino–thiazolo [4,5–D] pyrimidine analogues as anti–tumor epidermal growth factor receptor (EGFR) tyrosine kinase inhibitors. *Bioorganic & Medicinal Chemistry Letters* 19 (8): 2333–2337.

Lin, Wen–Huei et al. 1997. Dimerization of the N–terminal amphipathic –helix domain of the fungal immunomodulatory protein from *Ganoderma tsugae* (fip–gts) defined by a yeast two–hybrid system and site–directed mutagenesis. *Journal of Biological Chemistry* 272 (32): 20044–20048.

Lin, Wen–Hung et al. 2007. Improvement of sperm production in subfertile boars by *Cordyceps militaris* supplement. *American Journal of Chinese Medicine* 35 (4): 631–641.

Lin, X. X. et al. 2001. Effects of fermented *Cordyceps* powder on pulmonary in sensitized guinea pigs and airway inflammation in sensitized rats. *Zhongguo Zhong Yao Za Zhi* 26 (9): 622–625.

Lindequist, U. et al. 1989. Untersuchungen zur antiviralen Wirksamkeit von Ergosterolperoxid. *Pharmazie* 44: 579–580.

Lingham et al. 1998. Clavaric acid and steroidal analogues as RAS– and FPP–directed inhibitors of human farnesyl–protein transferase. *Journal of Medicinal Chemistry* 41 (23): 4492–4501.

List et al. 1957. Über das Vorkommen von Ergothionein im Schopftintling, *Coprinus comatus*. *Archiv der Pharmazie* 290 (11): 517–520.

Liu, Dong–Ze et al. 2007. A new cadinane sesquiterpene with significant anti–HIV–1 activity from the cultures of the Basidiomycete *Tyromyces chioneus*. *The Journal of Antibiotics* 60 (5): 332–334.

Liu, Dong–Ze et al. 2008. A new spiroaxane sesquiterpene from cultures of the Basidiomycete *Pholiota adiposa*. *Zeitschrift für Naturforschung B* 63 (1): 111–113.

Liu, Jikai. 2002. Biologically active substances from mushrooms in Yunnan, China. *Heterocycles* 57 (1): 157–167.

Liu, Jikai et al. 2004. DPPH radical scavenging activity of ten natural p–terphenyl derivatives obtained from three edible mushrooms indigenous to China. *Chemistry & Biodiversity* 1 (4): 601–605.

Liu, Qinghong et al. 2004. Isolation and characterization of a novel lectin from the wild mushroom *Xerocomus spadiceus*. *Peptides* 25 (1): 7–10.

Liu, Qinghong et al. 2006. First report of a xylose–specific lectin with potent hemagglutinating, antiproliferative and anti–mitogenic activities from a wild Ascomycete mushroom. *Biochimica et Biophysica Acta* 1760 (12): 1914–1919.

Liu, Xue–Ting et al. 2010. Antibacterial compounds from mushrooms I: A lanostane–type triterpene and prenylphenol derivatives from *Jahnoporus hirtus* and *Albatrellus flettii* and their activities against *Bacillus cereus* and *Enterococcus faecalis*. *Planta Medica* 76 (2): 182–185.

Liu, Y. Y. and S. X. Guo 2009. Nutritional factors determining sclerotial formation of *Polyporus umbellatus*. *Letters in Applied Microbiology*. 49 (2): 283–288.

Liu, Ya–Jun and Ke–Qin Zhang. 2004. Antimicrobial activities of selected *Cyathus* species. *Mycopathologia* 157 (2): 185–189.

References

Liu, Ying et al. 2007. Immunomodulating activity of *Agaricus brasiliensis* KA21 in mice and in human volunteers. *Evidence–Based Complementary and Alternative Medicine* 5 (2): 205–219.

Liu, Yu et al. 2002. Synthesis of organoselenium–modified –cyclodextrins possessing a 1,2–benzisoselenazol–3(2H)–one moiety and their enzyme–mimic study. *Helvetica Chimic Acta* 85 (1): 9–18.

Lo, Hui–Chen et al. 2004. The anti–hyperglycemic activity of the fruiting body of *Cordyceps* in diabetic rats induced by nicotinamide and streptozotocin. *Life Sciences* 74 (23): 2897–2908.

Lo, Hui–Chen et al. 2005. Effects of *Tremella mesenterica* on steroidogenesis in MA–10 mouse Leydig tumor cells. *Archives of Andrology* 51 (4): 285–294.

Lo, Tiffany Chien Ting et al. 2007. Pressurized water extraction of polysaccharides as secondary metabolites from *Lentinula edodes. Journal of Agricultural and Food Chemistry* 55 (10): 4196–4201.

Lorenzen, K. and Anke, T. 1998. Basidiomycetes as a source for new bioactive natural products. *Current Organic Chemistry* 2 (4): 329–364.

Lovy, A. et al. 1999. Activity of edible mushrooms against the growth of human T4 leukemia cancer cells and *Plasmodium falciparum. Journal of Herbs, Spices and Medicinal Plants.* 6 (4): 49–57.

Lu, L. 2002. Study on effect of *Cordyceps sinensis* and artemisinin in preventing recurrence of lupus nephritis. *Zhongguo Zhong Xi Yi Jie He Za Zhi* 22 (3): 169–171.

Lu, Mei–Kuang et al. 2006. Adenosine as an active component of *Antrodia cinnamomea* that prevents rat PC12 cells from serum deprivation–induced apoptosis through the activation of adenosine A2A receptors. *Life Sciences* 79 (3): 252–258.

Lu, Wei et al. 1985. Platelet aggregation potentiators from cho–rei. *Chemical and Pharmaceutical Bulletin* 33 (11): 5083–5087.

Lu, Xueming et al. 2010. Phytochemical characteristics and hypoglycaemic activity of fraction from mushroom *Inonotus obliquus. Journal of the Science of Food and Agriculture* 90 (2): 276–280.

Lubken et al. 2004. Hygrophorones A–G: Fungicidal cyclopentenones from *Hygrophorus* species (Basidiomycetes). *Phytochemistry* 65 (8): 1061–1071.

Lucas, E. H. et al. 1957. Tumor inhibitors in *Boletus edulis* and other Holobasidiomycetes. *Antibiotics & Chemotherapy* 7 (1): 1–4.

Lull, Cristina et al. 2005. Antiinflammatory and immunomodulating properties of fungal metabolites. *Mediators of Inflammation* 2005 (2): 63–80.

Lung, Ming–Yeou and Jie–Ching Tsai. 2009. Antioxidant properties of polysaccharides from the willow bracket medicinal mushroom, *Phellinus igniarius* (L.) Quel. (Aphyllophoromycetideae) in submerged culture. *International Journal of Medicinal Mushrooms* 11 (4): 383–394.

Luo, Du–Qiang et al. 2005. Activity in vitro and in vivo against plant pathogenic fungi of grifolin isolated from the Basidiomycete *Albatrellus dispansus. Zeitschrift für Naturforschung C* 60 (1): 50–56.

Luo, Hong et al. 2004. *Coprinus comatus:* A Basidiomycete fungus forms novel spiny structures and infects nematode. *Mycologia* 96 (6): 1218–1224.

Luo, Yangchao et al. 2009. Evaluation of antioxidative and hypolipidemic properties of a novel functional diet formulation of *Auricularia auricula* and hawthorn. *Innovative Food Science & Emerging Technologies* 10 (2): 215–221.

Lutzoni et al. 2001. Major fungal lineages are derived from lichen symbiotic ancestors. *Nature* 411 (6840): 937–1940.

Ma, Bing–Ji et al. 2005. An unusual nitrogenous terphenyl derivative from fruiting bodies of the Basidiomycete *Sarcodonn scabrosus. Zeitschrift für Naturforschung B* 60 (1): 565–568.

Ma, Bing–Ji et al. 2007. *Trametes versatilis,* a fungus highly producing eburicoic acid. *Zeitschrift für Naturforschung C* 62 (11–12): 909.

Ma, Wenzhe et al. 2004. Two new biologically

active illudane sesquiterpenes from the mycelial cultures of *Panaeolus retirugis*. *Journal of Antibiotics* 57 (11): 721–725.

Madley, Rebecca H. 2001. Medicinal mushrooms: A light in the dark. *Nutraceuticals World* October 2001.

Magnus et al. 1989. Conversion of indole–3–ethanol to fatty acid esters in *Craterellus cornucopioides*. *Phytochemistry* 28 (11): 2949–2954.

Mallick, Sanjaya Kumar et al. 2009. Macrophage stimulation by polysaccharides isolated from barometer earthstar mushroom, *Astraeus hygrometricus* (Pers.) Morgan (Gasteromycetideae). *International Journal of Medicinal Mushrooms* 11 (3): 237–248.

Mallick, Sanjaya Kumar et al. 2010. Antitumor properties of a heteroglucan isolated from *Astraeus hygrometricus* on Dalton's lymphoma bearing mouse. *Food and Chemical Toxicology* 48 (8–9): 2115–2121.

Manez et al. 1997. Effect of selected triterpenoids on chronic dermal inflammation. *European Journal of Pharmacology* 334 (1): 103–105.

Mannick, Elizabeth E. et al. 1996. Inducible nitric oxide synthase, nitrotyrosine, and apoptosis in *Helicobacter pylori* gastritis: Effect of antibiotics and antioxidants. *Cancer Research* 56 (14): 3238–3243.

Manojlovic, Nedeljko T. et al. 2005a. Antifungal activity of *Rubia tinctorum*, *Rhamnus frangula* and *Caloplaca cerina*. *Fitoterapia* 76 (2): 244–246.

Manojlovic, Nedeljko T. et al. 2005b. Antimicrobial metabolites from three Serbian *Caloplaca*. *Pharmaceutical Biology* 43 (8): 718–722.

Mao, Hui–Ling et al. 2007. Study on the extraction process of polysaccharide from *Agrocybe cylindracea*. *Zhong Yao Cai* 30 (2): 217–220.

Mao, Xian–Bing and Jian–Jiang Zhong. 2004. Hyperproduction of cordycepin by two–stage dissolved oxygen control in submerged cultivation of medicinal mushroom *Cordyceps militaris* in bioreactors. *Biotechnology Progress* 20 (5): 1408–1413.

Mao, Xiaolan. 1998. Economic fungi of China. Beijing: China Scientific Book Services.

Markhija, A. N. and J. M. Bailey et al. 1981. Identification of the antiplatelet substance in Chinese black tree fungus. *The New England Journal of Medicine* 304 (3): 175–176.

Marles, Robin J. and N. R. Farnsworth. 1995. Antidiabetic plants and their active constituents. *Phytomedicine* 2 (2): 137–189.

Maruyama, H. and T. Ikekawa. 2005. Combination therapy of transplanted meth–A fibrosarcoma in BALB/C mice with protein–bound polysaccharide EA6 isolated from enokitake mushroom *Flammunlina yelutipes* (W.Curt.: Fr.) Singer and surgical excision. *International Journal of Medicinal Mushrooms* 7 (1–2): 213–220.

Masaphy, S. et al. 1996. Degradation of atrazine by the lignocellulolytic fungus *Pleurotus pulmonarius* during solid–state fermentation. *Bioresource Technology* 56 (2–3): 207–214.

Masuda, Yuki et al. 2006. Macrophage J774.1 cell is activated by MZ–fraction (Klasma–MZ) polysaccharide in *Grifola frondosa*. *Mycoscience* 47 (6): 360–366.

Mata et al. 2001. Selection of strains of *Lentinula edodes* and *Lentinula boryana* adapted for efficient mycelial growth on wheat straw. *Iberoamericana de Micologia* 18 (3): 118–122.

Matsuda, M. et al. 1996. Laccarin, a new alkaloid from the mushroom, *Laccaria vinaceoavellanea*. *Heterocycles* 43 (3): 685–690.

Matsunaga, K. et al. 2003. Mass production of matsutake *(Tricholoma matsutake)* mycelia and its application to functional foods. *Bioindustry* 20 (1): 37–46.

Matsushima, Y. et al. 2009. Effects of *Psilocybe argentipes* on marble–burying behavior in mice. *Bioscience, Biotechnology, and Biochemistry* 73 (8): 1866–1868.

Matsushita, K. et al. 1998. ONO–4007 induces specific anti–tumor immunity mediated by tumor necrosis factor–alpha. *Anti–Cancer Drugs* 9 (3): 273–282.

References

Matsuura, Masanori et al. 2009. Idenitification of the toxic trigger in mushroom poisoning. *Nature Chemical Biology* 5 (7): 465–467.

Matsuzawa, Tsunetomo. 2006. Studies on antioxidant effects of culinary–medicinal bunashimeji mushroom *Hypsizygus marmoreus* (Peck) Bigel. (Agaricomycetideae). *International Journal of Medicinal Mushrooms* (8) 3: 245–250.

Mau, Jeng–Leun and Yu–Hsiu Teng. 1998. Nonvolatile taste components of three strains of *Agrocybe cylindracea*. *Journal of Agricultural and Food Chemistry* 46 (6): 2071–2074.

Mau, Jeng–Leun et al. 1998. Ultraviolet irradiation increased vitamin D2 content in edible mushrooms. *Journal of Agricultural and Food Chemistry* 46 (12): 5269–5272.

Mau, Jeng–Leun et al. 2002. Antioxidant properties of several medicinal mushrooms. *Journal of Agricultural and Food Chemistry* 50 (21): 6072–6077.

Mau, Jeng–Leun et al. 2004. Antioxidant properties of methanolic extracts from *Grifola frondosa, Morchella esculenta* and *Termitomyces albuminosus* mycelia. *Food Chemistry* 87 (1): 111–118.

Mavoungou, H et al. 1987. Anti–tumor activity of mycelia of *Agrocybe dura, Mycoacia uda* and *Phanerochaete laevis*. *Annales Pharmaceutiques Francaises* 45 (1): 71–77.

Mayell, M. 2001. Maitake extracts and their therapeutic potential: A review. *Alternative Medicine Review* 6 (1): 48–60.

McCay, Paul H. et al. Effect of subinhibitory concentrations of benzalkonium chloride on the competitiveness of Pseudomonas aeruginosa grown in continuous culture. *Microbiology* 156 (1): 30–38.

McMorris, Travor C. et al. 1999. Metabolism of antitumor acylfulvene by rat liver cytosol. *Biochemical Pharmacology* 57 (1): 83–88.

Meena et al. 2009. Antiarthritic activity of a polysaccharide–protein complex isolated from *Phellinus rimosus* (Berk.) Pilat (Aphyllophoromycetideae) in Freund's complete adjuvant–induced arthritic rats. *International Journal of Medicinal Mushrooms* 11 (1): 21–28.

Meisch et al. 1986. Characterization studies on cadmium–mycophosphatin from the mushroom *Agaricus macrosporus*. *Environmental Health Perspectives* 65: 29–32.

Melzig, M. F. et al. 1996. Screening of selected Basidiomycetes for inhibitory activity on neutral endopeptidase (NEP) and angiotensin–converting enzyme (ACE). *Pharmazie* 51 (7): 501–503.

Menser, Gary. 1977. *Hallucinogenic and poisonous mushroom field guide.* Berkeley: And/Or Press.

Mentel et al. 1994. In vitro antiviral effect of extracts of *Kuehneromyces mutabilis* on influenza virus. *Die Pharmazie* 49 (11): 859–860.

Michniewicz et al. 2005. The white–rot fungus *Cerrena unicolor* strain 137 produces two laccase isoforms with different physico–chemical and catalytic properties. *Applied Microbiology and Biotechnology* 69 (6): 682–686.

Mierau et al. 2003. Dacrymenone and VM 3298–2: New antibiotics with antibacterial and antifungal activity. *Zeitschrift für Naturforschung C* 58 (7–8): 533.

Mikiashvili, Nona A. and Omoanghe S. Isikhuemhen. 2009. Productivity and nutritional content of culinary–medicinal oyster mushroom *Pleurotus ostreatus* (Jacq.: Fr.) P. Kumm. (Agaricomycetideae) fruit bodies cultivated on substrates containing solid waste from anaerobic digested poultry litter. *International Journal of Medicinal Mushrooms* 11 (2): 207–213.

Mikiashvili, Nona A. et al. 2004. Lignocellulolytic enzyme activities of medicinally important Basidiomycetes from different ecological niches. *International Journal of Medicinal Mushrooms* 6 (1): 63–72.

Milton, J. M. et al. 1992. *Lepista nebularis:* Producer of nebularine. *The Mycologist* 6 (1): 44–45.

Mimura, H. et al. 1985. Purification, antitumor activity, and structural characterization of –1,3–glucan from *Peziza vesiculosa*. *Chemical & Pharmaceutical Bulletin* 33 (11): 5096–5099.

Min et al. 2000. Triterpenes from the spores of *Ganoderma lucidum* and their cytotoxicity against meth–A and LLC tumor cells. *Chemical and Pharmaceutical Bulletin* 48 (7): 1026–1033.

Misaki et al. 1981. Studies on interrelation of structure and antitumor effects of polysaccharides: Antitumor action of periodate–modified, branched (1 3)– –image–glucan of *Auricularia auricula–judae,* and other polysaccharides containing (1 3)–glycosidic linkages. *Carbohydrate Research* 92 (1): 115–129.

Miura et al. 2002. Systemic inflammatory response associated with augmentation and activation of leukocytes in *Candida*/indomethacin administered mice. *Biological & Pharmaceutical Bulletin* 25 (6): 816–822.

Mizuno, Masashi et al. 1999. Anti–tumor polysaccharide from the mycelium of liquid–cultured *Agaricus blazei* Murill. *International Union of Biochemistry and Molecular Biology* 47 (4): 707–714.

Mizuno, Takashi. 1999. The extraction and development of antitumor active polysaccharides from medicinal mushrooms in Japan (review). *International Journal of Medicinal Mushrooms* 1 (4): 9–30.

Mizuno, Takashi. 2000. Development of an antitumor biological response modifier from *Phellinus linteus* (Berk. Et Curt.) Teng (Aphyllophoromycetideae) (review). *International Journal of Medicinal Mushrooms* 2 (1): 21–34.

Mizuno, Takashi et al. 1990. Antitumor activity and some properties of water–soluble polysaccharides from "himematsutake," the fruiting body of *Agaricus blazei* Murill. *Agricultural and Biological Chemistry* 54 (11): 2889–2896.

Mizuno, Takashi et al. 1992a. Antitumor activity of some polysaccharides isolated from an edible mushroom, ningyotake, the fruiting body and the cultured mycelium of *Polyporous confluens*. *Bioscience, Biotechnology, and Biochemistry* 56 (1): 34–41

Mizuno, Takashi et al. 1992b. Antitumor–active polysaccharides isolated from the fruiting body of *Hericium erinaceum,* an edible and medicianl mushroom called yamabushitake or houtou. *Bioscience, Biotechnology, and Biochemistry* 56(2): 347–348.

Mizushina, Yoshiyuki et al. 1998. A mushroom fruiting body-inducing substance inhibits activities of replicative DNA polymerases. *Biochemical and Biophysical Research Communications* 249 (1): 17-22.

Mlinaric, A. et al. 2004. Anti–genotoxic activity of the mushroom *Lactarius vellereus* extract in bacteria and in mammalian cells in vitro. *Pharmazie* 59 (3): 217–221.

Mlinaric, A. et al. 2005. Screening of selected wood–damaging fungi for the HIV–1 reverse transcriptase inhibitors. *Acta Pharmaceutica* 55 (1): 69–79.

Moldavan, Mykhaylo G. et al. 1999. Effects of *Amanita* species extracts on neuron responses in the rat hippocampal stratum pyramidale (CA1 region) in vitro. *International Journal of Medicinal Mushrooms* 1 (4): 337–344.

Moldavan, Mykhaylo G. et al. 2001. Effects of some higher Basidiomycetes extracts on the neurons' activity. *Ukrayins'kyi Botanichnyi Zhurnal* 58 (2): 220–228.

Moldavan, Mykhaylo G. et al. 2007. Neurotropic and trophic action of lion's mane mushroom *Hericium erinaceus* (Bull.: Fr.) Pers. (Aphyllophoromycetideae) extracts on nerve cells in vitro. *International Journal of Medicinal Mushrooms* 9 (1): 15–28.

Moncalvo, Jean–Marc. 2005. Molecular systematics of *Ganoderma:* What is reishi? *International Journal of Medicinal Mushrooms* 7 (3): 353–534.

Montanini et al. 1999. Use of acetylcysteine as the life–saving antidote in *Amanita phalloides* (death cap) poisoning. Case report on 11 patients. *Arzneimittelforschung* 49 (12): 1044–1047.

Montenegro, Raquel Carvalho et al. 2004. Cytotoxic activity of pisosterol, a triterpene isolated from *Pisolithus tinctorius* (Mich.: Pers.) Coker &

Couch, 1928. *Zeitschrift für Naturforschung C* 59 (7–8): 519.

Montenegro, Raquel Carvalho et al. 2007. Pisoterol induces monocytic differentiation in HL–60 cells. *Toxicology in Vitro* 21 (5): 795–800.

Montenegro, Raquel Carvalho et al. 2008. Antitumor activity of pisosterol in mice bearing with S18 tumor. *Biological & Pharmaceutical Bulletin* 31 (3): 454–457.

Moody, A. R. and A. R. Weinhold. 1968. Stimulation of rhizomorph production by *Armillaria mellea* with lipid from tree roots. *Phytopathology* 62 (11): 1347–1350.

Moradali, Mohammad-Fata et al. 2008. Investigation of antimicrobial fatty acids from medicinal artist conk mushroom *Ganoderma applanatum* (Pers.) Pat. (Aphyllophoromycetideae) by TLC and spectroscopic detection. *International Journal of Medicinal Mushrooms* 10 (2): 149-154.

Mori, K. et al. 1987. Antitumor effects of edible mushrooms by oral administration. In *Cultivating Edible Fungi: International Symposium on Scientific and Technical Aspects of Cultivating Edible Fungi (Developments in Crop Science),* edited by P. J. Wuesst, D. J. Royse and R. B. Beelman. Amsterdam: Elsevier.

Mori, K. et al. 2008. Nerve growth factor–inducing activity of *Hericium erinaceus* in 1321N1 human astrocytoma cells. *Biological and Pharmaceutical Bulletin* 31 (9): 1727.

Morigiwa, A. et al. 1986. Angiotensin–converting enzyme inhibitory triterpenes from *Ganoderma lucidum*. *Chemical Pharmaceutical Bulletin* 34 (7): 3025–3028.

Morimoto et al. 2008. Oral administration of *Agaricus brasiliensis* S. Wasser et al. (Agaricomycetideae) extract downregulates serum immunoglobulin E levels by enhancing TH1 response. *International Journal of Medicinal Mushrooms* 10 (1): 15–24.

Morita et al. 1995. Production of two phytotoxic metabolites by the fungus *Alternaria cassiae.*

Bioscience, Biotechnology and Biochemistry 59 (9): 1792–1793.

Mothana et al. 2000. Ganomycins A and B, new antimicrobial farnesyl hydroquinones from the Basidiomycete *Ganoderma pfeifferi*. *Journal of Natural Products* 63 (3): 416–418.

Motoi et al. 2003. Structure and antitumor activity of 1,3–b–glucan from cultivated fruit bodies of culinary–medicinal mushroom *Hypsizygus marmoreus* (Peck) Bigel. (Agaricomycetideae). *International Journal of Medicinal Mushrooms* (5) 3: 263–276.

Muhlmann et al. 2006. Mycorrhiza of the host–specific *Lactarius deterrimus* on the roots of *Picea abies* and *Arctostaphylos uva–ursi*. *Mycorrhiza* 16 (4): 245–250.

Mukai et al. 2006. An alternative medicine, *Agaricus blazei,* may have induced severe hepatic dysfunction in cancer patients. *Japanese Journal of Clinical Oncology* 36 (12): 808–810.

Mukherjee, M. et al. 1993. Natural resistance of the mycelial culture of the mushroom, *Panaeolus papillonaceus,* towards growth inhibition by polyene antibiotics. *Current Microbiology* 27 (1): 1–4.

Mukherjee, M. and S. Sengupta. 1985. An inducible xylanase of the mushroom *Termitomyces clypeatus* differing from the xylanase/amylase produced in dextrin medium. *Journal of General Microbiology* 131: 1881–1885.

Muller et al. 1986. Screening of white–rot fungi for biological pretreatment of wheat straw for biogas production. *Applied Microbiology and Biotechnology* 24 (2): 180–185.

Muszynska et al. 2009. Indole compounds in fruiting bodies of some selected Macromycetes species and in their mycelia cultured in vitro. *Pharmazie* 64 (7): 479–480.

Mygind, Per H. et al. 2005. Plectasin is a peptide antibiotic with therapeutic potential from a saprophytic fungus. *Nature* 437 (7061): 975–980.

Nagai et al. 2006. Dilinoleoyl–phosphatidylethanolamine from *Hericium erinaceum* protects against

ER stress–dependent neuro–2A cell death via protein kinase C pathway. *The Journal of Nutritional Biochemistry* 17 (8): 530–535.

Nagao, Mie et al. 2009. Augmentation of sebaceous lipogenesis by an ethanol extract of *Grifola frondosa* (maitake mushroom) in hamsters in vivo and in vitro. *Experimental Dermatology* 18 (8): 730–733.

Nagao, T. et al. 1981. Chemoimmunotherapy with krestin (PSK) in acute leukemia. *Tokai Journal of Experimental and Clinical Medicine* 6 (2): 141–146.

Nair, M. S. R. and Marjorie Anchel. 1977. Frustulosinol, an antibiotic metabolite of *Stereum frustulosum:* Revised structure of frustulosin. *Phytochemistry* 16 (3): 390–392.

Najafzadeh et al. 2007. Chaga mushroom extract inhibits oxidative DNA damage in lymphocytes of patients with inflammatory bowel disease. *BioFactors* 31 (3–4): 191–200.

Nakamiya et al. 2005. Degradation of dioxins by cyclic degrading fungus, *Cordyceps sinensis. FEMS Microbiology Letters* 248 (1): 17–22.

Nakamura et al. 2003. Combined effects of *Cordyceps sinensis* and methotrexate on hematogenic lung metastasis in mice. *Receptors and Channels* 9 (5): 329–334.

Nakano, Takashi et al. 1996. Intratumoral administration of sizofiran activates langerhans cell and T–cell infiltration in cervical cancer. *Clinical Immunology and Immunopathology* 79 (1): 79–86.

Nakazato, Hiroaki et al. 1994. Efficacy of immunochemotherapy as adjuvant treatment after curative resection of gastric cancer. *The Lancet* 343 (8906): 1122–1126.

Nanba, Hiroaki. 1997a. Maitake D–fraction: Healing and preventive potential for cancer. *Journal of Orthomolecular Medicine* 12 (1): 43.

Nanba, Hiroaki et al. 1997b. Effect of maitake D–fraction on cancer prevention. *Annals of the New York Academy of Science* 833: 204–207.

Nanba, Hiroaki et al. 2000. Effect of maitake *(Grifola frondosa)* glucan in HIV–infected patients. *Mycoscience* 41 (4): 293–295.

Nano et al. 2002. In vitro tests to evaluate potential biological activity in natural substances. *Fitoterapia* 73 (2): 140–146. (may be in text as 2003)

Naoki et al. 1994. Pharmacological studies on *Cordyceps sinensis* from China. *Abstracts from the Fifth Mycological Congress.* Vancouver, BC, August 14–21.

Narisawa et al. 1992. Inhibitory effect of cryptoporic acid E, a product from fungus *Cryptoporus volvatus,* on colon carcinogenesis induced with N–methyl–N–nitrosourea in rats and with 1,2–dimethylhydrazine in mice. *Japanese Journal of Cancer Research* 83 (8): 830–834.

Ng, Tzi Bun et al. 2003. Calcaelin, a new protein with translation–inhibiting, antiproliferative and antimitogenic activities from the mosaic puffball mushroom *Calvatia caelata. Planta Medica* 69 (3): 212–217.

Ng, Tzi Bun et al. 2006. An agglutinin with mitogenic and antiproliferative activities from the mushroom *Flammulina velutipes. Mycologia* 98 (2): 167–171.

Ngai et al. 2005. Agrocybin, an antifungal peptide from the edible mushroom *Agrocybe cylindracea. Peptides* 26 (2): 191–196.

Nicholas et al. 2001. Cortamidine oxide, a novel disulfide metabolite from the New Zealand Basidiomycete (mushroom) *Cortinarius* species. *Journal of Natural Products* 64 (3): 341–344.

Niksic et al. 2004. Is *Phallus impudicus* a mycological giant? *Mycologist* 18 (1): 21–22.

Nitha, B. and Kainoor K. Janardhanan. 2005. Antioxidant, anti–inflammatory and antitumor activities of cultured mycelia of morel mushroom, *Morchella esculenta. Indian Journal of Medical Research* 121 (Supplement S): 133.

Nitha, B. and Kainoor K. Janardhanan. 2008. Aqueous–ethanolic extract of morel mushroom mycelium *Morchella esculenta,* protects cisplatin and gentamicin induced nephrotoxicity in mice. *Food Chemistry and Toxicology* 46 (9): 3193–3199.

Nitha, B. et al. 2007. Anti–inflammatory and anti–tumor activities of cultured mycelium of morel mushroom, *Morchella esculenta*. *Current Science* 92 (2): 235–239.

Noguchi et al. 2008. Effect of an extract of *Ganoderma lucidum* in men with lower uninary tract symptoms: A double–blind, placebo–controlled randomized and dose–ranging study. *Asian Journal of Andrology* 10 (4): 651–658.

Nozaki et al. 2010. Invariant V 14 natural killer T–cell activation by edible mushroom acidic glycosphingolipids. *Biological & Pharmaceutical Bulletin* 33 (4): 580–584.

Nukata et al. 2002. Neogrifolin derivatives possessing anti–oxidative activity from the mushroom *Albatrellus ovinus*. *Phytochemistry* 59 (7): 731–737.

Nussbaum et al. 1997. Reduction of anthranilic acid and related amino acids in fruit–bodies of *Hebeloma sacchariolens*. *Phytochemistry* 46 (2): 261–264.

Obara, Yutaro et al. 1999. Stimulation of neurotrophic factor secretion from 1321N1 human astrocytoma cells by novel diterpenoids, scabronines A and G. *European Journal of Pharmacology* 370 (1): 79–84.

Obara, Yutaro et al. 2001. Scabronine G–methylester enhances secretion of neurotrophic factors mediated by an activation of protein kinase C–zeta. *Molecular Pharmacology* 59 (5): 1287–1297.

Obuchi et al. 1990. Armillaric acid, a new antibiotic produced by *Armillaria mellea*. *Planta Medica* 56 (2): 198–201.

Odabasoglu, Fehmi et al. 2004. Comparison of antioxidant activity and phenolic content of three lichen species. *Phytotherapy Research* 18 (11): 938–941.

Odabasoglu, Fehmi et al. 2005. Antioxidant activity, reducing power and total phenolic content of some lichen species. *Fitoterpia* 6 (2): 216–219.

Odabasoglu, Fehmi et al. 2006. Gastroprotective and antioxidant effects of usnic acid on indomethacin–induced gastric ulcer in rats. *Journal of Ethnopharmacology* 103 (1): 59–65.

Ohga, S. et al. 2004. Utilization of pulsed power to stimulate fructification of edible mushrooms. *Mushroom Science Biotechnology* 16 (1): 343–351.

Ohmori, Toshihiro et al. 1988a. Component analysis of protein–bound polysaccharide (SN–C) from *Cordyceps ophioglossoides* and its effects on syngeneic murine tumors. *Chemical & Pharmaceutical Bulletin* 36 (11): 4505–4511.

Ohmori, Toshihiro et al. 1988b. Dissociation of a glucan fraction (CO–1) from protein–bound polysaccharide of *Cordyceps ophioglossoides* and analysis of its antitumor effect. *Chemical & Pharmaceutical Bulletin* 36 (11): 4512–4518.

Ohmori, Toshihiro et al. 1989. Isolation of galactosaminoglycan moiety (CO–N) from protein–bound polysaccharide of *Cordyceps ophioglossoides* and its effects against murine tumors. *Chemical & Pharmaceutical Bulletin* 37 (4): 1019–1022.

Ohno, Naohito et al. 2002. TH1–oriented immunomodulating activity of gel–forming fungal (1 3)–beta–glucans. *International Journal of Medicinal Mushrooms* 4 (1): 99–114.

Ohno, Naohito et al. 2003. Immunomodulating activity of a B–glucan preparation, SCG, extracted from a culinary–medicinal mushroom, *Sparassis crispa* Wulf.: Fr. (Aphyllophoromycetideae), and application to cancer patients. *International Journal of Medicinal Mushrooms* 5 (4): 383–392.

Ohsawa et al. 1992. Studies on constituents of fruit body of *Polyporous umbellatus* and their cytotoxic activity. *Chemical and Pharmaceutical Bulletin* 40 (1): 143–147.

Ohtomo, M. et al. 2001. In vivo and in vitro test study: Physiological activity in immune response system of representative Basidiomycetes. Unpublished research report provided to *Fungi Perfecti* from Tamagawa University, Japan.

Ohtsuka, S. et al. 1973. Polysaccharides having an anticarcinogenic effect and a method of producing them from species of *Basidiomycetes*. US Patent 1331513. Issued: September 26, 1973.

Ohtsuru et al. 2000. Screening of various mushrooms with inhibitory activity of adipocyte conversion. *Journal of the Japanese Society for Food Science and Technology* 47 (5): 394–396.

Ojemann et al. 2006. Tian ma, an ancient Chinese herb, offers new options for the treatment of epilepsy and other conditions. *Epilepsy & Behavior* 8 (2): 376–383.

Okamoto et al. 1994. Antimicrobial chlorinated orcinol derivatives from mycelia of *Hericium erinaceum*. *Phytochemistry* 34 (5): 1445–1446.

Okeke, B. C. et al. 1997. Comparative biotransformation of pentachlorophenol in soils by solid substrate cultures of *Lentinula edodes*. *Applied Microbiology and Biotechnology* 48 (4): 563–569.

Olberg S. and J. Andersen. 1999. Field attraction of beetles *(Coleoptera)* to the polypores *Fomes fomentarius* and *Phellinus* spp (fungi: Aphyllophorales) in northern Norway. *Entomologia Generalis* 24 (4): 217–36.

Opatz, Till et al. 2007. The creolophins: A family of linear triquinanes from *Creolophus cirrhatus* (Basidiomycete). *European Journal of Organic Chemistry* 2007 (33): 5546–5550.

Opatz, Till et al. 2008. Sterelactones: New isolactarane type sesquiterpenoids with antifungal activity from *Stereum* sp. IBWF 01060. *Journal of Antibiotics* 61 (9): 563–567.

Osmanova, Natalia et al. 2010. Azaphilones: A class of fungal metabolites with diverse biological activities. *Phytochemistry Reviews* 9 (2): 315–342.

Ostram. 1992. Another mushroom miracle. *New York Native* June 29: 34–35.

Ou, Hsin–Ting et al. 2005. The antiproliferative and differentiating effects of human leukemic U937 cells are mediated by cytokines from activated mononuclear cells by dietary mushrooms. *Journal of Agricultural and Food Chemistry* 53 (2): 300–305.

Outila et al. 1999. Bioavailability of vitamin D from wild edible mushrooms *(Cantharellus tubaeformis)* as measured with a human bioassay. *American Journal of Clinical Nutrition* 69 (1): 95–98.

Ouzouni, P. K. et al. 2009. Volatile compounds from the fruiting bodies of three *Hygrophorus* mushroom species from northern Greece. *International Journal of Food Science and Technology* 44 (4): 854–859.

Pacheco–Sanchez, Maribel et al. 2006. A bioactive (1 3)–, (1 4)–ß–D–glucan from *Collybia dryophila* and other mushrooms. *Mycologia* 98 (2): 180–185.

Pacheco–Sanchez, Maribel et al. 2007. Inhibitory effect of CDP, a polysaccharide extracted from the mushroom *Collybia dryophila,* on nitric oxide synthase expression and nitric oxide production in macrophages. *European Journal of Pharmacology* 555 (1): 61–66.

Paci et al. 2006. Pharmacokinetics, metabolism, and routes of excretion of intravenous irofulven in patients with advanced solid tumors. *Drug Metabolism & Disposition* 34 (11): 1918–1926.

Parish et al. 2004. A new ene–triyne antibiotic from the fungus *Baeospora myosura*. *Journal of Natural Prodcuts* 67 (11): 1900–1902.

Park, Cheol et al. 2005. Growth inhibition of U937 leukemia cells by aqueous extract of *Cordyceps militaris* through induction of apoptosis. *Oncology Reports* 13 (6): 1211–1216.

Park, Dong Ki et al. 2008. Immunoglobulin and cytokine production from mesenteric lymph node lymphocytes is regulated by extracts of *Cordyceps sinensis* in C57BI/6N mice. *Journal of Medicinal Foods* 11 (4): 784–788.

Park, E. J. et al. 1997. Antifibrotic effects of a polysaccharide extracted from *Ganoderma lucidum*, glycyrrhizin, and pentoxifylline in rats with cirrhosis induced by biliary obstruction. *Biological & Pharmaceutical Bulletin* 20 (4): 417–420.

Park, Hyuk–Gu et al. 2009. New method development for nanoparticle extraction of water–soluble –(1 3)–d–glucan from edible mushrooms, *Sparassis crispa* and *Phellinus linteus*. *Journal of Agricultural and Food Chemistry* 57 (6): 2147–2154.

Park, Sang Eun et al. 2009. Induction of apoptosis

and inhibition of telomerase activity in human lung carcinoma cells by the water extract of *Cordyceps militaris. Food and Chemical Toxicology* 47 (7): 1667–1675.

Park, Yoo Kyoung et al. 2004. Chaga mushroom extract inhibits oxidative DNA damage in human lymphocytes as assessed by comet assay. *BioFactors* 21 (1–4): 109–112.

Park, Young–Mi et al. 2005. In vivo and in vitro anti–inflammatory and anti–nociceptive effects of the methanol extract of *Inonotus obliquus. Journal of Ethnopharmacology.* 101 (1–3): 120–8.

Park, Young–Mi et al. 2004. Anti–inflammatory and anti–nociceptive effects of the methanol extract of *Fomes fomentarius. Biological & Pharmaceutical Bulletin* 27 (10): 1588–1593.

Pashinskii, V. G. et al. 1998. Antiulcer, adaptogenic and antitumour activities of a dry extract from *Inonotus obliquus* Pers Pil. *Rastitel' nye Resursy* 34 (1): 68–71.

Peintner, U. et al. 1998. The iceman's fungi. *Mycological Research.* 102 (10): 1153–1162.

Pemberton et al. 1994. Agglutinins (lectins) from some British higher fungi. *Mycological Research* 98 (3): 277–290.

Peng, Chiung–Chi et al. 2007. *Antrodia camphorata* extract induces replicative senescence in superficial TCC, and inhibits the absolute migration capability in invasive bladder carcinoma cells. *Journal of Ethnopharmacology* 109 (1): 93–103.

Pengsuparp, Thitima et al. 1995. Mechanistic evaluation of new plant–derived compounds that inhibit HIV–1 reverse transcriptase. *Journal of Natural Products* 58 (7): 1024–1031.

Penman et al. 1970. Messenger and heterogeneous nuclear RNA in HeLa cells: Differential inhibition by cordycepin. *Proceedings of the National Academy of Sciences* 67 (4): 1878–1885.

Pereverzev et al. 1993. The role of APUD–system cells and their mediators in the biological effects of adaptogens. *Inflammation Research* 38 (3–4): 188–190.

Petrova, Roumyana D. et al. 2005. Potential role of medicinal mushrooms in breast cancer treatment: Current knowledge and future perspectives. *International Journal of Medicinal Mushrooms* 7 (1–2): 141–146.

Petrova, Roumyana D. et al. 2007. Fungal substances as modulators of NF–kappaB activation pathway. *Molecular Biology Reports* 34 (3): 145–154.

Petrova, Roumyana D. et al. 2009. *Marasmius oreades* substances block NF–kappaB activity through interference with IKK activation pathway. *Molecular Biology Reports* 36 (4): 737–744.

Pettit et al. 2010. Antineoplastic agents. 556. Isolation and structure of coprinastatin 1 from *Coprinus cinereus. Journal of Natural Products* 73 (3): 388–392.

Pfister, Jurg R. 1988. Isolation and bioactivity of 2–aminoquinoline from *Leucopaxillus albissimus. Journal of Natural Products* 51 (5): 969–970.

Pilgrim, Horst et al. 1997. *Inonotus hispidus,* a source of new drugs. *Zeitschrift fur Mykologie* 62 (2): 169–94.

Piraino, Frank F. 2005. The development of the antiviral drug RC 28 from *Rozites caperata* (Pers.: Fr.) P. Karst. (Agaricomycetideae). *International Journal of Medicinal Mushrooms* 7 (3): 356.

Piraino, Frank F. and Curtis R. Brandt. 1999. Isolation and partial characterization of an antiviral, RC–183, from the edible mushroom *Rozites caperata. Antiviral Research* 43 (2): 67–78.

Pisha, Emily et al. 1995. Discovery of betulinic acid as a selective inhibitor of human melanoma that functions by induction of apoptosis. *Nature Medicine* 1 (10): 1046–1051.

Pohleven et al. 2009. Purification, characterization and cloning of a ricin B–like lectin from mushroom *Clitocybe nebularis* with antiproliferative activity against human leukemic T cells. *Biochimica et Biophysica Acta – General Subjects* 1790 (3): 173–181.

Pointing, S. B. et al. 2000. Optimization of laccase production by *Pycnoporus sanguineus* in submerged liquid culture. *Mycologia* 92 (1): 139–144.

Pokhrel, Chandra P. and Shoji Ohga. 2007. Submerged culture conditions for mycelial yield and polysaccharides production by *Lyophyllum decastes*. *Food Chemistry* 105 (2): 641–646.

Popova et al. 2009. Antibacterial triterpenes from the threatened wood–decay fungus Fomitopsis rosea. *Fitoterapia* 80 (5): 463–466.

Potron, M. et al. 1956. Champignons et diabete (Mushrooms and diabetes). *Concours Medical 36*, 3795–3796.

Poyedinok et al. 2005. The light factor in biotechnology cultivation of medicinal mushrooms. *International Journal of Medicinal Mushrooms* 7 (3): 369–378.

Preuss et al. 2007. Enhanced insulin–hypoglycemic activity in rats consuming a specific glycoprotein extracted from maitake mushroom. *Molecular and Cellular Biochemistry* 306 (1–2): 105–113.

Pringle et al. 2009. The ectomycorrhizal fungus *Amanita phalloides* was introduced and is expanding its range on the west coast of North America. *Molecular Ecology* 18 (5): 817–833.

Pujol et al. 1990. Research of antifungal substances secreted by higher fungi in culture. *Annales Pharmaceutiques Francaises* 48 (1): 17–22.

Puttaraju et al. 2006. Antioxidant activity of indigenous edible mushrooms. *Journal of Agricultural and Food Chemistry* 54 (26): 9764–9772.

Pyo, Paul et al. 2008. Possible immunotherapeutic potentiation with D–fraction in prostate cancer cells. *Journal of Hematology and Oncology* 1 (25).

Qi, Ge et al. 2009. Effects of *Ganoderma lucidum* spores on sialoadenitis of nonobese diabetic mice. *Chinese Medical Journal* 122 (5): 556-560.

Qin, Xiang–Dong and Ji–Kai Liu. 2004. Natural aromatic steroids as potential molecular fossils from the fruiting bodies of the Ascomycete *Daldinia concentrica*. *Journal of Natural Products* 67 (12): 2133–2135.

Qin, Xiang–Dong et al. 2006. Concentricolide, an anti–HIV agent from the Ascomycete *Daldinia concentrica*. *Helvetica Chimica Acta* 89 (1): 127–133.

Qing, C. et al. 2004. Effects of albaconol from the Basidiomycete *Albatrellus confluens* on DNA topoisomerase II–mediated DNA cleavage and relaxation. *Planta Medica* 70 (9): 792–796.

Qiu, G. and Wu, A. R. 1986. Chinese materia medica with antiatopy effect. *Abstracts of Chinese Medicine* 1: 113.

Quack et al. 1978. Antibiotics from Basidiomycetes. V. Merulidial, a new antibiotic from the Basidiomycete *Merulius tremellosus* Fr. *Journal of Antibiotics* 31 (8): 737–741.

Quang, Dang Ngoc et al. 2004. Thelephantins I–N; P–terpenyl derivatives from the inedible mushroom *Hydnellum caeruleum*. *Phytochemistry* 65 (8): 1179–1184.

Quang, Dang Ngoc et al. 2005. Antimicrobial azaphilones from the xylariaceous inedible mushrooms. *International Journal of Medicinal Mushrooms* 7 (3): 452–455.

Quang, Dang Ngoc et al. 2006. Inhibitory activity of nitric oxide production in RAW 264.7 cells of daldinals A–C from the fungus *Daldinia childiae* and other metabolites isolated from inedible mushrooms. *Journal of Natural Medicines*. 60 (4): 303–307.

Rabinovich, Maia et al. 2007. Copper– and zinc–enriched mycelium of *Agaricus blazei* Murrill: Bioaccumulation and bioavailability. *Journal of Medicinal Food* 10 (1): 175–183.

Rafati et al. 2009. Enhancement of indole alkaloids produced by *Psilocybe cubensis* (Earle) Singer (Agaricomycetideae) in controlled harvesting light conditions. *International Journal of Medicinal Mushrooms* 11 (4): 419–426.

Rahouti et al. 1999. Growth of 1044 strains and species of fungi on 7 phenolic lignin model compounds. *Chemosphere* 38 (11): 2549–2559.

Raman, N. et al. 1993. Mycorrhizal status of plant species colonizing a magnesite mine spoil in India. *Biology and Fertility of Soils* 16 (1): 76–78.

Rana et al. 2008. Evaluation of antibacterial potential of two species of genus *Agaricus* L: Fr. (Agaricomycetideae) from India. *International Journal of Medicinal Mushrooms* 10 (4): 163–169.

Rankovic, Branislav et al. 2007. Evaluation of antimicrobial activity of the lichens *Lasallia pustulata, Parmelia sulcata, Umbilicaria crustulosa* and *Umbilicaria cylindrica. Mikrobiologya* 76 (6): 817–821.

Rankovic, Branislav et al. 2010. Antioxidant and antimicrobial properties of the lichens *Anaptychya ciliaris, Nephroma parile, Ochrolechia tartarea* and *Parmelia centrifuga. Central European Journal of Biology* 5 (5): 649–655.

Rapior et al. 2002. The anise–like odor of *Clitocybe odora, Lentinellus cochleatus* and *Agaricus essettei. Mycologia* 94 (3): 373–376.

Rasser, Falk et al. 2000. Secondary metabolites from a *Gloeophyllum* sp. *Phytochemistry* 54 (5): 511–516.

Rasser, Falk et al. 2002. Terpenoids from *Bovista* sp. 96042. *Tetrahedron* 58 (39): 7785–7789.

Reade et al. 1983. Investigation of white–rot fungi for the converstion of poplar into a potential feedstuff for ruminants. *Canadian Journal of Microbiology* 29 (4): 457–463.

Reay, Marie. 1977. Ritual madness observed: a discarded pattern of fate in Papua New Guinea. *The Journal of Pacific History* 12: 55-79.

Rebhun et al. 2005. Use of agro–industrial waste for production of laccase and manganese peroxidase from white–rot Basidiomycetes. *International Journal of Medicinal Mushrooms* 7 (3): 459–460.

Rempel et al. 2002. Characterization of the recognition of blood group B trisaccharide derivatives by the lectin from *Marasmius oreades* using frontal affinity chromatography–mass spectrometry. *Glycoconjugate Journal* 19(3): 175–180.

Ren, G. et al. 2006. Evaluation of cytotoxic activities of some medicinal polypore fungi from China. *Fitoterapia* 77 (5): 408–410,

Ribeiro, Barbara et al. 2007. Phenolic compounds, organic acids profiles and antioxidative properties of beefsteak fungus *(Fistulina hepatica). Food and Chemical Toxicology* 45 (10): 1805–1813.

Richter et al. 2003. A comparison of mycorrhizal and saprotrophic fungus tolerance to creosote in vitro. *International Biodeterioration & Biodegradation* 51 (3): 195–202.

Robbins, Tom 1976. Superfly: The Toadstool That Conquered The Universe. *High Times* (December).

Robbins, William J. et al. 1945. A survey of some wood–destroying and other fungi for antibacterial activity. *Bulletin of the Torrey Botanical Club* 72 (2): 165–190.

Rosa, Luiz Henrique et al. 2003. Screening of Brazilian Basidiomycetes for antimicrobial activity. *Memorias do Instituto Oswaldo Cruz.* 98 (7): 967–974.

Rosecke, Joachim et al. 2000. Volatile constituents of wood–rotting Basidiomycetes. *Phytochemistry* 54 (8): 747–750.

Rouhana–Toubi, A. et al. 2009. Ethyl acetate extracts of submerged cultured mycelium of higher Basidiomycetes mushrooms inhibit human ovarian cancer cell growth. *International Journal of Medicinal Mushrooms* 11 (1): 29–37.

Roupas et al. 2010. Mushrooms and agaritine: A mini–review. *Journal of Functional Foods* 2 (2): 91–98.

Royse, et al. 2003. Influence of precipitated calcium carbonate ($CaCO_3$) on shiitake *(Lentinula edodes)* yield and mushroom size. *Bioresouce Technology* 90 (2): 225–228.

Rubel, William and David Arora. 2008. A study of cultural bias in field guide determinations of mushroom edibility using the iconic mushroom, *Amanita muscaria,* as an example. *Economic Botany* 62 (3): 223–243.

Rukachaisirikul et al. 2004. 10–membered macrolides from the insect pathogenic fungus *Cordyceps militaris* BCC 2816. *Journal of Natural Products* 67 (11): 1953–1955.

Russo et al. 2007. Putrescine–1,4–dicinnamide from *Pholiota spumosa* (Basidiomycetes) inhibits cell growth of human prostate cancer cells. *Phytomedicine.* 14 (2–3): 185–191.

Ruttimann–Johnson, Carmen and Richard T. Lamar. 1997. Binding of pentachlorophenol to humic substances in soil by the action of white rot fungi. *Soil Biology and Biochemistry* 29 (7): 1143–1148.

Ryan and Bumpus. 1989. Biodegradation of 2,4,5–trichlorophenoxyacetic acid in liquid culture and in soil by the white rot fungus *Phanerochaete chrysosporium*. *Applied Microbiology and Biotechnology* 31 (3): 302–307.

Rym, K. H. et al. 1999. Antiviral effect of water soluble substance from *Elfvingia applanata* alone and in combinations with interferons against vesicular stomatitis virus (New Jersey serotype). *The Korean Journal of Mycology* 27 (2): 175-179

Ryong et al. 1989. Antiatherogenic and antiatherosclerotic effects of mushroom extracts revealed in human aortic intima cell culture. *Drug Development Research* 17 (2): 109–117.

Rzymowska, J. 1998. The effect of aqueous extracts from Inonotus obliquus on the mitotic index and enzyme activities. *Bollettino Chimico Farmaceutico* 137 (1): 13–15.

Saar et al. 1991. Ethnomycological data from Siberia and northeast Asia on the effect of *Amanita muscaria*. *Journal of Ethnopharmacology* 31 (2): 157–173.

Sabotic et al. 2009. Aspartic proteases from Basidiomycete *Clitocybe nebularis*. *Croatica Chemica Acta* 82 (4): 739–745.

Sack et al. 1997. Novel metabolites in phenanthrene and pyrene transformation by *Aspergillus niger*. *Applied Environmental Microbiology* 63 (7): 2906–2909.

Sadava et al. 2009. Effect of Ganoderma on drug–sensitive and multidrug–resistant small–cell lung carcinoma cells. *Cancer Letters* 277 (2): 182–189.

Samorini, Giorgio. 1995. Traditional use of psychoactive mushrooms in Ivory Coast? *Eleusis* 1 (1): 22–27.

Sanford et al. 1990. Stimulation of vascular cell proliferation by beta–galactoside specific lectins. *The FASEB Journal* 4 (11): 2912–2918.

Sano et al. 2002. Inhibitory effects of edible higher Basidiomycetes mushroom extracts on mouse type IV allergy. *International Journal of Medicinal Mushrooms* 4 (1): 35–39.

Sapkota, Kumar et al. 2010. Enhancement of tyrosine hydroxylase expression by Cordyceps militaris. *Central European Journal of Biology* 5 (10): 214–223.

Sarikurkcu et al. 2008. Evaluation of the antioxidant activity of four edible mushrooms from the Central Anatolia, Eskisehir – Turkey: *Lactarius deterrimus, Suillus collitinus, Boletus edulis, Xerocomus chrysenteron*. *Biosource Tecnology* 99 (14): 6651–6655.

Sasaki et al. 1971. Antitumor polysaccharides from some polyporaceae, *Ganoderma applanatum* (Pers.) Pat and *Phellinus linteus* (Berk. Et Curt) Aoshima. *Chemical and Pharmaceutical Bulletin* 19 (4): 821–826.

Sasek et al. 2000. The Utilization of Bioremediation to reduce Soil Contamination: Problems and Solutions. *Nato Science Series IV, Earth & Environmental Sciences,* Vol. 19.

Sasek, V. et al. 1998. Screening for efficient organopollutant fungal degraders by decolourisation. *Czech Mycology* 50; 303–311.

Sato, Mayumi et al. 2002. Dehydrotrametenolic acid induces preadipocyte differentiation and sensitizes animal models of noninsulin–dependent diabetes mellitus to insulin. *Biological and Pharmaceutical Bulletin* 25 (1): 81.

Sato, Shin et al. 2004. Microbial scission of sulfide linkages in vulcanized natural rubber by a white rot Basidiomycete, *Ceriporiopsis subvermispora*. *Biomacromolecules* 5 (2): 511–515.

Scheibner, K. et al. 1997. Screening for fungi intensively mineralizing 2, 4, 6–trinitrotoluene. *Applied Microbiology and Biotechnology* 47 (4): 452–457.

Scheibner, Manuela et al. 2008. Novel peroxidases of *Marasmius scorodonius* degrade –carotene. *Applied Microbiology and Biotechnology* 77 (6): 1241–1250.

Schlegel et al. 2000. Piptamine, a new antibiotic produced by *Piptoporus betulinus* Lu 9–1. *Journal of Antibiotics* 53 (9): 973–974.

Schurr, Theodore G. 1995. Aboriginal Siberian use of *Amanita muscaria* in shamanistic practices: Neuropharmacological effects of fungal alkaloids ingested during trance induction, and the cultural patterning of visionary experience. *Curare* 18 (1): 31–65.

Seeger, Ruth and Elisabeth Bunsen. 1980. Degranulation of rat mast cells in vitro by the fungal cytolysins phallolysin, rubescenslysin and fascicularelysin. *Naunyn–Schmiedebergs Archives of Pharmacology* 315 (2): 163–166.

Seeger, Ruth and Pete Schweinshaut. 1981. Vorkommen von Caesium in Höheren Pilzen. *The Science of the Total Environment* 19 (3): 253–276.

Sekiya et al. 2005. Inhibitory effects of triterpenes isolated from chuling (*Polyporous umbellatus* FRIES) on free radical–induced lysis of red blood cells. *Biological and Pharmaceutical Bulletin* 28 (5): 817–821.

Sekizawa et al. 2002. Panepophenanthrin, from a mushroom strain, a novel inhibitor of the ubiquitin–activating enzyme. *Journal of Natural Products* 65 (10): 1491–1493.

Serck–Hanssen, K. and Wikstrom C. 1978. Novel 7–phenylheptan– 3–ones from the fungus *Phellinus tremulae*. *Phytochemistry* 17 (9): 1678–1679.

Sezginturk et al. 2005. Detection of benzoic acid by an amperometric inhibitor biosensor based on mushroom tissue homogenate. *Food Technology and Biotechnology* 43 (4): 329–334.

Shamtsyan et al. 2005. Immunomodulating activity of *Bjerkandera* sp. *International Journal of Medicinal Mushrooms* 7 (3): 462–463.

Shao et al. 2005. A new cytotoxic lanostane triterpenoid from the Basidiomycete *Hebeloma versipelle*. *The Journal of Antibiotics* 58 (12): 828–831.

Sharma, V. P. and S. R. 2009. Molecular identification and cultivation of the black poplar culinary–medicinal mushroom *Agrocybe aegerita* (V. Brig.) Singer (Agaricomycetideae). *International Journal of Medicinal Mushrooms* 11 (1): 87–91.

Sharma, V. P. et al. 2008. Effect of various supplements on lignocellulolytic enzyme production and yield of culinary–medicinal mushroom *Flammulina velutipes* (W. Curt.: Fr.) Singer (Agaricomycetideae). *International Journal of Medicinal Mushrooms* 10 (1): 87–92.

Shavit, Elinoar and Efrat. 2010. Lead and arsenic in *Morchella esculenta* fruitbodies collected in lead arsenate contaminated apple orchards in the northeastern United States: A preliminary study. *Fungi* 3 (2): 11–18.

Sheena et al. 2003. Antibacterial activity of three macrofungi, *Ganoderma lucidum, Navesporus floccosa* and *Phellinus rimosus* occurring in south India. *Pharmaceutical Biology* 41 (8): 564–567.

Shen, Jin–Wen et al. 2009. Activity of armillarisin B in vitro against plant pathogenic fungi. *Zeitschrift für Naturforschung C* 64 (11–12): 790–792.

Shen, Qing et al. 2002. Molecular phylogenetic analysis of *Grifola frondosa* (maitake) reveals a species partition separating eastern North American and Asian isolates. *Mycologia* 94 (3): 472–482.

Shi, Lin–Mei and Zha–Jun Zhan. 2007. Structural revision of 19, 20–epoxycytochalasin D and its cytotoxic activity. *Journal of Chemical Research* 3: 144–145.

Shi, Yu–Ling et al. 2002a. Genoprotective activities of mushrooms. *Seventh International Mycological Congress Book of Abstracts* #167.

Shi, Yu–Ling et al. 2002b. Mushroom–derived preparations in the prevention of H2O2–induced oxidative damage to cellular DNA. *Teratogenesis, Carcinogenisis, and Mutagenesis* 22 (2): 103–111.

Shibata, H. et al. 1998. Molecular properties and activity of amino–terminal truncated forms of lipase activator protein. *Bioscience, Biotechnology, and Biochemistry* 62 (2): 354–357.

Shibata, K. et al. 1969. Laboratory and clinical studies on minocycline in the surgical field. *Japanese Journal of Antibiotics* 22 (6): 458–462.

Shibata, S. et al. 1968. Antitumor studies on some extracts of Basidiomycetes. *GANN: Japanese Journal of Cancer Research* 59 (2): 159–161.

Shibata, Yasuhiro et al. 2005. Administration of extract of mushroom *Phellinus linteus* induces prostate enlargement with increase in stromal component in experimentally developed rat model of benign prostatic hyperplasia. *Urology* 66 (2): 455–460.

Shimada, Shoichiro et al. 2004. Inhibitory activity of shiitake flavor against platelet aggregation. *Biofactors* 22(1–4): 177–179.

Shimada, Yasuhiko et al. 2003. Dietary eritadenine and ethanolamine depress fatty acid desaturase activities by increasing liver microsomal phosphatidylethanolamine in rats. *The Journal of Nutrition* 133 (3): 758–765.

Shimizu, S. et al. 2002. Activation of the alternative complement pathway by *Agaricus blazei* Murill. *Phytomedicine* 9 (6): 536–545.

Shin, Kuk Hyun et al. 2003. Anti–tumour and immuno–stimulating activities of the fruiting bodies of *Paecilomyces japonica,* a new type of *Cordyceps* sp. *Phytotherapy Research* 17 (7): 830–833.

Shin, Kwang Soo and Yeo Jin Lee. 2000. A novel extracellular peroxidase of the white rot Basidiomycete *Coriolus hirsutus. Mycologia* 92 (3): 537–544.

Shiu, W. C. T. et al. 1992. A clinical study of PSP on peripheral blood counts during chemotherapy. Phytotherapy Research 6 217–218.

Shnyreva, Alla V. et al. 2010. Extracts of medicinal mushrooms *Agaricus bisporus* and *Phellinus linteus* induce proapoptotic effects in the human leukemia cell line K562. *International Journal of Medicinal Mushrooms* 12 (2): 167–175.

Shon, Yun–Hee and Kyung–Soo Nam. 2002. Cancer chemoprevention inhibitory effect of soybeans fermented with Basidiomycetes on 7,12–dimethylbenz[A]anthracene/12–O–tetradecanoylphorbol–13–acetate–induced mouse skin carcinogenesis. *Biotechnology Letters* 24 (10): 1005–1010.

Shon, Yun–Hee and Kyung–Soo Nam. 2004. Inhibition of cytochrome P450 isozymes and ornithine decarboxylase activities by polysaccharides from soybeans fermented with *Phellinus igniarius* or *Agrocybe cylindracea. Biotechnology Letters* 26 (2): 159–163.

Shuvy et al. 2008. Intrahepatic CD8+ lymphocyte trapping during tolerance induction using mushroom derived formulations: A possible role for liver in tolerance induction. *World Journal of Gastroenterology* 14 (24): 3872–3877.

Sia, G. M. and J. K. Candlis. 1999. Effects of shiitake *(Lentinus edodes)* extract on human neutrophils and the U937 monocytic cell line. *Phytotherapy Research* 13 (2): 133–137.

Silberborth, Sven et al. 2000. The irpexans, a new group of biologically active metabolites produced by the Basidiomycete *Irpex* sp. *Journal of Antibiotics* 53 (10): 1137–1144.

Silberborth, Sven et al. 2002. Gerronemins A–F, cytotoxic biscatechols from a *Gerronema* species. *Phytochemistry* 59 (6): 643–8.

Silva, Fabricio S. et al. 2009. In vitro pharmacological screening of macrofungi extracts from the Brazilian northeastern region. *Pharmaceutical Biology* 47 (5): 384–389.

Siu et al. 2004. Pharmacological basis of 'yin–nourishing' and 'yang–invigorating' actions of *Cordyceps,* a Chinese tonifying herb. *Life Sciences* 76 (4): 385–395.

Slane et al. 2004. Screening of wood damaging fungi and macrofungi for inhibitors of pancreatic lipase. *Phytotherapy Research* 18 (9): 758–762.

Sliva, Daniel 2003. *Ganoderma lucidum* (reishi) in cancer treatment. *Integrative Cancer Therapies* 2 (4): 358–364.

Smania, A. et al. 1999. Antimicrobial activity of steroidal compounds isolated from *Ganoderma applanatum* (Pers.) Pat. (Aphyllophoromycetideae) fruitbody. *International Journal of Medicinal Mushrooms* 1 (4): 325–330.

Smania, A. et al. 2003. Toxicity and antiviral activity of cinnabarin obtained from *Pycnoporus sanguineus* (Fr.) Murr. *Phytotherapy Research* 17 (9): 1069–1072.

Smania, E. F. A. et al. 2003. Antifungal activity of sterols and triterpenes isolated from *Ganoderma annulare*. *Fitoterapia* 74 (4): 375–377.

Smith, Terence A. 1977. Tryptamine and related compounds in plants. *Phytochemistry* 16 (2): 171–175.

Sokovic et al. 2006. Antimicrobial activity of essential oils and their components against the three major pathogens of the cultivated button mushroom, *Agaricus bisporus*. *European Journal of Plant Pathology* 116 (3): 211–224.

Solomko et al. 2005. The selection of alternative substrates for medicinal mushroom cultivation. *International Journal of Medicinal Mushrooms* 7 (3): 466.

Son et al. 2006. Macrophage activation and nitric oxide production by water soluble components of *Hericium erinaceum*. *International Immunopharmacology* 6 (8): 1363–1369.

Song, C. H. et al. 1998. Anti–complementary activity of endopolymers produced from submerged mycelial culture of higher fungi with particular reference to *Lentinus edodes*. *Biotechnology Letters* 20 (8): 741–744.

Song, Nan–Kyu et al. 2000. Identification of nitric oxide synthase in *Flammulina velutipes*. *Mycologia* 92 (6): 1027–1032.

Song, Yun Seon et al. 2004. Anti–angiogenic and inhibitory activity on inducible nitric oxide production of the mushroom *Ganoderma lucidum*. *Journal of Ethnopharmacology* 90 (1): 17–20.

Songulashvili et al. 2007. Basidiomycetes laccase and manganese peroxidase activity in submerged fermentation of food industry wastes. *Enzyme and Microbial Technology* 41 (1–2): 57–61.

Sontag et al. 1999. Montadial A, a cytotoxic metabolite from *Bondarzewia montana*. *Journal of Natural Products* 62 (10): 1425–1426.

Sorimachi, K. et al. 1990. Anti–viral activity of water–soluble lignin derivatives in vitro. *Agricultural and Biological Chemistry* 54 (5): 1337–1339.

Sorimachi, K. et al. 2001. Inhibition by *Agaricus blazei* Murill fractions of cytopathic effect induced by western equine encephalitis (WEE) virus on VERO cells in vitro. *Bioscience, Biotechnology, and Biochemistry* 65 (7): 1645–1647.

Sostrin, Ben. 2002. Mamalu o wahine (woman's mushroom). *MushRumors* 41 (3).

Spoerke, Barry H. and David G. Rumack. 1994. *Handbook of mushroom poisoning: Diagnosis and treatment*. Boca Raton: CRC Press.

Stadler, Marc et al. 1994. Fatty acids and other compounds with nematicidal activity from cultures of Basidiomycetes. *Planta Medica* 60 (2): 128–132.

Stadler, Marc et al. 2005. Novel analgesic triglycerides from cultures of *Agaricus macrosporus* and other Basidiomycetes as selective inhibitors of neurolysin. *Japanese Journal of Antibiotics* 58 (12): 775–786.

Stamets, Paul. 2005. Notes on nutritional properties of culinary–medicinal mushrooms. *International Journal of Medicinal Mushrooms* 7 (3): 103–110.

Stanikunaite, Rita et al. 2007. Evaluation of therapeutic activity of hypogeous Ascomycetes and Basidiomycetes from North America. *International Journal of Medicinal Mushrooms* 9 (1): 7–14.

Stanikunaite, Rita et al. 2008. Lanostane–type triterpenes from the mushoom *Astraeus pteridis* with antituberculosis activity. *Journal of Natural Products* 71 (12): 2077–2079.

Stanley et al. 2005. *Ganoderma lucidum* suppresses angiogenesis through the inhibition of secretion of VEGF and TGF–beta1 from prostate cancer cells. *Biochemical and Biophysical Research Communications* 330 (1): 46–52.

Stavinoha, W. B. et al. 1995. Study of the antiinflammatory efficacy of *Ganoderma lucidum*. In B.-K. Kim, & Y.S. Kim (editors), *Recent Advances in* Ganoderma lucidum *research*. Seoul: The Pharmaceutical Society of Korea.

Stefer et al. 2003. A pervaporation–bio–hybridreactor (PBHR) for improved aroma biosynthesis with submerged culture of *Ceratocystis fimbriata.* *Communications in Agricultural and Applied Biological Sciences* 68 (2A): 247–252.

Steffen, Kari T. et al. 2002. Removal and mineralization of polycyclic aromatic hydrocarbons by litter–decomposing Basidiomycetous fungi. *Applied Microbiology and Biotechnology* 60 (1–2): 212–217.

Steffen, Kari T. et al. 2003. Degradation of benzo[a] pyrene by the litter–decomposing Basidiomycete *Stropharia coronilla:* Role of manganese peroxidase. *Applied and Environmental Microbiology* 69 (7): 3957–3964.

Steinkraus, D. C. and J. B. Whitfield. 1994. Chinese caterpillar fungus and world record runners. *American Entomologist* Winter 1994: 235–239.

Steyn, D. G. 1966. The treatment of cases of *Amanita phalloides* and *Amanita capensis* poisoning. *South African Medical Journal* 40 (5): 405–406.

Sublette, K. et al. 1992. Degradation of munition wastes by *Phanerochaete chrysosporium. Applied Biochemistry and Biotechnology* 34–35: 709–723

Su, Chen–Yi et al. 1999. Predominant inhibition of ganodermic acid S on the thromboxane A_{2-} dependent pathway in human platelets response to collagen. *Biochimica et Biophysica Acta – Molecular and Cell Biology of Lipids* 1437 (2): 223–234.

Su, Huey–Jen et al. 2000. New lanostanoids of *Ganoderma tsugae. Journal of Natural Products* 63 (4): 514–516.

Suay et al. 2000. Screening of Basidiomycetes for antimicrobial activities. *Antoine van Leeuwenhoek* 78 (2): 129–140.

Sugano et al. 1982. Anticarcinogenic actions of water–soluble and alcohol–insoluble fractions from culture medium of *Lentinus edodes* mycelia. *Cancer Letters* 17 (2): 109–114.

Sugiyama et al. 1992. Isolation of plasma cholesterol–lowering components from ningyotake (*Polyporus confluens*) mushroom. *Journal of Nutritional Science and Vitaminology* 38 (4): 335–342.

Sumba, Julius David. 2005. GACOCA formulation of East African wild mushrooms show promise in combating Kaposi's sarcoma and HIV / AIDS. *International Journal of Medicinal Mushrooms* 7 (3): 473–474.

Sun, Jie et al. 2004. Novel antioxidant peptides from fermented mushroom *Ganoderma lucidum. Journal of Agricultural and Food Chemistry* 52 (21): 6646–6652.

Sun, Jun–En et al. 2008. Antihyperglycemic and antilipidperoxidative effects of dry matter of culture broth of *Inonotus obliquus* in submerged culture on normal and alloxan–diabetes mice. *Journal of Ethnopharmacology* 118 (1): 7–13.

Sun, Yongxu et al. 2010a. Purification, structural analysis and hydroxyl radical–scavenging capacity of a polysaccharide from the fruiting bodies of *Russula virescens. Process Biochemistry* 45 (6): 874–879.

Sun, Yongxu et al. 2010b. Water–soluble polysaccharide from the fruiting bodies of *Chroogomphis rutilus* (Schaeff.: Fr.) O. K. Miller: Isolation, structural features and its scavenging effect on hydroxyl radical. *Carbohydrate Polymers* 80 (3): 720–724.

Suzuki, Ikukatsu et al. 2001. Antihypertensive effect of *Lyophyllum decastes* Sing. in spontaneously hypertensive rats. *International Journal of Medicinal Mushrooms* 3 (2–3): 231.

Suzuki, Takuo et al. 2006. Screening of novel nuclear receptor agonists by a convenient reporter gene assay system using green fluorescent protein derivatives. *Phytomedicine* 13 (6): 401–411.

Swanson and Fahselt 1997. Effects of Ultraviolet on polyphenolics of *Umbilicaria* America. *Canadian Journal of Botany* 75 (2) 284–289.

Szallasi et al. 1999. A non–pungent triprenyl phenol of fungal origin, scutigeral, stimulates rat dorsal root ganglion neurons via interaction at vanilloid receptors. *British Journal of Pharmacology* 126 (6): 1351–1358.

Taichi, Usui et al. 1983. Isolation and characterization of antitumor active –d–glucans from the fruit bodies of *Ganoderma applanatum*. *Carbohydrate Research* 115 (2): 273–280.

Taira, Kentaro et al. 2005. Novel antimutagenic factors derived from the edible mushroom *Agrocybe cylindracea*. *Mutation Research* 586 (2): 115–123.

Takahashi et al. 1992. 5–Lipoxygenase inhibitors isolated from the mushroom *Boletopsis leucomelas* (Pers.) Fayod. *Chemical & Pharmaceutical Bulletin* 40 (12): 3194–3196.

Takakura, Yoshimitsu et al. 2009. Tamavidins–novel avidin–like biotin–binding proteins from the tamogitake mushroom. *FEBS Journal* 276 (5): 1383–1397.

Takazawa et al. 1982. An antifungal compound from "shiitake" *(Lentinus edodes)*. *Yakugaku Zasshi* 102 (5): 489–491.

Takei et al. 2005. Ergosterol peroxide, an apoptosis–inducing component isolated from *Sarcodon aspratus* (Berk.) S. Ito. *Bioscience, Biotechnology, and Biochemistry* 69 (1): 212–215.

Talpur, N. A. et al. 2002. Antihypertensive and metabolic effects of whole maitake mushroom powder and its fractions in two rat strains. *Molecular and Cellular Biochemistry* 237 (1–2): 129–136.

Talukdar, R. et al. 2007. Pancreatic stellate cells: New target in the treatment of chronic pancreatitis. *Journal of Gastroenterology and Hepatology* 23 (1): 34–41.

Tamaki et al. 2007. Studies on the deodorization by mushroom *(Agaricus bisporus)* extract of garlic extract–induced oral malodor. *Journal of Nutritional Science and Vitaminology* 53 (3): 277–286.

Tan, Jian–Wen et al. 2002. Lepidolide, a novel seco–ring–A cucurbitane triterpenoid from *Russula lepida* (Basidiomycetes). *Zeitschrift für Naturforschung C* 57 (11–12): 963–965.

Tan, Jian–Wen et al. 2003. Lepidamine, the first aristolane–type sesquiterpene alkaloid from the Basidiomycete *Russula lepida*. *Helvetica Chimica Acta* 86 (2): 307–309.

Tan, Jian–Wen et al. 2004. Nigricanin, the first

ellagic acid derived metabolite from the Basidiomycete *Russula nigricans*. *Helvetica Chimica Acta* 87 (4): 1025–1028.

Tansuwan et al. 2007. Antimalarial benzoquinones from an endophytic fungus, *Xylaria* sp. *Journal of Natural Products* 70 (10): 1620–1623.

Taupp, Daniela E. et al. 2008. Stress response of *Nidula niveo–tomentosa* to UV–A light. *Mycologia* 100 (4): 529–538.

Tay et al. 2004. Evaluation of the antimicrobial activity of the acetone extract of the lichen *Ramalina farinacea* and its (+)–usnic acid, norstictic acid, and protocetraric acid constituents. *Zeitschrift für Naturforschung C* 59 (5–6): 384.

Teichert et al. 2007. Brunneins A–C, –carboline alkaloids from *Cortinarius brunneus*. *Journal of Natural Products* 70 (9): 1529–1531.

Tepkeeva et al. 2009. Cytostatic activity of peptide extracts of medicinal plants on transformed A549, H1299, and HeLa cells. *Bulletin of Experimental Biology and Medicine* 147 (1): 48–51.

Terakawa et al. 2008. Immunological effect of active hexose correlated compound (AHCC) in healthy volunteers: A double–blind, placebo–controlled trial. *Nutrition and Cancer* 60 (5): 643–651.

Terrazas–Siles et al. 2005. Isolation and characterization of a white rot fungus *Bjerkandera* sp. strain capable of oxidizing phenanthrene. *Biotechnology Letters* 27 (12): 845–851.

Thompson G. and R. Medve. 1984. Effects of aluminum and manganese on the growth of ectomycorrhizal fungi. *Applied Environmental and Public Health Microbiology* 48 (3): 556–560.

Thormann, Markus N. et al. 2002. The relative ability of fungi from *Sphagnum fuscum* to decompose selected carbon substrates. *Canadian Journal of Microbiology* 48 (3): 204–211.

Toshiro et al. 2003. Antihypertensive effect of gamma–aminobutyric acid–enriched *Agaricus blazei* on mild hypertensive human subjects. *Nippon Shokuhin Kagaku Kogaku Kaishi* 50 (1): 167–173.

Trejo–Hernandez et al. 2001. Residual compost of *Agaricus bisporus* as a source of crude laccase for enzymic oxidation of phenolic compounds. *Process Biochemistry* 36 (7): 635–639.

Tringali et al. 1989. An antitumor principle from *Suillus granulatus. Journal of Natural Products* 52 (4): 844–845.

Tsai et al. 2008. Antioxidant properties of ethanolic extracts from culinary–medicinal button mushroom *Agaricus bisporus* (J. Lange) Imbach (Agaricomycetideae) harvested at different stages of maturity. *International Journal of Medicinal Mushrooms* 10 (2): 127–137.

Tsukamoto, S. et al. 2003. Tricholomalides A−C, new neurotrophic diterpenes from the mushroom *Tricholoma* sp. *Journal of Natural Products* 66 (12): 1578–1581.

Tuomela, Marja et al. 1998. Mineralization and conversion of pentachlorophenol (PCP) in soil inoculated with the white–rot fungus *Trametes versicolor. Soil Biology and Biochemistry* 31 (1): 65–74.

Tuomela, Marja et al. 2002. Degradation of synthetic ^{14}C–lignin by various white–rot fungi in soil. *Soil Biology and Biochemistry* 34 (11): 1613–1620.

Tura, Daniel et al. 2009. Medicinal species from genera *Inonotus* and *Phellinus* (Aphyllophoromycetideae): Cultural–morphological peculiarities, growth characteristics, and qualitative enzymatic activity tests. *International Journal of Medicinal Mushrooms* 11 (3): 309–328.

Uchida, Atsushi. 1995. Method for treatment of chronic fatigue syndrome. US Patent 5424300. Issued: June 13, 1995.

Ueda, Keiko et al. 2008. An endoplasmic reticulum (ER) stress–suppressive compound and its analogues from the mushroom *Hericium erinaceum. Bioorganic & Medicinal Chemistry* 16 (21): 9467–9470.

Ukawa, Yuuichi et al. 2002. Effect of hatakeshimeji (*Lyophyllum decastes* Sing.) mushroom on serum lipid levels in rats. *Journal of Nutritional Science and Vitaminology* 48 (1): 73–76.

Ukawa, Yuuichi et al. 2007. Oral administration of the extract from hatakeshimeji (*Lyophyllum decastes* Sing.) mushroom inhibits the development of atopic dermatitis–like skin lesions in NC/NGA mice. *Journal of Nutritional Science and Vitaminology* 53 (3): 293–296.

Ullrich et al. 2004. Novel haloperoxidase from the agaric Basidiomycete *Agrocybe aegerita* oxidizes aryl alcohols and aldehydes. *Applied and Environmental Microbiology* 70 (8): 4575–4581.

Umezawa et al. 1995. Total synthesis of (±)–, (–)–, and (+)–oudemansin X. *Chemical & Pharmaceutical Bulletin* 43 (7): 1111–1118.

Unyayar, Ali et al. 2005. Cytotoxic activities of *Funalia trogii* (Berk.) Bond. Et. Singer ATCC 200800 bioactive extract on HeLa cells and fibroblast cells. *International Journal of Medicinal Mushrooms* 7 (3): 478–479.

Unyayar, Ali et al. 2006. Evaluation of cytotoxic and mutagenic effects of *Coriolus versicolor* and *Funalia trogii* extracts on mammalian cells. *Drug and Chemical Toxicology* 29 (1): 69–83.

Van, Q. et al. 2009. Anti–inflammatory effect of *Inonotus obliquus, Polygala senega* L., and *Viburnum trilobum* in a cell screening assay. *Journal of Ethnopharmacology* 125 (3): 487–493.

Van Aken, Benoit et al. 1997. Biodegradation of 2, 4, 6–trinitrotoluene (TNT) by the white–rot Basidiomycete *Phlebia radiata. Biotechnology Letters* 19 (8): 813–817.

Van Aken, Benoit et al. 1999. Transformation and mineralization of 2,4,6–trinitrotoluene (TNT) by manganese peroxidase from the white–rot Basidiomycete *Phlebia radiata. Biodegradation* 10 (2): 83–91.

Van Hamme, Jonathan D. et al. 2003. Dibenzyl sulfide metabolism by white rot fungi. *Applied and Environmental Microbiology* 69 (2): 1320–1324.

Vartiamäki et al. 2009. Effect of application time on the efficacy of *Chondrostereum purpureum* treatment against the sprouting of birch in Finland. *Canadian Journal of Forest Research* 39 (4): 731–739.

Vecchi et al. 2009. ACE inhibitory tetrapeptides from *Amaranthus hypochondriacus* 11S globulin. *Phytochemistry* 70 (7): 823–952.

Verhagen et al. 1996. The ubiquity of natural absorbable organic halogen production among Basidiomycetes. *Applied Microbiology and Biotechnology* 45 (5): 710–718.

Vinogradov, Evgeny et al. 2004. The isolation, structure, and applications of the exocellular heteropolysaccharide glucuronoxylomannan produced by yellow brain mushroom *Tremella mesenterica* Ritz.:Fr. (Heterobasidiomycetes). *International Journal of Medicinal Mushrooms* 6 (4): 361–372.

Volc, J. et al. 1985. Glucose–2–oxidase activity in mycelial cultures of Basidiomycetes. *Folia Microbiologica* 30 (2): 141–147.

Wachtel–Galor, S. et al. 2004. *Ganoderma lucidum* ('lingzhi'); acute and short–term biomarker response to supplementation. *International Journal of Food Sciences and Nutrition* 55 (1): 75–83.

Wagenfuhr et al. 1989. Industrial Patent DD 271 078 A1. Issued: August 23, 1989.

Wall, R. E. 1990. The fungus *Chondrostereum purpureum* as a silvicide to control stump sprouting in hardwoods. *Northern Journal of Applied Forestry* 7 (1): 17–19.

Wang, F. and J. K. Liu. 2005. Two new steryl esters from the Basidiomycete *Tricholomopsis rutil*. *Steroids* 70 (2): 127–130.

Wang, Hexiang and Tzi Bun Ng. 2000. Isolation of a novel ubiquitin–like protein from *Pleurotus osteatus* mushroom with anti–human immunodeficiency virus, translation–inhibitory and ribonuclease activities. *Biochemical and Biophysical Research Communications* 276 (2): 393–812.

Wang, Hexiang and Tzi Bun Ng. 2001. Isolation and characterization of velutin, a novel low–molecular–weight ribosome–inactivating protein from winter mushroom *(Flammulina velutipes)* fruiting bodies. *Life Sciences* 68 (18): 2151–2158.

Wang, Hexiang and Tzi Bun Ng. 2006. A laccase from the medicinal mushroom *Ganoderma lucidum*. *Applied Microbiology and Biotechnology* 72(3): 508–513.

Wang, Hexiang and Tzi Bun Ng. 2007. An antifungal peptide from red lentil seeds. *Peptides* 28 (3): 547–552.

Wang, Hexiang et al. 2000. A new lectin with highly potent antihepatoma and antisarcoma activities from the oyster mushroom *Pleurotus ostreatus*. *Biochemical and Biophysical Research Communications* 275 (3): 810–816.

Wang, Hexiang et al. 2002. Isolation of a new heterodimeric lectin with mitogenic activity from fruiting bodies of the mushroom *Agrocybe cylindracea*. *Life Sciences* 70 (8): 877–885.

Wang, Jinn Chyi et al. 2005. Hypoglycemic effect of extract of *Hericium erinaceus*. *Journal of the Science of Food and Agriculture* 85 (4): 641–646.

Wang, Nan et al. 2000. Detecting in 9 extracellular enzyme activities of *Agrocybe aegerita* strains. *Mycosystema* 19 (4): 540–546.

Wang, Po–Hui et al. 2004. Fungal immunomodulatory protein from *Flammulina velutipes* induces interferon–Y production through P38 mitogen–activated protein kinase signaling pathway. *Journal of Agricultural Food Chemistry* 52 (9): 2721–2725.

Wang, Xi and Leslie C. Plhak. 2004. Monoclonal antibodies for the analysis of gossypol in cottonseed products. *Journal of Agricultural and Food Chemistry* 52 (4): 709–712.

Wang, Ying et al. 2005. Phelligridimer A, a highly oxygenated and unsaturated 26–membered macrocyclic metabolite with antioxidant activity from the fungus *Phellinus igniarius*. *Organic Letters* 7 (21): 4733–4736.

Wang, Ying et al. 2007. Structures, biogenesis, and biological activities of Pyrano[4,3–c]isochromen–4–one derivatives from the fungus *Phellinus igniarius*. *Journal of Natural Products* 70 (2): 296–299.

Wang, Yuxin et al. 2003. Manganese–lignin peroxidase hybrid from *Bjerkandera adusta* oxidizes polycyclic aromatic hydrocarbons more actively in the absence of manganese. *Canadian Journal of Microbiology* 49 (11): 675–682.

Wangun, Hilaire V. Kemami and Christian Hertweck. 2007. Squarrosidine and pinillidine: 3,3'–fused bis(styrylpyrones) from *Pholiota squarrosa* and *Phellinus pini*. *European Journal of Organic Chemistry* 2007 (20): 3292–3295.

Wangun, Hilaire V. Kemami et al. 2004. Anti–inflammatory and anti–hyaluronate lyase activities of lanostanoids from *Piptoporus betulinus*. *Journal of Antibiotics* 57 (11): 755–8.

Warner et al. 2004. *Marasmius oreades* lectin induces renal thrombotic microangiopathic lesions. *Experimental and Molecular Pathology* 77 (2): 77–84.

Wasser, Solomon P. and Alexander L. Weis. 1999. Therapeutic effects of substances occurring in higher Basidiomycetes mushrooms: A modern perspective. *Critical Reviews in Immunology* 19 (1): 65–96.

Wasson, R. Gordon et al. 2008. *The Road to Eleusis: Unveiling the Secret of the Mysteries*. Berkeley: North Atlantic Books.

Watanabe, Hideaki and Masahisa Nakada. 2008. Biomimetic total synthesis of (−)–erinacine E. *Journal of the American Chemical Society* 130 (4): 1150–1151.

Watanabe, N. et al. 1990. A novel n6–substituted adenosine isolated from mi huan jun *(Armillaria mellea)* as a cerebral–protecting compound. *Planta Medica* 56 (1): 48–52.

Watanabe, Reiko et al. 2002. A novel dipeptide, N––glutamyl boletine, and a cyclic iminium toxin from the mushroom *Tylopilus* sp. (Boletaceae). *Tetrahedron Letters* 43 (11): 2043–2046.

Weckesser et al. 2007. Screening of plant extracts for antimicrobial activity against bacteria and yeasts with dermatological relevance. *Phytomedicine* 14 (7–8): 508–516.

Wei et al. 2009. Isolating a cytoprotective compound from *Ganoderma tsugae*: Effects on induction of NRF–2–related genes in endothelial cells. *Bioscience, Biotechnology, and Biochemistry* 71 (8): 1757–1763.

Weil, David A et al. 2006. Manganese and other micronutrient additions to improve yield of *Agaricus bisporus*. *Bioresource Technology* 97 (8): 1012–1017.

Wells, Kenneth. 1994. Jelly fungi, then and now! *Mycologia* 86 (1): 18–48.

Weng et al. 2010. Ganodermasides A and B, two novel anti–aging ergosterols from spores of a medicinal mushroom. *Bioorganic and Medicinal Chemistry* 18 (3): 999–1002.

Werner, Andrew R. and Robert B. Beelman. 2002. Growing high–selenium edible and medicinal button mushrooms (*Agaricus bisporus* (J. Lge) Imbach) as ingredients for functional foods or dietary supplements. *International Journal of Medicinal Mushrooms* 4 (2): 169–174.

Wilhelm et al. 2004. New peptaibols from *Mycogone cervina*. *Journal of Natural Products* 67 (3): 466–468.

Willenborg et al. 1990. Effects of environmental stress factors on ectomycorrhizal fungi in vitro. *Canadian Journal of Botany* 68 (8): 1741–1746.

Winter et al. 2002. The mushroom *Marasmius oreades* lectin is a blood group type B agglutinin that recognizes the gal 1, 3gal and gal 1, 3gal 1, 4GlcNAc porcine xenotransplantation epitopes with high affinity. *The Journal of Biological Chemistry* 277 (17): 14996–15001.

Withers and Umezawa. 1991. Cyclophellitol: A naturally occurring mechanism–based inactivator of beta–glucosidases. *Biochemical and Biophysical Research Communications* 177 (1): 532–537.

Won, Shen-Jeu et al. 1992. *Ganoderma tsugae* mycelium enhances splenic natural killer cell activity and serum interferon production in mice. *The Japanese Journal of Pharmacology* 59 (2): 171-176.

Wood et al. 2004. Clitolactone: A banana slug anti-feedant from *Clitocybe flaccida*. *Mycologia* 96 (1): 23–25.

Wu, Geng–Shu et al. 1997. Inhibitive effect of *Umbellatus polyporus* polysaccharide on cachexic manifestation induced by toxohormone–L in rats. *Zhongguo Zhong Xi Yi Jie He Za Zhi* 17 (4): 232–233.

Wu, Jian Yong et al. 2007. Inhibitory effects of ethyl acetate extract of *Cordyceps sinensis* mycelium on various cancer cells in culture and B16 melanoma in C57BL/6 mice. *Phytomedicine* 14 (1): 43–49.

Wu, Liping et al. 2003. Purification and activities of an alkaline protein from mushroom *Coprinus comats*. *Wei Sheng Wu Xue Bao* 43 (6): 793–798.

Wu, Ming–Der et al. 2008. Maleimide and maleic anhydride derivatives from the mycelia of *Antrodia cinnamomea* and their nitric oxide inhibitory activities in macrophages. *Journal of Natural Products* 71 (7): 1258–1261.

Wu, Qin et al. 2010. Chemical characterization of *Auricularia auricula* polysaccharides and its pharmacological effect on heart antioxidant enzyme activities and left ventricular function in aged mice. *International Journal of Biological Macromolecules* 46 (3): 284–288.

Wu, Shimin et al. 2005a. Characteristic volatiles from young and aged fruiting bodies of wild *Polyporus sulfureus* (Bull.: Fr.) Fr. *Journal of Agricultural and Food Chemistry* 53 (11): 2524–2528.

Wu, Shimin et al. 2005b. Volatile compounds from the fruiting bodies of beefsteak fungus *Fistulina hepatica* (Schaeffer: Fr.) Fr. *Food Chemistry* 92 (2): 221–226.

Wu, Shu–Jing et al. 2007. *Armillariella mellea* shows anti–inflammatory activity by inhibiting the expression of NO, iNOS, COX–2 and cytokines in THP–1 cells. *American Journal of Chinese Medicine* 35 (3): 507–516.

Wu, Tao et al. 2004. Chitin and chitosan value–added products from mushroom waste. *Journal of Agricultural and Food Chemistry* 52 (26): 7905–7910.

Wu, Tian–Shung et al. 2001. Cytotoxicity of *Ganoderma lucidum* triterpenes. *Journal of Natural Products* 64 (8): 1121–1122.

Wunch et al. 1997. Screening for fungi capable of removing benzo[a]pyrene in culture. *Applied Microbiology and Biotechnology* 47 (5): 620–624.

Xiao et al. 2007. Clinical experience in treatment of *Amanita* mushroom poisoning with glossy *Ganoderma* decoction ( ) and routine Western medicines. *Chinese Journal of Integrative Medicine* 13 (2): 147–147.

Xie, Chun et al. 2006. Vialinin B, a novel potent inhibitor of TNF– production, isolated from an edible mushroom, *Thelephora vialis*. *Bioorganic and Medical Chemistry Letters* 16 (20);: 5424.5426.

Xie, Qiang–Min et al. 2006. Effects of cryptoporus polysaccharide on rat allergic rhinitis associated with inhibiting eotaxin mRNA expression. *Journal of Ethnopharmacology* 107 (3): 424–430.

Yadav, J. S. and C. A. Reddy. 1993a. Degradation of benzene, toluene, ethylbenzene and xylenes (BTEX) by the lignin–degrading Basidiomycete *Phanerochaete chrysosporium*. *Applied and Environmental Microbiology* 59 (3): 756–762.

Yadav, J. S. and C. A. Reddy. 1993b. Mineralization of 2,4–dichlorophenoxyacetic acid (2,4–D) and mixtures of 2,4–D and 2,4,5–trichlorophenoxyacetic acid by *Phanerochaete chrysosporium*. *Applied and Environmental Microbiology* 59 (9): 2904–2908.

Yaghoubi, Kamel et al. 2008. Variable optimization for biopulping of agricultural residues by *Ceriporiopsis subvermispora*. *Bioresource Technology* 99 (10): 4321–4328.

Yagi, Fumio et al. 2000. Hemagglutinins (lectins) in fruit bodies of Japanese higher fungi. *Mycoscience* 41 (4): 323–330.

Yamac, Mustafa and Fatma Bilgili. 2006. Antimicrobial activities of fruit bodies and/or mycelial cultures of some mushroom isolates. *Pharmaceutical Biology* 44 (9): 660–667.

Yamac, Mustafa et al. 2008. Hypoglycemic effect of *Lentinus strigosus* (Schwein.) Fr. crude exopolysaccharide in streptozotocin–induced diabetic rats. *Journal of Medicinal Food* 11 (3): 513–517.

Yamada et al. 1984. Structure and antitumor activity of an alkali–soluble polysaccharide from *Cordyceps ophioglossoides. Carbohydrate Research* 125 (1): 107–115.

Yamaguchi et al. 2000. Inhibitory effects of water extracts from fruiting bodies of cultured *Cordyceps sinensis* on raised serum lipid peroxide levels and aortic cholesterol deposition in atherosclerotic mice. *Phytotherapy Research* 14 (8): 650–652.

Yamamoto, K. et al. 2007. Antitumor activities of low molecular weight fraction derived from the cultured fruit body of *Sparassis crispa* in tumor–bearing mice. *Journal of the Japanese Society for Food Science Technology* 54 (9): 419–423.

Yamamoto, K. et al. 2009. Anti–angiogenic and anti–metastatic effects of –1,3–D–glucan purified from hanabiratake, *Sparassis crispa. Biological & Pharmaceutical Bulletin* 32 (2): 259–263.

Yamamoto, T. et al. 1981. Inhibition of pulmonary metastasis of Lewis lung carcinoma by a glucan, schizophyllan. *Invasion & Metastasis* 1 (1): 71–84.

Yamamoto, Yoshikazu et al. 1993. Using lichen tissue cultures in modern biology. *The Bryologist* 96 (3): 384–393.

Yan, R. et al. 1987. Treatment of chronic hepatitis B with wulingdan pill. *Abstracts of Chinese Medicine* 2 (188): 380–383.

Yano, T. et al. 1991. Polysaccharide–induced protection of carp, *Cyprinus carpio* L., against bacterial infection. *Journal of Fish Diseases* 14 (5): 577–582.

Yang, Byung–Keun et al. 2002. Hypoglycemic effect of a *Lentinus edodes* exo–polymer produced from a submerged mycelial culture. *Bioscience, Biotechnology, and Biochemistry* 66 (5): 937–942.

Yang, Byung–Keun et al. 2007. Hypoglycemic effects of *Ganoderma applanatum* and *Collybia confluens* exo–polymers in streptozotocin–induced diabetic rats. *Phytotherapy Research* 21 (11): 1066–1069.

Yang, Na et al. 2005. Molecular character of the recombinant antitumor lectin from the edible mushroom *Agrocybe aegerita. Journal of Biochemistry* 138 (2): 145–150.

Yang, Q. Y., editor. 1999. *Advanced Research in PSP.*

Hong Kong: Hong Kong Association for Health Care Ltd.

Yang, Wei–Min et al. 2003. Albaconol from the mushroom *Albatrellus confluens* induces contraction and desensitization in guinea pig trachea. *Planta Medica* 69 (8): 715–719.

Yang, Yan et al. 2009. Structural analysis of a bioactive polysaccharide, PISP1, from the medicinal mushroom *Phellinus igniarius. Bioscience, Biotechnology, and Biochemistry* 73 (1): 134–139.

Yassin, Majed and Jamal A. Mahajna. 2003. Submerged cultured mycelium extracts of higher Basidiomycetes mushrooms selectively inhibit proliferation and induce differentiation of K562 human chronic myelogenous leukemia cells. *International Journal of Medicinal Mushrooms* 5 (3): 277–292.

Yassin, Majed et al. 2008. Substances from the medicinal mushroom *Daedalea gibbosa* inhibit kinase activity of native and T315I mutated Bcr–Abl. *International Journal of Oncology* 32 (6): 1197–1204.

Yateem, A. et al. 1998. White rot fungi and their role in remediating oil contaminated soil. *Environment International* 24 (1–2): 181–187.

Yatsuzuka et al. 2007. Effect of usuhratake (*Pleurotus pulmonarius*) on sneezing and nasal rubbing in BALB/C mice. *Biological and Pharmaceutical Bulletin* 30 (8): 1557.

Ye, Mao et al. 2005. Grifolin, a potential antitumor natural product from the mushroom *Albatrellus confluens*, inhibits tumor cell growth by inducing apoptosis in vitro. *FEBS Letters* 579 (16): 3437–3443.

Ye, Mao et al. 2007. Grifolin, a potential antitumor natural product from the mushroom *Albatrellus confluens*, induces cell–cycle arrest in G1 phase via the ERK1/2 pathway. *Cancer Letters* 258 (2): 199–207.

Yen, Gow-Chin and Jun-Yi Wu. 1999. Antioxidant and radical scavenging properties of extracts from *Ganoderma tsugae. Food Chemistry* 65 (3): 375-379.

Yesil, O. F. et al. 2004. Level of heavy metals in some edible and poisonous macrofungi from Batman of southeast Anatolia, Turkey. *Journal of Environmental Biology* 25 (3): 263–268.

Yesilada, O. et al. 2002. Decolourisation of textile dye astrazon red FBL by *Funalia trogii* pellets. *Biosource Technology* 81 (2): 155–157.

Ying, Jiangzhe et al. 1987. *Icones of Medicinal Fungi from China*. Beijing: Science Press.

Yoo, Hwa–Seung et al. 2004. Effects of *Cordyceps militaris* extract on angiogenesis and tumor growth. *Acta Pharmalogica Sinica* 25 (5): 657–665.

Yoon, Sang Yeon et al. 1994. Antimicrobial activity of *Ganoderma lucidum* extract alone and in combination with some antibiotics. *Archives of Pharmaceutical Research* 17 (6): 438–442.

Yoon, Seon–Joo et al. 2003. The nontoxic mushroom *Auricularia auricula* contains a polysaccharide with anticoagulant activity mediated by antithrombin. *Thrombosis Research* 112 (3): 151–158.

Yoshida, Isao et al. 1996. Polysaccharides in fungi. XXXVII. Immunomodulating activities of carboxymethylated derivatives of linear (1 3)– –D–glucans extracted from the fruiting bodies of *Agrocybe cylindracea* and *Amanita muscaria*. *Biological & Pharmaceutical Bulletin* 19 (1): 114–121.

Yoshikawa, Kazuko et al. 2001. A benzofuran glycoside and an acetylenic acid from the fungus *Laetiporus sulphureus* Var. Miniatus. *Chemical and Pharmaceutical Bulletin* 49 (3): 327.

Yoshikawa, Kazuko et al. 2005. Lanostane triterpenoids and triterpene glycosides from the fruit body of *Fomitopsis pinicola* and their inhibitory activity against cox–1 and cox–2. *Journal of Natural Products* 68 (1): 69–73.

Yoshikawa, Kazuko et al. 2008. Novel abietane diterpenoids and aromatic compounds from *Cladonia rangiferina* and their antimicrobial activity against antibiotics resistant bacteria. *Chemical and Pharmaceutical Bulletin* 56 (1): 89–92.

Yoshikawa, Noriko et al. 2004. Antitumour activity of cordycepin in mice. *Clinical and Experimental Pharmacology and Physiology* 31 (Supplement S2): S51–S53.

Yoshioka, Yuko et al. 1985. Antitumor polysaccharides from *P. ostreatus* (Fr.) Quel.: Isolation and structure of a –glucan. *Carbohydrate Research* 140 (1): 93–100.

You et al. 1994. Combined effects of chuling *(Polyporous umbellatus)* extract and mitomucin C on experimental liver cancer. *American Journal of Chinese Medicine* 22 (1): 19–28.

Youn et al. 2009. Potential anticancer properties of the water extract of *Inonotus obliquus* by induction of apoptosis in melanoma B16–F10 cells. *Journal of Ethnopharmacology* 122 (2): 221–228.

Yu, Hui Mei et al. 2006. Comparison of protective effects between cultured *Cordyceps militaris* and natural *Cordyceps sinensis* against oxidative damage. *Journal of Agricultural and Food Chemistry* 54 (8): 3132–3138.

Yu, Hyung Eun et al. 2007. Characterization of a novel ß–hydroxy– ß–methyl glutaryl coenzyme A reductase–inhibitor from the mushroom *Pholiota adiposa*. *Biotechnology and Bioprocess Engineering* 12 (6): 618–624.

Yu, Linghong and Huailing Wei. 2000. The hypnotic and sedative actions of the spores of *Ganoderma lucidum* (Curt.: Fr.) P. Karst (Aphyllophoromycetideae) in mice. *International Journal of Medicinal Mushrooms* 2 (4): 344–349.

Yu, Lugang et al. 1993. Reversible inhibition of proliferation of epithelial cell lines by *Agaricus bisporus* (edible mushroom) lectin. *Cancer Research* 53 (19): 4627–4632

Yu, Lugang et al. 1999. Edible mushroom *(Agaricus bisporus)* lectin, which reversibly inhibits epithelial cell proliferation, blocks nuclear localization sequence–dependent nuclear protein import. *The Journal of Biological Chemistry* 274 (8): 4890–4899.

Yu, Rongmin et al. 2004. Isolation and biological properties of polysaccharide CPS–1 from cultured *Cordyceps militaris*. *Fitoterapia* 75 (5): 465–472.

Yuan, Dan et al. 2004. An anti–aldosteronic diuretic component (drain dampness) in *Polyporus sclerotium*. *Biological and Pharmaceutical Bulletin* 27 (6): 867–870.

Yuan, Zuomin et al. 1998. Hypoglycemic effect of water–soluble polysaccharide from *Auricularia auricula–judae* Quel. on genetically diabetic KK–Ay mice. *Bioscience, Biotechnology, and Biochemistry* 62 (10): 1898–1903.

Yue, Grace Gar–Lee et al. 2008. Effects of *Cordyceps sinensis*, *Cordyceps militaris* and their isolated compounds on ion transport in Calu–3 human airway epithelial cells. *Journal of Ethnopharmacology* 117 (1): 92–101.

Yue–Qing, Zhou et al. 2005. A comparison study of the anticancerous activity and mechanism of ethanolic extracts from different *Ganoderma lucidum* (W.Curt.: Fr.) Lloyd strains. *International Journal of Medicinal Mushrooms* 7 (3): 488–489.

Yun, Bong–Sik et al. 2000a. Curtisians A–D, new free radical scavengers from the mushroom *Paxillus curtisii*. *Journal of Antibiotics* 53 (2): 114–122.

Yun, Bong–Sik et al. 2000b. Two P–terphenyls from mushroom *Paxillus panuoides* with free radical scavenging activity. *Journal of Microbiology and Biotechnology* 10 (2): 233–237.

Yun, Bong–Sik et al. 2001. Suillusin, a unique benzofuran from the mushroom *Suillus granulatus*. *Journal of Natural Products* 64 (9): 1230–1231.

Yun, Bong–Sik et al. 2002a. New tricyclic sesquiterpenes from the fermentation broth of *Stereum hirsutum*. *Journal of Natural Products* 65 (5): 786–788.

Yun, Bong–Sik et al. 2002b. Sterins A and B, new antioxidative compounds from *Stereum hirsutum*. *Journal of Antibiotics* 55 (2): 208–210.

Yurekli, F. et al. 1999. Plant growth hormone production from olive oil mill and alcohol factory wastewaters by white rot fungi. *World Journal of Microbiology and Biotechnology* 15 (4): 503–505.

Zadržil, F. et al. 1982. "Palo podrido"—decomposed wood used as feed. *Applied Microbiology and Biotechnology* 15 (3): 167–171.

Zaidman, Ben–Zion and Jamal A. Mahajna. 2005. Secondary metabolites from edible and medicinal mushrooms as molecular therapy for prostate cancer. *International Journal of Medicinal Mushrooms* 7 (3): 485.

Zaidman, Ben–Zion et al. 2007. Adverse effects of mycelia and culture broth extracts from *Bjerkandera adusta* (Willd.: Fr.) P. Karst. and *Hypholoma fasciculare* (Huds.: Fr.) P. Kumm. on breast and prostate cancer cells. *International Journal of Medicinal Mushrooms* 9 (1): 39–46.

Zaidman, Ben–Zion et al. 2008. *Coprinus comatus* and *Ganoderma lucidum* interfere with androgen receptor function in LNCaP prostate cancer cells. *Molecular Biology Reports* 35 (2): 107–117.

Zang, M. 1984. Mushroom distribution and the diversity of habitats in Tibet, China. *Journal of American Amateur Mycology* 6 (2): 15–20.

Zechlin, Lothar et al. 1981. Antibiotika aus Basidiomyceten, XII. Cristatsäure, ein modifiziertes Farnesylphenol aus Fruchtkörpern von *Albatrellus cristatus*. *Liebigs Annalen der Chemie* 1981 (12): 2099–2105.

Zenkova, Valentina A. et al. 2003. Antimicrobial activity of medicinal mushrooms from the genus *Coprinus* (Fr.) S. F. Gray (Agaricomycetideae). *International Journal of Medicinal Mushrooms* 5 (1): 37–42.

Zhan, Zha–Jun and Jian–Min Yue. 2003. New glycosphingolipids from the fungus *Catathelasma ventricosa*. *Journal of Natural Products* 66 (7): 1013–1016.

Zhang, Guoking et al. 2006. Hypoglycemic activity of the fungi *Cordyceps militaris*, *Cordyceps sinensis*, *Tricholoma mongolicum*, and *Omphalia lapidescens* in streptozotocin–induced diabetic rats. *Applied Microbiology and Biotechnology* 72 (6): 1152–1156.

Zhang, Guoking et al. 2010. Helvellisin, a novel alkaline protease from the wild Ascomycete mushroom *Helvella lacunose. Journal of Bioscience and Bioengineering* 109 (1): 20–24.

Zhang, Guoqing et al. 2009. A novel lectin with antiproliferative activity from the medicinal mushroom *Pholiota adiposa. Acta Biochimica Polonica* 56 (3): 415–421.

Zhang, Guowei et al. 2010. Diuretic activity and kidney medulla AQP1, AQP2, AQP3, V_2R expression of the aqueous extract of sclerotia of *Polyporus umbellatus* FRIES in normal rats. *Journal of Ethnopharmacology* 128 (2): 433–437.

Zhang, Jie et al. 1994. Antitumor active protein–containing glycans from the Chinese mushroom songshan lingzhi, *Ganoderma tsugae* mycelium. *Bioscience, Biotechnology, and Biochemistry* 58 (7): 1202–1205.

Zhang, Jing and Xiao Zhang Feng. 1997. Sesquiterpene hydroxylactone from *Lactarius subvellereus. Phytochemistry* 46 (1): 157–159.

Zhang, Jingsong et al. 2005. Bioactive components of *Ganoderma lucidum* (W.Curt.: Fr.) Lloyd can induce apoptosis of tumor cells. *International Journal of Medicinal Mushrooms* 7 (3): 487.

Zhang, Ling et al. 2009. Antihypertensive effect of 3,3,5,5–tetramethyl–4–piperidone, a new compound extracted from *Marasmius androsaceus. Journal of Ethnopharmacology* 123 (1): 34–39.

Zhang, Mei et al. 2001. Evolution of mushroom dietary fiber (nonstarch polysaccharides) from sclerotia of *Pleurotus tuber–regium* (Fries) Singer as a potential antitumor agent. *Journal of Agricultural and Food Chemistry* 49 (10): 5059–5062.

Zhang, Min et al. 2008. Dietary intakes of mushrooms and green tea combine to reduce the risk of breast cancer in Chinese women. *International Journal of Cancer* 124 (6): 1404–1408.

Zhang, Weiyun et al. 2005. Immunomodulatory and antitumor effects of an exoploysaccharide fraction from cultivated *Cordyceps sinensis* (Chinese caterpillar fungus) on tumour–bearing mice. *Biotechnology and Applied Biochemistry* 42 (1): 9–15.

Zhang, Weiyun et al. 2008. Effects of the exopoly-saccharide fraction (EPSF) from a cultivated *Cordyceps sinensis* on immunocytes of H22 tumor bearing mice. *Fitoterapia* 79 (3): 168–173.

Zhang, Xia et al. 2004. Dynamical influence of *Cordyceps sinensis* on the activity of hepatic insulinase of experimental liver cirrhosis. *Hepatobiliary and Pancreatic Diseases International* 3 (1): 99–101.

Zhang, Yanjun et al. 2002. Cyclooxygenase inhibitory and antioxidant compounds from the mycelia of the edible mushroom *Grifola frondosa. Journal of Agricultural and Food Chemicals* 50 (26): 7581–7585.

Zhang, Yanjun et al. 2003. Cyclooxygenase inhibitory and antioxidant compounds from the fruiting body of an edible mushroom, *Agrocybe aegerita. Phytomedicine* 10 (5): 386–390.

Zhao, Chenguang et al. 2003. An antitumour lectin from the edible mushroom *Agrocybe aegerita. Biochemical Journal* 374 (2): 321–327.

Zhao, Hang and Wenquan Liang. 2004. Studies on the extraction process of *Cryptoporus volvatus* oil by orthogonal design method. *Zhong Yao Cai* 27 (5): 373–374.

Zhao, Xiao–Yan et al. 2004. Inhibitory effects of cryptoporous polysaccharide on airway constriction, eosinophil release, and chemotaxis in guinea pigs. *Acta Pharmacologica Sinica* 25 (4): 503–507.

Zhao, Yongxun et al. 2007. Anti–tumor function of polysaccharides from *Pholiota adiposa* mycelium. *Acta Edulis Fungi* 14 (2): 49–54.

Zheng, Chang–Ji et al. 2006. Atromentin and leucomelone, the first inhibitors specific to enoyl–ACP reductase (FabK) of *Streptococcus pneumoniae. Journal of Antibiotics* 59 (12): 808–812.

Zheng, Shang–Zheng et al. 2004. Two new polyporusterones from *Polyorus umbellatus. Natural Product Research* 18 (5): 403–407.

Zheng, Wei–Fa et al. 2007. Sterol composition in field–grown and cultured mycelia of *Inonotus obliquus. Yao Xue Xue Bao* 42: 750–756.

561

Zheng , Wei–Fa et al. 2009. Accumulation of anti-oxidant phenolic constituents in submerged cultures of *Inonotus obliquus*. *Bioresource Technology* 100 (3): 1327–1335.

Zhou, D. H. and L. Z. Lin. 1995. Effect of jinshu-bao capsule on the immunological function of 36 patients with advanced cancer. *Chung Kuo Chung Hsi I Chieh Ho Tsa Chih* 15 (8): 476–478.

Zhou, H. P. et al. 1989. Anti–aging effect of the polysaccharides from *Auricularia auricula* and *Tremella fuciformis*. *Zhongguo Yaoke Daxue Xuebao* 20 (5): 303–306.

Zhou, Shufeng ewt al. 2005. Clinical Trials for Medicinal Mushrooms: Experience with Ganoderma lucidum (W.Curt.:Fr.) Lloyd (Lingzhi Mushroom). *International Journal of Medicinal Mushrooms* 7 (1–2): 111–118.

Zhu et al. 2000. Effects of extracts from sporo-derm–broken spores of *Ganoderma lucidum* on HeLa cells. *Cell Biology and Toxicology* 16 (3): 201–206.

Zjawiony et al. 2005. *Merulius incarnates* Schwein., a rare mushroom with highly selective antimicrobial activity. *International Journal of Medicinal Mushrooms* 7 (3): 365–366.

Zorn et al. 2003. Cleavage of beta, beta–carotene to flavor compounds by fungi. *Applied Microbiology and Biotechnology* 62 (4): 331–336.

Zou et al. 2005. Optomization of nutritional factors of exopolysaccharide production by submerged cultivation of the medicinal mushroom *Oudemansiella radicata*. *World Journal of Microbiology and Biotechnology* 21 (6–7): 1267–1271.

Zusman et al. 1997. Role of apoptosis, proliferating cell nuclear antigen and p53 protein in chemically induced colon cancer in rats fed corncob fiber treated with the fungus Pleurotus ostreatus. *Anticancer Research* 17 (3C) 2105–2113.

Abbott, Sean, and R.S. Currah. *The Larger Cup Fungi and Other Ascomycetes of Alberta : An Annotated Checklist.* Edmonton: Devonian Botanic Garden, University of Alberta, 1989.

Allegro, John Marco. *The Sacred Mushroom and the Cross: A Study of the Nature and Origins of Christianity within the Fertility Cults of the Ancient Near East.* London: Hodder & Stoughton Ltd, 1970.

Allen, Eric, Duncan Morrison and Gordon Wallis. *Common Tree Diseases of British Columbia.* Victoria, BC: Pacific Forestry Center, 1996.

Andre, Alestine and Alan Fehr. *Gwich'in Ethnobotany: Plants Used by the Gwich'in for Food, Medicine, Shelter and Tools.* Tsiigehtchic, N.W.T: Gwich'in Social and Cultural Institute and Aurora Research Institute, 2001.

Arora, David. *Mushrooms Demystified.* Berkeley, CA: Ten Speed Press, 1986.

Arthur, James. *Mushrooms and Mankind—The Impact of Mushrooms on Human Consciousness and Religion.* Escondido, CA: The Book Tree, 2000.

Barron, George. *Mushrooms of Ontario and Eastern Canada (Lone Pine Field Guides).* Edmonton, Alberta, Canada: Lone Pine Publishing, 1999.

Benjamin, Denis R. *Mushrooms Poisons and Panaceas: A Handbook for Naturalists, Mycologists, and Physicians.* New York: W.H. Freeman & Company, 1995.

Bennet, J. W., K. G. Wunch, and B. D. Faison. "Use of Fungi Biodegradation" In *Manual of Environmental Microbiology,* edited by Criston J. Hurst, 960—971. Washington D.C.: ASM Press, 2002.

Blanchette, Robert A., Brian D. Compton, Robert L. Gilbertson, and Nancy J. Turner. "Nineteenth Century Shaman Grave Guardians Are Carved *Fomitopsis Officinalis* Sporophores." *Mycologia* 84 (1992): 119-124.

Boericke, William. *Boericke's New Manual of Homeopathic Materia Medica with Repertory.* New Delhi: B Jain Publishers, 2008.

Boik, John. *Natural Compounds in Cancer Therapy: Promising Nontoxic Antitumor Agents From Plants & Other Natural Sources.* Princeton, MN: Oregon Medical Press, 2001.

Bortenschlager, Sigmar, and Klause Oggel, editors. *The Iceman and his Natural Environment: Palaeobotanical Results (The Man in the Ice).* Vienna: Springer, 2000.

Bossenmaier, Eugene F. *Mushrooms of the Boreal Forest.* Saskatoon: University Extension Press, University of Saskatchewan, 1997.

Boulet, Bruno. *Les champignons des arbres de l'est de l'Amérique du Nord.* Sainte-foy: Publications du Québec, 2003.

Brodie, Harold J. *Fungi Delight of Curiosity.* Toronto: University of Toronto Press, 1989.

Brodo, Irwin, Stephen Sharnoff, and Sylvia Sharnoff. *Lichens of North America.* New Haven: Yale University Press, 2001.

Buhner, Stephen H. *Sacred and Herbal Healing Beers: The Secrets of Ancient Fermentation.* Boulder, CO: Siris Books, 1998.

———. *Sacred Plant Medicine.* Rochester, VT: Bear & Company, 2006.

———. *Herbal Antibiotics: Natural Alternatives for Treating Drug-Resistant Bacteria (Storey Medicinal Herb Guide).* Pownal, VT: Storey Books, 1999.

Buller, Reginald. *Researches on Fungi Volumes 1-6.* London: Longmans, Green & Co., 2010.

But, Paul P. H., and Hson-Mou Chang. *Pharmacology and Applications of Chinese Materia Medica: Volume I.* Translated by Lai-Ling Wang, Sih-Cheng Yao, and Shem Chang-Shing Yuen. New Jersey: World Scientific, 2001.

Chang, Shu-Ting, and Phillip G. Miles. *Mushrooms: Cultivation, Nutritional Value, Medicinal Effect, and Environmental Impact.* Boca Raton, FL: CRC Press, 2004.

Chang, S. T., and W. A. Hayes. *The Biology and Cultivation of Edible Mushrooms.* New York: Academic Press, 1978.

Chappell, Peter. *Emotional Healing with Homeopathy: Treating the Effects of Trauma.* Berkeley, CA: North Atlantic Books, 2003.

Chatroux, M. D., and Sylvia C. *Materia Poetica : Homeopathy In Verse.* Oregon: Poetica Press, 1998.

Chatroux, M. D., and Sylvia C. *Botanica Poetica.* Oregon: Poetica Press, 2004.

Christensen, Clyde M. *Molds, Mushrooms & Mycotoxins.* Minnesota: Universitiy of Minnesota Press, 1975.

Cochran, K. W., and E. H. Lucas. "Chemoprophylaxis of Poliomyelitis in Mice Through the Administration of Plant Extracts." *Antibiotics Annual* (1959): 104-9.

Cooke, R. C. *Fungi.* London (St. James Place): Collins, 1981.

Czarnecki, Jack. *A Cook's Book of Mushrooms: With 100 Recipes for Common and Uncommon Varieties.* New York: Artisan, 1995.

Deshmukh, S. K., and M. K. Rai, editors. *Biodiversity of Fungi: Their Role in Human Life.* Enfield, NH: Science Publishers, 2005.

Didukh, Maryna, Eviatar Nevo, and Solomon P. Vassar. et al. *Impact of the Family Agaricaceae (F>.) Cohn on Nutrition and Medicine.* Ruggell: A.R.G. Gantner, 2004.

Evenson, Vera S. *Mushrooms of Colorado and the Southern Rocky Mountains.* Englewood, CO: Westcliffe Publishers, 1997.

Findlay, W. P. K. *Fungi-Folklore, Fiction, & Fact.* Richmond, UK: Richmond Publishing, 1982.

Fine, Gary A. *Morel Tales: The Culture of Mushrooming.* Cambridge: Harvard University Press, 1998.

Freedman, Louise. *Wild about Mushrooms: The Cookbook of the Mycological Society of San Francisco. Myco Society of San Francisco.* Berkeley, CA: Aris Books, 1987.

Friedman, Sara Ann. *Celebrating the Wild Mushroom: A Passionate Quest.* New York: Dodd, Mead, 1986.

Friend, Tim. *Third Domain: The Untold Story Of Archaea And The Future Of Biotechnology* Washington D.C.: Joseph Henry Press, 2007.

Gadd, Geoffrey M. *Fungi in Bioremediation.* Cambridge: Cambridge University Press, 2001.

Gartz, Jochen. *Magic Mushrooms Around the World: A Scientific Journey Across Cultures and Time-The Case for Challenging Research and Value Systems.* Los Angeles: LIS Publications, 1996.

Gregg, Susan. *The Complete Illustrated Encyclopedia of Magical Plants.* Beverly, MA: Fair Winds Press, 2008.

Gurudas. *The Spiritual Properties of Herbs.* San Rafael: Cassandra Press, 1988.

Haard, Karen, and Richard Haard. *Poisonous and Hallucinogenic Mushrooms.* Seattle, WA: Homestead Book Co., 1977.

Hadeler, Hajo. *Medicinal Mushrooms You Can Grow for Health, Pleasure and Profit: A Handbook For Beginners.* Sechelt, BC: Cariaga Publishing House, 1995.

Halpern Georges M. *Cordyceps: China's Healing Mushroom.* New York: Avery Press, 1999.

Halpern, Georges M., and Andrew H. Miller. *Medicinal Mushrooms.* New York: M. Evans and Co., 2002.

Heinrich, Clark. *Magic Mushrooms in Religion & Alchemy.* Rochester, VT. Park Street Press, 2002.

Hobbs, Christopher. *Medicinal Mushrooms: An Exploration of Tradition, Healing and Culture.* Santa Cruz, CA: Botanica Press, 1995.

Hudler, George W. *Magical mushrooms, mischievous molds.* Princeton, NJ: Princeton University Press, 1998.

Jones, W.A. *The Savoury Mushroom: Cooking with Wild and Cultivated Mushrooms.* Vancouver, BC: Raincoast Books, 2000.

Jones, Kenneth. *Shiitake: the Healing Mushroom.* Rochester, VT: Healing Arts Press, 1995.

———. *Cordyceps: Tonic Food of Ancient China.* Seattle, WA: Sylvan Press, 1997.

Kaul, T. N. *Biology and Conservation of Mushrooms.* Enfield, NH: Science Publishers, 2002.

Keane, Kahlee, and Dean Howarth. *The Standing People: Field Guide of Medicinal Plants for the Prarie Provinces.* Saskatoon, Saskatchewan: Root Woman & Dave: Save our Species, 2009.

Keewaydinoquay. *Puhpohwee for the People: A Narrative Account of Some Use of Fungi Among the Ahnishinaubeg.* Cambridge, MA: Botanical Museum of Harvard University, 1978.

Klán, Jaroslav, and Bohumil Van ura. *Mushrooms and Fungi.* London: Hamlyn, 1981.

Larsen, Stephen. *The Shaman's Doorway: Opening the Mythic Imagination to Contemporary Consciousness.* New York: Harper & Row, 1976.

Letcher, Andy. *Shroom: A Cultural History of the Magic Mushroom.* New York: Ecco, 2007.

Leto, Steven. "Magical Potions: Entheogenic Themes in Scandinavian Mythology," *Shaman's Drum* 54 (2000): 64.

Marles, Robin et al. *Aboriginal Plant Use in Canada's Northwest Boreal Forest.* Vancouver: UBC Press, 2000.

Marley, Greg A. *Mushrooms for Health: Medicinal Secrets of Northeastern Fungi.* Camden, ME: Down East, 2009

Matsumoto, Kosai. *The Mysterious Reishi Mushroom: Its Powers for Health and Longevity and in the Treatment of cancer and Other Incurable Diseases.* Santa Barbara, CA: Woodbridge Press Pub. Co., 1979.

McIlvaine, Charles, and Robert K. Macadam. One Thousand American Fungi: Toadstools, Mushrooms, Fungi: How to Select and Cook the Edible; How to Distinguish and Avoid the Poisonous. New York: Dover Publications, 1973.

McKenna, Terence K. *Food of the Gods: The Search for the Original Tree of Knowledge: A Radical History of Plants, Drugs, and Human Evolution.* New York: Bantam Books, 1993.

McNeil, Raymond. *Le Grand Livre des Champignons du Québec et l'Est du Canada.* Waterloo, Québec: Éditions M. Quintin, 2006.

McCune, Bruce, and Linda Geiser, et al. *Macrolichens of the Pacific Northwest.* Corvallis: Oregon State University Press, 2009.

Miller, Orson K., and Hope Miller. *North American Mushrooms: A Field Guide to Edible and Inedible Fungi.* Guildford, CN: Falcon Guide, 2006.

Mohammed, Gina H., and Nathalie Gagné. *Catnip and Kerosene Grass: What Plants Teach Us About Life.* Sault Ste. Marie, Ontario: Candlenut Books, 2002.

Money, Nicholas P. *Mr. Bloomfield's Orchard: The Mysterious World of Mushrooms, Molds, and Mycologists.* New York: Oxford University Press, 2002.

Moore, David. *Slayers, Saviors, Servants, and Sex: An Exposé of Kingdom Fungi.* New York: Springer, 2001

Morgan, Adrian. *Toads and Toadstools: The Natural History, Folklore, and Cultural Oddities of a Strange Association.* Berkeley, CA: Celestial Arts, 1995.

Mori, Kisaku. *Mushrooms as Health Foods.* Tokyo: Japan Publications, 1974.

Mourning Dove, Heister Dean Guie, Lucullus Virgil McWhorter, and Luther Standing Bear. *Coyote Stories.* Caldwell, Idaho: The Caxton Printers, Ltd., 1933.

Mulders, Evelyn. *Western Herbs for Eastern Meridians & Five Element Theory.* Lake Country, BC: E. Mulders, 2006.

Pace, Giuseppe. *Mushrooms of the World.* Willowdale, Ontario: Firefly Books, 1998.

Parker, Loni, and David T. Jenkins. *Mushrooms, A*

Separate Kingdom. Birmingham: Oxmoor House, 1979

Plischke, John. *Good Mushroom, Bad Mushroom: Who's Who, Where to Find Them, and How to Enjoy Them Safely*. Pittsburgh, PA: St. Lynn's Press, 2011.

Powell, Simon G. *The Psilocybin Solution: The Role of Sacred Mushrooms in the Quest for Meaning*. Rochester, VA: Park Street Press, 2011. Available online at www.lycaeum.org/books/books/psilocybin-solution.

Rätsch, Christian. The Dictionary of Sacred & Magical Plants. Santa Barbara, CA: ABC-CLIO, 1992.

———. *The Encyclopedia of Psychoactive Plants: Ethnopharmacology and its Applications*. Rochester, VT: Park St Press, 2005.

Rice, Miriam, and Dorothy M. Beebee. *Mushrooms for Color*. Eureka, CA: Mad River Press, 1980.

———. *Mushrooms for Dyes, Paper, Pigments & Mycostix™*. Forestville, CA: Mushrooms for Color Press, 2007.

Rogers, Robert Dale. *Sundew, Moonwort: Medicinal Plants of the Prairies*. Edmonton, Alberta: Robert Dale Rogers, 1999-2001.

Rogers, Robert Dale, and Capital Health Authority. *Herbal Drug Interactions: Professional Reference Guide*. Edmonton, Alberta: Capital Health Authority and Robert Rogers, 2003.

Rogers, Robert Dale, and Karamat Wilderness Ways (Firm). *Rogers' Herbal Manual*. Edmonton, Alberta: Karamat Wilderness Ways, 2000.

Rolfe, R. T., and F. W. Rolfe. *The Romance of the Fungus World: An Account of Fungus Life in its Numerous Guises, both Real and Legendary*. Philadelphia: J.B. Lippincott Co., 1928.

Šašek, Václav, John A. Glaser, P. Baveye, and NATO. *The Utilization of Bioremediation to Reduce Soil Contamination: Problems and Solutions*. Dordrecht: Boston: Kluver Academic Publishers, 2003.

Schaechter, Moselio. *In the Company of Mushrooms: A Biologist's Tale*. Cambridge, MA: Harvard University Press, 1997.

Schalkwijk-Barendsen, Helene M.E. *Mushrooms of Western Canada*. Edmonton, Alberta: Lone Pine, 1991.

Schenk, George. *Moss Gardening: Including Lichens, Liverworts, and other Miniatures*. Portland, OR: Timber Press, 1997.

Schüffler, Anja, and Timm Anke. "Secondary Metabolites of Basidiomycetes." *The Mycota* 15 (2009): 209–31.

Sept, J. Duane. *Common Mushrooms of the Northwest: Alaska, Western Canada, and the Northwestern United States*. Sechelt, BC: Calypso Pub., 2006

Shulgin, Alexander T., and Ann Shulgin. *Tikhal: The Continuation*. Berkeley, CA: Transform Press, 1997.

Singh, Jagjit, and K. R. Aneja. *From Ethnomycology to Fungal Biotechnology: Exploiting Fungi from Natural Resources for Novel Products*. New York: Kluwer Academic/Plenum Publishers, 1999.

Smith, Alexander H. *A Field Guide to Western Mushrooms*. Ann Arbor: University of Michigan Press, 1975.

Spahr, David L. *Edible and Medicinal Mushrooms of New England and Eastern Canada*. Berkeley, CA: North Atlantic Books, 2009.

Spoerke, David G., and Barry H. Rumack. *Handbook of Mushroom Poisoning: Diagnosis and Treatment*. Boca Raton, FL: CRC Press, 1994.

Stamets, Paul. *Growing Gourmet and Medicinal Mushrooms*. Berkeley, CA: Ten Speed Press, 2000.

———. *Psilocybin Mushrooms of the World: An Identification Guide*. Berkeley, CA: Ten Speed Press, 1996.

———. *Mycelium Running: How Mushrooms Can Help Save the World*. Berkeley, CA: Ten Speed Press, 2005.

Stamets, Paul, and C. Dusty Wu Yao. *MycoMedicinals. An Informational Treatise on Mushrooms*. Olympia, WA: MycoMedia, 2002.

Stephenson, Steven L. *The Kingdom Fungi: The Biology of Mushrooms, Molds, and Lichens*. Portland, OR: Timber Press, 2010.

Strassman, Rick, et al. *Inner Paths to Outer Space: Journeys to Alien Worlds Through Psychedelics and other Spiritual Technologies.* Rocheseter, VT: Park Street Press, 2008.

Teeter, Donald F. *Amanita Muscaria: Herb of Immortality.* Manor, TX: Ambrosia Society, 2005. Ebook available at www.ambrosiasociety.org.

Trudell, Steve, Jospeh Ammirati, and Marsha Mello. *Mushrooms of the Pacific Northwest.* Portland, OR: Timber Press, 2009.

Turner, Nancy. *Plants of Haida Gwaii.* Victoria, BC: Sono Nis Press, 2003.

Turner, W. B. *Fungal Metabolites.* New York: Academic Press, 1971.

Twentyman, Ralph. *The Science and Art of Healing.* Edinburgh: Floris Books, 1989.

Vermeulen, Frans. *Fungi: Kingdom Fungi.* Haarlem, Netherlands: Emyrss, 2007.

Vitt, Dale H., Janet E. Marsh, and Robin B. Bovey. *Mosses, Lichens & Ferns of Northwest North America.* Edmonton, Alberta: Lone Pine, 1988

Voitk, Andrus. *A Little Illustrated Book of Common Mushrooms of Newfoundland and Labrador.* Rocky Harbour, NL: Gros Morne Co-operating Association with Andrus Voitk, 2007.

Wang, Huijun, and Shuqin Fan. *Icones of Medicinal Fungi from China.* Beijing: Science Prcss, 1987.

Wasser, S. P. "Medicinal Mushrooms as a Source of Antitumor and Immunomodulating Polysaccharides." *Applied Microbiology and Biotechnology* 60 (2002) 258-74.

Wasson, Valentia Pavlovna, and Robert Gordon Wasson. *Mushrooms, Russia, and History.* New York: Pantheon Books, 1957. Online at www.newalexandria.org/archive.

Wasson, R. Gordon. *Soma, The Divine Mushroom of Immortality.* New York: Harcourt, Brace & World, 1968.

Wasson, R. Gordon, Albert Hoffmann, and Carl A.P. Ruck. *The Road to Eleusis: Unveiling the Secret of the Mysteries.* New York: Harcourt, Brace, Jovanovich, 1978.

Watling, Roy, and Natural History Museum (London, England). *Fungi.* Washington, D.C.: Smithsonian Books, 2003.

Weaver, William Woys. *Sauer's Herbal Cures: America's First Book of Botanic Healing, 1762-1778.* New York. Routledge, 2001.

Willard, Terry. *Reishi Mushroom: Herb of Spiritual Potency and Medical Wonder.* Issaquah, WA: Sylvan Press, 1990.

Williamson, B. L. *Reflections on the Fungaloids.* Ottawa: Algrove Pub., 2002.

Fungal Essence Resources

Bailey Flower Essences: www.baileyessences.com

Bloesem Remedies: Bram Zaalberg Nederland: www.bloesem-remedies.com

BrynaHerb Essences: info@brynaherb.uk

Canadian Forest Tree Essences: www.essences.ca

Findhorn Essences: www.findhornessences.com

Korte PHI Essences: www.kortephi.com or PO Box 192, Gibson's, B.C. V0N 1V0

Miriana fortem: www.mirianaflowers.com

Petit Fleur Essences: www.aromahealthtexas.com

Phi Essences BV (formerly Korte PHI): www .Phiessences.com

Prairie Deva Flower Essences: www.selfhealdistributing.com

Silvercord: www.silvercord-essences.co.uk

Tree Frog Farm: www.treefrogfarm.com

Interesting Companies, Journals, and Websites

Alberta Mycological Society: www.wildmushrooms.ws

International Journal of Medicinal Mushrooms: www.begellhouse.com/journals

Functional Fungi LLC: www.FunctionalFungi.com

Gourmet Mushrooms, Inc: www.GourmetMushroomsInc.com

HYY: www.houseofyinyang.com

George Barron: www.uoguelph.ca/~gbarron/species

MushroomScience: www.mushroomscience.com

Matsutake info: www.matsiman.com

Mycorant: www.mycorant.com

Healing Mushrooms:
www.healing-mushrooms.net

Mush-World: www.mushworld.com

NAMA: www.namyco.org

Nikken: www.Nikken.com

Fungi Perfecti: www.fungi.com

Mushroom Observer:
www.mushroomobserver .com

Tom Volk: www.tomvolkfungi.net

Aloha Medicinals: www.alohamedicinals.com

Econet: www.myco.html

International Mycological Network:
www.fungi.net

Michael Wood: www.mykoweb.com

Cartoons:
www.bsu.edu/classes/ruch/msa/tansey

Fungi Magazine: www.fungimag.com

Mycologia Journal: www.mycologia.org

Amanita muscaria: www.ambrosiasociety.org

Michael Kuo: www.mushroomexpert.com

Bryce Kendrick: www.mycolog.com

Pacific Northwest Key Council:
www.svims.ca/council

Matchmaker—Mushrooms of the Pacific Northwest: www.pfc.forestry.ca/biodiversity/
matchmaker/index_e.html

The Mushroom Journal:
www.mushroomthejournal.com

Med Mushrooms and Cancer: www.icnet.uk/
labs/med_mush/med_mush.html

Cornell University: www.mycology.cornell.edu

Know Your Mushrooms:
www.sphinxproduction .com

Just Mushroom Stuff:
www.justmushroomstuff.com

Wild Mushroom Products:
www.darcyfromtheforest.com

Everything Mushrooms:
www.everythingmushrooms.com

Everything Lichens: www.lichen.com

Lichens: http://web.uvic.bc/~stucraw/index.html

Ways of Enlichenment:
http://waysofenlichenment .net/

John Plischke III: 51, 52, 53, 65, 91, 101, 102, 115, 117, 119, 125 (above and below), 128 (above and below right), 131, 133, 137, 140, 141, 143 (below left and right), 145, 173, 190 (below right), 200, 201, 225 (four lower photos) 237 (above), 242, 244, 245, 247 (far right; both middle and below), 253 (above), 265, 271, 279 (below right), 284, 293 (all photos), 297, 298, 299, 301, 302, 303, 305, 311 (above), 323 (middle right, below left, below right), 327, 328 (middle right, below left), 339, 365, 370, 373 (above), 382, 386 (above, below right), 393, 419, 427, 430, 432, 437

April Braemar: 333 (above)

Jeanette Gasser: 229 (below left)

Chris Kolzac: 401

Paul Kroeger: 359, 360 (middle right, below right)

Jim Malenzcak: 35 (middle right)

Ali-Sun Morgan: 105, 106 (below left and right), 360 (above and below left)

Denise O'Reilly: 275 (above)

Martin Osis: 11 (above), 56, 63, 165 (below left, middle right), 205 (above right), 208, 217 (left), 255 (above left), 320, 323 (above left)

Bill Richards: 253 (below left and right)

Christine Roberts: 165 (left), 312

John and Shelley Stobee: 205 (below), 287

John Thompson: 160, 185, 333 (below left), 328 (above left, below right), 345 (above)

Burton Yang: 176 (above and below right)

Dusty Yao-Stamets: 153

All other photographs by Robert Rogers

571

ROBERT DALE ROGERS has been a student of native plants and fungi from the Canadian prairies for more than forty years. He is a retired clinical herbalist, amateur mycologist, and professional member of the American Herbalist Guild.

Robert is the author of seven volumes of native and cultivated plants called *Sundew, Moonwort: Medicinal Plants of the Prairies.* He has written *Rogers' Herbal Manual,* which accompanies a seven-volume video series with Mors Kochanski on edible and medicinal plants of the boreal forest. Robert coauthored *Herbal Drug Interactions,* a publication of Capital Health and the Royal Alexandra Hospital.

Robert teaches plant medicine at Grant MacEwan University and the Northern Star College of Mystical Studies in Edmonton (www.northernstarcollege.com). He is a consultant to the herbal, mycological and nutraceutical industries, and is currently vice president of the Alberta Mycological Society, chair of the medicinal mushroom committee of the North American Mycological Association, and on the editorial board of the *International Journal of Medicinal Mushrooms.*

He lives in Edmonton, Canada with his beautiful wife, Laurie. You may contact him directly at scents@telusplanet.net. You can also check out their websites at www.scentsofwonder.ca or www.selfhealdistributing.com.